The International Handbook of Black Community Mental Health

Endorsements

"This Handbook is a landmark in our understanding of the mental health issues which challenge African-heritage populations in Europe (particularly in the UK and the Netherlands) and in North America – countries which imposed slavery on African populations. The racism which survives today is a perpetuation of the values which supported slavery: issues of labelling and victim-blaming continue, and take their toll on minority populations. The 40 activists, clinicians and scholars who contribute chapters to this handbook are well qualified and experienced in their specialist fields and bring their unique insights and knowledge on Black Community Mental Health issues to a Handbook which will be of great value for students, trainees, academics and practitioners from multidisciplinary backgrounds. The authors have also been ably guided and organised by the Handbook's three editors (two from the US, one from the UK). Overall, there is much quality in the writing, many insights, and bases for further action."

Dr. Alice Sawyerr, PhD Psychology, FHEA, CPsychol, CSci, AFBPsS, Lecturer at the University of Oxford, Consultant Chartered Psychologist (BPS), Consultant Systemic Family Psychotherapist (AFT and UKCP) and BPS registered Expert Witness in Family Court Cases in UK.

"As far as I am aware this is the first publication of its kind on the experiences and provision of services to the BME community. This in itself is something of a sad statement to make in 2020 after many years of campaigning, analysis, research and policy intervention (I know I have been involved in many of them over the years) we have yet to produce a publication specifically on the issues pertaining to BME mental health. For producing this work the editors should be congratulated. The challenges within these pages are not only for members of the BME community to read, reflect and act. This book is essential reading for any Mental Health practitioner who wishes to understand and practice in a system which is beneficial to all regardless of race."

Lord Victor O. Adebowale, CBE

The International Handbook of Black Community Mental Health

EDITED BY

RICHARD MAJORS
University of Colorado–Colorado Springs, USA

KAREN CARBERRY
Orri – Intensive Day Treatment for Eating Disorders, UK

THEODORE S. RANSAW
Michigan State University, USA

Foreword by Professor Joseph L. White, "The Father of Black Psychology"
Prologue by Professor Alvin Poussaint, MD, Emeritus Harvard Medical School

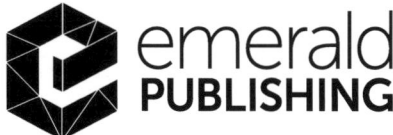

United Kingdom – North America – Japan – India – Malaysia – China

Emerald Publishing Limited
Howard House, Wagon Lane, Bingley BD16 1WA, UK

First edition 2020

Copyright © 2020 Emerald Publishing Limited

Reprints and permissions service
Contact: permissions@emeraldinsight.com

No part of this book may be reproduced, stored in a retrieval system, transmitted in any form or by any means electronic, mechanical, photocopying, recording or otherwise without either the prior written permission of the publisher or a licence permitting restricted copying issued in the UK by The Copyright Licensing Agency and in the USA by The Copyright Clearance Center. Any opinions expressed in the chapters are those of the authors. Whilst Emerald makes every effort to ensure the quality and accuracy of its content, Emerald makes no representation implied or otherwise, as to the chapters' suitability and application and disclaims any warranties, express or implied, to their use.

British Library Cataloguing in Publication Data
A catalogue record for this book is available from the British Library

ISBN: 978-1-83909-965-6 (Print)
ISBN: 978-1-83909-964-9 (Online)
ISBN: 978-1-83909-966-3 (Epub)

Printed and bound by CPI Group (UK) Ltd, Croydon, CR0 4YY

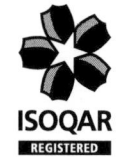

ISOQAR certified
Management System,
awarded to Emerald
for adherence to
Environmental
standard
ISO 14001:2004.

Certificate Number 1985
ISO 14001

INVESTOR IN PEOPLE

To Professor Joseph White

My elder, mentor and friend.

Professor White was 'The Father of Black Psychology' and was one of the founding members of the Association of Black Psychology. Professor White was a scholar, pioneer, trailblazer, but even more than that he was good friend, always there when you needed him for encouragement or advice; as well he was a very kind person, humorous and, just a down to earth decent human being, who will be truly missed by all of us who knew him. And Joe yes, we will try hard to 'keep the faith' just as you used to tell us all to do.

And to:

Professor Reginald Jones

My elder, mentor and friend.

Professor Jones was a quiet, sweet and gentle human being with a quick disarming big smile; you truly will be missed.

Professor Jones was the 'architect'/designer, an editor of numerous articles and books (e.g. his well-known and popular *Black Psychology* series) on Black psychology and he was an influential Publisher of the Black Psychology Movement. He organised and structured the Black Psychology academic movement like no one else. He brought together all the top Black psychologist/academics in the world to help make Black Psychology a scientific field and a legitimate area of scholarship after Joseph White developed/created Black Psychology as a discipline. He was the founder of Cobb & Henry Publishers, one of the first Black academic presses in the USA, Cobb & Henry. Cobb & Henry was the publisher for many of his groundbreaking Black psychology publications.

His classic Black Psychology anthologies and his psychology books were published in a variety of different areas (e.g. special education and the gifted, racial identity, tests and measurements, mental health cognition and intelligence, personality and Black development and aging in children, adolescents and adults) which provided the academic platform for what we know today as Black Psychology.

Contents

List of Tables and Figures	*xi*
About the Editors	*xiii*
About the Authors	*xv*
Foreword *Joseph L. White*	*xxix*
Prologue *Alvin Poussaint*	*xxxi*
Prelude *Eugene Ellis*	*xxxv*
Acknowledgements	*xxxvii*

**Black Mental Health and the New Millennium:
Historical and Current Perspective on Cultural Trauma
and 'Everyday' Racism in White Mental Health Spaces —
The Impact on the Psychological Well-being of
Black Mental Health Professionals**
Richard Majors — 1

Structure of the Book
Karen Carberry — 27

Part I: Race Relations

**Chapter 1 Systemic Racism: Big, Black, Mad and Dangerous
in the Criminal Justice System**
Sharon Walker — 41

**Chapter 2 In the Name of Our Humanity: Challenging Academic
Racism and its Effects on the Emotional Wellbeing of
Women of Colour Professors**
Philomena Essed and Karen Carberry — 61

Chapter 3   Racial Battle Fatigue: The Long-term Effects of Racial Microaggressions on African American Boys and Men
William A. Smith, Rodalyn David and Glory S. Stanton   83

Chapter 4   Racism in Academia: (How to) Stay Black, Sane and Proud as the Doctoral Supervisory Relationship Implodes
Sharon Walker   93

Chapter 5   Implicit Provider Bias and its Implications for Black/African American Mental Health
Andra D. Rivers Johnson   113

Part II: Policy

Chapter 6   Thirty Years of Black History Month and Thirty Years of Overrepresentation in the Mental Health System
Patrick Vernon   137

Chapter 7   Race and Risk – Exploring UK Social Policy and the Development of Modern Mental Health Services
Patricia Clarke   149

Chapter 8   Remaining Mindful about Children and Young People
Mhemooda Malek and Simon Newitt   163

Part III: Interventions

Chapter 9   Cultural Competencies in Delivering Counselling and Psychotherapy Services to a Black Multicultural Population: Time for Change and Action
Nicholas Banks   181

Chapter 10   Social and Emotional Education and Emotional Wellness: A Cultural Competence Model for Black Boys and Teachers
Richard Majors, Llewellyn E. Simmons and Cornelius Ani   199

Chapter 11   ASD and Cultural Competence: An ASD Multicultural Treatment- Led Model
Mary Henderson and Richard Majors   239

Chapter 12   Moving Young Black Men Beyond Survival Mode: Protective Factors for Their Mental Health
Ivan Juzang   257

Chapter 13 African Americans and the Vocational Rehabilitation Service System in the United States: The Impact on Mental Health
Julie Vryhof and Fabricio E. Balcazar 275

Chapter 14 Targeted Intervention in Education and the Empowerment and Emotional Well-being of Black Boys
Cheron Byfield and Tony Talburt 293

Part IV: Theory and Practice

Chapter 15 Toward Positions of Spiritual Reflexivity as a Resource: Emerging Themes and Conversations for Systemic Practice, Leadership, and Supervision within Black Mental Health
Maureen Greaves 309

Chapter 16 'Marginal Leaders': Making Visible the Leadership Experiences of Black Women in a Therapeutic Service for Disenfranchised Young People
Romana Farooq and Tânia Rodrigues 329

Chapter 17 Forty Years in the Wilderness: A Review of Systemic Barriers to Reducing the Over-representation of Black Men in the UK Psychiatric System
Gail Coleman-Oluwabusola 343

Chapter 18 Oppositional and Defiant Behaviours Among Black Boys in Schools: Techniques to Facilitate Change
Steve Clarke 361

Chapter 19 Black Therapists – White Families, Therapists' Perceptions of Cultural Competence in Clinical Practice
Karen Carberry and Belinda Brooks-Gordon 379

Chapter 20 Transracial Adoption and Mental Health
Nicholas Banks 405

Chapter 21 Dementia and its Impact on Minority Ethnic and Migrant Communities
David Truswell 423

Chapter 22 Mental Health/Illness Revisited in People of African-Caribbean Heritage in Britain
Florence Gwendolyn Rose and Tony Leiba 441

x   Contents

Chapter 23   Researching African-Caribbean Mental Health in the UK: An Assets-based Approach to Developing Psychosocial Interventions for Schizophrenia and Related Psychoses
Dawn Edge, Amy Degnan and Sonya Rafiq   455

Chapter 24   'Lone Wolf' Case Study Considerations of Terrorist Radicalisation from the Black Experience
Nicholas Banks   471

Part V: Clinical Practice

Chapter 25   Spotlight on Sensory Processing Difficulties
Lisa Prior and Tiffany Howl   489

Chapter 26   Forced Marriage as a Representation of a Belief System in the UK and its Psychological Impact on Well-being
Doreen Robinson and Reenee Singh   505

Chapter 27   Systemic Family Therapy with Transgenerational Communities in Haiti and the Dominican Republic
Karen Carberry, Jean Gerald Lafleur and Genel Jean-Claude   527

Chapter 28   Engaging with Racialized Process in Clinical Supervision: Political or Personal
Isha Mckenzie-Mavinga   557

Part VI: Recommendations

Chapter 29   Recommendations
Patrick Vernon   571

Glossary   575

Index   577

List of Tables and Figures

Figures

Chapter 12

| Fig. 1. | The MEE Eight Variables Model. Developed by MEE Productions Inc. | 261 |
| Fig. 2. | The Evolution of Resiliency Factors. Developed by MEE Productions Inc. | 268 |

Chapter 17

| Fig. 1. | Proposed Development of Persecutory Frameworks for Black Men Experiencing Persecutory Delusions in the UK. | 351 |

Chapter 18

| Fig. 1. | An Algorithm of the PSOR Model. | 372 |

Chapter 19

| Fig. 1. | Therapists' Age Range. | 386 |

Chapter 26

| Fig. 1. | Genogram 1 Nadira. | 510 |
| Fig. 2. | Genogram Kavitha. | 513 |

Chapter 27

Fig. 1.	Pastor Jean Gerald Lafleur (left); Pastor David Badio (centre); and Pastor Genel Jean-Claude (right). Haitian Pastors - Community Elders and Gatekeepers	540
Fig. 2.	Abisola Ifasawo and Alison Greenaway - UK Haiti Mission Team 2015	542
Fig. 3.	Karen Carberry (left) delivering Community based transgenerational Systemic Family Therapy with Pastor Jean Gerald Lefleur (out of picture shot)	549

Tables

Chapter 19

Table 1.	The Cultural Background of Therapists.	386
Table 2.	Dates in which First Generation Parents Migrated to the UK.	387
Table 3.	Parents' Occupation on Arrival in the UK.	387
Table 4.	Therapist's Occupation.	387
Table 5.	Therapist's Therapeutic Qualifications.	387
Table 6.	Association of Significant Independent Variables on the Dependent Variable.	389
Table 7.	Relevant Findings.	391

Chapter 25

Table 1.	Indicators of SPD.	495
Table 2.	Ways to Explain SPD to Others.	497
Table 3.	Strategies to Try.	499

Chapter 27

Table 1.	The Timeline Below Illustrates an Overview of Systemic Family Therapy with Communities of Transgenerational Families in Haiti and the Dominican Republic Between 2012 and 2017.	538

About the Editors

Richard Majors, PhD, is a Counselling Psychologist, Honorary Professor at the University of Colorado in the United States, and Distinguished Fellow and Director of the Applied Centre Emotional Literacy Leadership and Research (ACELLR), who has been living and working in the UK for over 20 years. He is the founder and former deputy editor of the *Journal of African American Studies* (formerly the *Journal of African American Men*, the first refereed journal on Black men in the United States), one of the largest ethnic journals in the United States.. He also is a former Clinical Fellow in Psychiatry at the Harvard Medical School. While at Harvard, he co-founded the National Council of African American Men, one of the first umbrella groups in the United States for African American males. He was a Senior Research Associate at the prestigious Urban Institute in Washington, DC for two years. In 1996/1997 prior to moving to the UK, he was appointed a Leverhulme Visiting Fellow for Research in England. In 2000 he was appointed a Canterbury Fellow at the University of Canterbury, New Zealand.

He wrote the lead psychological expert statement, in the UK high court for the landmark case, *SG* vs *St. Gregorys Science School*, which successfully overturned previous policy and legislation that prevented Black children from being able to wear culture-specific hairstyles in school. He has also met with members of the Clinton Administration to discuss youth policy. He has authored/co-authored seven books and dozens of scholarly articles. His book *Cool Pose: The Dilemmas of Black Manhood in America* (1992) was submitted for Pulitzer Prize by the publisher and was on the publisher bestsellers' list in 1992. *Cool Pose* is considered a classic in the field and is one of the most cited books in race relations and gender in the United States. Previously, in the UK, he was selected to be on a Ministerial Working Group on Education and Gangs. He was selected in 2015 to receive the Warrior Award from the International Colloquium on Education for his longstanding service, research and leadership on education globally. In 2016, he was shortlisted, for the Medical Livewire Global Award for his work in the field of psychology. He was again honoured in 2018 by Medical Livewire for his outstanding work in the field of psychology and this time was bestowed with their prestigious award 'Psychology Professional of The Year'. In 2019, he received the Expert Witness Award from *Lawyer Monthly Magazine*, in recognition of his specialised knowledge and experience within the area of Trans-cultural Psychology.

Karen Carberry, M.Sc., Dip.Psych., Black British Family and Systemic Psychotherapist, Consultant Family Therapist of Orri – Specialist Day Treatment for Eating Disorders, AFT Registered Systemic Supervisor and a Fellow of the Asian Academy of Family Therapy (AAFT). Karen was recently appointed Consultant Clinical Supervisor of HOPE Bereavement Support in Leeds, UK; who offer supportive counselling, therapeutic groups for women and families around child loss and miscarriage; coaching and raising mental health awareness regarding the impact of bereavement within BME communities. Karen gained her Master's Degree from the Institute of Family Therapy in London and Birkbeck College, University of London. In addition to her clinical inpatient work in Child and Adolescent Mental Health Services (CAHMS) and adult psychiatry, Karen has managed several family centres and contact centres for divorced/estranged parents and their children. Karen also has extensive clinical specialism in working with all parties affected by adoption. As a practitioner-scholar, she has been involved in a variety of academic activities both nationally and internationally, and written book reviews for various publishers. Karen has presented papers, lectures and conducted a number of master classes/seminars in the UK, Jamaica, Indonesia, Haiti, Singapore, and the Dominican Republic amongst other countries.

Theodore S. Ransaw received his Bachelor's and Master's Degrees in Communication Studies and his Ph.D. Degree in Education from the University of Nevada, Las Vegas. His Doctorate is in Curriculum and Instruction with a focus on Multicultural and International Education. Currently, he is a K-12 Outreach Specialist in the College of Education at Michigan State University (MSU) and Core Faculty in African and African-American Studies, also at MSU. His research centers on cognition of identity and schooling. He looks at what fathers do to help their children get ahead in school, the relationship between Black male identity and educational outcomes, and the role student identity plays in education. He also served as a director of four mentorship programs at three at-risk schools and as an achievement gap specialist for males of color. He is a certified education coach and an education consultant. He has co-edited the *Handbook of Research on Black Males* (2018) and has authored *The Art of Being Cool: The Pursuit of Black Masculinity* (2013).

About the Authors

Cornelius Ani, MBBS, MSc, MRCP, FRCPsych, FHEA, MD, is a Consultant Child and Adolescent Psychiatrist in Surrey, UK, is an Honorary Clinical Senior Lecturer at Imperial College London, and is an Associate Lecturer in Child and Adolescent Mental Health (CAMH) at the University of Ibadan, Nigeria. His research includes projects in Africa, Asia, UK and North America. He was instrumental in setting up the first post-graduate training in CAMH in West Africa. He conducted the first systematic study on aggressive behaviour among Nigerian primary school students and supervised the first school-based intervention study to reduce aggression among Nigerian students.

Fabricio E. Balcazar, Ph.D., is a Professor with the Department of Disability and Human Development at the University of Illinois at Chicago. His primary interest is in developing methods for enhancing and facilitating consumer empowerment and personal effectiveness among individuals with disabilities. He has published more than 80 peer-reviewed journal articles and co-edited a book entitled *Race, Culture and Disability: Issues in Rehabilitation Research and Practice*. He is a Fellow of the American Psychological Association (APA) and the former President of Division 27 of the APA, Society for Community Research and Action.

Nicholas Banks, PhD, at the time of wring this chapter, is a Senior Lecturer in Psychology at the Institute of Psychology, University of Wolverhampton, UK. He has an active forensic private practice with international connections in Africa and the Middle East. He was a Lecturer in Social Work (psychology, child development and communicating with children) at the University of Birmingham, UK for 10 years. He was a Senior Lecturer in Counselling and Psychotherapy for almost two years at the University of Nottingham, UK (counselling and special educational needs). He is a Chartered Clinical Psychologist. He has worked as an Educational Psychologist. He has research interests in attachment, fostering and adoption, parenting skills, abuse issues, substance abuse related to parenting, black children and families, issues of identity and counselling and psychotherapy, special educational needs and autism. He published the first evidence-based British book on cross-cultural counselling (Avebury Publishers).

Belinda Brooks-Gordon, Ph.D., is a Reader in Psychology and Social Policy, Birkbeck, University of London. She was awarded the Doctoral Degree at the University of Cambridge, UK. She is the Caribbean-born British daughter of an

Irish migrant mother, and her teenage years were spent in West Africa. This led to an interest in migration, integration, and its impact on one's sense of self and racial identity. She is the Director of the Family and Systemic Therapy Course at Birkbeck and the Institute of Family Therapy. She was therefore enthusiastic about the original research in this chapter when Karen first suggested it as a topic to explore. Like many supervisors, she felt that she learned more than she imparted in its gestation and delivery.

Cheron Byfield, Dphil, was awarded the Doctoral degree at the University of Oxford, UK. She has been working with Black boys since 1999 when she co-founded Excell3 and its subsidiary 'the National Black Boys Can Association'. Through the network of over 30 locally based Black Boys Can projects which they established throughout the country, they raised the academic aspirations and achievement of well in excess of 10,000 Black boys taking a holistic approach to supporting them by not only working with the boys, but also training and empowering their parents, training and challenging educational institutions, engaging the community and lobbying the political machinery to effect change for black boys. They established partnerships with leading universities including the universities of Oxford and Cambridge and through their innovative programme that have been successful in supporting many students to gain access and obtain Bachelor's, Master's and Doctorate degrees from these institutions.

Patricia Clarke obtained an MA/DiPSW from the University of Nottingham in 1996. She has worked in the independent sector: the Sheffield African Caribbean Mental Health Association although has spent most of her career working within statutory services. Following qualification as an approved mental health professional (AMHP) in 1999, she has delivered training to AMHPS and members of multi-disciplinary teams. She remains passionate about delivering quality training and has devised and delivered training regarding: risk assessment, supervision, safeguarding, and mental health law.

Steve Clarke is a former Principal Educational Psychologist who works in the North West of England. He obtained his Ph.D. in 1996 and his thesis was on the application of a Personal Construct Psychology approach with young people who experience social, emotional and mental health difficulties. He is now in private practice and continues to use his expertise to promote better outcomes for young people with social, emotional and mental health difficulties.

Gail Coleman-Oluwabusola is a Consultant Clinical Psychologist and Head of Psychology in an Independent Mental Health Hospital in South Manchester, UK. Prior to qualifying as a clinical psychologist, she worked in NHS mental health services, proactively engaging with Black communities and researching inequalities. She also co-chaired the North West 'Race' and Culture special interest group of the British Psychological Society. She began training for her Doctorate in Clinical Psychology in 1998 at the University of Liverpool, UK. She qualified in 2002. At this time, her thesis focussed on the experiences of Black men in the UK psychiatric system. Since qualifying she has worked in the NHS, independent forensic settings and government departments often with a focus on Black and Minority Ethnic Communities. She is currently an Honorary Lecturer in the Department of Clinical Psychology at Sheffield University, UK. She continues to lecture and provide training for NHS and social care staff on the trauma of racism.

Rodalyn David was a Graduate Research Assistant in the Department of Education, Culture, and Society at the University of Utah and a Doctoral student during the writing of this chapter.

Amy Degnan, PhD, is a Trainee Clinical Psychologist with the Greater Manchester Mental Health NHS Foundation Trust. After completing her PhD in 2017, she was awarded the Doctor of Philosophy Degree in Clinical Psychology at The University of Manchester. Her research interests are in the fields of psychosis and improving access to culturally appropriate and effective psychological interventions for underserved or disadvantaged groups. Her PhD explored the social network characteristics and psychological processes related to engagement with mental health services in Black African and Caribbean people with non-affective psychosis. She completed this research whilst managing a three-year National Institute for Health Research (NIHR) funded Health Service and Delivery Research (HS&DR) trial to develop and test the feasibility of a Culturally adapted Family Intervention (CaFI) for Black Caribbean people with non-affective psychosis and their families. She is currently conducting research to explore the psychological mechanisms in the development of 'negative symptoms' in psychosis. Once qualified, she plans to continue the research whilst practicing as a Clinical Psychologist in the National Health Service (NHS).

Dawn Edge has a PhD in Medical Sociology from the University of Manchester, awarded in 2003. She is a Professor. She is a Senior Lecturer in the Division of Psychology and Mental Health in the School of Health Sciences. She has a focus on driving Equality, Diversity & Inclusion (ED&I). Reflecting on her strong commitment to integrating research, policy and practice and to public service, she is actively engaged in working with communities to improve health and wellbeing – especially among those who are marginalised, socially excluded, and experience inferior access to health and care. Formerly, a Non-Executive Director of two NHS Mental Health Trusts in the North West of England, she has also held secondments to the national Care Standards Improvement Partnership (CSIP) and its precursor, the National Institute for Mental Health in England (NIMHE). NIMHE was established by the Department of Health (DH) to improve the lives of people who experience mental health problems, to promote mental health and resilience, reduce stigma and tackle inequalities. She was awarded an NHS North West Doctoral Training Fellowship to undertake a Master's of Research (MRes) in Social Science (Salford, 2000) and PhD in Mental Health (Manchester, 2003). Her postdoctoral research was facilitated by winning a Faculty of Medical & Human Science 'Stepping Stones' Award (University of Manchester, 2006–2010).

Philomena Essed is a Professor of Critical Race, Gender and Leadership Studies at the Antioch University's Graduate School of Leadership and Change and an Affiliated Researcher for the University of Utrecht's Graduate Gender Program. She holds a PhD from the University of Amsterdam and Honorary Doctorate Degrees from the University of Pretoria (2011) and Umeå University (2015). In 2011, The Queen of the Netherlands honoured her with a Knighthood. Well known for introducing the concepts of *everyday racism* and *gendered racism*, she also pioneered in developing theory on *social and cultural cloning*. The now classical 1984 (in Dutch) *Alledaags Racisme* (English version, *Everyday Racism*, 1990) has been republished in 2018. Other books include *Understanding Everyday Racism*; *Diversity: Gender, Color and Culture* and co-edited volumes: *Race Critical Theories*; *Refugees and the Transformation of Societies; A Companion to Gender Studies* ('outstanding' 2005 CHOICE award); *Clones, Fakes and Posthumans: Cultures of Replication, (2012), Dutch Racism* (2014), and *Relating Worlds of Racism* (2019). Her current focus is on dignity and ethics of care as experience and practice in leading change.

Romana Farooq is a Principal Clinical Psychologist and a Clinical Lead in the National Health Service in the United Kingdom. She was awarded the Doctorate in Clinical Psychology from the University of Leeds, UK. She specialises in working with children, young people and their families who have experienced human rights based violations, trafficking, forced criminality and exploitation. She has been involved in shaping, developing and delivering services for children and young people subject to sexual exploitation, sexual violence or displaying harmful sexual behaviour. She also has experience of working with grassroots communities and third sector organisations to bring about meaningful community engagement with statutory services. She has worked extensively with marginalised communities in particular Black, Asian and Minority Ethnic groups, escaping gender-based violence or political violence. Recently, she was awarded the British Psychological Society Early Career Award for outstanding contribution to services working with children, young people and their families. The award is presented to clinical psychologists who have shown significant skill within five years of qualifying. She is also an Expert Member on the Government Advisory Group on Child Exploitation.

Maureen Greaves is the Director of Mustard Seed Associates CIC, and practices as a Consultant Systemic Psychotherapist and as a Supervisor. She also works as an Independent Social Worker, a Leadership Coach and a Training Facilitator. Her extensive experience within child and adolescent mental health services in the UK, for over 25 years, has enriched her knowledge and skills within the field of mental health. As a Black Christian woman and current Independent Systemic Doctoral researcher, she is passionate about aspects of spirituality and mental health, particularly relevant within the African Caribbean community. She is interested in the use of reflexivity (with a spiritual orientation) and is curious as to how this might shape psychological healing and self-acceptance and also how *spiritual* reflexivity could contribute to the dominant discourse within healthcare in collaborative ways. The epistemological lens of Christianity is used as a backdrop for personalised and considered contributions to the field, to bring to the forefront her recognised bias in thinking and application to practice. There is potential to use spiritual reflexivity as a framework for including concepts of spiritual capital within practice and organisational development, using a strengths-based model. Spirituality is applicable to both faith-based practitioners and black community members alike and provides opportunity for a more comprehensive discussion and exploration.

Mary Henderson is a BABCP Accredited Psychotherapist, holds COSCA Diploma in Counselling at The Centre of Therapy and Counselling Studies in Glasgow, Scotland. She has been privileged to work across the lifespan both within Adult Improving Access to Psychological Therapies and Child and Adolescent Mental Health (CAMHS) within many NHS Trusts across England and delivered CBT through private insurance work and by way of online therapy within NHS Trusts. Through her work, she was drawn to working with black minority ethnic children, young people and adults became increasingly aware of their struggle. When invited to help write this chapter on ASD Assessment and cultural competence, she was delighted to draw on her assessment and therapeutic intervention experience from working in CAMHS. Her chapter highlights the need for an implementation of a specific culturally competent model to be utilised when assessing for ASD and for a more radical early assessment programme to be established, especially for those within a BME population.

Tiffany Howl BSc (Hons), MSc, PGCert, PGDip, is a BABCP accredited Cognitive Behavioural Psychotherapist, DBT Therapist, Clinical Supervisor and Mindfulness Teacher. As a psychology graduate she began her career at the African Caribbean Community Initiative in Wolverhampton where she worked for 3 years, initially as a trainee Counsellor and then as a Psychological Wellbeing Practitioner, providing clinical services to the black community where historically, access to psychological therapies were scarce. Tiffany graduated with a Master's degree in Health Psychology in 2016 and went on to obtain a Postgraduate Diploma in Evidence Based Psychotherapies (CBT) in 2017. She is experienced with working with both adults and children within the NHS, third sector and private sector. Tiffany has further training in Schema Focused Therapy and third-wave CBT approaches including Acceptance and Commitment Therapy, Dialectic Behavioural Therapy and Mindfulness based Cognitive Therapy. Tiffany is a qualified CBT Clinical Supervisor. When approached to contribute a chapter on Sensory Processing Disorder with consideration of cultural competence in delivery, both Howl and Prior pooled their experiences to produce their chapter in this Handbook.

Genel Jean-Claude, Pastor, was born in L'Azile, Haiti. He did his primary studies at the Evangelical Baptist School of Bellevue, L'Azile. After primary studies, his parents decided to send him to Port-au-Prince for high school studies at the Louis Joseph Janvier College of Carrefour, a town in the Haitian capital. In 2002, under the direction of God, he emigrated to Santo Domingo, Dominican Republic. After two years outside of his country, he went back to Haiti to marry the pretty Emanie Almaus. With his beautiful wife, God granted him four beautiful children, who are Manigerlly, Germanley, Betsaleel, and Berukhia. Always under the direction of God, the Tabernacle of the Witnesses of Christ was born in June 2004 with him as a founding pastor. He was awarded a Degree in theology at Bible School World Grace Mission, Inc. Santo Domingo, and, with the passion for theology, he decided to enrol at the National Evangelical University of the Dominican Republic, where he obtained a license in theology. With 14 years of pastoral ministry, he can see the mighty hand of God miraculously day by day, which is the joy of his heart. He has a vision to open this ministry in Haiti with the objective of seeking lost souls for God. They have a lot of vision for children, young people more precisely, because they believe in the integral development of being. By the grace of God, he speaks French, Spanish, Creole, and a little English. He thanks God for this privilege, Alleluia!!

Andra D. Rivers Johnson is a 1984 Graduate from the Allegheny College in Meadville, Pennsylvania where she received her B.A. Degree in Sociology. In 1988, she received her M.S.S.A. Master of Science in Social Administration Degree from the Case Western Reserve University's Mandel School of Applied Social Science in Cleveland, Ohio. She is currently a 2020 graduation candidate for the Doctor of Social Work DSW degree from the University of Southern Suzanne Dworak-Peck School of Social Work. Andra is a Licensed Independent Social Worker with supervisor endorsement in the state of Ohio; she is a licensed Clinical Social Worker in the states of Indiana and Wisconsin, and also a licensed Chemical Addictions Counselor in the state of Indiana. She has more than 30 years of clinical experience working with children, adolescents, adults, couples, families and groups in inpatient, outpatient, community-based, home-based, hospital-based, military and veterans' affairs, criminal justice, outreach, and private practice settings. Her background working extensively with diverse populations include racial, ethnic, gender, religious, sexual orientation, lifestyle, elderly populations, and people with disabilities. As a veteran of the United States Army and retiree from the Department of Veterans Affairs, she remains committed to meeting the mental health and substance use disorder needs and challenges faced by active duty military, veterans, and their families. Andra has presented on "Paradigm Shift: Mental Health and AODA through the Lens of Black/African Americans, focusing on the psychosocial and cultural responses of Black/African Americans to mental health and AODA issues, to venues in America's southwest, Midwest and southern states. Her private practice, Four Rivers & Associates LLC, is based in Roanoke, Indiana, and focuses primarily on providing clinical supervision, consultation services, and advocacy for heart health equity for Black women with heart disease.

Ivan Juzang is the founder and president of MEE Productions Inc., a market research, health communications and social marketing firm that specializes in culturally relevant behavior health messages for hard-to-reach, low-income, and underserved audiences. He earned a Bachelor of Science Degree in Mechanical Engineering from Carnegie Mellon University and created MEE during his final year at the Wharton Graduate School of the University of Pennsylvania. He has more than 25 years of practical, first-hand experience working in low-income urban communities across America. His company gained national prominence in 1992 with the release of its primary research study, *The MEE Report: Reaching the Hip Hop Generation,* which focused on previously unexplored cultural and communication dynamics of urban teens. Over the years, he has helped mental and public health agencies engage low-income communities and youth affected by trauma and who use negative coping behaviors (including opioids) to escape their realities. Over the years, he has extensive experience with strengthening protective factors of youth and young adults affected by trauma by developing and implementing behavior health intervention campaigns around mental health issues. His expertise includes promoting and strengthening protective factors that allow young people to address their most challenging personal issues by seeking positive coping behaviors or treatment. MEE's 2010 study, *Moving Beyond Survival Mode: Promoting Mental Wellness and Resiliency as a Way to Cope with Urban Trauma,* explored issues related to stress and trauma, and promoting mental wellness in low-income African American communities. Among his publications on Black males are *Tackling America's Opioid Epidemic from the Ground Up* (2015), and *Heard Not Judged: Insights into the Talents, Realities and Needs of Young Men of Color* published in 2016 and funded by the Open Society Foundations and the California Endowment. He has served on the boards of many of the most influential national foundations and non-profit organizations including: The National Campaign to Prevent Teen and Unplanned Pregnancy and The Alan Guttmacher Institute.

Jean Gerald Lafleur, Pastor, was born in Port-au-Prince, Haiti. He left for Jamaica to study at the Christ for the Nations Institute in 1996. Upon completion of his studies and due to Divine Intervention, he migrated to Antigua where he met and married his lovely wife, Elsa Eleanor Gordon. Together, he along with his wife, an anointed Prophetic psalmist, has been pastoring Restoration Ministries, Antigua for approximately 17 years. As a man who has a tremendous Apostolic and Prophetic grace on his life, he has mentored and fathered many sons over the years. On October 12, 2003, he with the support of his wife established Restoration Ministries Haiti, and continues to give oversight to the same. With a vision of making a global impact, he has travelled to over 30 countries around the world including North and South America, Asia and the Caribbean. He is the current President of the Haggai Institute Alumni Association in Antigua and one of the founding members of Kingdom Connections also in Antigua. Apostle Lafleur is a humanitarian at heart with a passion to see spiritual, physical and developmental growth in the lives of the people of his native land, Haiti and the world. "Friends of Haiti" in Antigua and "Restoration Ministries Foundation" in Jacmel are two organizations he has founded in an effort to assist in building homes, coordinating feeding programs and sponsorships for the educational needs of the children there. Apostle Jean Gerald Lafleur and Pastor Elsa Lafleur are the proud parents of two handsome and energetic boys, Jeremiah and Elisha.

Tony Leiba, PhD, is an Emeritus Professor of London South Bank University. Within London South Bank University, he contributes to the Department of

Mental Health Studies and is available for consultation on mental health education and practice within the Faculty of Health and Social Care. He teaches and researches mental health care, inter-professional education and training, research methods, evidence-based practice and conflict management. Research activities include: collaborative research with users and carers and supervising MPhil/PhD students. With regard to inter-professional education and training, he facilitates team-working away days to enable staff to reflect on how they are learning and working together. He visits Kobe University in Japan to work with the Faculty of Health Sciences in their development of undergraduate inter-professional education and training programs.

Mhemooda Malek, M.Sc., currently works in national regulation of higher education and has previously worked in mental health policy, research and engagement of minority communities in policy and planning of services. Malek's Master's Degree was awarded at the University of Bristol. Growing up in England as both a first generation migrant and also the child of first generation migrants from a former British colony, inequalities experienced by marginalized communities at the grassroots level have been all too familiar. Malek's career in policy research, service delivery and development has revealed the lack of sufficient meaningful progress on achieving race equality in the systems and structures that impact our everyday lives, including our physical and mental health. The multi-layered, embedded, historical and political nature of injustice can remain hidden from view unless one has the capacity and inclination to unravel and understand its complex terrain. Children and young people have a right to accessible knowledge and support that can enable recognition of the impact of structural racism and other inequalities, the process of internalizing injustice and building resilience. Malek's work is informed by the belief that empowering individuals and communities is a key integral part of challenging the systems and politics that perpetuate inequalities.

Isha Mckenzie-Mavinga obtained the Doctor of Psychotherapy by Professional Studies Degree from the Metanoia Institute and Middlesex University. While introducing transcultural process to several counselling courses, She found that students were reticent to address black issues. It turned out that they had a variety of powerful feelings about racism that silenced them and they also felt unsupported in their fears ability to develop a dialogue in this area. So, she set up black issues workshops to facilitate the impact of racism on their interactions and facilitate their learning in this area. This became her research area for Doctoral study. She had previously set up therapeutic services at the African Caribbean Mental health Association, in Brixton, where previously patients were only accessing befriending and legal support. After that, she published some papers and two books on the subject of black issues and racism. These were followed by workshops to encourage therapeutic dialogue about black issues and racism.

Simon Newitt, Ph.D., is the Chief Executive of Off the Record (Bristol), a youth mental health charity. His Doctoral Degree was awarded at the University of

Central Lancashire, UK. While working in NHS Child and Adolescent Mental Health Services on the national five-year Delivering Race Equality in Mental Healthcare Programme, he grew concerned by and interested in the way ideological power and structural racism was being administered through public service design, recycling the social exclusion and oppression that the state's efforts at 'inclusion' purported to address. As a result, he undertook a three-year Participatory Action Research project with a small group of young Black British men aged 15–24 in the inner city neighbourhood of St Pauls, Bristol. The collaboration challenged how he understood social research as well as constructs of mental health, race, masculinity, power and marginalization. Recognizing the need for a more socially conscious mental health provision, he established Project Zazi, a small team working creatively and experimentally with young people in Bristol to unpick the psychocultural effects of internalized racism.

Lisa Prior has worked for the past five years as a Senior CAMHS Practitioner in Blackpool working with young people with a range of difficulties including Sensory Processing Disorder. She studied BSc Hons Occupational Therapy at the University of Cumbria and later studied with Tiffany Howl, completing their PG Dip CYP IAPT CBT at the Greater Manchester Cognitive Behaviour Therapy Training Centre.

Sonya Rafiq (MRes) is currently a PhD Student in Psychology and Mental Health at the University of Manchester. She was awarded the Master's Degree at the University of Manchester, England. Her areas of interest include adverse life experiences, culture, and Severe Mental Illness. Black, Asian and Minority Ethnic groups often experience high rates of lifetime adversity. She is interested in how these experiences and their culture shape their mental health problems, and how psychological therapy can be adapted to take into account these variables.

Doreen Robinson is a qualified Social Worker and Systemic Family Psychotherapist. She has experience of over thirty years of clinical practice with a variety of cultural groups across London and adjacent counties. She has worked in areas of community work, child protection, fostering and adoption, mental health with adults, children and families both within voluntary and statutory child and health services. Doreen was a member of staff in the Asian Service at the Tavistock Clinic of the Tavistock and Portman NHS Trust and a founder member of the South Camden Community Cahms Team where she is the Lead Systemic Psychotherapist. She provides systemic consultation to community groups including a Peer Mentoring Scheme that she helped create.
Doreen teaches systems theory and practice on a number of post graduate courses at the Tavistock and Portman NHS Trust.

Tânia Rodrigues, PhD, is a Consultant Clinical Psychologist working in forensic and mental health settings in the United Kingdom. She completed her clinical training in Psychology at the University of the Western Cape, South Africa, and has 15 years' post-qualification experience, specializing in the assessment and treatment of psychiatric and psychological disorders. She started her career in South Africa and worked predominantly with trauma and sexual violence against women. In the UK, she worked as the Lead Clinical Psychologist for several low/medium secure male and female mental health and learning disability services as well as Clinical Service Lead for Female Services within one of the leading private mental health organizations. More recently, she has returned to working in the community with young people either in care or on the edge of care, their families and carers and exposed to significant trauma due to child sexual exploitation, trafficking and displacement due to war.

Florence Gwendolyn Rose, PhD, MSc, BA Open (Hons), RGN, RNT, RHV. She is a retired Nurse Lecturer from Greenwich University, London and the Open University. As a Health Visitor, her work include working with a range of families from different cultural backgrounds. She worked as a youth leader and a trainer for many years. Her youth work involves working with young black people. Her work as public health nurse (Health Visitor) involves working with families from different cultural background. The research for her PhD was prompted by the discrimination she experienced in her professional life and the inability to speak out against discrimination and oppression without disastrous consequences. Her recent healing projects as a result of her research and published book on promoting Health and Spiritual Healings been prompted by inequality and oppression especially of African-Caribbean people in the UK. In the promoting of these issues, it has been further highlighted that there is a close link between spirituality, mental health and Illness. She celebrates 50 years on the UK nursing register and has come to realise that writing about the issues of discrimination and oppression will reach more people than she as a lone person can achieve. Her personal healing journey came to the forefront in 1998 when she wrote a book on relationships and continued following the death of her mother in 2002. Her professional healing journey started when she started her nurse training in 1967 and developed further when she was called to the ministry in 1983 and was ordained as a missionary. Following her ordination, she went on to train as a Health Visitor (known at its inception as a sanitary missionary) and a teacher. Her career as a nurse spans all levels of teaching nursing, health care and promoting health. In 2003, as she recovered from the death of her mother, she embarked on research into Spiritual Healing. She gained a PhD and subsequently published the book on Health Promotion-Spiritual Healing. Other publications are Relationships, "Black and Ethnic Minority Elders: Who cares?" published in an international nursing journal, and articles on Diabetes, Dementia, and Cholesterol published in the Christian journal *Focus*. She currently serves as Lay Preacher for the URC. She is a motivational speaker and recently retired as the Director of Coaching and Development Consultancy. She is currently writing a book on *Where Is God in Dementia?*

Llewellyn E. Simmons, PhD, is currently the Director of Academics at the Ministry of Education and a Senior Fellow of the Applied Centre for Emotional Literacy Leadership and Research (ACELLR). He is a former Assistant

Professor of the University of Dayton. He has a long range of community activism nationally and internationally. Most notably, a national activism in Bermuda, inspired by an international brotherhood in the United States of America sparked the establishment of 100 Blackman Plus of Bermuda. In addition, he co-founded the Venturilla Summer School for Boys and is the Vice President for the Audacia Resettlement Works, an organization for African refugees. The three principles governing his actions are: Freedom–Justice–Equity. It is out of these three that Life–Liberty–Pursuit of Happiness is realized. As an international educator, he is committed to building Black Communities and Community Wealth on the foundation of: Economics, Political Development, Social Justice, Media, and Education. He has numerous publications to his credit. Most recent publications are *National Development: Conflated Concepts as False Narratives* and *Inquiry: An Emancipatory Pedagogical Strategy for Bermuda Schools*. His most recent presentation and developing manuscript presented at the Colloquium for Black Males is titled "The Educational Trajectory of Bermuda's Black Males: Stopping Bullets and Building Community Wealth." Works in progress include "A Social Emotional Learning Curriculum – Preschool to Senior" and "Bermuda's Covenant." Internationally, he has imparted these principles and practices where he is called to be a servant leader. He is a former Bermuda National footballer and Somerset Trojan; one of only two goalkeepers to become Bermuda's Most Valuable Player; a College Most Valuable Player; Former Bermuda Track Field 110-meter hurdles champion and many, many Football Championships locally and internationally. He is an avid reader, researcher, and scholar.

Reenee Singh is a Consultant Family and Couples Systemic Psychotherapist. She is the Director of the London Intercultural Couples Centre at the Child and Family Practice, the Co-director of the Tavistock Family Therapy and Systemic Research Centre and the Editor of the *Journal of Family Therapy*.

William A. Smith is a Full Professor and the Department Chair in the Department of Education, Culture and Society at the University of Utah. He also holds a joint appointment in the Ethnic Studies Program (African American Studies division) as a Full Professor. He has served as the Associate Dean for Diversity, Access, & Equity in the College of Education (2007–2014) as well as a Special Assistant to the President at the University of Utah & its NCAA Faculty Athletics Representative (2007–2013). He is the Co-editor (with Philip Altbach & Kofi Lomotey) of the book, *The Racial Crisis in American Higher Education: The Continuing Challenges for the 21st Century* (2002). In 2018, he received the College of Education's Faculty Service Award for Outstanding Research and Scholarship. His research primarily focuses on his theoretical contribution of Racial Battle Fatigue which is the cumulative emotional, psychological, physiological, and behavioral effects that racial micro-level aggressions and macro-level aggressions (microaggressions and macroaggressions) have on People of Color. His work has appeared in such prestigious journals: *The International Journal of Qualitative Studies in Education, Journal of Negro Education, Harvard Educational Review,*

Educational Administration Quarterly, American Educational Research Journal, and *American Behavioral Scientist,* among others. He received his Undergraduate and Master's Degrees from Eastern Illinois University (BA in Psychology and MS in Guidance and Counseling) and his Ph.D. from the University of Illinois at Urbana–Champaign (educational policy studies, sociology/social psychology of higher education).

Glory S. Stanton is a Graduate of the University of Utah, where she earned her B.S. Degree in Health Promotion and Education (Provider Health emphasis) and a minor in Sociology. She was a student researcher working under the mentorship of Dr. William A. Smith, Ph.D., Professor at the University of Utah, in the Departments of Ethnic Studies and Education, Culture and Society. Her undergraduate research focus was understanding the impact that racial battle fatigue had on the biopsychosocial effects of Black men living in predominately White communities. She is currently pursuing her Master's Degree at Vanderbilt University, where her graduate research focuses on racial battle fatigue in Black men as it relates to bioethics and human rights law. She plans to pursue her Juris Doctorate Degree upon graduation and begin her career in law.

Tony Talburt is a senior lecturer and author with interests in the political history of Africa and its Diaspora and also International Politics. He has over 30 years of teaching experience in schools, colleges and universities in Ghana, Jamaica and the UK and worked for a number of years as education and curriculum advisor at Excell3 in Birmingham, UK. He is a graduate from the University of the West Indies (Mona Campus) with a B.A. Degree in History with Social Science and also obtained his M.A. Degree in international Studies from the University of Warwick. His PhD was obtained from the London South Bank University in International Politics. Some of his recent books include: *History on the Page: Adventures in Black British History*, London: New Generation Publishers (2012), *Andrew Watson: The World's First Black Football Superstar*, Hertfordshire: Hansib Publishers (2017), and as Co-editor of *Fight for Freedom: Black Resistance and Identity*, Accra: Sub-Saharan Press (2017).

David Truswell has worked in community-based mental health services in the UK for over 30 years developing services for people with complex care needs and enduring mental health problems in a career spanning the voluntary sector, local authority services, and the NHS at a senior level. He has two Master's level Degrees, including a distinction level MBA. From 2009 to 2011, he was the Dementia Implementation Lead for Commissioning Support for London, working with commissioners across London to improve dementia services. He is currently the Chair of the Dementia Alliance for Culture and Ethnicity (www.demace.com), a UK alliance of local and national voluntary organisations working with dementia and an independent writer and researcher on dementia support and services for Black and minority ethnic communities. He is also the Director of somfreshthinking limited, a healthcare consultancy working on service redesign and change management in health and social care services.

Patrick Vernon (LLM Warwick University) OBE, PhD, is the Associate Director for Connected Communities at the Centre for Ageing Better. He is a Clore and Winston Churchill Fellow, a Fellow of Goodenough College, a Fellow at Imperial War Museum, and a former Associate Fellow for the Department of History of Medicine at Warwick University. He is a former Director of Black Thrive in Lambeth, a Non-Executive Director of Camden and Islington Mental Health Foundation Trust, Health Partnership Coordinator for National Housing Federation, a former member of Healthwatch England, NHS England Equality Diversity Council, an Advisory board member for Time to Change and a former member of the Labour and the Government Ministerial Advisory for Mental Health. He is also the founder of Every Generation Media and 100 Great Black Britons, which develops education programmes, publications and films on cultural heritage and family history. He was made Pioneer of the Nation for Cultural History by the Queen in 2003. He is a leading expert on African and Caribbean genealogy in the UK. In 2017, he was a guest editor for *Black History Month* magazine, and in 2018 he led the campaign for Windrush Day and amnesty for the Windrush Generation. He was awarded an OBE in 2012 for his work tackling health inequalities for UK ethnic minority communities, is patron of the ACCI mental health charity in Wolverhampton, Santé, a refugee project in Camden and was awarded an honorary Doctor of Letters by Wolverhampton University in 2018. In 2018, he was selected as one of the 1,000 Evening Standard Progressive Londoners for his campaign for Windrush Day and 2019 by the Independent Happy List for fundraising efforts regarding Windrush Justice Fund.

Julie Vryhof, M.U.Ed, Union University, Doctoral Student at the University of Illinois of Chicago. She is currently a PhD student in Disability Studies at the University of Illinois at Chicago. She has the Master's Degree in Urban Education from Union University and worked for four years as a Special Education Teacher in elementary schools in Memphis, TN. Her research interests are at the intersections of disability, schooling and race in the USA particularly has public and charter schools supports students of colors with disabilities who have experienced adjudication.

Sharon Walker, PhD, is a Senior Lecturer with London Metropolitan University (England), qualified in Social Work in 1992 with an MSc Degree in Social Policy and Social Work Studies and has completed three additional Master's Degrees. She worked for HM Prison Service developing therapeutic drug treatment programs and conducted similar work in prisons across Europe. She returned to social work management for a short time prior to becoming a Senior Lecturer in Social Work and commenced a Professional Doctorate in Systemic Practice. Her original research was developing a pedagogy for social work students using a relationship-based approach. However, her personal experiences of academia led her to focus on race and the disproportionality of mental health amongst black communities. Her publications reflect both her original area of research and her subsequent interest in race, culture and mental ill health of black people in social systems. She has a Phd by publication awarded by London Metropolitan University.

Foreword

Joseph L. White

I have been affectionately and respectfully called, 'The Father of Black Psychology'. As a clinical psychologist and activist, I had been a mentor to many young people and former graduate students like Dr Majors over the years. Since meeting Richard in Washington, DC at the American Psychological Association annual conference in the mid-1980s, it has been an absolute pleasure to watch him grow from being a graduate student to becoming a very good clinician/therapist and an internationally well-known and respected academic psychologist, particularly in the field of masculinity and gender. His book *Cool Pose* is considered a classic in the field and is one of the most cited books in race relations and gender in the US.

When I started studying and teaching psychology, the deficit model of psychology was the predominant lens/model in which white traditional 'worldview' psychology interpreted and viewed black people and our culture. The deficit model suggested that African-Americans were somehow deficient/inferior to whites with respect to intelligence, various abilities, family structure, and other factors.

Implicit in this concept of cultural deprivation is the notion that the dominant white middle-class culture is the normative standard and the so-called 'correct' culture. What emerged as normal or abnormal was always in comparison with that of white European-Americans. For many white social scientists and psychologists, 'different' became synonymous with 'deficient' rather than with simply being different. Thus, any behaviours, customs, experiences, values, and lifestyles that differed from the Euro-Americans norm were seen as deficient. Due to the inadequate exposure to Euro-American values, norms, customs, and lifestyles, African-Americans were seen as 'culturally deprived' and in need of cultural enrichment.

These racist and stereotypical views were indeed biased and flawed, and were not based on any reliable scientific data, but they were still allowed to flourish without scientific scrutiny. Over my life as a psychologist, scholar, administrator, and activist, I did my very best to challenge and fight such injustices and correct these racist ideologies, falsehoods, and stereotypes that have been unfairly targeted against our people unscientifically for years. In fact, it was these racist ideologies that inspired me to write my 1970 article, 'Towards a Black Psychology', and to challenge the prevailing hegemonic bias. I argued for the importance of developing a black psychology that would counter biased and racist analyses, for more scientific data, and for a non-pathological/more balanced view of African-American culture, rather than focussing on pathology.

Therefore, the Afrocentric or multicultural models of psychology is a much better or more appropriate model for understanding African-Americans and people of African descent than eurocentrism. These models assume that all cultures have strengths and limitations and rather than being viewed as deficient, any differences between cultural/ethnic groups should be viewed as simply different. Black psychology over the years, has played a vital role in providing evidence-based data/models about African-Americans and African-American culture that are more accurate, reliable, and scientific and thereby challenge stereotypes and racist ideology.

Much like myself in developing a distinct and non-biased culturally based psychology, Richard Majors, Karen Carberry, and Theodore S. Ransaw in *The International Handbook of Black Community Mental Health* shift the paradigm of thinking in Black Mental Health, by bringing awareness to important, sensitive, and taboo/controversial subjects in mental health, which many whites are not comfortable discussing. Some of the areas the authors deal with in their book are racism/discrimination in mental health (e.g., institutional, everyday racism, implicit bias and micro-aggression, racialised white/black supervisory relationships, and the overrepresentation of black men in the mental health system). In their book they also deal with subjects like: the impact of dementia on African-American population communities, sensory processing issues, autism, learning disabilities, among other areas. The authors not only deal with 'problems' in mental health, they also seek and propose solutions to address many of the problems identified above. The authors believe focussing on these topical areas in mental health will educate their audience about how various forms of challenges/discriminations impact people of colour's black mental health. They introduce new therapeutic models and cultural competence methodologies and they share new emotional literacy and emotional wellness technologies, just to mention only a few solutions that are offered in their book.

This book addresses one of the most important issues of our time and does so in a compelling way. I think this outstanding book is very timely and will go a long way towards raising awareness challenging systems and structures and creating more favourable positive outcomes for people of colour who access mental health services. As such, I highly recommend this book and hopes this book receives the wide readership and distribution it deserves.

Professor Joseph White
Clinical Psychologist
University of California – Irvine
Department of Psychology, Psychiatry and Comparative Culture

Prologue

Alvin Poussaint

Racist incidents have proliferated dramatically under the current political zeitgeist. Unfortunately, all forms of racism have flourished, including 'Everyday Racism' (Essed,1991), institutional racism and micro-aggressions among other forms of both overt/covert forms of racism, as chronicled here in *The International Handbook of Black Community Mental Health*. While I am alarmed by this situation, I am particularly distressed by the manifestation of extreme racist violence often perpetrated by paranoid/delusional individuals towards people of colour. I have been passionate about fighting the malignancy of extreme racism my entire career.

As a psychiatrist, I was involved in the 1969 petitioning of the American Psychiatric Association (APA) to include extreme racism in the Diagnostic and Statistical Manual of Mental Disorders (DSM). Despite such efforts, the APA continues to resist considering extreme racism as a mental health disorder.

Extreme racists' violence should be considered in the context of behaviour described by Gordon Allport (1954) in *The Nature of Prejudice*. Allport's 5-point scale categorises increasingly dangerous acts. It begins with verbal expression of antagonism, progresses to avoidance of members of disliked groups, then to active discrimination against them, to physical attacks, and finally to extermination (lynching, massacre, and genocide). That fifth point on the scale, the acting out of extermination fantasies, is readily classifiable as delusional behaviour. Similarly, Sullaway and Dunbar (1996) used a prejudice rating scale to assess and describe levels of prejudice. They found associations between highly prejudiced people and other indicators of psychopathology. The subtype at the extreme end of their scale is a paranoid/delusional prejudice disorder.

The psychiatric profession's primary index for diagnosing psychiatric symptoms, the DSM, does not list racism, prejudice, or bigotry in its text or index. The association's officials rebuffed the criteria outlined above, arguing that so many Americans are racist that even extreme racism is normative and better thought of as a social aberration, or a 'social problem' like sexism and ageism, than an indication of individual psychopathology. Other mental health professionals disagree. Still, many psychiatrists believe that a diagnosis of mental illness would serve as an excuse and absolve perpetrators of personal responsibility for their gruesome acts. Others believe a psychiatric diagnosis would open doors to an insanity defence plea that might lead to exoneration. In fact, such fears do not hinder diagnosing mental disorders in capital murder defendants. Raising these extraneous issues evades the point.

Currently there is meagre support for including extreme racism under any diagnostic category. To continue perceiving it as normative and not pathological is to lend it legitimacy. Clearly, anyone who scapegoats a whole group of people and seeks to eliminate them to resolve his or her internal conflicts meets criteria for a delusional disorder, a major psychiatric illness.

A growing number of psychiatrists, psychologists, mental health professionals, and academics believe extreme racism should be classified in the DSM as a mental disorder. Like all others who experience delusions, extreme racists do not think rationally. Healthcare professionals have observed and worked with people of colour who have been victimised and traumatised by racism. In some parts of the world, these numbers have grown and given the current political zeitgeist many observers feel they will rise.

Anecdotally, I have known psychiatrists who have treated patients who projected their own behaviours and fears onto people of colour as scapegoats. Often, their strong racist feelings were tied to fixed belief systems, reflecting symptoms of mental dysfunction. Take paranoid disorder, for example, where sufferers often project unacceptable feelings and ideas onto other people and groups. Mental health professionals must collectively challenge the resistance to accepting such symptoms as serious mental illness.

Using the DSM's structure of diagnostic criteria for delusional disorder, I suggest the following subtype:

> Prejudice type: A delusion whose theme is that a group of individuals, who share a defining characteristic, in one's environment have a particular and unusual significance. These delusions are usually of a negative or pejorative nature, but also may be grandiose in content. When these delusions are extreme, the person may act out by attempting to harm, and even murder, members of the despised group(s).

Extreme racist delusions can also occur as a major symptom in other psychotic disorders, such as schizophrenia and bipolar disorder. Persons suffering such delusions have serious social dysfunction that impairs their ability to work with others and maintain employment.

Interventions with afflicted individuals may prevent tragedies like those in Charleston, Douglas, and Parkland High School from happening in the future. The shooters involved in these massacres subscribed to some form of racist ideology. Surely, adding 'extreme racism' to the classification system of the DSM should be viewed as a matter of urgency.

In Europe and the international community, there has been some progress towards racism becoming classified as a mental disorder. The *Oxford Handbook of Personality Disorders*, last revised in 2012, has in their classification system:

'pathological bias'. Pathological bias is defined as having extreme racist and supremacist views that could lead one to commit acts of violence against a person or persons of another race. Also, the ICD-10 (International Classification of Diseases) uses what they refer to as 'Z' codes; 'Z' codes theoretically could be used to classify racist acts. Z 55 – Z 65 cover 'Persons with potential health hazards related to socioeconomic and psychosocial circumstances'. For example, Z 62 deals with, 'Problems related to social upbringing'. There is also Z 60 and Z 64, which refer to 'Problems related to social environment and psychosocial circumstances', respectively. It would seem that both descriptions could fit the perpetrators and victims of racism. It's time for the DSM to follow suit with similar changes.

I applaud Majors, Carberry, and Ransaw, the editors of this new book, *The International Handbook of Black Community Mental Health*, for arguing and advocating not only for the importance of including extreme racism in the DSM but for highlighting the less extreme and often more subtle and sophisticated forms of racism that people of colour endure. While these forms may be less extreme and overt, nevertheless they can be just as devastating. As the editors rightfully argue, racism takes on different forms and levels. Racism does not have to be extreme for someone to experience victimisation and traumatisation. The editors point out that much is said about institutional racism in the UK and Europe, where many of the chapter authors reside, while other less extreme, more subtle and sophisticated forms of racism are ignored: everyday racism (Essed, 1991), implicit biased racism, racial battle fatigue (Smith, 2008), and microaggressions (Pierce, 1970) in everyday life impact staff within the workforce across all professions.

These types of racism are finally being given more serious consideration and more research is being conducted in UK, Europe and worldwide to access their impact on mental health, victimisation, traumatisation, bullying, harassment, and other interactions.

The authors of this book provide rich and detailed testimonials on people's lives with case studies of people of colour who have been affected by various forms of racism in their daily lives. These experiences have affected their mental health through inequalities in mental health access and services, graduate student retention, and supervisory experiences in academia, staffing, and promotions. Disparities are reflected in the over-representation of Black men hospitalised, incarcerated, and involved in mental health services, and the lack of services for those with learning disabilities and vocational challenges.

The editors discuss these critical problematic areas and offer solutions: they explore new policy recommendations and provide concrete ideas about cultural competence, emotional literacy and emotional wellness, case study methodologies, mindfulness strategies, and the introduction of new technologies for psychosocial intervention with people of colour who have schizophrenia and related psychoses. I applaud their work. This insightful book will prove valuable for individuals who seek a better understanding of the challenges people of colour face in mental health.

References

Sullaway, M., & Dunbar, E. (1996). Clinical manifestations of prejudice in psychotherapy: Toward a strategy of assessment and treatment. *Clinical Psychology: Science and Practice*, *2*, 296–309.

Professor Alvin Poussaint, MD, Emeritus Harvard Medical School

Prelude
Eugene Ellis

Black individuals who enter into a mental wellbeing service or a learning environment are in search of a competent resource that can support them through a process of change and development. Frequently, however the lens through which they are seen is not sufficiently variable enough to take into account the cultural diversity of the society in which they live, nor does the lens take into account the social construct of race and how hostile forces of discrimination and oppression can confine and define ones sense of self and wellbeing and also ones position in society.

If you begin to research mental health outcomes for BME communities, and as you will no doubt find reading the chapters to come, you will quickly discover that there are countless studies which document an enduring institutional insensitivity to the social forces of culture and race, which are fundamental dimensions for every human being and therefore should be integrated into a general clinical and educational approach.

The central aim of this book is to move away from a culture-blind and colour-blind approach to mental wellbeing and education, and bring together knowledge, practice and experience that will both illustrate and illuminate the latest thinking and practice in these very important areas.

The editors of this book have brought together important thinkers from the United Kingdom, Europe and across the United States to produce what is a significant contribution towards addressing black mental wellbeing. This book provides a wealth of knowledge and experience from a wide range of perspectives including such diverse areas as culturally competent assessment and treatment of ASD and sensory processing difficulties, targeted interventions for young black boys in education, psychological wellbeing in transracial adoption, a focus on the importance of religious and spiritual awareness, the dynamics of supporting individuals and families through the impact of racism and exploring gender discourses within the South Asian forced marriage system. Research and solutions are also presented for reducing the overrepresentation of black men in the UK psychiatric system and shedding light on race equality within learning institutions.

This book is written for therapists, educators and policymakers as well as anyone who wants to understand and develop culturally competent practice and intervention in their organisations. In a wide range of chapters, over 40 authors share their wisdom and bring their expertise to life. Readers will come away with new theoretical frameworks, useful language and terminology, in-depth knowledge about specific cultural populations and practical interventions and strategies. In the end, BME populations in mental health services and education will benefit the most from this book when the societal context of their lives, both external and internal, is more fully understood and welcomed as an important part of their lives.

Acknowledgements

Richard Majors

I would first like to acknowledge these historical "Freedom Fighters"/Activists and Elders: Nat Turner, John Brown, Denmark Vesey, Gabriel Prosser, Malcolm X, Harriet Tubman, Charles Deslondes, Toussaint Louverture, Jean-Jacques Dessalines, Nanny of Maroons and all the other historical Freedom Fighters/Activist and Elders who had the courage to stand up and fight racism inequalities and social justice, in spite of... and in many instances paying the ultimate price - giving up their lives so that my life and my people's lives would be better. My dear Brothers and Sisters...Thank you from the bottom of my heart...

I also would like to recognise and salute our modern "Freedom Fighters"/Activists whose actions, research, writings and speeches challenged Eurocentric/white hegemonic racist ideology/pseudo-science and by doing so, they helped to lay the pathway directly or indirectly for the creation of the Black psychology movement, Afrocentic ideology and the Association of Black Psychologists. They are: First and foremost, Professor Joseph White and the founding members of the Association of Black Psychologists, Dr. Bobby E. Wright, Professor Charles W. Thomas, Kobi Kazembe Kambon aka Joseph Baldwin, Na'im Akbar, Adelbert Jenkins, Daudi Ajani ya Azibo, John Henrik, Clarke Molefi, Kete Asante, Dr. Yosef Ben-Jochannan, Professor Cheikh Anta Diop and Maulana Karena among others of course... I thank each and every one of you from the bottom of my heart...

I would like to acknowledge here as well my family and friends. I am deeply indebted to many people, without their contribution, love, support or encouragement in my life this book would not have been completed: First and foremost, I would like to thank my Mother Fannie Sue Majors, Grandmother Lillian A. McGill, Father Richard Majors, Daisy Majors and the late Mrs Viola Scott, Eugene and the Scott family, who all accepted me and took me under her/their wing during a vulnerable time when my grandmother passed away, I will always be grateful to each and every one of you. I know the value of role models and I want to thank my "dream team of role models": the Love family, Mr James, Mr John Derek, Roy Cochran, R. Weingarten, Gary, Rollie Barnet, J. Koenig Aunts: Ruth and Marie and Uncles: Charles, Claude, George and Wally. I was so fortunate and blessed during my childhood to have such special relatives and people and role models in my life like each one of you were to me ...your words, behaviors, actions, and wisdom influenced, shaped, guided and made me the person I am today. I could never ever thank each of you enough... Thank you... Love you all.

I am also indebted to my sisters and brother: my big sister Lynn Johnson, Holly Small, Lisa Majors, Chan Majors, Tish Majors Brown, Stacey Wallace, Theda Lewis and her daughter and my late niece Clovella Layvonne Richardson. I would like to honor other family members who have passed: Doug and Vincent Small.

I am indebted to the late friends and colleagues who had a major influence on my life: Dr. Stuart Jones, Dr. Joseph White, Dr. Reginald Jones, Dr. Jack Easley, Dr. Eugene Link, Dr. Ron Fitzgerald and Michael Love, MayPearl Fields and Jean Matthew Elmore, Hollis Head Jr, Shedon Julius, Vera Michell, Dr. Arthur Nikelly, Nontombo Philups, and Eddie "Bongo" Folk... Thank you all I love each and every one of you dearly.

I would also like to honor other late friends and colleagues who impacted my life: Chip and Michael Dickerson, Kevin Cadle, Rosalie Tabin, Bill Hampton C.P. Gause, Dr. Peter Stubing and the Richardson family: Mrs Gertrude, Howard and Jeffery Richardson who were kind enough to allow me to stay in their lovely home while in college... Thank you.

I would like to recognise all my nieces and nephews and David, and all my cousins and relatives in the Midwest.

I am equally deeply appreciative of the support, love and guidance of my very good friends: Charles Hughes my uncle, Eugene Scott, Lew Simmons, George Brown, Dorian and Darryl Howard, Douglas, Spike and Sister Milton, Micheal Winston, Ducey boy and Wendy Henderson, Phil, Yemane Tewelde, Hugh Hall, Thomas Mutunga, elder Boniface Kikwau, Israel and Seth Adedzi, Lawrence Quayson, Eric Orr, Greg Young, Roland McKenzie, Cornelius Ani, Will Levan, Greg Foster, Cliff Stroughter, Abe and Denise Lee, Lorenzo Thornton, Douglas Jenkins, Ian Millard, Andrew Shelley, David Munro, Sharon Walker, John Oguchkwu, Thad Branch, Sobe Chukwu, Altie Daniel, Joe Jackson, John Barnes, Diane Watt, Nehemiah Nixon, Bob Hall, Tony White, Steve Clarke, Rose Genas, Sheldon Lee, Darryl Hutson, Ronald Hall, Rodney Jackson, Sharon Walker, Sandy Parker and all my Southside and Northside "Cool pose" childhood friends.

Finally, I like to recognise the following for their guidance/support in graduate school and during my fellowship time: Dr J. McVicker Hunt, Dr. Klaus Witz, Dr. Terry Denny, Dr. Steve Tozier, Dr. Ralph Page, Dr. Philup Jones, Dr. Norman Denzin, Dr. Harry Triandis, Robert Sprague, Dr. Ken Monterio, Dr. Elaine Copeland and Dr. Alvin Poussaint.

I like to give a special thank you to Darrell for all his unwavering administrative assistance over the years on my various projects, without his support I would have not have had the success on this project as well as others... Thank you so much Darrell.

I want to recognise and thank all my students in Psychology of African Africans (P337) the first course of its at the time at the university, for all your contributions and support and for making me a better teacher.

I would like to give a special thanks to my co-editors, first Karen Carberry whose hard work, dedication to our project and expert project management skills made this project possible and secondly to my other co-editor, Ted Ransaw for his keen insights and steadfast contribution throughout the project. I would also like to thank Dr. Gary Sailes for his support and assistance to this project and Patrick Vernon for his policy contributions to our book. And finally this project would not have been completed without the unyielding support, expertise and guidance of both our commissioning and content editors Emma Leverton and Sophie Barr at Emerald Publishing, and Rajachitra at Cenveo. Thank you each and every one of you.

Karen Carberry

The place in which I currently stand is due to many people. The first is by the grace of God, who has brought me through a mighty long way, who reminds me during times of challenge. 'But you are a chosen people, a royal priesthood, a holy nation, God's special possession, that you may declare the praises of him who called you out of darkness into his wonderful light' 1 Peter 2:9.

I want to thank my parents, Mr Helmet (Hugh) Carberry and Mrs Dorrel (Cherry) Carberry nee Palmer, a Jamaican couple who have been together for nearly 60 years. They arrived in the United Kingdom in the early 1960s and their experience and journey in England has, like so many Jamaicans, been extraordinary. They met in the UK, developed a life together in marriage and have taught their four children the importance of education, and remaining true to our sense of self in our bi-cultural experience. Thank you Mum for telling off the Careers Advisor at school, who suggested that, I could only aspire to work on the checkout in the supermarket. Although cashiers hold a noble job, God had other plans for me. Our parents have taught us by observing their lives that all our talents are transferable. Arriving in the Windrush era, and employed through many different professions, my father's retirement from the Civil Service ended with a royal invitation and attendance at the Queens Garden party with his wonderful wife. As Sir Michael Caine would say 'Not a lot of people know that!'. Mum and Dad, humbly I salute you.

I want to thank my two brothers Dennis and Jason, and Jason's wife Patricia Carberry for their support through these mission trips to Haiti and the Dominican Republic. My wonderful sister Sharon Carberry who unselfishly transcribed many hours of data to help me with my studies, reflections and the chapter on working with Haitian families.

I want to acknowledge the late Pastor Harrold of Pilgrim Union Church God for her love and wisdom under which I came to know the Lord Jesus Christ and her daughter Hope; the late Evangelist, Sister Barbara Howe, who went home to be with the Lord in 2018, who led the missionary team. Sister Barbara who invited me to be part of the team, and taught me how to serve in the community; and her husband Evangelist Brother Wilfred Howe for raising funds towards my mission trips to Haiti and whetting my appetite for Haiti by leading our church's contribution in the relief programme following the earthquake in 2010. Little did we know what God had in store for us.

Honour to Pastor Christie John-Baptiste of Kingsway International Christian Church, and Director of the charity, Support A Nation. Pastor Christie is an incredible Evangelist who introduced me to Haiti in 2011/2012 and has mentored me through all of these mission trips. Thank you and your leading, friendship, opportunities for mission and support with the mission prayer team.

xl   Acknowledgements

Pastor Jean Gerald Lafleur, Pastor David Badio, Pastor Fedony Charles and the Haitian community in Morne Ogre and Jacmel; young people's translator Reginald Des-sources, Jean Louis, together with the congregation of Restoration Ministry. Rev Genel Jean-Claude of Iglasia Taburnacle in Santo Domingo, the Dominican Republic and respective congregation. You are all so special in my heart. Thank you for welcoming me into your lives and teaching me another level of bi-cultural experience allowing me to develop my craft in systemic community family therapy. Thank you for all your gifts, and testimonies, of how your lives have changed, allowing me to share your stories.

I would like to thank my friend Alison Greenaway, who has come along on mission each year, and her children. Hannah Greenaway, Lucinda Greenaway, Nathan Greenaway and husband Chris Greenaway. My spiritual daughter Abisola Ifasawo, and my dear friend Yvonne Akinmuboni accompanying me, and for their contribution to the mission trips which I had the honour to lead between 2014 and 2017. Thank you for your support and service.

I would like to thank Three Counties Church in Haslemere for their love and support for the work in Haiti and the Dominican Republic and for welcoming Pastor Gerald and his wife Pastor Elsa Lafleur on the visit to the United Kingdom. My pastor (now retired) Jonathon Carter and his wife Hazel for support and who have provided teaching on walking in faith, being a child of Christ and lover of our communities. Cheryl Taylor, Clem and June Burford, thank you for your kindness and emotional retreats. Mr and Mrs Colin Coomer for their generosity, support and interest in Haitian children and families.

Mr Neil Law, my former Therapy Services manager at the Priory Southampton, for his encouragement and opportunities to promote the work in Haiti through the Priory organisation. And Libby Payne, retired Clinical Director of CiC, Kate Nowlan for their support and encouragement for this book.

Ms Maimunah Mosli, of **PPIS** Family Therapy, and the Board of Directors for their kindness in inviting me to Singapore to first present on the therapeutic work with the lovely community in Haiti. I was very heartened to hear from the fieldworkers who work in disaster zones and attended my workshop that validated their practitioner experiences. Kerrie Jones, Clinical Director of Orri, colleague and friend who tirelessly works with me & Orri team in the clinical trenches.

I would like to thank the eminent Ros Draper, trailblazer and one of the main leaders in the field of systemic family therapy, who fortunately also happens to be my clinical supervisor for the last 10 years. Ros has supported me during my family therapy training, foray into mission work in Haiti and the Dominican Republic and financial gifts for the Haitian community. Thank you for your feedback on the chapter on family therapy in Haiti and the Dominican Republic.

My co-author Dr Belinda Gordon-Brooks of Birkbeck College, University of London who supervised my master's thesis and showed unwavering belief in my work. We did it! Professor Philomena Essed thank you for the honour of co-authoring our chapter, together with your encouragement and kindness throughout this project.

Audrey Murray, Pastor Patsy Ferreria and her Pastor, Everette Brown whose congregation has financially contributed to my mission trips; Dr Rev Gwen Rose,

Acknowledgements   xli

United Reformed Church in Catford; Elaine Cato and Jenifer Shields of New Life Assembly and the Psalmody School, under whose tutelage I was prepared to grow a little more in confidence in my relationship with the Lord. This little group of strong, Christian Black women who, along with Maureen Greaves, gave up their time to pray and come alongside me, through thick and thin for over 10 years, unwavering in their unconditional love. Thank you (SOS) Sisters on Service. Thank you Professor Joanna Bennett for your call to action and zeal for Justice. We continue to stand with you.

I would like to mention a special thank you to Mrs Viv Church, Mr Daniel Ollivierre for their prompt and scholarly attention to detail and support of this project. My beautiful daughter Cherelle Gordon-Lewis and her husband Matthew Gordon-Lewis who collected and filled their apartment with goods for the lovely families in Haiti.

Dr Deborah Gabriel of Black British Academics for her encouragement and without whom I would not have become acquainted with co-editor Dr Richard Majors. Dr Majors thank you for your inspirational lead and opportunity to work together. It has been quite a journey. Dr Theodore S. Ransaw our co-editor and friend from across the pond, thank you for your kindness and encouragement to me throughout this project. Thank you also to Jen McCall, Emma Leverton, Sophie Barr and the team at Emerald Publishing. Rajachitra you are a blessing.

An enormous thank you to all the authors who have contributed to this Handbook, it has been an absolute honour to work with you. I am so happy to have had so many people encourage me on this journey. Your names are not forgotten, but written on my heart.

Theodore S. Ransaw

I would like to acknowledge Associate Provost and Associate Vice President Theodore 'Terry' Curry, and his staff, Associate Provost and Associate Vice President Hiram Fitzgerald, Assistant Vice President Charles Rivers, Dean Christopher Long, Dean Steve Esquith, Dean Sherman Garnett, Dean Robert Floden, for their leadership, Distinguished Professor Emeritus Robert L. Green for his mentorship, Executive Director Larry Gould for sharing his knowledge, Dr Jawanza Kunjufu for his decades of work supporting people of African descent, Dr William Cross for his expertise on Black consciousness, Dr Michael Stitt for his work on advancing the scholarship of African storytelling and Dr Raymond Moody for his tireless research on the psychology of consciousness.

Black Mental Health and the New Millennium: Historical and Current Perspective on Cultural Trauma and 'Everyday' Racism in White Mental Health Spaces — The Impact on the Psychological Well-being of Black Mental Health Professionals

Richard Majors

Roger Kline in his report *Snowy White Peaks* (2014) reported that in the National Health Service (NHS) the proportion of senior managers who are Black and Minority Ethnic (BME) had not increased since 2008 – but had fallen over the previous three years. Such data suggest that discrimination is still a problem within the NHS. Kline also found the NHS treats BME staff less favourably than white staff in their recruitment, promotion and career progression. Kline's findings suggest that NHS discriminatory practices favour white applicants and are a predictor of patient care. Kline also reported that these same BME staff were significantly more likely to be bullied at work. Much like those BME Kline reported in his study who were bullied, I was a victim of bullying in the NHS as well, so much so I decided to no longer work for the NHS and work privately. This is not an uncommon occurrence for people of colour – my colleagues who work for the NHS often complain how difficult it is to work in the NHS due to the constant bullying, harassment, abuse, and negative racialised interactions/communications between Blacks and whites (e.g. daily and constant insulting micro-aggressions in the workplace/training institutions, see further description of micro-aggression below) (Guttridge, 2020). The bullying is not always blatant but more often it is 'coded'/nonverbal – a look, stare, stance or being the last one in the queue constantly for admin support/ assistance, e.g. typing up assessments, letters, etc. Or it's the support staff's unwillingness ever it seems to help you in the same way they do with white staff who they often cannot do enough for. If you are a person of colour working in the NHS your work/contributions are valued less and you are usually criticised more. Many Black colleagues for these reasons despise working for the NHS. Beside Kline's research, where is the evidence for such claims? You see it with your own eyes every day how your white colleagues are treated and how you and your Black colleagues are treated! Every person of colour (and white ones too if they being honest) who are reading this will understand exactly what I am saying, if they have ever worked in the NHS.[1] I would be remiss here if I did not as well mention the inequalities around *racialised work references*, supervisors do for whites versus references that they do for Black workers. People of colour constantly complain of unfair differential/racialised references they receive when compared with white colleagues for comparable work. White supervisors know they are often only providing people of colour low/biased racialised references, so do their managers, and no one say anything or does anything about it! These differential/racialised references stay with the Black candidate for the rest of their working career and lives and these differential/racialised references can ruin careers or, at the very least, be a barrier to future employment options and climbing up the ladder. Differential/racialised references are both unethical and immoral. And much more research needs to be carried out on these racialised injustices in the workplace that people of colour have complained about for years, while NHS supervisors and management turn their backs and constantly deny it happens or is happening.

Hence, although I commend Kline's report and effort to address the inequality and widespread discrimination in its various forms against BME staff in the NHS, I believe he did not go far enough. There are not just discrimination and inequalities in e.g. bullying and *differential work referencing* concerning people of colour who work in the NHS, but across the board in services, provisions, resources and in the treatment of people of colour in mental health, particularly when relating to Black males who unfairly oftentimes end up in the criminal justice system, because they more often than not do not have access to traditional mental health mainstream services, or they fear altogether using traditional mental health services because they believe the services to be racial/gender biased. Is it possible this bias and police overzealous behaviour towards Black males, when held in police custody with mental health issues, die disproportionately after use of force or restraint than receive the medical help they deserve and need? No wonder Black males are more likely to be over-represented in mental health facilities and hospitals. (see Sharon Walker's chapter for in this book further discussion).

There are also high levels of inequalities and discrimination towards people of colour in most of the academic/graduate training institutions in the UK for those people of colour who want to work in mental health. Such students are less likely to have support of any kind, be encouraged, they receive less financial support, by the way of teaching or research assistantships when compared to whites, white

---

[1] First and foremost, the authors of this book and I want to show our gratitude towards the NHS as our book nears completion. We applaud the efforts and courage of the NHS and the NHS Volunteer Responders that are involved in the COVID-19 pandemic and the dangerous and unpredictable climates you work in every day. We all stand shoulder to shoulder with you. Nevertheless, the sad truth is that the problems addressed in this chapter do in fact exist and need to be eradicated. We hope that, in the future, these issues will be addressed with the same fervour, energy and passion with which the current crisis is being tackled as we strive towards a better world and society for all races.

supervisors/academics tend to disapprove of them doing 'Black research', which they feel oftentimes is not legitimate, is unimportant or they are ignorant of cultural research, or 'fear' this kind of research being done altogether. Because of the lack of support/encouragement, lack of a diverse teaching/supervisory staff and cultural competence model at the teaching institution or university in question, many people of colour in our Black community never graduate to work in their chosen profession – mental health – because they are either 'pushed out' or dropped by the department.

As such, in this book we felt it was important for us to put a 'face' on many of these people of colour who were merely a statistic in Kline's book. These people of colour who are constantly victims of discrimination and racism in Kline's book are real people and human beings whose voices must be heard. It was important for us to tell some of the stories of these people of colour and to put a 'face' on their lives. Therefore, this book chronicles the rich stories, ethnographies and anecdotes of people of colour and their racialised/discriminatory interactions and communications with white authority figures in mental health that have had a devastating impact on their lives.

Everyday Racism

Discrimination and inequalities regarding people of colour are often perpetuated by white management, academic staff, colleagues and support staff, in both overt and covert racist ways e.g. implicit bias, in 'everyday' interactions/communications such as bullying and racial 'micro-aggression'. These forms of discrimination and racism work both on an institutional level and on a personal level, but we believe it is the day-to-day, personal level or 'everyday' form of racism rather than institutional racism that is more degrading, demoralising and devastating and deteriorates one's mental health more over time.

Therefore, institutional racism does not go far enough in explaining the often hostile 'everyday' racialised interactions/communications between whites and Blacks that affect the relationships between people of colour and white authority figures.

We believe racial micro-aggressions can be more profound and vicious than 'institutional racism' (the 'comfortable/safe' form of racism that has become so over-used) in which no one ever seems accountable because 'the institution did it!'. It seems that this form of 'virtual racism' – that is, racism that is out there somewhere in a cloud – cannot be traced back to individuals, despite the fact that systems, structures, policies and governance (e.g. institutional racism) are created, run, operated and maintained by individuals – with names, I might add! That is, they place racism in institutions as inanimate lifeless structures. Yet when an individual or group is guilty of a racist act in the workplace, they hide behind the 'institution'. Very rarely is the person(s) made accountable or responsible because they hide behind the cloak of the 'institution', so nothing is ever resolved because the faceless/nameless entity is somehow not really a person but the 'institution'. So oftentimes no one is ever held responsible for the act. Nevertheless, while racial micro-aggressions are offensive and often hostile or vicious (whether intentionally or not), at least the victim can 'place/identify' the wrongdoer, which is the first important/critical step to rectifying/healing.

Hence, our book, *The International Handbook of Black Community Mental Health*, is the first book to go beyond institutional racism in health care and address the destructive racialised communications/micro-aggressions ('personal level' racism) in both mental health/academic settings between Black mental health providers/ Black graduate students training to be mental health providers and white authority figures. These white hegemonic/white privilege driven destructive racialised communications impact services relationships, treatment outcomes and graduation rates. Thus, one of the primary goals of our book was to move beyond institutional racism as an inappropriate model/political non- accountable driven model of racism and begin to examine racism in mental health on a more personal level: 'everyday racism', implicit bias and micro-aggression, and the devastating impact it has on people's lives. We believe personal level racism is a more adequate model for understanding how racism impact and affect treatment, stereotypes, inequalities, resources, access to mental health services, misdiagnoses, among other areas.

Because of the various forms of discrimination, racism and inequalities found within an organisation, together with a lack of cultural competence among white managers and staff in mental health services, mental health provisions and services for people of colour have been in crisis for a long time. The Care Quality Commission (2011) has highlighted the need to address inequalities in mental health service provision for people of colour. No wonder, then, that people of colour in the UK are four times more likely to be sectioned and detained under the Mental Health Act, die in police custody, are more likely to be diagnosed with mental health problems and be admitted to hospital for mental illness. According to the mental health charity Mind, young African-Caribbean men are more likely to face negative experiences when they use mental health services, resulting in poor mental health outcomes (Tugwell, 2017). People of colour living in the UK have lower rates of common mental disorders than other ethnic groups but are more likely to be misdiagnosed and diagnosed with severe mental illness (Tugwell, 2017). They are more likely to enter mental health services via the courts or the police rather than from primary care, which is the main route to treatment for other groups. They are similarly over-represented in high- and medium-secure units and prisons and criminalised rather than being medicalised for mental health issues. Research reveals that 56% of patients in mental health units who have been sectioned are Black, which is more than any other ethnic group (reinforcing the myth of Black men as 'big, bad and dangerous' – see Majors, 2001 for further discussion). People of colour tend to receive higher levels of psychotropic medication rather than being offered talking therapies such as psychotherapy (Tugwell, 2017). In comparison, white patients are often presented with a variety of cognitive and behavioural therapies aimed at not developing a dependency on medication, because there is more focus on promoting continuity and stability in managing their mental illness. Therefore, white patients often report positive clinical experiences that are situated around self-help, empowerment and wellness (Arday, 2018).

The lack of access to talking therapy may affect suicide rates among people of colour. In the UK, whites have higher rates of suicide than African-Caribbeans. However, recent research reports that suicide rates, particularly among young African-Caribbean men, are increasing (Bhui & McKenzie, 2008; Samaritans, 2018; *see Columbia Suicide Prevention questionnaire/protocol in the addendum to this chapter*). In the UK and internationally, programmes focussing on suicidal prevention in the Black community are expanding. One of the successful international suicide prevention organisations, Choose Life International, is developing a range of national and international seminars and conferences, as well as telephone and face-to-face counselling, to reduce the number of suicides in the Black community.

Racialising and Biased Roots of Schizophrenia

One of the most disturbing issues in the Black community is the over-/misdiagnosis of schizophrenia, particularly in Black males, by white mental health providers, who lack the cultural competence, knowledge and training to diagnose people of African descent correctly or adequately. African-Caribbean people are 3–5 times more likely than any other group to be diagnosed and admitted to hospital for schizophrenia in the UK and they are 17 times more likely than white males to be diagnosed for schizophrenia or bipolar disorder even when they do not suffer with such mental health disorders (Davie, 2014).

Black men are more likely to be over-diagnosed with schizophrenia not only because of ignorance, a lack of knowledge, training and cultural competence but also for political reasons and for social control. The Diagnostic and Statistical Manual (DSM) was created by the American Psychiatric Association (APA) to classify/diagnose mental health disorders. In the mid-to-late 1960s, schizophrenia as a diagnosis began to become more gender-specific, politicised and disproportionately applied to African-American men. While the Black man's symptoms might have played a part in the diagnoses, it is very clear that such diagnoses in the 1960s had more to do with their connection to the civil rights protest/city riots in that decade and Black men's involvement in parties and organisations like the Black Panther Party and Nation of Islam. Black men were unfairly viewed in society as violent and dangerous. Thus, this biased diagnosis of 'racialised aggression' reflected the political zeitgeist. During this period of race-based diagnoses, the APA changed the paranoid subtype of schizophrenia to a disorder of masculinised belligerence.

Professor Jonathan Metzl in his book *The Protest Psychosis: How Schizophrenia Became a Black Disease* (2010) said Black men during this time were viewed by the APA, as reflected in the DSM, as hostile and aggressive, and 'delusional', for their participation in protest activities and for belonging to political organisations. Metzl said that such diagnoses of schizophrenia were therefore politically driven. (These interpretations have historical roots in the Eugenics movement, *see Even the Rats Were White* by Robert Guthrie).

Hence, in the 1960s, many Black men were diagnosed with schizophrenia because of racism and the political period they lived in and not because of their clinical symptoms (Guthrie, 1968; Metzl, 2010; Thomas & Sillen, 1972).

There is an underlying assumption that Black men are 'big, bad and dangerous'. This stereotype still prevails within society and is reflected in mental health services, provisions, diagnoses and treatment. Therefore, institutions and therapists are less likely to empathise with Black men or feel comfortable offering them 'talking therapy', because they are often 'feared' by organisations and therapist who provide therapeutic services. As such, treatment for Black males tends to be ad hoc and crisis oriented.

Race-based or politically driven over-diagnosis of schizophrenia continued throughout the 1980s and the 1990s. A number of articles from leading psychiatric and medical journals showed that doctors diagnosed the paranoid subtype of schizophrenia in

African-American men 5–7 times more often than in white men groups. Sadly, during this time pharmaceutical companies jumped on the 'racial stereotype' bandwagon, showing the 'so called angry Black men' protesting in the streets to promote antipsychotic drug sales (Metzl, 2010). White and Parham (1990) propose a Black psychology/Afro-centric psychology to prevent over-diagnoses and racial stereotyping of people of African descent in mental health. (See Professor Joseph White's 'the Father of Black Psychology' Foreword in this book for further discussion on this subject.)

Roots of Mistrust

Biased, political and race-based diagnoses of Black men have historical roots. During slavery, slaves who escaped bondage were called crazy or mad by plantation owners. In the 1850s, psychologists felt that slaves who ran away from their white masters did so because of a mental illness called 'drapetomania'. Drapetomania is considered the beginning point for scientific racism. Medical journals of the time also described a condition called 'dysaesthesia aethiopis', which was a form of madness characterised by 'rascality' and disrespect for the master's property. Brutal beatings were considered to be the 'cure' (Metzl, 2010).

Because of this traumatic history and ill treatment, Black males often do not feel comfortable accessing formal/traditional mental health services for help and support and therefore tend to reject any idea that they have 'mental illness'. They see mental health as more politically driven even today. Thus, they view such mental health labels/services as nothing more than 'stitch-up jobs' to hurt and pathologise them. Because of feelings of being 'stitched up', Black males have developed a 'cultural paranoia' (Grier & Cobb, 1968) and a 'cultural mistrust' (Terrell & Terrell, 1981) when around whites. Given this backdrop it is understandable that people of colour do not trust white hegemonic, Eurocentric mental health services – they are not comfortable with them and therefore often will refuse; if they do hesitantly access services, they usually soon disengage, resulting in a further deterioration of mental health.

Both 'cultural paranoia' and 'cultural mistrust' are considered acts of justified suspicion (being on constant guard) that Blacks often use when engaging with whites, particularly white authority figures (see the 'Cool Pose' theory, Majors & Bilson (1992) for examples of how both 'cultural paranoia' and 'cultural mistrust' are manifested in everyday life). Both behaviours are employed by Black individuals to protect themselves and make them less vulnerable when around whites, given white people's hegemonic power to hurt Black people. Both 'cultural paranoia' and 'cultural mistrust' are considered by Black psychiatrists and psychologists to be examples of positive cultural adaptive strategies rather than pathology. Nevertheless, while 'Cool Pose' can be viewed as a positive cultural adaptive strategy, it can also be problematic. Because of constant trauma, racial micro-aggression and impact of everyday racism, Black males adopt a 'Cool Pose' (Majors & Billson, 1992) as mentioned above. The 'Cool Pose' is a defence par excellence and is an expression of cultural masculine identity, which works very well in most situations to help Black males counter racism. But there is a flip side, it can work so well, it can be hard to shut down. That is, many Black males become so conditioned to keeping up their guard due to racism, that even without a particular threat they still may keep their 'Cool Pose' guard switched on regardless, which can cause its own stress – secondary extreme stress. I have termed this conditioned strength, *"the problem of selective indiscrimination"* (Majors,1987; Majors & Billson 1992). That is, because of the constant perception of a perceived threat of white racism and mistrust of whites, many Black males' Cool Poses stay switched on as a way to protect themselves, which can be harmful to their psychological well-being.

Much like cultural paranoia and cultural mistrust, Richard Majors and Janet Mancini Bilson in *Cool Pose: The Dilemmas of Black Manhood in America* (1992) describe how Blacks adopt a 'Cool Pose' as a defense when they feel threatened or sense mistrust by white hegemonic forces, as a way to protect, empower, preserve self-esteem and 'keep whites off guard'.

People of colour attempt to mediate the psychological impact of everyday racism and racial micro-aggressions by developing such coping/adaptive strategies as cultural paranoia, cultural mistrust and Cool Pose (Majors, 1992). Nevertheless, 'everyday racism' and racial micro-aggression can cause trauma and be very damaging to the mental health and well-being of people of colour as mentioned above. The mistrust, constant threat or the anticipation of threat of interracial interactions (with whites) can create a healthy mistrust/paranoia in many and in others it may create a state of 'Black anxiety/Black extreme anxiety' due to constant/perceived threat of white interracial interaction(s) and resultant stress. This Black anxiety/Black extreme anxiety has a historical context. That is, the historical baggage of slavery and its intergenerational 'memory' along with the de facto discrimination over many years has created Black anxiety/Black extreme anxiety ('Black racialised anxiety') in many people of colour. People of colour learn early in their lives that whites wield/yield a lot of power to maintain, control, hurt and punish 'for those people of colour who do not stay in line, be defined by them or do not obey' (see Bobby Wright's Mentacidal argument). These historical 'control' institutions towards people of colour are maintained and reinforced today by white privilege/white hegemony, everyday racism (personal-level racism), institutional racism and racial micro-aggressions (e.g. racialised interaction/communications both in the workplace and in society). Given the impact of different forms of racism on people of colour, the well-known psychiatrist Professor Alvin Poussaint in the Preface to this book, argues for the importance of the American Psychiatry Association (APA) adding 'extreme racism' (white directed racism) as an official category in the DSM (*The Diagnostic and Statistical Manual of Mental Disorders*). I would argue in addition to extreme racism, different forms/levels of 'Black anxiety'/'Black extreme anxiety' be considered for inclusion to the DSM as well due to the psychological impact of white-related stress. Both forms of these kinds of racism are due to actions of white aggression, whether direct or indirect, and therefore these behaviours are on a continuum of white psychopathologic behaviours.

Joseph White and Thomas Parham in *The Psychology of Blacks: An African American Perspective* (1990) argue for the need for a Black/African-American psychology (e.g. Afro-centric) to prevent 'deficient-specific interpretations', inferior diagnoses, stereotyping and pathologising people of African descent. They also argue for the importance of a Black/African-American psychology to promote the uniqueness, cultural values and world views of people of African descent (*see also Jones, Black Psychology, 2004*).

Wade Boykins, a well-known American psychologist, has developed a sociocultural/psychosocial model in education that is applicable to positive Black mental health. We believe his cultural model, which focusses on 'verve', prevents mental illness, promotes resiliency and leads to positive healthy outcomes and 'wellness' for people of colour (Boykins & Bailey, 2000). Ransaw (2019) also argues for the importance of developing an emancipatory education framework to counter oppressive ideologies towards people of colour and promote the uniqueness of Black culture.

While both cultural paranoia and cultural mistrust act as positive adaptive strategies over a long period, constant exposure to toxic environments and climates and 'everyday' racialised interactions and communications can lead to trauma and pathology.

Everyday racism usually takes the form of racial micro-aggression because of the constant insults and acts of humiliation that wear victims down. Racial micro-aggressions and negative racialised interactions between whites and Blacks can come from anyone, but they more often than not come from white authority figures and whites in power. The centrality of whiteness/white hegemonic privilege drives racial micro-aggressions towards Black staff/therapists and Black service users in mental health settings every day. Racial micro-aggressions and negative racialised interactions and communications also affect students of colour in universities as well. As stated earlier, many graduate students of colour who attend universities to train as providers, therapists and academics disproportionately either drop out or are pushed out of graduate school because of the lack of personal support or support to allow Black graduates to conduct research on and write their theses and dissertations on Black topics. Constant micro-aggressions, and offensive remarks by academic staff or white academic staff, wear people down and over time contribute towards a variety of mental health problems among people of African descent (see Sharon Walker's chapter in this book). Micro-aggression in mental health is reflective of everyday life for people of colour. Examples of micro-aggressions in the workplace/academia are not only prevalent there, but in everyday public life as well, including when a woman clutches her purse in fear when a Black man walks past her on a street, or when she sees a Black man coming along the street and she quickly crosses over so that she does not have to walk past him. Or when security guards follow Black men in stores but not white people, thinking the Black men are not there to buy anything but rather to steal (Lowe, 2015).

Racial and Cultural Trauma

Micro-aggressions over an extended period of time can lead to traumatisation and symptoms resembling post-traumatic stress disorder (PTSD) in reaction to the constant and daily degrading insults that can cause a sense of hopelessness. As Smith (2010) states,

> "The accumulation of emotional and physiological symptoms resulting from subtle and overt forms of racial verbal and non-verbal micro-aggressions at the societal, interpersonal, and

institutional level can lead to traumatic psychological and physiological stress symptoms."

No wonder, given the impact of racial micro-aggressions, that people of colour often suffer from race-/culture-specific PTSD. While people of colour like anyone else can suffer from PTSD, the trauma tends to be in the past and finite. We therefore believe PTSD is limited when seeking to understand victims' feelings of ongoing, day-to-day threat and danger. Therefore, PTSD does not capture the racialised aspects of continuous trauma that people of colour often face. We believe a more racial-/cultural-specific trauma model would be more appropriate and nuanced for understanding and interpreting PTSD-specific features/stress among people of African descent. Therefore, we prefer a framework that considers models such as continuous traumatic stress (CTS), post-traumatic slave syndrome (PTSS) (DeGruy, 2005), battered race syndrome (Ratliff, 2014) and racial battle fatigue (see Smith's chapter in this book). All of these racialised trauma-related frameworks consider that daily encounters with white hegemonic racism and the day-to-day impact of 'everyday racism' first posited by Essed (1991) and other conditions created by white hegemonic forces, such as persistent poverty and unemployment, hyper-vigilance, hopelessness, environmental racism, living in squalid, gang-infested and crime-ridden neighbourhoods, can cause stress, anger, anxiety, hopelessness, depression and suicides in addition to other mental health challenges (see Majors & Gordon, 1994, for further discussion).

Let's look briefly at each of these models that help to explain racial and cultural trauma. The first framework I would like to address is continuous traumatic stress (CTS). CTS is a model developed in the 1980s by a group of mental health professionals working in apartheid-era South Africa, who were attempting to provide psychological support to victims of political violence within a context of ongoing state racial repression. CTS as a framework helps us to understand the psychological impact of people of colour living in high-stress environments where there is a realistic threat of present and future danger. Threats of harm for many people of colour never go away, and this creates an internal 'state of emergency' (Vitelli, 2013). People experiencing CTS are usually more preoccupied with what could happen to them in the present or the future ('anticipatory anxiety') than with the past.

The second framework is Post Traumatic Slave Syndrome (PTSS), (DeGruy, 2005), which focusses on historical and intergenerational trauma. PTSS argues that centuries of slavery, systemic racism and oppression have resulted in the development of multi-generational adaptive behaviours. PTSS can also cause trauma in the next generation, for example, 'transgenerational trauma' (Sullivan, 2013). The child may internalise their family's experience of trauma or the PTSS may be a result of parental rearing styles (e.g. strict authoritarian rearing). Another major way that stress can be transmitted across generations is biologically, through the uterine environment. Exposure to harmful stimuli at this stage can have detrimental effects. Empirical evidence has shown that trauma experienced by a mother during pregnancy can affect her offspring's physiology and psychology (Yehuda & Lehrner, 2018). We are also aware of the very real dangers and concerns regarding how Black women are treated in pregnancy, together with overall care for Black, Asian, minority ethnic (BAME) women. Recent statistics illustrated within the fifth MBRRACE-UK (2018) annual report of the Confidential Enquiries into Maternal Deaths and Morbidity highlight the high mortality rate of Black women in pregnancy in the UK. Results from 2014 to 2016 show that Black women in the UK are five times more likely to die in childbirth compared with white women (MBRACE, 2018). Therefore, the exposure to generational trauma for the Black child is ongoing, both before and after birth, affecting their attachment and emotional and social development.

Battered race syndrome (Ratliff, 2014) compares the abusive relationship between a man and a woman in battered woman syndrome and the 400-year abusive relationship between America and African-Americans and stress/traumatisation.

Finally, racial battle fatigue (Smith, 2010, see his chapter in this book) is a term coined in 2003 by Smith to explain the social and psychological stress African-American males have endured historically at the hands of whites. Smith believes stress develops from having to constantly deal with blatant racism and micro-aggressions. His work helps us to better understand combat stress and the racial undertones, nuances and extreme stress African-Americans historically endure from whites.

Racial micro-aggressions (e.g. 'personal-level racism') that can lead to trauma/pathology then help us to understand the various kinds of racialised interactions and communications that white staff often have with both service users and people of African descent who work in white mental health establishments (e.g. managers, mental health providers, team leaders, staff, therapists and support staff) as well as the Black graduate students' negative racialised experiences/supervisory relationships at universities.

Many of the clinical authors of this book who have worked in local mental health establishments have been targets of vicious racial micro-aggression attacks. These attacks have been both overt and covert and also non-verbal, taking the form of degrading insults, isolation, humiliation, name-calling, rolling of the eyes, staring. Additionally, support staff are often reluctant to provide the same kind of support that's provided for white colleagues/staff in the office and if they are provided support, they are the last ones in the queue to receive help or support from support staff e.g. support staff are often unwilling to type up their documents, assessments or letters. These are just a few examples of other forms of 'subtle' racialised micro-aggressions that people of colour have to deal with on a daily basis when working with white colleagues either in mental health or academic spaces. When people of colour complain about this treatment, they feel the white establishment does nothing at all. Thus, people of colour tend to be reluctant to complain because of office 'stigma/politics', indirect retaliation, being ostracised, fear of losing their job or being 'blacklisted', or fear of losing opportunities in the future for promotion or being phased out because they made a complaint. These racial micro-aggressions by white mental health providers create a toxic and hostile working climate that communicates very clearly to people of colour who work in mental health: 'you are not welcome or wanted here'.

These behaviours seem to have increased significantly in the UK following the vote on Brexit (Booth, 2019).

No wonder, with such alarming levels of care and inferior level of treatment, many people of colour in the UK distrust white personnel, staff and mainstream mental health services, and therefore are reluctant to engage with them (Sinusi, 2018). Many people of colour feel that mental health services in this country are not there to provide help or support but rather are a mechanism to stigmatise them and delay their recovery. People of colour often feel white mental health providers yield significant power over them and make culturally insensitive decisions that hurt or harm. We place health care providers/managers at the centrality of hegemonic 'whiteness' (Grey, Sewell, Shapiro, & Ashraf, 2013). The Black community often feels white mental health providers and managers are biased, stereotype them, fear them, regarding them as more aggressive or dangerous than others (particularly young Black males). They do not believe white providers and managers are properly trained (or feel the need to be), or are capable or culturally competent to deliver adequate mental health services to the Black community (Abbott, 2014). In our experience, white therapists are often not comfortable serving people of colour and refrain from doing so when there they have a choice to serve audiences they are more comfortable with, especially in relation to Black males. Many Black service users view providers and managers and therapeutic agencies/organisations as inflexible white space that reinforces white Eurocentric models of health care which are dismissive of Black culture and values (Mind, 2013) – see Professor Joseph White's Foreword on the history of 'deficit psychology' and the importance of Black/Afro-centric psychology to understanding people of colour.

Cultural Competence

One specific strategy to improve services and access is cultural competence. As discussed, many of the problems in mental health are due to a lack of appreciation and understanding of cultural competence. Cultural competence is the ability to relate effectively with individuals from various groups and backgrounds. Culture can be defined as the behaviours and non-verbal behaviours (see Andrews & Majors, 2004; Majors, 1991), customs, identities, attitudes, racial identities, lifestyle, values, experiences and beliefs shared by a group of people. For example, the author of this work, during many visits to East Africa, while working in indigenous villages, learnt that when certain tribal members described or explained particular mental health problems they would do it somatically rather than mentally. For example, rather than describe depression as a mental condition they might say 'I have a headache'. Some cultures did not recognise or know how to describe symptoms associated with stress, depression or certain mental health problems in traditional western ways (Arday, 2018).

Because of cultural mistrust of white health providers, people of colour often engage with their social networks and friends in spiritual ways, such as praying or seeking community support, rather than accessing local mental health services. Therefore, culture can influence such things as social networks, customs, beliefs, dress, language, religious orientation, customs and foods people eat, among many other things (Pedersen, 2002). Cultural competence is also a tool that helps us interpret culture-specific nonverbal behaviours, nuances and subtleties (Majors & Gordan, 1994).

From a mental health point of view, culture influences how people from different backgrounds (e.g. racial) address emotional and mental distress, seek help, use support and cope with various problems. Individuals, institutions and mental health organisations and providers would benefit greatly from applying cultural competence models if they are to offer culturally appropriate services, preventions, outreach, assessments and interventions. Cultural competence also promotes self-awareness of the health care provider. Self-awareness is the first step for mental health providers towards understanding personal and cultural values, biases, stereotypes and beliefs. This self-awareness should help individuals appreciate, connect and empathise with patients who may not be from their own culture. Through a cultural competence framework, staff and service providers are challenged to continually examine their own beliefs, and to work with mutual transformation as they develop their skills, and appropriately apply interventions that are culture and context centred, and authentic to what is sometimes called the BAME clients' and families' value system (Pedersen, 2002). The government and the NHS must improve access to better health care and dismantle the legacy of inequalities and endorse policy driven actions that make use of a culture-specific applicable framework that is so critical for improving mental health equity in people of colour.

People of colour express a desire for greater diversification regarding service providers. People of colour therapists and service providers tend to be more empathetic towards understanding the plights and experiences of other ethnic people of colour (Arday, 2018). As Grey et al. (2013) and MIND (2013) found, people with an ethnic background who have experienced racial discrimination in health care have a preference for ethnic similarity regarding health care providers. They feel people of colour who are service providers are more empathetic, do not fear them, overreact or misdiagnose them when compared with white service providers (White & Parham, 1990). As such, health care must become more diversified and culturally competent to meet a vastly growing world population of people of colour. Therefore, policies, modalities, methodologies, strategies, programmes and training material targeted towards people of colour must become more culturally relevant, cognizant and sensitive if they are to meet the needs of this population and prevent an even greater or deeper crisis in mental health than there is now. In addition, financial resources must be provided for white health care providers to undertake compulsory continuing professional development training. Cultural competence training should move beyond its current status among many white service providers as an unimportant 'tick box exercise'.

Conclusion

Given this sad portrayal and status of mental health in the Black communities, *The International Handbook of Black Community Mental Health* can be depicted as a response to the plethora of challenges experienced by people of colour. We therefore have developed this book to inform, challenge, change attitudes, educate, raise awareness and influence and shape policy that will hopefully improve mental health services, eradicate inequality, discrimination, negative racialised communications/micro-aggressions and improve the treatment of people of colour who access mental health services.

Tangible actions must be reflected through diversifying health care staff within mental health services, and developing culturally sensitive systems and culturally appropriate interventions for both Black providers and service users, if things are genuinely to change.

People of colour experience mental health differently. These experiences are often situated within and tinged by racist connotations. Given these negative racial ascriptions, people of colour are often misdiagnosed, treated differently within mental health services and consistently experience poorer satisfaction and less productive outcomes (Vernon, 2011).

This *Handbook* includes not only statistics and discussions in traditional areas of mental health but also but puts a 'face' on Kline's (2014) victims in the NHS by presenting and highlighting rich stories, ethnographies and anecdotes of personalised trauma experienced and endured by people of colour, not only within mental health settings but among students involved in academia/graduate training in our universities. We shift the paradigm of academic mental health books to moving beyond statistics and theory-laden text as mentioned above to hearing about people's lives and their described experiences of everyday racism and micro-aggressions. In doing so, we challenge sensitive and taboo/controversial subjects many individuals are not comfortable dealing with or talking about.

The covert subtleties of everyday racism, micro-aggression and implicit bias, particularly in academia, and their detrimental impacts are steeped in oppressive practice, with the blame often put on the person of colour (Sue et al., 2007). Racial micro-aggression is a more adequate model than institutional racism for understanding race dynamics and racialised interactions/communications such as those between white authority figures/management and black providers/service users and supervisory/supervisee negative cross-cultural communications.

In this book, not only do we look at the entire family life cycle of people of colour and mental health, we also address the over-representation of Black men in the mental health system and other inequalities in mental health services. We recommend applying emotional literacy and emotional wellness and cultural competence strategies and models for both people of colour and Black males to address racism, discrimination and inequalities, and to improve their lives. By not just focussing on 'problems' inherent in mental health, the editors and contributors in this book looked at on solutions: offering new frameworks, methodologies and therapeutic models that seek to redress many of the problems found in the mental health service and universities. Thus, *The International Handbook of Black Community Mental Health* is a timely and essential tool, which we hope will play its part in helping to both enhance white providers' knowledge and insight into Black mental health, develop knowledge towards providing a better experience and service for Black providers and service users, and improve the experiences and lives of people of colour who access mental health services. The time for change is now.

References

Abbott, D. (2014, May 15). Mental health and the BME community in London. Retrieved from https://www.dianeabbott.org.uk/news/speeches/news?p=102993

Andrews, V., & Majors, R. (2004). African American nonverbal culture in black psychology. In R. L. Jones (Ed.), *Black psychology* (4th ed., pp. 269–294). Berkeley, CA: Cobb & Henry Publishers.

Arday, J. (2018). Understanding mental health: What are the issues for black and ethnic minority students at university? *Social Sciences, 7*, 1–35.

Bhui, K., & McKenzie, K. (2008). Rates and risk factors by ethnic group for suicides within a year of contact with mental health services in England and Wales. *Psychiatric Services, 59*, 414–420.

Booth, R. (2019, May 20). Racism on the rise since Brexit vote nationwide study reveals. *The Guardian* [UK]. Retrieved from https://www.theguardian.com/world/2019/may/20/racism-on-the-rise-since-brexit-vote-nationwide-study-reveals

Boykins, A. W., & Bailey, C. (2000). Rhythmic-movement facilitation of learning in working-class Afro-American children. *The Journal of Genetic Psychology, 149*, 335–347.

Care Quality Commission. (2011, April 6). Care Quality Commission looks ahead as last count me in census is published. Retrieved from https://www.cqc.org.uk/news/releases/care-quality-commission-looks-ahead-last-count-me-census-published

Davie, E. (2014, October 28). It's time to tackle mental health inequality among black people. The Guardian [UK]. Retrieved from https://www.theguardian.com/healthcare-network/2014/oct/28/tackle-mental-health-inequality-black-people

DeGruy, J. (2005). *Post traumatic slave syndrome: America's legacy of enduring injury and healing*. New York, NY: Uptone Press.

Essed, P. (1991). *Understanding everyday racism: An interdisciplinary theory*. Newbury Park, CA: Sage.

Grey, T., Sewell, H., Shapiro, G., & Ashraf, F. (2013). Mental health inequalities facing UK minority ethnic populations: Causal factors and solutions. *Journal of Psychological Issues in Organizational Culture, 3*, 146–157.

Grier, W. & Cobb, P. (1968). *Black rage*. New York, NY: Basic Books.

Guthrie, R. (1968). *Even the rats were white*. Boston, MA: Addison-Wesley.

Guttridge, R. (2020, March 13). A third of black or minority ethnic Walsall Manor Hospital staff say they were bullied or harassed by colleagues. *Express & Star* [UK]. Retrieved from https://www.expressandstar.com/news/health/2020/03/13/a-third-of-black-or-minority-ethnic-walsall-manor-hospital-staff-say-they-were-bullied-or-harassed-by-colleagues/

Jones, R. (2004). *Black psychology*. Hampton, VA: Cobb & Henry.

Kline, R. (2014). The "snowy white peaks" of the NHS: A survey of discrimination in governance and leadership and the potential impact on patient care in London and England. Hendon: Middlesex University. Retrieved from https://www.england.nhs.uk/wp-content/uploads/2014/08/edc7-0514.pdf

Lewis-Fernández, R., Aggarwal, N. K., Hinton, L., Hinton, D. E., & Kirmayer, L. J. (Eds.). (2015). *DSM-5 handbook on the cultural formulation interview*. Washington, DC: American Psychiatric Publishing.

Lowe, F. (2015). A day in the life of black men: Microaggressions, a subtle form of racism. Retrieved from https://medium.com/@northstarnewstoday/a-day-in-the-life-of-black-men-microaggressions-a-subtle-form-of-racism-777d8dec3770

Majors, R. (1991). Nonverbal behaviors and communication styles among African Americans. In R. L. Jones (Ed.), *Black psychology* (3rd ed., pp. 269–294). Berkeley, CA: Cobb & Henry Publishers.

Majors, R. (2001). *Educating our black children: New directions and radical approaches*. London: Routledge Falmer.

Majors, R., & Bilson, J. (1992). *Cool pose: The dilemmas of black manhood in America*. New York, NY: Lexington Books.
Majors, R., & Gordan, J. (1994). *The American black male: His present status and his future*. Chicago, IL: Nelson Hall.
MBRRACE. (2018, November). Saving lives, improving mothers' care: Lessons learned to inform maternity care from the UK and Ireland confidential enquiries into maternal deaths and morbidity 2014–16. Retrieved from https://www.npeu.ox.ac.uk/downloads/files/mbrrace-uk/reports/MBRRACE-UK%20Maternal%20Report%202018%20-%20Web%20Version.pdf
Metzl, J. (2010). *The protest psychosis: How schizophrenia became a black disease*. Boston, MA: Beacon Press.
Mind. (2013). Mental health crisis care: Commissioning excellence for black and minority ethnic groups. Retrieved from https://www.mind.org.uk/media/494422/bme-commissioning-excellence-briefing.pdf
Pedersen, P. B. (2002). The making of a culturally competent counsellor. *Online Readings in Psychology and Culture, 10*. doi:10.9707/2307-0919.1093
Ransaw, T. (2019). The black founders of emancipatory education: Frederick Douglas, W.E.B Dubois, Brooker T. Washington, Carter G. Woodson, Molefi Asante, Jawanza Kunjufu, William Cross and Richard Majors. In T. Ransaw, C. P. Gause, & R. Majors (Eds.), *The handbook of research on black males: Quantitative, qualitative and interdisciplinary* (pp. 299–324). East Lansing, MI: Michigan State University Press.
Ratliff, B. (2014). *Battered race syndrome*. Irvine, CA: Point of View Publishing.
Samaritans. (2018, December). Suicide statistics report. Retrieved from https://www.nspa.org.uk/resources/samaritans-suicide-report-2018
Sinusi, V. (2018, May 15). These black women felt excluded by mainstream mental health charities – So they started their own. *INews*. Retrieved from https://inews.co.uk/culture/black-women-mental-health-charities/
Sue, D. W., Nadal, K. L., Capodilupo, C. M., Lin, A. I., Torino, G. C., & Rivera D. P. (2007). Racial microaggressions against Black Americans: implications for counselling. *Journal of Counselling & Development, 86*, 330–338.
Sullivan, S. (2013). Inheriting racist disparities in health: Epigenetics and the transgenerational effects of white racism. *Critical Philosophy of Race, 1*, 190–218.
Terrell, F., & Terrell, S. L. (1981). An inventory to measure cultural mistrust among blacks. *The Western Journal of Black Studies, 5*, 180–184.
Thomas, T., & Sillen, S. (1972). *Racism and psychiatry*. New York, NY: Citadel Press.
Toward an understanding of misandric microaggressions and racial battle fatigue among African Americans in historically White institutions. In E. M. Zamani--Gallaher and V. C. Polite (Eds.) *The state of the African American male*. East Lansing, MI: Michigan State University Press.
Tugwell, G. (2017, September 10). Let's talk about the black mental health crisis in the UK. *Maroon News*. Retrieved from https://www.maroon-news.co.uk/single-post/2017/09/10/Let%E2%80%99s-talk-about-the-black-mental-health-crisis-in-the-UK
Vernon, P. (2011). Put race equality in mental health back on the agenda. *The Guardian* [UK]. Retrieved from https://www.guardian.co.uk/society/joepublic/2011/mar/01/race-equality-mental-health
Vitelli, R. (2013, May 29). When the trauma doesn't end: How can people learn to live with chronic traumatic stress? *Psychology Today*. Retrieved from https://www.psychologytoday.com/gb/blog/media-spotlight/201305/when-the-trauma-doesnt-end
White, J. L., & Parham, T. A. (1990). *The psychology of blacks: An African American perspective*. Upper Saddle River, NJ: Prentice Hall.
Yehuda, R., & Lehrner, A. (2018). Intergenerational transmission of trauma effects: Putative role of epigenetic mechanisms. *World Psychiatry, 17*, 243–257.

Addenum

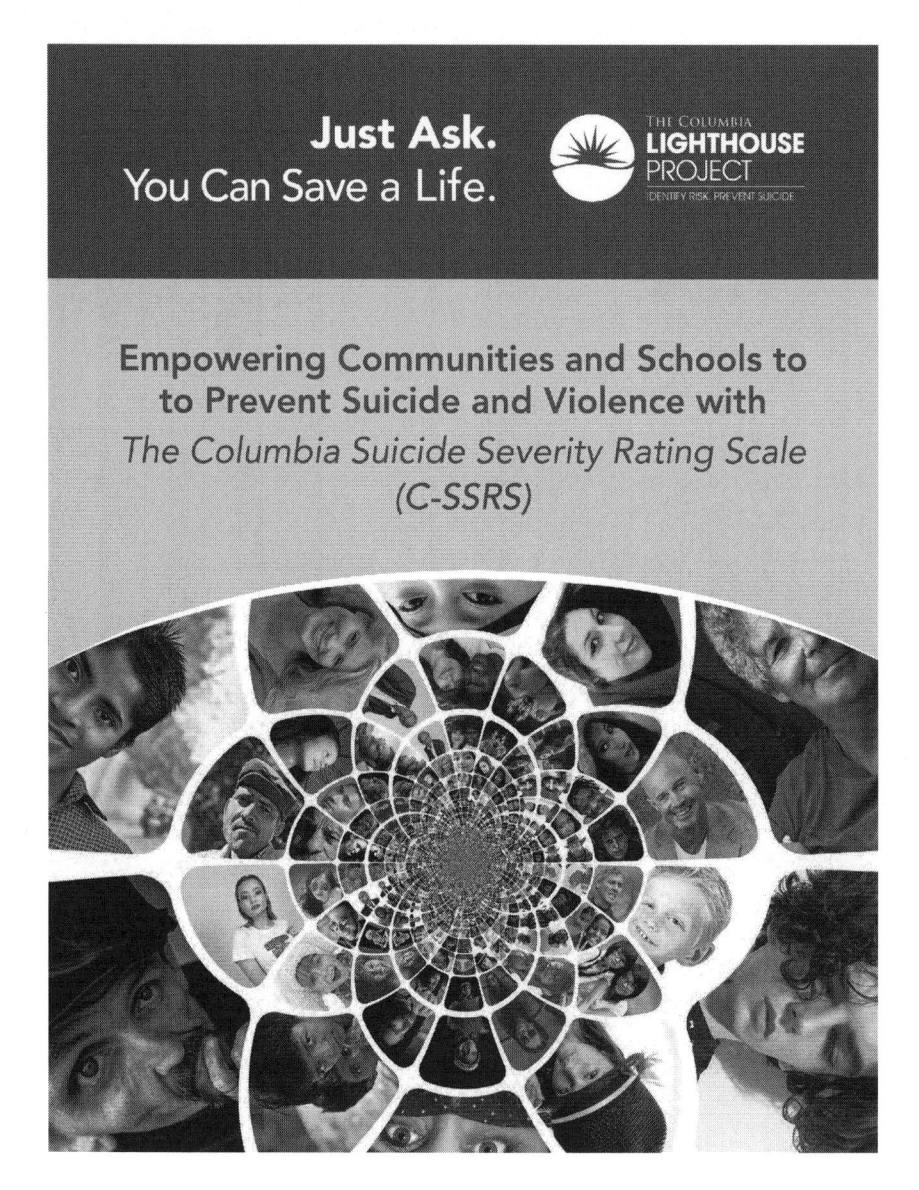

Just Ask. You Can Save a Life.

THE COLUMBIA
LIGHTHOUSE
PROJECT
IDENTIFY RISK. PREVENT SUICIDE

Empowering Communities and Schools to to Prevent Suicide and Violence with
The Columbia Suicide Severity Rating Scale (C-SSRS)

The C-SSRS: A Few Simple Questions to Find People at Risk and Prevent Suicide

~80% of school shooters had a history of suicidal thoughts or behavior

*Vossekuil, B. et al. National Threat Assessment Center, Washington DC 2002.

Just ask a few questions to find people who need help before it's too late, **Prevent violence before it starts.**

What is The Columbia Suicide Severity Rating Scale (C-SSRS) Screener?

The C-SSRS is a few simple questions about suicidal thoughts and behavior that empower communities, families and individuals to find people who are at risk and prevent tragedies before they happen. The C-SSRS tells the teacher, parent or peer who needs a next step, and provides setting-specific recommendations.

- **Simple:** You can ask as few as two to six questions, with no mental health training required to ask them.

- **Effective:** Experience shows that the scale uniquely identifies those who would otherwise be missed.

- **Efficient:** Use of the scale redirects resources to where they are needed most, preventing unnecessary interventions that are often costly, traumatic, and lead to disengagement from the needed care. The C-SSRS provides evidence-based thresholds to connect those at risk to the right level of care.

- **Free:** It's available at no cost.

- **The Most Evidence-Supported:** The scale originated in a NIMH adolescent suicide attempter treatment study, and generated an unprecedented amount of research that validates the questions' value.

Regarding the C-SSRS, "We found another big piece of the school shooting puzzle – an antibiotic for suicide. This ... could fundamentally change the game for early identification and intervention."
Ryan Petty, parent of a Marjory Stoneman Douglas High School shooting victim from Parkland, FL

MYTHS vs. FACTS

"Asking a depressed person about suicide may put the idea in their heads"	▶ Asking does **not** suggest suicide, or make it more likely. ▶ Open discussion is more likely to be experienced as relief than intrusion. ▶ Depressed students who get screened are less distressed and suicidal than high-risk students who are not screened (Gould et al, 2005).
"There's no point in asking about suicidal thoughts… if someone is going to do it, they won't tell you"	▶ Many will be honest when asked, even if they would never bring it up. ▶ Ambivalence, contradictory statements and behavior are common. ▶ Many give hints to friends or family, even if they don't tell a clinician.
"Someone that makes suicidal threats won't really do it, they are just looking for attention"	▶ Those who talk about suicide or express thoughts about wanting to die are most at risk of a real suicide attempt. ▶ 80% of people who die by suicide gave some indication or warning first.

"If implemented to the extent of its capacity across the country, the Columbia has the potential to keep the 64 million children in our schools safe physically and mentally by helping prevent school violence."

James Shelton, Former Deputy Secretary, U.S. Department of Education

---

Youth and Suicide

- Approximately 16% of US high school students report seriously considering suicide
- Each year, 8% make one or more suicide attempts (CDC, 2015)
- 25% of teachers report being approached by an at-risk student
- An estimated 51,518 U.S. adolescents are hospitalized each year for self-inflicted injuries, resulting in total annual costs of approximately $477,580,000 (CDC, 2010)
- Suicide is the second leading cause of death among U.S. college students, and less than 20% of students who die by suicide received any campus-based mental health services

Black Mental Health and the New Millennium   19

A Critical Protection Strategy for Whole Communities

- In schools and on college campuses, the C-SSRS creates a tight/comprehensive network of support, when it is used by teachers, coaches, public safety officers, student life staff, resident advisors, and most critically, peers.
- The C-SSRS has been successfully implemented in many schools and systems across the US (e.g., every teacher in Tennessee) and abroad (every school teacher in Israel).

Putting these simple questions in everybody's hands creates a common language and a linking of systems.

This facilitates care delivery and enages the whole community in helping to prevent tragedy.

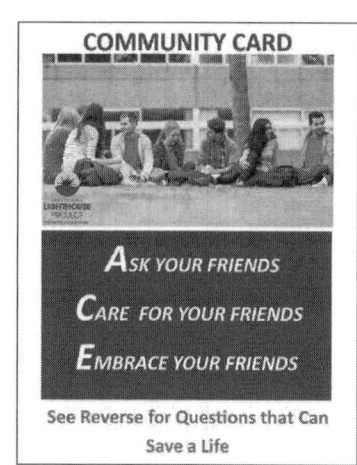

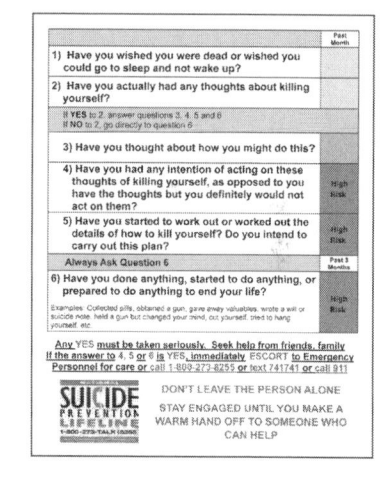

COMMUNITY CARD

ASK YOUR FRIENDS

CARE FOR YOUR FRIENDS

EMBRACE YOUR FRIENDS

See Reverse for Questions that Can Save a Life

	Past Month
1) Have you wished you were dead or wished you could go to sleep and not wake up?	
2) Have you actually had any thoughts about killing yourself?	
If YES to 2, answer questions 3, 4, 5 and 6 If NO to 2, go directly to question 6	
3) Have you thought about how you might do this?	
4) Have you had any intention of acting on these thoughts of killing yourself, as opposed to you have the thoughts but you definitely would not act on them?	High Risk
5) Have you started to work out or worked out the details of how to kill yourself? Do you intend to carry out this plan?	High Risk
Always Ask Question 6	Past 3 Months
6) Have you done anything, started to do anything, or prepared to do anything to end your life? Examples: Collected pills, obtained a gun, gave away valuables, wrote a will or suicide note, held a gun but changed your mind, cut yourself, tried to hang yourself, etc.	High Risk

Any YES must be taken seriously. Seek help from friends, family
If the answer to 4, 5 or 6 is YES, immediately ESCORT to Emergency
Personnel for care or call 1-800-273-8255 or text 741741 or call 911

SUICIDE PREVENTION LIFELINE
1-800-273-TALK (8255)

DON'T LEAVE THE PERSON ALONE
STAY ENGAGED UNTIL YOU MAKE A
WARM HAND OFF TO SOMEONE WHO
CAN HELP

> Having a common language to talk about difficult topics such as suicide fosters an essential protective and promotive factor for all youth - social and psychological connectedness to school or "the belief held by students that adults and peers in the school care about their learning as well as about them as individuals..." *(CDC, 2009)*

Build Connections by Simply Asking

Just asking the questions can be a positive action. When we ask a student, an elder, a partner how they're doing, it signals that someone cares about them. This simple action promotes connectedness – a critical protective factor against suicide and violence.

The C-SSRS creates a common language. Having a common language with clear definitions of suicidal thoughts and behaviors is critical for developing school safety and response protocols. Schools distribute the Columbia Community Cards to teachers, coaches, parents and students, so that everyone is empowered to ask about suicide:

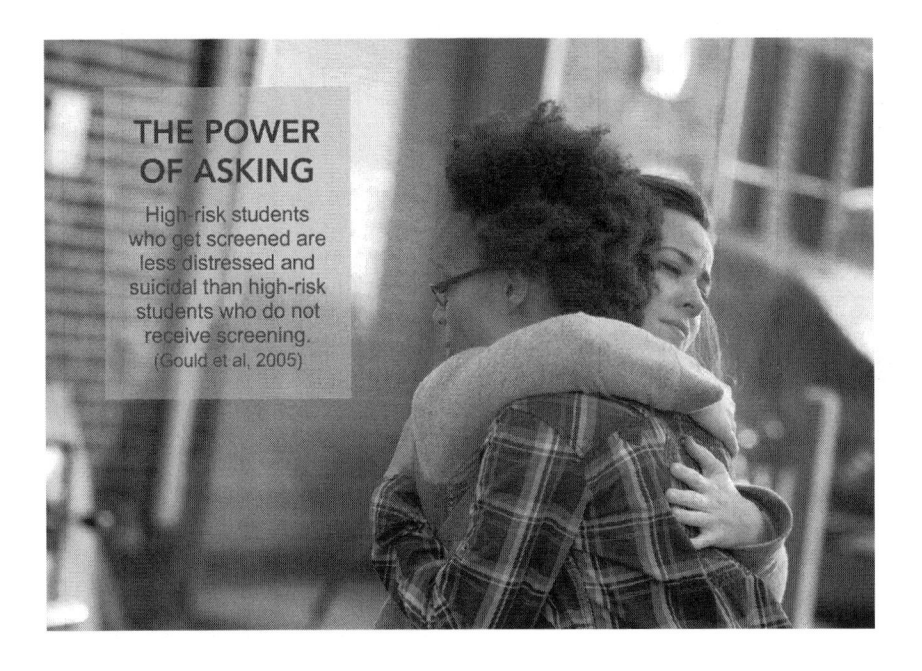

THE POWER OF ASKING
High-risk students who get screened are less distressed and suicidal than high-risk students who do not receive screening.
(Gould et al, 2005)

Steps You Can Take

68% of school shooters and 85% of youth firearm suicides get their guns from a parent or other family member's home

Firearms
- Keep firearms locked in a safe and ammunition stored in a separate location.
- Biometric locks are best because youth often know safe combinations or can find keys.
- Ask a friend or family member to store a firearm for you while you work on becoming healthy again.
- Check out a local shooting club or local police precinct to see if they have temporary storage options.

Medications
- Never keep lethal doses of any medication on hand. Work with your doctor and pharmacist to make sure you have a safe dosage in your home.
- Consider keeping medications locked in a safe place or have a responsible adult monitor use.
- Properly dispose of medications you no longer need.

THE C-SSRS IN ACTION
Saving Lives: Preventing Suicide & Violence

Follow this link or scan this code to watch a short demonstration of how to ask questions with the C-SSRS screener

https://tinyurl.com/CSSRSDemoVideo

After putting the C-SSRS in everybody's hands, the U.S. Marine Corps **had a 22% reduction in the number of service member suicides.**

At Centerstone, one of the largest behavioral healthcare providers in the United States, the suicide rate among its Tennessee patients **was lowered by 65% within the first 20 months of implementation.**

Utah **reversed an almost decade-long increase** in suicide deaths.

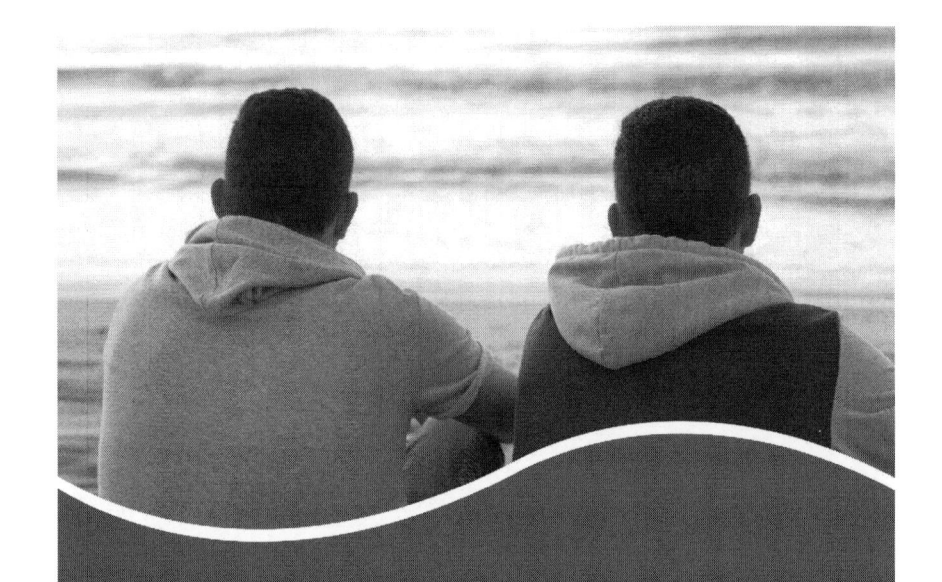

The Columbia Lighthouse Project
is dedicated to improving suicide risk assessment prevention across all sectors of society. The suicide assessment method developed in collaboration with other academic medical centers, the Columbia Suicide Severity Rating Scale, is used extensively in healthcare and education systems, state-wide suicide prevention programs, military, as well as academic and industry research in the US and abroad.

In order to help integrate the C-SSRS into your prevention protocols, **we will:**
- Help select the right screening tool and modify it for your setting
- Answer questions about how to use the tool and provide hands-on support
- Direct you to resources that can bolster your suicide prevention efforts

For support, copies of the tool, or additional information, please visit
cssrs.columbia.edu

Identify risk. Prevent suicide. Together, we can make a difference.

"We all have the potential to use the C-SSRS to save a life."

– Keita Franklin, Director
U.S. Department of Defense Suicide Prevention Office

The C-SSRS has been endorsed, recommended, or adopted by:

World Health Organization | FDA | SAMHSA
Department of Defense | CDC | NIH | Action Alliance

Identify risk. Prevent suicide.
Together, we can make a difference.
www.cssrs.columbia.edu

THE COLUMBIA
LIGHTHOUSE PROJECT
IDENTIFY RISK. PREVENT SUICIDE.

COLUMBIA-SUICIDE SEVERITY RATING SCALE (C-SSRS)

Lifetime Recent

Version 1/14/09 m9/12/17

Posner, K.; Brent, D.; Lucas, C.; Gould, M.; Stanley, B.; Brown, G.; Fisher, P.; Zelazny, J.; Burke, A.; Oquendo, M.; Mann, J.

Disclaimer:

This scale is intended to be used by individuals who have received training in its administration. The questions contained in the Columbia-Suicide Severity Rating Scale are suggested probes. Ultimately, the determination of the presence of suicidal ideation or behavior depends on the judgment of the individual administering the scale.

Definitions of behavioral suicidal events in this scale are based on those used in **The Columbia Suicide History Form**, developed by John Mann, MD and Maria Oquendo, MD, Conte Center for the Neuroscience of Mental Disorders (CCNMD), New York State Psychiatric Institute, 1051 Riverside Drive, New York, NY, 10032. (Oquendo M. A., Halberstam B., & Mann J. J., Risk factors for suicidal behavior: Utility and limitations of research instruments. In M.B. First [Ed.] Standardized Evaluation in Clinical Practice, pp. 103–130, 2003.)

For reprints of the C-SSRS contact Kelly Posner, Ph.D., New York State Psychiatric Institute, 1051 Riverside Drive, New York, New York, 10032; inquiries and training requirements contact posnerk@nyspi.columbia.edu
© 2008 The Research Foundation for Mental Hygiene, Inc.

SUICIDAL IDEATION		
Ask questions 1 and 2. If both are negative, proceed to "Suicidal Behavior" section. If the answer to question 2 is "yes", ask questions 3, 4 and 5. If the answer to question 1 and/or 2 is "yes", complete "Intensity of Ideation" section below.	Lifetime: Time He/She Felt Most Suicidal	Past 1 month
1. Wish to be Dead Subject endorses thoughts about a wish to be dead or not alive anymore, or wish to fall asleep and not wake up. *Have you wished you were dead or wished you could go to sleep and not wake up?* If yes, describe:	Yes ☐ No ☐	Yes ☐ No ☐
2. Non-Specific Active Suicidal Thoughts General non-specific thoughts of wanting to end one's life/die by suicide (e.g., *"I've thought about killing myself"*) without thoughts of ways to kill oneself/associated methods, intent, or plan during the assessment period. *Have you actually had any thoughts of killing yourself?* If yes, describe:	Yes ☐ No ☐	Yes ☐ No ☐
3. Active Suicidal Ideation with Any Methods (Not Plan) without Intent to Act Subject endorses thoughts of suicide and has thought of at least one method during the assessment period. This is different than a specific plan with time, place or method details worked out (e.g., thought of method to kill self but not a specific plan). Includes person who would say, *"I thought about taking an overdose but I never made a specific plan as to when, where or how I would actually do it…and I would never go through with it."* *Have you been thinking about how you might do this?* If yes, describe:	Yes ☐ No ☐	Yes ☐ No ☐
4. Active Suicidal Ideation with Some Intent to Act, without Specific Plan Active suicidal thoughts of killing oneself and subject reports having <u>some intent to act on such thoughts</u>, as opposed to *"I have the thoughts but I definitely will not do anything about them."* *Have you had these thoughts and had some intention of acting on them?* If yes, describe:	Yes ☐ No ☐	Yes ☐ No ☐
5. Active Suicidal Ideation with Specific Plan and Intent Thoughts of killing oneself with details of plan fully or partially worked out and subject has some intent to carry it out. *Have you started to work out or worked out the details of how to kill yourself? Do you intend to carry out this plan?* If yes, describe:	Yes ☐ No ☐	Yes ☐ No ☐

INTENSITY OF IDEATION		
The following features should be rated with respect to the most severe type of ideation (i.e., 1-5 from above, with 1 being the least severe and 5 being the most severe). Ask about time he/she was feeling the most suicidal.		
Lifetime - *Most Severe Ideation:* _____ _____ 　　　　　　　　　　　　　*Type # (1-5)*　　　　　*Description of Ideation* Recent - *Most Severe Ideation:* _____ _____ 　　　　　　　　　　　　　*Type # (1-5)*　　　　　*Description of Ideation*	Most Severe	Most Severe
Frequency *How many times have you had these thoughts?* 　(1) Less than once a week　(2) Once a week　(3) 2-5 times in week　(4) Daily or almost daily　(5) Many times each day	_____	_____
Duration *When you have the thoughts how long do they last?* 　(1) Fleeting - few seconds or minutes　　　　　　(4) 4-8 hours/most of day 　(2) Less than 1 hour/some of the time　　　　　　(5) More than 8 hours/persistent or continuous 　(3) 1-4 hours/a lot of time	_____	_____
Controllability *Could/can you stop thinking about killing yourself or wanting to die if you want to?* 　(1) Easily able to control thoughts　　　　　　　(4) Can control thoughts with a lot of difficulty 　(2) Can control thoughts with little difficulty　　(5) Unable to control thoughts 　(3) Can control thoughts with some difficulty　　(0) Does not attempt to control thoughts	_____	_____
Deterrents *Are there things - anyone or anything (e.g., family, religion, pain of death) - that stopped you from wanting to die or acting on thoughts of suicide?* 　(1) Deterrents definitely stopped you from attempting suicide　(4) Deterrents most likely did not stop you 　(2) Deterrents probably stopped you　　　　　　　　　　　　(5) Deterrents definitely did not stop you 　(3) Uncertain that deterrents stopped you　　　　　　　　　　(0) Does not apply	_____	_____
Reasons for Ideation *What sort of reasons did you have for thinking about wanting to die or killing yourself? Was it to end the pain or stop the way you were feeling (in other words you couldn't go on living with this pain or how you were feeling) or was it to get attention, revenge or a reaction from others? Or both?* 　(1) Completely to get attention, revenge or a reaction from others　(4) Mostly to end or stop the pain (you couldn't go on 　(2) Mostly to get attention, revenge or a reaction from others　　　　living with the pain or how you were feeling) 　(3) Equally to get attention, revenge or a reaction from others　　(5) Completely to end or stop the pain (you couldn't go on 　　　　and to end/stop the pain　　　　　　　　　　　　　　　　　　living with the pain or how you were feeling) 　　　　　　　　　　　　　　　　　　　　　　　　　　　　　　　　(0) Does not apply	_____	_____

© 2008 Research Foundation for Mental Hygiene, Inc.　　　C-SSRS—Lifetime Recent (Version 1/14/09)

SUICIDAL BEHAVIOR (Check all that apply, so long as these are separate events; must ask about all types)	Lifetime	Past 3 months

Actual Attempt:
A potentially self-injurious act committed with at least some wish to die, *as a result of act*. Behavior was in part thought of as method to kill oneself. Intent does not have to be 100%. If there is **any** intent/desire to die associated with the act, then it can be considered an actual suicide attempt. **There does not have to be any injury or harm**, just the potential for injury or harm. If person pulls trigger while gun is in mouth but gun is broken so no injury results, this is considered an attempt.
Inferring Intent: Even if an individual denies intent/wish to die, it may be inferred clinically from the behavior or circumstances. For example, a highly lethal act that is clearly not an accident so no other intent but suicide can be inferred (e.g., gunshot to head, jumping from window of a high floor/story). Also, if someone denies intent to die, but they thought that what they did could be lethal, intent may be inferred.
Have you made a suicide attempt?
Have you done anything to harm yourself?
Have you done anything dangerous where you could have died?
    What did you do?
    Did you_____ as a way to end your life?
    Did you want to die (even a little) when you____?
    Were you trying to end your life when you____?
    Or Did you think it was possible you could have died from____?
Or did you do it purely for other reasons / without ANY intention of killing yourself (like to relieve stress, feel better, get sympathy, or get something else to happen)? *(Self-Injurious Behavior without suicidal intent)*
If yes, describe:
	Yes No
	☐ ☐
	
	Total # of Attempts
	_____
		Yes No
		☐ ☐
		
		Total # of Attempts
		_____

Has subject engaged in Non-Suicidal Self-Injurious Behavior?	Yes No ☐ ☐	Yes No ☐ ☐
Interrupted Attempt: When the person is interrupted (by an outside circumstance) from starting the potentially self-injurious act *(if not for that, actual attempt would have occurred)*. Overdose: Person has pills in hand but is stopped from ingesting. Once they ingest any pills, this becomes an attempt rather than an interrupted attempt. Shooting: Person has gun pointed toward self, gun is taken away by someone else, or is somehow prevented from pulling trigger. Once they pull the trigger, even if the gun fails to fire, it is an attempt. Jumping: Person is poised to jump, is grabbed and taken down from ledge. Hanging: Person has noose around neck but has not yet started to hang - is stopped from doing so. **Has there been a time when you started to do something to end your life but someone or something stopped you before you actually did anything?** If yes, describe:	Yes No ☐ ☐ Total # of interrupted _____	Yes No ☐ ☐ Total # of interrupted _____
Aborted or Self-Interrupted Attempt: When person begins to take steps toward making a suicide attempt, but stops themselves before they actually have engaged in any self-destructive behavior. Examples are similar to interrupted attempts, except that the individual stops him/herself, instead of being stopped by something else. **Has there been a time when you started to do something to try to end your life but you stopped yourself before you actually did anything?** If yes, describe:	Yes No ☐ ☐ Total # of aborted or self-interrupted _____	Yes No ☐ ☐ Total # of aborted or self-interrupted _____
Preparatory Acts or Behavior: Acts or preparation towards imminently making a suicide attempt. This can include anything beyond a verbalization or thought, such as assembling a specific method (e.g., buying pills, purchasing a gun) or preparing for one's death by suicide (e.g., giving things away, writing a suicide note). **Have you taken any steps towards making a suicide attempt or preparing to kill yourself (such as collecting pills, getting a gun, giving valuables away or writing a suicide note)?** If yes, describe:	Yes No ☐ ☐ Total # of preparatory acts _____	Yes No ☐ ☐ Total # of preparatory acts _____

	Most Recent Attempt Date:	Most Lethal Attempt Date:	Initial/First Attempt Date:
Actual Lethality/Medical Damage: 0. No physical damage or very minor physical damage (e.g., surface scratches). 1. Minor physical damage (e.g., lethargic speech; first-degree burns; mild bleeding; sprains). 2. Moderate physical damage; medical attention needed (e.g., conscious but sleepy, somewhat responsive; second-degree burns; bleeding of major vessel). 3. Moderately severe physical damage; *medical* hospitalization and likely intensive care required (e.g., comatose with reflexes intact; third-degree burns less than 20% of body; extensive blood loss but can recover; major fractures). 4. Severe physical damage; *medical* hospitalization with intensive care required (e.g., comatose without reflexes; third-degree burns over 20% of body; extensive blood loss with unstable vital signs; major damage to a vital area). 5. Death	*Enter Code* _____	*Enter Code* _____	*Enter Code* _____
Potential Lethality: Only Answer if Actual Lethality=0 Likely lethality of actual attempt if no medical damage (the following examples, while having no actual medical damage, had potential for very serious lethality: put gun in mouth and pulled the trigger but gun fails to fire so no medical damage; laying on train tracks with oncoming train but pulled away before run over). 0 = Behavior not likely to result in injury 1 = Behavior likely to result in injury but not likely to cause death 2 = Behavior likely to result in death despite available medical care	*Enter Code* _____	*Enter Code* _____	*Enter Code* _____

Structure of the Book

Karen Carberry

At the time of this Handbook going into production the world has been globally afflicted by the COVID-19 pandemic. Not only has the coronavirus infiltrated every race and socio-economic status across the world, it has also emphasised the historical disparity across racial lines. With 40% of minority ethnic employees in post, tabloids galvanised the nation to support the NHS staff, initially depicted as all white teams at the front-line of the attack against the virus. In quick succession, we observed that despite pleading for effective protective equipment, Black, Asian and minority ethnic doctors, nurses and consultants described as BAME, were the first to meet their demise after contracting the virus in the line of duty. (Weaver, 2020; Siddique, 2020). Personally, with a history spanning 3 generations employed within the NHS, it has been a worrying time.

With the national 'lock-down' in place, only NHS employees, together with special teachers caring for children of NHS staff, were deemed to be included as 'essential key-workers' who could travel. Ferrying staff to work, transportation services revealed that the first bus drivers who contracted the disease through their front-line working conditions, were also men of colour (McDonald & Topham, 2020). Reports also suggest that a whopping 34% of patients admitted to critical care, were from BAME communities, who account for just 14% of the national population (Icnac, 2020 p.4; Croxford,2020). Why is this happening? We know from our Handbook that racism and micro-aggression are contributory factors to developing stress related conditions, such as anxiety, and high blood pressure, which is prevalent within the BAME community. Research also posits that a compromised immune system perpetuated by early adversity, such as bullying, together with the ecological fight-or-flight response, negatively affect the immune system (Morey et al., 2015 pp. 2, 4).

Across the UK and United States black people and minority ethnic families epitomised the highest percentage of those both contracting and dying from the condition. Reports that black men wearing masks to protect themselves from the virus, and in a quest to venture out to shop for essentials, have been asked to leave supermarkets - prohibited from buying food for themselves and their families (Yan, 2020). In this unprecedented time in which the global pandemic has affected every political, social and financial infrastructure, the way in which Black communities and people of colour are treated has not wavered. Even in a pandemic where everyone is suggested to be at equal risk, bigotry, racism and unfairness prevails (Hirsch, 2020).

The structure of this book therefore, not only illuminates the current, and historical discrepancies, narratives and challenges emblematic of men and women and their collective experiences; there are models for transgenerational solutions, evidence based practice, cause for celebration and strategies for for thriving and over-coming for families and their communities. The structure of the Handbook holds the keys for moving forward at such a time as this, in globally re-building equitable structures with exciting new paradigms accessible through our e-book and hardback versions.

The International Handbook of Black Community Mental Health has 40 contributors and 29 chapters. There are six parts in total: Part I – Race Relations; Part II – Policy; Part III – Interventions; Part IV – Theory and Practice; Part V – Clinical Practice; and Part VI – Recommendations. Each chapter of the book specifically emphasises and integrates core cultural competencies.

Part I – Race Relations

Our first section on Race Relations comprises 5 chapters, beginning with the flagrant racialisation of black men in 'Chapter 1: Systemic Racism: Big, Black, Mad and Dangerous in the Criminal Justice System' by *Dr Sharon Walker*. In this chapter, discussions focus largely on the experiences of black men, who are more likely than black women to encounter the phenomena of a mental health diagnosis, detention and death in a forensic setting. The chapter briefly explores reasons for the over-representation of black people with mental health issues before Dr Walker offers her own theoretical interpretation, which is a combination of systemic racism influenced by post-colonial conceptualisation.

Turning to women's experiences, 'Chapter 2: In the Name of Our Humanity: Challenging Academic Racism and its Effects on the Emotional Wellbeing of Women of Colour Professors' is written by Professor *Philomena Essed* and *Karen Carberry*. The hiring of women of colour faculty is not without unwritten presuppositions. We are expected to tolerate racism and to draw from cultural experience in catering to students of colour or when it fulfils institutional needs such as bringing 'colour' to all white committees. Yet, the normative profile of university teachers demands detachment with a focus on high output in terms of students and publications. This chapter further illustrates the phenomena of microaggressions and 'every-day racism in universities'; institutions that are responsible for educating our mental health practitioners, clinicians and policymakers. The chapter addresses its effect on emotional wellbeing together with techniques and strategies to strengthen emotional resilience. Tools for emotional wellbeing to assist in overcoming the stresses of bias and prejudice are explored and shared, which include fully utilising employment assistance programme agencies.

'Chapter 3: Racial Battle Fatigue: The Long-Term Effects of Racial Microaggressions on African American Boys and Men', by *Professor William A. Smith*, *Rodalyn David* and *Glory S. Stanton*, further deepens the discussion on the nuances of racism and its cumulative exhaustive effect, often unseen, but nonetheless deeply destructive. African American males experience acute or chronic stress from discriminatory treatment and racial micro-aggressions, decreasing their biopsychosocial health. Racial micro-aggressions include, but are not limited to, merciless and mundane exclusionary messages, being treated as less than fully human, and civil and human rights violations. Racial micro-aggressions are key to understanding increase in racial battle fatigue (Smith, 2010) resulting from the psychological and physiological stress that racially marginalised individuals/ groups experience in response to specific race-related interactions between them and the surrounding dominant environment. Today, racial micro-aggressions continue to contribute to the negative workplace experiences of African American boys and men in schools, at work and in society. This chapter focusses on the definition, identification and long-term effects of racial micro-aggressions and the resultant racial battle fatigue in anti-black misandric environments.

Recursively reflecting back on University education, the students' perspective is covered in 'Chapter 4: Racism in Academia: (How to) Stay Black, Sane and Proud as the Doctoral Supervisory Relationship Implodes'. This chapter intends to provide an exploration of the experience of three black doctoral students, including the author, *Dr Sharon Walker*, as their PhD journeys come to a premature end. Dr Walker discusses how, as a black woman in academia, one can be perceived through a dysconscious racial lens purposed to maintain white privilege.

'Chapter 5: Implicit Provider Bias and its Implications for Black/African American Mental Health' by *Andra D. Rivers Johnson* expounds upon the role of implicit provider bias in US mental health care, as it is an important issue that continues to be of concern in the twenty-first century for the Black/African American community. Access to mental health and quality care remains elusive as members of this social group lack access to mental health screening, diagnosis and attention due to institutional and cultural barriers. Supporting the position that implicit and explicit provider bias exists in the mental health profession, this chapter explores how implicit provider bias is an intractable institutional barrier that prevents Black/African Americans from accessing mental health and quality care. A review of the implications related to mental health outcomes with Black/African American clients is also explored, followed by a brief overview of the Black/African American cultural responses to implicit provider bias. The author examines various ways to help identify, address and eliminate implicit provider bias using evidence-based personal and community engagement strategies that promote mental health wellness within the Black/African American community. Implications for best practices in Black/African American mental health are addressed to eradicate the risk of unethical or medical malpractice with Black/African American clients, reduce the mental health disparity experienced by Blacks/African Americans and create mental health equity for this population.

Part II – Policy

Three chapters written by leading writers with a convergence on racism, discrimination and inequalities in policy, provides insightful discussion and guidance for all parties.

Renowned author and activist, *Dr Patrick Vernon OBE* clearly and succinctly expounds this argument in 'Chapter 6: Thirty Years of Black History Month and

Thirty Years of Overrepresentation in the Mental Health System', which is a jaw-dropping account and an overview of the impact of the British social and mental health policy and its antecedent history, which has had far reaching consequences on the mental health of the black community in the UK.

The chapter explores current policy, new trends in psychosis and mental ill health within the black community, and examines whether the current austerity measures has exacerbated an increase in mental illness and social exclusion; making recommendations for future policy development in tackling racial inequality and the impact on black communities if current mental health and other aspects of society remain unchanged in a post Brexit Britain.

Narratives of the 'expert by experience' - the client, client, the Approved Mental Health Professional (AMPH) and social care practitioners are voiced within 'Chapter 7: Race and Risk – Exploring UK Social Policy and the Development of Modern Mental Health Services' by *Patricia Clarke*. The chapter offers an opportunity to consider the policy context within the provision of mental care within the UK and the inter-relationship with BME communities. Diminishing resources, the impact of 'austerity', plus discrimination and poor care continues to compromise safety and wellbeing. The emergence of a new social policy context in which legislation promotes safeguarding for all users of statutory health services may offer the prospect of improving the service's user experience and safety for all.

In continuing the theme of safety, 'Chapter 8: Remaining Mindful about Young People' by *Mhemooda Malek* and *Dr Simon Newitt*, a key issue explored is the long-needed attention to meaningfully identifying and addressing the mental health and wellbeing of children and young people from BME communities. This attention is needed across policy, research, planning and the provision of services, and some of the consequences of the lack of due focus to date are explored. Consideration is given to services provided by the voluntary and community sector, including a case study of an initiative aiming to develop culturally sensitive approaches to engaging and working with young people.

This section clearly illustrates the inextricable linkage of how policy is recursively linked to the application and outcome of unhelpful/helpful service interventions within BME communities. In order to ameliorate these concerns it necessitates interventions that challenge the status quo; hence galvanising scholars and practitioners in Part III, to develop theories, apply to practice novel service interventions.

Part III – Interventions

This section has six chapters, aimed both at understanding and challenging many of the problems described previously in mental health services, provisions and training. This section deals with cultural competencies, inequalities in patient services, social emotional wellness in education, Autistic Spectrum Disorder (ASD) and issues that affect black males, who get caught up in the mental health system. Not only do the contributors in this section share their innovative insights, ideas, development of knowledge production, community interventions and practices, they also share methods that positively support and empower BAME communities in a culturally competent manner.

In determining essential clinical training for working therapeutically, 'Chapter 9: Cultural Competencies in Delivering Counselling and Psychotherapy Services to a Black Multi-cultural Population: Time for Change and Action' by *Dr Nicholas Banks* considers provision in counselling and associated mental health support services and the need for multi-cultural competencies (MCC) in delivering ethical services to multi-cultural populations. The author suggests that an effective means of supporting the needs of mental health professionals may be through the training of MCC supervisors who are then able to train mental health professionals to become more culturally competent and promote more appropriate services to people of colour. The author in a sense ratifies, positively enhances and augments the new *DSM-5 Handbook on the Cultural Formulation Interview* (Lewis-Fernández, Aggarwal, Hinton, L., Hinton, D. E., & Kirmayer, 2015), further challenging training institutions and mental health practitioners to recalibrate their training and therapeutic models in order to prepare and adequately train the therapeutic community to be culturally competent in order to meet the psychology needs of the BAME community.

The theme of cultural competence in training is expanded internationally within the school teaching profession in 'Chapter 10: Social and Emotional Education and Emotional Wellness: A Cultural Competence Model for Black Boys and Teachers', co-authored by *Dr Richard Majors, Dr Llewellyn E. Simmons and Dr Cornelius Ani*. The authors examine teachers' emotional literacy and anxiety in their relationships with young black males in school and discuss the importance of developing an emotional literacy/cultural competence model called 'Teacher Empathy' to remedy teacher's lack of emotional literacy and problems communicating with black boys. Therefore, their model focusses on how teachers can develop relationships and communicate more effectively with black males. The aim/goal of their model/curriculum (see the Addendum to the Introduction for samples of their curriculum and toolkit) is to improve academic performance, motivate, reduce exclusions and help both black males and teachers, regulate and manage their behaviours more effectively for more positive outcomes.

Special needs assessment and diagnosis often overrides the influence of cultural traditions and cultural norms, which may affect the correct assessment and treatment. 'Chapter 11: ASD & Cultural Competence: An ASD Multi-cultural Treatment Led Model' by *Mary Henderson* and *Dr Richard Majors* address this impasse, noting that, although there are clear guidelines in relation both to the criteria and assessment of ASD, there appears to be an absence of strict cultural competency guidelines in the assessment. The authors provide clear examples through case studies, educating the reader regarding the possibility of stigma in certain cultures where a mental health diagnosis such as ASD can be considered negatively, potentially preventing clinicians from seeing the whole picture. Safe practice is developed with the clinician in mind with this competency mode.

'Chapter 12: Moving Young Black Men beyond Survival Mode: Protective Factors for Their Mental Health' by *Ivan Juzang* continues with the theme of protection and prevention. This chapter focusses on preventing or reducing mental health issues among young black men in low-income, urban communities as a way to counter the risk factors (social determinants) that keep them in survival mode.

Using a 'protective factors framework' with black males as an inoculation against the stressors they will face early on in life, will arm them with the skills needed to thrive even in the face of repeated exposure to extreme poverty and adverse childhood experiences. The author explains how protective factor interventions should be studied and evaluated, and raises the question of why potential 'population health' interventions that can provide better outcomes in a cost effective, culturally relevant way are not being funded and published. Promoting protective factors to cope with stress and trauma is not a new recommendation, yet a protective factors framework to address and prevent black youth violence has not been implemented in scale and evaluated.

Developing evaluative equitable support for those who are disabled is discussed in 'Chapter 13: African Americans and the Vocational Rehabilitation Service System in the United States: The Impact on Mental Health' by *Professor Fabricio E. Balcazar* and *Julie Vryhof*. It provides a comprehensive description of the Vocational Rehabilitation Service System, created in 1973 in the USA to help people with disabilities access necessary support and services to return to work and live independently. The programme receives federal funds and operates in all 50 states and territories. The programme is designed to allow consumers to develop a rehabilitation plan in collaboration with a vocational rehabilitation counsellor and receive necessary services and support to meet their rehabilitation goals. Unfortunately, there are serious issues with access to services and rehabilitation success for minority individuals in the programme, particularly African Americans. The chapter first provides a brief overview of the Rehabilitation Act and its purpose, then introduces some of the research that has been conducted to evaluate the programme over the years, with particular emphasis on the outcomes for African Americans, before examining a series of studies conducted by the authors in the state of Illinois. The chapter concludes with some suggestions about ways in which the system could be improved and ways to empower African Americans pursuing rehabilitation and independent living goals, including peer-support and supported employment.

Emotional literacy, in recent years, has been gaining momentum as a model that can support and improve the lives of adults and children; and 'Chapter 14: Targeted Intervention in Education and the Empowerment and Emotional Well-Being of Black Boys' by *Dr Cheron Byfield* and *Dr Tony Talburt* considers why so many black boys in UK schools still fail to achieve high levels of academic attainment, decades after this issue was raised in the 1970s and, more importantly, what steps can be taken to help raise their academic performance and improving their overall emotional wellbeing and mental health in schools. This chapter briefly examines some of the targeted intervention strategies employed by Excell3, the umbrella organisation that runs the National Black Boys Can Project. The fundamental philosophy underpinning their approach is that all black boys, regardless of their socioeconomic backgrounds, can, if appropriately supported, raise their levels of academic success, social aspirations and self-esteem. For nearly two decades, Black Boys Can Projects have been engaged in developing and carrying out specific interventions, designed to help boys re-think how they approach their education, personal development and career goals.

Part IV – Theory and Practice

This section comprises 10 chapters and focusses on the reconstruction of the black community proposing theoretical models, practice and emerging themes that support, help and empower both Windrush survivors and people of colour, whom the mental health system has failed over the years. They also provide ethnographic insights into obstacles and strengths, at both the micro- and macro-level, experienced/used by black female leadership in the mental health services.

Faith is one aspect of life that people of colour draw strength from in a race-conscious society, and therefore an important contribution within 'Chapter 15: Towards a Position of Spiritual Reflexivity as a Resource: Emerging Themes and Conversations for Systemic Practice, Leadership, and Supervision within Black Mental Health' by *Maureen Greaves*. This chapter represents a body of practice-based research that acknowledges and explores the increasing presence of spirituality in systemic supervision and leadership coaching. The coexistence of inspiration and challenge showcase the resourcefulness of spirituality, referenced through paying attention to the spiritual aspects of *knowing*; particularly within the organisational domains which surround black mental health. Personal contributions are considered through the lens of Christianity, while appreciating the applicability of multi-faith and agnostic professionals alike.

The theme of leadership continues through 'Chapter 16: "Marginal Leaders": Making Visible the Leadership Experiences of Black Women in a Therapeutic Service for Disenfranchised Young People' by *Dr Romana Farooq* and *Dr Tânia Rodrigues*. Although women are obtaining and maintaining leadership positions in health, education and social care services, women from BAME backgrounds remain a minority and on the margins. In particular, services working therapeutically with marginalised and oppressed communities often fail to represent the population they serve. In this chapter, the authors outline the development of an innovative therapeutic service for disenfranchised young people with black women as leaders. The authors reflect on how they developed a leadership style drawing on Afrocentric practice, social justice, emancipatory practice and community psychology as they attempted to bring about system change. They also draw on ideas of 'marginality' to make visible their experience of 'be-coming' leaders, and the challenges that they experienced on several different levels: personal, professional, institutional, political and cultural. They also examine how race, gender and class intersect in black women's leadership experiences, and how they tackle stereotyping in the making of black female leaders. Finally, the chapter examines how black female leaders make creative use of their marginal positions to influence and reflect a radical standpoint on self, children, young people, families and community.

In 2019, the UK looked back in history with the nation concurrently honouring the 70th anniversary of the NHS and 70 years since the landing of the Empire Windrush carrying many first generations from the Caribbean. Amongst all the celebrations are the many years of trauma and disappointment in the NHS mental health services the Windrush generation helped to build. It is thus pertinent to include 'Chapter 17: 40 Years in The Wilderness: A Review of Systemic Barriers to Reducing The Over-representation of Black Men in the UK Psychiatric System' by

Dr Gail Coleman-Oluwabusola, which briefly summarises research over the past four decades (and prior) associated with black men and mental health in the UK.

Early interventions and understanding of self are key constructs for black boys to take them through to adulthood. In 'Chapter 18: Oppositional and Defiant Behaviours Among Black Boys in Schools: Techniques to Facilitate Change by *Dr Steve Clarke*. The author presents a Personal Construct Psychology derived approach, as a methodology for working with those who are struggling to cope with the education system. which offers a way through the conceptual confusion clouding thinking about aspects of black boys lives that concern us, often leaving institutions lacking the energy and ability to loosen their thinking and move in the direction of rewarding new attitudes and behaviours.

Research on attitudes within therapeutic relationships are further discussed in 'Chapter 19: Black Therapists – White Families: Positive Outcomes. Therapists' Perceptions of Cultural Competence in Clinical Practice by *Karen Carberry* and *Dr Belinda Brooks-Gordon*. A culturally competent counsellor, using positive aspects of themselves, offers White clients the opportunity to 'risk take', challenge previously held assumptions and transform themselves in counselling; skilful handing of therapy will prevent clients from feeling shame for some of the emotions associated with the early white racial identity statuses. In addition to the theory maps that black therapists employ, awareness of the convergence of multiple cultural contexts and collective identities empowers trainees to deal with families from different ecological niches, and raises consciousness about professional and personal biases. Results suggest that black therapists are able to significantly perceive the statuses of their White clients and their own racial identity, in order to addresses the importance of taking into account the cultural context when working with, for example, interracial couples, particularly when one partner is more or less understanding of the other person's reality in a race conscious society. The use of reflexivity and socialisation maps in processing some of the difficult emotions associated with cross-cultural and interracial therapy is explored.

The cross-cultural theme in family dynamics continues in 'Chapter 20: Transracial Adoption and Mental Health' by *Dr Nicholas Banks*. The author considers historical and current perspectives on transracial adoption, mainly, but not exclusively, from a British perspective. The term 'transracial adoption' refers to the adoption of children who are from a different ethnicity than that of the adoptive parents (e.g. white parents and black children). In this chapter, the focus is on children of black British origin, including African-Caribbean, black African children and children of mixed 'race' with a black parent. The term black children is used as a generic term unless otherwise specified. Mixed 'race' families, where one parent is black and one parent is white, are seen as a 'variant of the black family'.

As one moves through the mid to latter years of the family life cycle, we can observe the various challenges of mental health continuing. 'Chapter 21: Dementia and its Impact on Minority Ethnic and Migrant Communities' by *David Trusswell* clarifies that is often assumed that dementia is an illness that has its greatest impact on the economically developed regions of the world due to the greater human longevity in those regions. The stereotypic picture of an older person living with Alzheimer's disease, the most common form of dementia, is of a white European or North American man or woman. Dementia is often regarded as a less dominant health concern for the world's economically underdeveloped regions and for minority ethnic and migrant populations within the developed world. This chapter challenges this stereotype, looking at the impact of dementia in economically underdeveloped countries and on minority ethnic and migrant communities living in the developed world.

Remaining with the elderly, 'Chapter 22: Mental Health/Illness Revisited in People of African-Caribbean Heritage in Britain' by *Dr Florence Gwendolyn Rose* and *Professor Tony Leiba* examines mental health in the older Windrush community based on case studies from the African-Caribbean mental health project called 'Hagar', followed by an analysis of the case studies and a comparative analysis of Fannon's theory on racism. The conclusion is that health care providers must acknowledge the presence of institutional racism in mental health services and the need to change and include more culturally sensitive 'talking and other therapies'.

Another pioneering study in this section is 'Chapter 23: Researching African-Caribbean Mental Health in the UK: An Assets-based Approach to Developing Psychosocial Interventions for Schizophrenia and Related Psychoses' by *Dr Dawn Edge*, *Dr Amy Degnan* and *Sonya Rafiq*, Their research highlights that, in the UK, people of African-Caribbean origin experience significantly higher rates of diagnosis with schizophrenia and related psychoses than all other ethnic groups. Schizophrenia care for African-Caribbeans is characterised by inferior access, experiences and outcomes and by fear and mistrust of mental health services. Findings indicate that adopting an assets-based approach to working collaboratively with African-Caribbeans enhances engagement of people often labelled 'hard-to-reach'. Community-partnered participatory research of this type has implications for developing, implementing and evaluating more accessible and acceptable interventions for both mental and physical health in the global health arena.

Mental health concerns of hard-to-reach people include those who are involved in domestic and international terrorism. This seminal 'Chapter 24: "Lone Wolf" Case Study Considerations of Terrorist Radicalisation from the Black Experience – Impact on Mental Health' by *Dr Nicholas Banks* uses two case studies of individuals who converted to Islam, became radicalised and carried out terrorist acts: Richard Reid in the UK; and Carlos Bledsoe in the USA. Issues of religion, mental health and radicalisation are explored from the black experience. Attachment-related principles are applied to the case study examples at the end of the chapter to explore the psychological and social vulnerability of the case study individuals.

Part V – Clinical Practice

The fifth section discusses best practice and highlights clinical models in four chapters, focussing on the most important values and beliefs of people of colour, within clinical examples of practice in order to deliver the best and most culturally competent care.

Acknowledging the works and opposing stand points of the Sensory Integration Community, Ayres and APA, 'Chapter 25: Spotlight on Sensory Processing Difficulties' by *Lisa Prior* and *Tiffany Howl* begins this section with current thinking about sensory processing difficulties, and discusses implications for current assessment, treatment options and provision. An experiential perspective is then presented from Prior's work as an occupational therapist in Child and Adolescent Mental Health Services (CAMHS), identifying commonly recognised presentations (which can indicate sensory processing difficulties including ASD, Attention deficit hyperactivity disorder (ADHD), 'fussy eater', 'emotional dysregulation' and 'meltdowns') to detail how these difficulties can be assessed and formulated with use of the sensory profile. The chapter also provides practical examples of how to screen for these difficulties, explain them to young people, parents and schools and manage them through sensory activities and environmental adaptations. Through contributions from Howl's experiences working in the African Caribbean Community Initiative and as a Specialist Psychological Wellbeing Practitioner improving access to psychological therapies for the 'hard-to-reach' population, consideration is given to adapting these resources with the intention of them being more acceptable and accessible for use in work within BAME communities. The chapter concludes with questions about future implications for service provisions for people with sensory processing difficulties and how raised awareness of these difficulties might impact on other evidence based diagnoses and treatments such as Cognitive Behaviour Therapy (CBT) (drawing on the authors recent learning on the Children and Young People (CYP), Improving Access to Psychological Therapies (IAPT), (CBT course), for anxiety presentations.

Marital and family relationships can also be quite complex to treat, and 'Chapter 26: Forced Marriage as a Representation of a Belief System in the UK and it's psychological impact on well-being Families' by *Doreen Robinson* and *Dr Reenee Singh* is the first of two chapters in our Handbook focussing on working with the family and community beliefs systems therapeutically. In this chapter, the authors describe the belief system of Izzat, which is central among South Asian families. The idea of forced marriage is based upon the concept of Izzat, or honour, which is a cornerstone of family life in South Asian communities. The closest English translations to Izzat and Sharam are honour and shame, respectively. The authors argue that Izzat and Sharam are mechanisms that safeguard patriarchal customs, such as arranged marriage, which are familiar to them as they write from their respective backgrounds as two Asian women. The authors illustrate the concept of Izzat through two vignettes and explicate theoretical ideas, based on Izzat, to include Boszormenyi-Nagy's ideas about belief systems. These ideas resonate with the strong influence of Izzat upon South Asian family and community systems, which authors have met in practice. They further explore the continuum of marriage to include forced, arranged and consensual marriage within the context of Izzat, and also consider issues of cultural competence and expertness and how these interplay with strongly held belief systems such as Izzat, concluding with some clinical implications and pointers for practice.

Historically the Caribbean has a large Asian-Caribbean population in which belief systems postulated within the previous chapter hold true - particularly regarding the aspect of partriachy. The international perspective on working with families moves to the 2010 earthquake in Haiti, which indelibly provides an insight into the effects of trauma and loss, and the faith-testing dilemmas faced by families and communities. Stories of these concerns and responses are contained in 'Chapter 27: Systemic Family Therapy with Transgenerational Communities in Haiti and the Dominican Republic' by *Karen Carberry, Pastor Jean Gerald Lafleur* and *Rev. Genel Jean-Claude*. This chapter highlights collaborative methods for community mobilisation with Pastors as community gatekeepers to address transgenerational trauma and wellbeing. Through the lens of natural disaster, political history and the interplay of subtle and overt racism, this model highlights the need for knowledge of spiritual belief systems and cultural nuances in order to develop, apply and utilise clinical expertise in transgenerational family therapy with Haitian families to assist in the reconstruction of mental health in black communities.

With a plethora of cutting edge evidence based practice, and culturally based research and interventions (organisational, clinical, pastoral and and therapeutic) the authors illuminate a range of and different types of cross-cultural relationship styles requiring management and supervision. With vignettes, and testimonies regarding the positive effects of culturally competent practice, the chapter demonstrates an urgency and an increased demand from academics to decolonise the education, leadership and clinical training methodologies and practice in Universities and training institutions (John, 2019).

This *Handbook* raises many questions regarding the interactions and communications styles of white supervisors, for example, cross-cultural supervision, and some of the experiences of the negative impact on students of colour in academia. Therefore, it is befitting to conclude with 'Chapter 28: Engaging with Racialized Process in Clinical Supervision. Political or Personal' by lecturer and international supervisor *Dr Isha McKenzie-Mavinga*, which deals with uncomfortable feelings that often occur between the supervisor and supervisee dyad, namely the radicalised process that occurs in therapeutic work and clinical supervision, which shows up in ways that the supervisor acknowledges/addresses the impact of racism in the therapeutic space. The author recommends that taking action on the racialised interaction/space means beginning to restore harmony against current and historic anti-oppressive practice. Cultural competence training for such white supervisors may offer a first step in seeking redress.

Part VI – Recommendations

The final section provides recommendations towards a 10-point action plan for change between 2020 – 2030 addressing the various mental health issues raised and examined in the previous sections. *The International Handbook of Black Community Mental Health* is a timely and essential national and international tool, with evidenced-based formulations and interventions to effectively infiltrate the mental health framework, including policies, education, the criminal justice service, clinical training and mental health services in order to effectively reconstruct the transgenerational health of the black community and people of colour. As we battle to live, strive, survive and thrive into a new century in 2020, now is the time to utilise and apply the contents of this Handbook for a paradigm change.

References

Croxford, R. (2020, April 12). Coronavirus: Ethnic Minorities'Are a third of patients'. Available at https://www.bbc.co.uk/news/uk-52255863. Accessed on 12 April 2020.

Hirsch, A. (2020, April 9). If coronavirus does not discriminate how come black people are bearing the brunt. The Guardian. Retrieved from https://www.theguardian.com/commentisfree/2020/apr/08/coronavirus-black-people-ethnic-minority-deaths-pandemic-inequality-afua-hirsch

Intensive Care National Audit & Research Centre. (2020, April 4). ICNARC report on COVID-19 in critical care, P4, London, United Kingdom. Retrieved from https://www.icnarc.org/About/Latest-News/2020/04/04/Report-On-2249-Patients-Critically-Ill-With-Covid-19.

Jan, T. (2020, April 9). Two Black Men say they were kicked out of Walmart for wearing protective masks. Others worry that it will happen to them. The Washington Post. Retrieved from https://www.washingtonpost.com/business/2020/04/09/masks-racial-profiling-walmart-coronavirus/

John, G. (2019). *Decolonising curriculum*. First BELMAS annual educational leadership lecture, University College London, UK, 7 October. Retrieved from https://www.belmas.org.uk/Annual-Lecture-2019.

McDonald, H. & Topham, G. (2020, April 6). Colleagues of bus drivers who died of coronavirus call for better protection. The Guardian. Retrieved from https://www.theguardian.com/world/2020/apr/06/colleagues-bus-drivers-died-coronavirus-better-protection

Morey, J. N., Boggero, I. A., Scott, A. B., & Segerstrom, S. C. (2015). Current Directions in Stress and Human Immune Function. Current opinion in psychology, 5, 13–17.

Siddique, H. (2020, April 10). UK Government urged to investigate Coronavirus deaths of BAME doctors. The Guardian. Retrieved from https://www.theguardian.com/society/2020/apr/10/uk-coronavirus-deaths-bame-doctors-bma

Smith, W. A. (2010). Toward an understanding of misandric microaggressions and racial battle fatigue among African Americans in historically White institutions. In E. M. Zamani-Gallaher and V. C. Polite (Eds.) *The state of the African American male* (pp. 265–277). East Lansing, MI: Michigan State University Press.

Weaver, M. (2020, April 9). Doctor who pleaded for more PPE dies of Coronavirus. *The Guardian* Retrieved from https://www.theguardian.com/world/2020/apr/09/consultant-who-pleaded-for-more-nhs-hospital-ppe-dies-of-coronavirus.

Part I

Race Relations

Chapter 1

Systemic Racism: Big, Black, Mad and Dangerous in the Criminal Justice System

Sharon Walker

Introduction

I have written elsewhere about the issue of black academics in the UK experiencing mental ill health (Walker, in press). Yet, it is only one emerging area in an existing phenomenon of black people disproportionately diagnosed with a mental illness in other institutions such as the criminal justice system (CJS). The Black Manifesto (2010) states:

> we can objectively measure structural inequalities, discrimination and disparities in the criminal justice system, employment, education, poverty, health and housing. Disparate outcomes for Black and Minority Ethnic people in the UK have NOT been eliminated and, in fact in some areas, have increased. (p. 2)

The Black Manifesto note Britain's pride in its historic contributions to setting global standards for democracy and the rule of law yet it has not managed as a country to reduce racism or the over representation of black people with mental ill health. Findings from the Angiolini Report of the Independent Review of Deaths and Serious Incidents in Police Custody (2017) highlighted evidence of racial disproportionality in police restraint deaths. Indeed, during a 12-day period in 2017, Shane Bryant, 29; Rashan Charles, 20; Edson da Costa, 25; and Darren Cumberbatch aged 32, died following arrest. Newspaper reports suggest the official investigation into the death of Cumberbatch underplays the deterioration in his mental health whilst in contact with the police (*The Guardian*, 2017). As there was alleged use of force and Cumberbatch was taken to hospital with injuries, a referral should have been made immediately to the Independent Police Complaints Commission however this did not happen until 10 days later, by which time Cumberbatch had succumbed to his injuries. Cumberbatch and the three other men were black. These racialised deaths have continued despite the documented history – which when publicised are often portrayed as isolated incidents – of black people dying in forensic settings as a consequence of the use of force or restraint. Well documented is also the over representation of black people detained under the Mental Health Act yet underrepresented in community treatment such as counselling or therapy (Cabinet Office; Race Disparity Audit, 2017), indicating the lack of support and intervention preventing deterioration in the mental health of black people. Dyer (2017) suggests this is the country's 'dirty secret' that needs to be addressed.

I refer to 'black people' as those who identify their origins as Black British, Black Caribbean or Black African. Although Asian people face discrimination, they are not significantly disproportionally over represented in mental health or criminal justice statistics, which is the focus of this chapter. Still, many studies are not so discerning and do use the term Black and Minority Ethnic (BME) without making the distinctions between Black and Asian. However, these broader definitions are in line with that used in the government document Delivering Race Equality in Mental Health Care (Department of Health, 2005) which includes:

> all people of minority ethnic status in England. It does not only refer to skin colour but to people of all groups who may experience discrimination and disadvantage, such as those of Irish origin, those of Mediterranean origin and East European migrants. (p. 11)

I also use the term racism as oppose to discrimination. Race is the basis for the oppressive behaviour based on colour or ethnicity whereas discrimination can occur on the basis of any type of perceived difference, for example, gender or disability. Stokely and Hamilton (1967) suggest 'By "racism" we mean the predication of decisions and policies on considerations of race for the purpose of subordinating a racial group and maintaining control over that group' (p. 20). My interest in the wellbeing of black people in the CJS is borne out of my experience as a black woman working within police custody suites in East London in the late 1990s, assessing people with mental health and substance misuse issues. This was followed by 10 years with HM Prison Service and National Offender Management Service as one of the few black female senior managers. I have subsequently developed my own thinking about the reasons for the over representation of black people with mental health issues and their experience in the CJS. Nonetheless, the process of writing this chapter has been an unexpected emotional toil. Reading report after report about black men who have been diagnosed with a mental illness, detained, injured and killed in twenty-first century Britain has been an emotional challenge. Knowing that this occurs at the hands of the police who have a duty to serve and protect and nursing staff that have a duty of care makes it even more appalling. The notion that successive governments have failed to implement recommendations from reviews and inquiries that might have saved lives is nothing short of diabolical. Despite the knowledge emergent from research, reports, reviews and recommendations, there is a continuance of the disproportionality faced by black people in mental health and CJS.[1]

---

[1] At the time of publication, COVID-19 had created a pandemic. The intensive care national audit office (2020) found one third of people stricken by the virus were BME, despite making up only 17% of the UK population. Similarly, in the US, 23% of the population in Cook County, Illinois are black yet 58% of COVID-19 deaths were of black people.

As I write I wonder what difference this chapter can make in the midst of the existing plethora of text that have failed to ignite a response from those with the power to end this phenomenon of what is essentially a legitimised racialisation of mental health and lawful killing of black men. That said, I continue, believing that I have a duty to contribute to the discourse until these experiences are no longer a 'dirty secret' which remain unresponded to. In this chapter my discussions focus largely on the experiences of black men as they are more likely than woman to encounter the phenomena of a mental health diagnosis, detention and death in a forensic setting. I will briefly explore reasons given by other researchers for the over representation of black people with mental health issues before offering my own theoretical interpretation which is a combination of systemic racism influenced by post-colonial conceptualisation.

Over-representation in Mental Ill Health and Custody

Sharpley, Hutchinson, McKenzie, and Murray (2001) note how after the large-scale migration of people from the Caribbean to the UK in the 1950s, only a decade later research indicated an over representation of those migrants being diagnosed with schizophrenia. To contextualise the scale of the over representation, Xanthos (2008) states that in any given country schizophrenia typically affects 1% of the population. Yet Hickling (2005) identified a 6- to 18-fold elevated rate of diagnosis amongst the black population in the UK. A larger scale study reported a year later found a ninefold increase in the risk of black people developing schizophrenia with an increased risk of 1.4 for South Asians when compared to the white British population (Fearon et al., 2006). Tortelli et al. (2015) found statistically significant higher incidence rates in the black Caribbean group, present across all major psychotic disorders, including schizophrenia and bipolar disorder. Stevenson and Rao (2014) found despite

> controlling for the social and economic factors known to influence wellbeing, there appears to be a residual, non-random difference – with people from Black and Minority Ethnic (BME) communities reporting lower levels of wellbeing than their White counterparts. (p. 12)

Since 2005, the Care Quality Commission conducted an annual census in relation to people from specific ethnic backgrounds experiencing mental ill health. Their last survey concluded that people from Ethnic Minorities remain disproportionately represented on mental health wards with no signs of this reducing (Care Quality Commission, 2011). The census identified that rates of hospital detention were between 19% and 32% above average for people with mental ill health from black Caribbean, black African and mixed white/black groups. This was two times higher than the average for 2010. Supporting these findings, the Health and Social Care Information Centre (2016) found Black or Black British people were the highest proportion of ethnic minority groups who had spent time in mental health hospitals in the year 2014/2015.

Self-isolation, illness, fear of death and increased risk of being stopped by police under the UK COVID-19 Bill will undoubtedly exacerbate the mental health of black people.

The over representation of mental ill health amongst black people also permeates throughout each juncture of the CJS. The Ministry of Justice (2015) state:

> In general, Black, Asian and Minority Ethnic (BAME) groups appear to be overrepresented at most stages throughout the CJS, compared with the White ethnic group ... with little change in relative positions between ethnic groups. (p. 7)

Thornicroft (2006) found 10% of black patients in forensic settings have not committed a crime, they have been admitted to these units from general psychiatric wards. A decade later the European Commission against Racism and Intolerance Report (ECRI, 2016) noted an increase whereby black people are 50% more likely to be referred to the psychiatric services via the police than white people. Singh et al. (2014) argue that ethnicity acts as a predictor of the high levels of mental health detention amongst black people. A variety of reports and research demonstrate this point. For example, the Bradley report (2013) identified

> BME communities are 40% more likely than White Britons to access mental health services via a CJS gateway (Bradley, 2009). Black people, in particular, are more likely to experience higher compulsory admission rates to hospital, greater involvement in legal and forensic settings and higher rates of transfer to medium and high security. (p. 4)

The findings from the Bradley report echo what was reported 10 years prior in the Bennett Inquiry (2003). They reported that black patients are more likely to be restrained, more likely to be secluded and more likely to be prescribed medication than any other group. These patients are also less likely to be given psychological treatment rather than physical treatment. Fitzpatrick, Kumar, Nkansa-Dwamena, and Thorne (2014) noted

> The most egregious inequalities in mental health care continues to be the overrepresentation of black men at the 'hard end' of services at point of arrest, in prison and within secure treatment. In its most extreme form this is represented by repetition of deaths in custody under restraint. (p. 8)

INQUEST (2015) suggests deaths of people in mental health detention make up 60% of the overall death in any type of custodial setting. They posit the high incidence of these deaths are amongst black people and are concerned that institutional racism is a contributory factor.

Findings from INQUEST's casework demonstrate the disproportionate number of people from BME communities die in or after detention in police custody following the use of force. From 1990 to 2017 there have been a total of 94 BME deaths in police custody, 13 of which have been shootings within the Metropolitan Police Service. In other constabularies in England and Wales there have been

76 BME deaths; three of which have been shootings. During the same period there have been 247 self-inflicted BME deaths and 203 non- self-inflicted deaths (excluding natural deaths) in prisons in England and Wales (INQUEST, 2017). The Angiolini Report confirmed

> The Government has acknowledged that there is 'significant over-representation of Black, Asian and minority ethnic (BAME) individuals in the criminal justice system' and that 'disproportionate number of people who have died following the use of force were from BAME communities'. (p. 84)

The combination of these statistics demonstrates the over represented of black people in relation to mental health, the CJS and the likelihood of death (excluding natural causes) when in the CJS. A variety of reasons for this racialisation of mental health have been offered by different researchers.

Reasons for Over Representation

Sharpley et al. (2001) found theories explaining the reasons for increased rates of black people diagnosed with mental health issues ranged from genetic predisposition, migration factors, cannabis use, social disadvantage to racism. Singh et al. (2014) suggest racial discrimination still remains the most studied variable in mental health disadvantage for Black Caribbean's. Alarcon (2009) argues the cultural needs of black people and their behaviour is misunderstood and misinterpreted, resulting in misplaced diagnosis. Comparison studies have been conducted in attempt to support or contest this theory. Studies have looked at the rates of mental health diagnosis of black people in their country of origin, compared to the rates of black people in the UK who have a mental health diagnosis. For example, Hickling and Rodgers-Johnson (1995) looked at the incidence of schizophrenia in Jamaica, Bhugra et al. (1996) focussed on Trinidad and Mahy, Mallett, Leff, and Bhugra (1999) looked at Barbados. Each found the rate of schizophrenia in the respective country was equitable to the incidence of schizophrenia amongst the British white population in the UK. Thus, the over representation could be concluded as being connected to a phenomenon experienced by black people once they arrive or are born in the UK. Hickling, McKenzie, Mullen, and Murray (1999), a Jamaican psychiatrist and his colleagues examined the same patients as his white counterparts yet they only agreed on the diagnosis of 55% of cases. Still, other research has suggested the over representation is not necessarily due to a cultural misdiagnosis. For example, Fung, Jones, and Bhugra (2009) found that factors such as age, sex, socioeconomic status, social isolation, genetic factors, infections, stress, substance misuse and discrimination, appeared to be related to the over representation. These factors tended not to have been accounted for in the early research of the 1960s and 1970s, largely as a consequence of poor patient record keeping and inadequate methodology in the research (Pinto, Ashworth, & Jones, 2008; Tortelli et al., 2015). However, there has since been much support for the notion that the experiences of racism and discrimination increase the risk of mental ill health within the black community. Bhui et al. (2005) identified a strong association between perceived discrimination in the workplace by black people and the development of mental health disorders. Pinto et al. (2008) posits a combination of isolation and exclusion, both within society and within the family, contributes to the incidence mental ill health in black people. However, they concluded racism itself may contribute to social exclusion, increasing the vulnerability to schizophrenia. The ECRI noted the allegations of discrimination that black people have made against the police and by the mental health services. ECRI suggest high levels of coercion rather than care typify the black patient experience. The Black Manifesto (2010) found 40% of patients in Broadmoor, Ashworth and Rampton high security psychiatric hospitals were of African-Caribbean origin and the average stay for these patients was more than nine years, longer than the stay of white patients.

Big, Bad and Dangerous

Rather than the behaviour of black people being misunderstood and misinterpreted resulting in misplaced diagnosis, there is also an ideology that a stereotype of black men being big, bad and dangerous pervades the mental health and CJSs with the consequence of higher rates of schizophrenia attributed particularly to black men. The Angiolini Report (2017) argues

> The stereotyping of young Black men as 'dangerous, violent and volatile' is a longstanding trope that is ingrained in the minds of many in our society. People with mental health needs also face the stereotype of the mentally ill as 'mad, bad and dangerous'. (p. 88)

The construction of the black man as 'big, bad and dangerous' is not only dehumanising, but creates the risk of over use of force when those who have the power to retrain is seeing a vulnerable and mentally ill man as a threat. The report further states

> It is not uncommon to hear comments from police officers about a young Black man having 'superhuman strength' or being 'impervious to pain' and, often wholly inaccurately, as the 'biggest man I have ever encountered'. Such perceptions increase the likelihood of force and restraint being used against an individual who may be unwell. The detainee is effectively dehumanised. (Angiolini Report, 2017, p. 88)

The notion of 'Big, bad and dangerous' is not new. It was evident in the case three black men who died in the 1980s and 1990s whilst detained in Broadmoor. The three men of concern were Michael Martin who died in 1984, Joseph Watts died in 1988 and Orville Blackwood died in 1991 following the use of restraint and the forcible injection of tranquillising medication. All three had a diagnosis of schizophrenia (INQUEST, 2015). The Special Hospital Service Authority (SHSA, 1993) was tasked to investigate the circumstances of Blackwood's death and review the circumstances of the deaths of Martin and Watts. Crichton (1994) states the impression given of these men during the inquiry by staff at Broadmoor was that they were 'big, black and dangerous' so much so the committee investigating Blackwood's death used the phrase in the title of their report. The stereotype of the black male with mental health issues continues to exist. The Angiolini Report (2017) notes that during the review into the death of Sean Rigg in 2008 after being restrained by police, an officer described Rigg's behaviour as possibly related to mental health, but also 'other reasons, especially with people you come across in Brixton' (p. 87). The reference to Brixton (in Lambeth, South London) appears to have been in regarding the 26% black population and assumptions about smoking cannabis. The Independent Inquiry into the death of David 'Rocky' Bennet who died in 1998 in a secure psychiatric hospital after being restrained stated

> Psychiatrists sometimes make a diagnosis of 'drug induced psychosis' which, as far as African-Caribbean's are concerned, nearly always relates to the use of cannabis. There appears to be no clear medical basis for this diagnosis. (Norfolk & Cambridgeshire Strategic Health Authority, 2003, p. 41)

As such, when a psychiatrist makes a diagnosis based on a stereotype there is the risk that this misdiagnosis will lead to the wrong treatment. The Angiolini Report (2017) also stated 'racial stereotyping needs to be investigated within the context of a wider picture of related deaths and non-fatal incidents where race may have been a factor' (p. 87). Coupled with the racial stereotyping is the lack of response to the recommendations made in reports to change process that are related to the deaths of these men.

Inertia Following Inquires

Despite the racialised stereotype, Cummins (2015) notes the inquiries into Martin and Watts concluded that there was 'no direct evidence of racism at Broadmoor' (p. 16). Yet, the SHSA inquiry contested this and stated that staff and management did not seem to appreciate how subtle forms of racism operate. Crichton reports the inquiry found *by omission* (my emphasis) a racial institutional bias against ethnic minorities. The inquiry identified there was no equal opportunities policy, no statistics kept on the numbers of black patients and a colour-blind approach was taken which ignored the issues of black patients. The report states 'The experience of Afro-Caribbean inner-city youngsters is not fully understood by Eurocentric psychiatry and those who work in the psychiatric system. It is important that differences are recognised and catered for' cited in Crichton (1994). Several years later, the review into the death of Sean Rigg as referred to in the Angiolini Report (2017) raised comparable concerns regarding the race blind approach. It stated

The lack of reference to race throughout is not a sign of non-discrimination, but rather an indication of malaise and/or a lack of confidence about how to address racial issues appropriately. (p. 88)

The 'malaise' mentioned continues regarding the recommendations in the Blackwood inquiry. Crichton and Sheppard (1996) highlight the inquiry team requested to be reassembled to consider how their recommendations were being followed up. The SHSA did not invite them back; it was later recognised there was an 'absence of any formal procedure for follow up of those recommendations or explanation for their non-implementation' (Downham & Lingham, 2009, p. 63). An absence of action was noted in the Bennett Inquiry about issues raised in the SHSA (1993) report into Blackwood and the issues emerging from the Bennett Inquiry (Norfolk & Cambridgeshire Strategic Health Authority, 2003):

that Inquiry also wrote a chapter on the problems of racism which contains information on many of the general matters that we have heard during the course of this Inquiry and set out in this report. While we recognise that it takes time to implement reforms and to act upon recommendations, we express our grave concern at the apparent lack of reaction by anybody in authority to attempt to implement these and other recommendations made in that report. (p. 63)

The Bennett Inquiry also identified the needs of black patients were not adequately met and the issues they highlight in the report had been known to the National Health Service (NHS) for years. The following is a summary of black people who died whilst in psychiatric custody. The list is taken from The Institute of Race Relations, and includes those who died following the death of Orville Blackwood in 1991 until the Inquiry into David Rocky Bennett in 2003:

- *28/8/91 Orville Blackwood (31)*. Orville was found dead in a secure unit of Broadmoor top security hospital after being given a tranquilliser injection.
- *8/1/92 Mark Fletcher (21)*. Mark was detained by police and then sectioned under the Mental Health Act and transferred to a Psychiatric hospital where collapsed after being restrained and given an injection into his spine.
- *6/92 Munir Yusef Mojothi (26)*. Munir was a psychiatric patient, he was given an injection of droperidol and then transferred to Clifton hospital, where he was given another injection and an intravenous dose of the drug was given by a doctor.
- *23/6/92 Jerome Scott (27)*. Jerome collapsed and died on his way to hospital in a police van. Two psychiatrists administered an intravenous injection. Jerome was held down by police and then injected with two different anti-psychotic drugs.
- *30/1/94 Rupert Marshall (29)*. Rupert died in Horton psychiatric hospital, Epsom after being restrained and injected with an anti-psychotic drug.

- *10/8/94 Jonathan Weekes.* Jonathan died in hospital, he had depression. It was later revealed that Jonathan was receiving eight different drugs this information was not available to the inquest.
- *30/10/1998 David 'Rocky' Bennett*, restrained by four nurses for over 30 minutes.

The Institute of Race Relations (2004) interviewed Richard Stone, member of the Bennett Inquiry panel, he stated:

> If the government does not respond to our recommendation that they acknowledge institutional racism in the mental health service they will get away without doing anything. Furthermore, my concern is that there will be more deaths resulting from restraint in the prone position unless recommendation nine – the three-minute time limit for such restraint – is implemented as a matter of urgency. We can't wait for more research. (p. 1)

Delivering Race Equality (2005) was a five-year action plan established the government following the Bennett Inquiry. The aim was to address these deep-seated race related issues and produce services that were more sensitive to the black community. However, this failed to happen and the initiative was abandoned with many of the recommendations outstanding. The roll call of black people who died between Blackwood and Bennett may not have been as extensive if some of the recommendations had been implemented. MIND (2013) conducted research into the number of deaths due to the use of restraints, they state,

> Shockingly, since Rocky Bennett's death there have been at least 13 restraint-related deaths of people detained under the Mental Health Act 1983. Eight of these occurred in a single year (2011). More than 15 years since Rocky Bennett's death, we are still no closer to implementing the lessons learned from his death and people are still dying as a result of physical restraint. (p. 3)

The MIND (2013) report further noted

> It is totally unacceptable that the lessons learnt as a result of the tragic deaths of Orville Blackwood, Michael Martin, Joseph Watts and David Bennett continue to be ignored and people using mental health services still remain at high risk of injury and even death as result of the use of physical restraint. (p. 4)

Following the failure of Delivering Race Equality (2005), other national initiatives aimed to address racial inequalities such as the Mental Health Task Force (2015) and The Ministerial Advisory Group on Mental Health Strategy (2017) have been set up. These national initiatives have coexisted alongside local initiatives such Lambeth Black Health and Wellbeing Commission, formed following the death of Sean Rigg. The Commission found 26% of the population in Lambeth was from African or Caribbean descent, yet 70% of the residents in secure psychiatric settings in the area were black (2014). Despite these national and local schemes – many of which only last the lifespan of a government term in office – statistics from the Race Disparity Audit (2017) demonstrate little has changed for the plight of black people. This raises important questions regarding why successive governments have failed to nationally implement the recommendations from these inquiries despite the number of deaths that continue to occur. It also raises questions about how these (mainly) black men have been constructed as big, bad and dangerous, diagnosed with schizophrenia, held in forensic mental health settings and detained longer than their white counterparts or killed. Many would argue it is a result of institutionalised racism but I contend this provides only a partial explanation.

Why Institutional Racism is Not the Answer

Institutional Racism is the term often used to explain racism that is inherent in institutions. The term was defined by Stokely and Hamilton (1967) with reference to racism in America.

> Institutional racism refers to particular and general instances of racial discrimination, inequality, exploitation, and domination in organisational or institutional contexts, such as the labour market or the nation-state. (p. 3)

However, the term was not widely introduced into discourse in England until over 30 years later when the Home Office (1999) inquired into the racially motivated murder of Stephen Lawrence. The chair of the inquiry, William Macpherson then defined Institutional Racism as:

> […] the collective failure of an organisation to provide an appropriate or professional service to people because of their colour, culture or ethnic origin. It can be seen or detected in processes, attitudes and behaviour which amount to discrimination through unwitting prejudice, ignorance, thoughtlessness and racist stereotyping, which disadvantage minority ethnic people. (para 6.34)

When unpicking Macpherson's definition, there are a number of points to consider. The phrase, 'the collective failure of an organisation' indicates no-one is at fault or is accountable for the racism that exists in the organisation or institution. As a collective failure, it can be assumed that a collective response is required for change. This itself is problematic as it averts liability from those leading the organisation who ultimately have decision-making powers on how the institution is run, what is permissible, what policies are in place and the sanctions for not adhering to those policies.

Souhami (2012) questions if the term Institutional racism works conceptually as an instrument for change. She argues:

> While the concept provoked an urgent reaction, its central ambiguities confronted police services with profound difficulties in responding ... it inadvertently focused attention on internal police culture. Consequently, despite the Inquiry's intention that the term would divert attention away from a preoccupation with overt racism among police staff, this is precisely where reform activity was directed. (p. 1)

Souhami (2012) goes further to suggest that 'the concept not only failed to direct attention to the dynamics of institutional discrimination but, through the activity it elicited, in fact sustained them' (p. 1). I contend the problem is sustained *in part* due to individuals not being found culpable for their racist actions. Stokely and Hamilton (1967) note racism takes two forms: individual and institutional. They argue that institutional racism is more subtle and covert and as it originates within recognised institutions in society. However, Deloria (1982) argues the institution should be seen as having the personality – or what I understand as organisational culture – and suggests this is what needs to change. He states that attempts to change individual are futile 'personality substantially affects how individual members of the institution respond to external phenomena, and not the other way around' (Deloria, 1982, p. 51). However, the task to change becomes more complex when the institution claims to be unaware of the racist and discriminatory culture. Macpherson's definition refers to 'discrimination through unwitting prejudice'. The word 'unwitting' suggests the racism is emanating from a place of unknowing or unintentionality, further excusing the individuals and institution from responsibility. Paradies, Bastos, and Priest (2016) suggests the concept of bias is often referred to within health care contexts to describe unconscious forms of discrimination, known as implicit bias. My concern is the extent to which racist behaviours are excused as unwitting, ignorance, thoughtlessness implicit bias, which all contribute to the perpetuation of racism but without accountability. The Independent Inquiry into the death of David Bennett (2003) stated 'there was a real difference between unconscious misunderstanding and deliberate racism' (p. 23). I would suggest much of the construction of the big, bad and dangerous black man that went on with staff in the mental health services was *conscious* racist stereotyping. Cummins (2015) argued that patients such as Blackwood had the insight to believe his period in detention was extended due to racist stereotyping not because his mental health justified it (p. 17). Blackwood was detained in Broadmoor for a significantly longer period than if he had been detained in prison for his original offence. The stereotype of him being big, bad and dangerous fed into how he was perceived, treated and ultimately killed. Cummins (2015) argues that 'Psychiatry, along with the CJS agencies has played a key role in creating the racist stereotype of the psychically aggressive violent black male' (p. 22). Here Cummins is clearly asserting the institutions – medical as in psychiatry and the CJS –are at fault without holding the individuals who created and perpetuated the stereotypes to account. I am not arguing that institutional racism is the single reason for the over representation of black people with diagnosed as schizophrenic, or the over representation of black people with mental health issues in the CJS, or why more black people than any other racial group die whilst detained. Rather I am arguing that systemic racism provides a more adequate explanation for these phenomena.

Systemic Racism

'Deaths of people from BAME communities, in particular young Black men, resonate with the Black community's experience of systemic racism'. Angiolini Report (2017, p. 84). The report espouses the term 'systemic racism' diverging from the expression 'Institutionalised racism' but no definition of systemic racism is offered. Feagin (2001) provides us with a discourse relating to systemic racism in America. He posits a meaning of systemic racism whereby

> Systemic racism includes the complex array of anti-black practices, the unjustly gained political economic powers of whites, the continuing economic and other resource inequalities along racial lines and the white racist ideologies and attitudes created to maintain and rationalise white privilege and power. Systemic here means that the core racist realities are manifested in each of societies major parts ... the economy, education religion, the family – reflects the fundamental reality of systemic racism. (p. 6)

Feagin (2006) proposes that systemic racism becomes embedded in each aspect of society and perpetuated by social processes that reproduce not only racial inequality but also the fundamental racist relationship between the racially oppressed and the racial oppressors. Feagin suggests these processes are historical and can be traced back to slavery when the relationships between the oppressors (privileged white people) and the oppressed (black people) began. He identifies various points in American history post-slavery and post-segregation to demonstrate how embedded systemic racism is and continues to be in society. I consider myself a systemic thinker; seeing through a systemic lens (Von Bertalanffy, 1968). Campbell (2000) explains:

> Systemic thinking is a way to make sense of the relatedness of everything around us. In its broadest application, it is a way of thinking that gives practitioners the tools to observe the connectedness of people, things and ideas; everything is connected to everything else. (p. 7)

The concept of connections are inherent in Feagins argument of systemic racism and are aligned with the phenomena in England experienced by black men in the criminal justice and mental health systems. The connection between the people who are killed by restraint is that they are black men seen as big, bad and/or mad and dangerous. The institutions they die in namely forensic mental health or criminal justice are connected; often black men are referred from a criminal justice setting into a secure mental health setting. There are similarities in the circumstances surrounding their death. There is a pattern in the process following their death; an inquiry, recommendations are made and ignored and initiatives are abandoned. Another death takes place and the pattern repeats itself. Von Bertalanffy (1968) discussed how general systems seeks to maintain an equilibrium by a continuous inflow and outflow, a building up and breaking down of components, where patterns are repeated to achieve a steady state. From a systemic perspective, the same is true of human systems which strive to maintain a balance, equilibrium or the status quo in society and between interpersonal relationships. Not everyone within the system may benefit from the equilibrium state, however, whilst the majority does benefit or is at least not disadvantaged, the system will continue to reproduce itself in the same way. To understand how Feagin's position relates not only to systemic racism in America but also to England is to understand the parallels between countries in that there is a culture of privileges associated with 'whiteness' and disadvantages associated with being black that is traced back to slavery and colonialism. I will use the example of the historical relationship between England and Jamaica, where my parents migrated from, to explore the longstanding culture of racism, disadvantage and the relationship between the oppressor and oppressed which Feagin speaks of.

Colonisation; Native, Object and Possession

Jamaica became a British Colony when the country was seized from Spain in 1655. The colonisation became formal in 1670, when the Treaty of Madrid (also known as the Godolphin Treaty) was signed. The treaty decreed that Spain recognised *English Possessions* in the Caribbean Sea 'all those lands, islands colonies and places, whatsoever situated in the West Indies' (National Humanities Centre, n.d., p. 6). Immediately what comes to my mind is Jamaica as an *object* to be fought over while the word *possession* dehumanises the people who inhabit the country. Jamaica became one of the biggest slave markets and slave destinations in the world to provide a slave trade meeting the labour force required to extract sugar from sugarcane. This exemplifies the beginning of the relationship between the oppressor and the oppressed.

With the abolition of the slave trade, Britain sent migrants of colour importing workers from China and India (1850–1866) – then a British Colony – under contracts of indenture to support the workforce which had become depleted by the loss of slavery. However, living and working conditions were not much better than when people were enslaved, therefore the Chinese Government brought their citizens out of the indentured contracts (Rajkumar, 2013). For the Indians and Jamaicans colonised by the British, they had little option but to remain. World War I brought with it the prospect of being a paid soldier, therefore my grandfather was one of the 10,280 men from Jamaica to volunteer to join the British

West Indies Regiment (BWIR), segregated from white soldiers. The SS Verdala transported soldiers from Jamaica during March 1916, inadequate clothing and heating resulted in more than 600 soldiers suffering from exposure and frostbite leaving 106 men to have amputations (Bourne, 2014). The training camps in England had substandard accommodation whereby men from the BWIR developed further frostbite and pneumonia. In addition to this, the soldiers were initially denied a pay rise given to other British troops on the basis they were classified as natives (Peatfield, n.d.). By the end of war, almost as many black men had died from illness; 1,071 as had died in action; 1,185 (Peatfield, n.d.). This demonstrates the lack of value placed on the life of the black soldier, not perceived as equal to that of their white counterparts; viewed as 'native'.

Following the destruction from World War II and the need for nurses to work in the newly established National Health Service (NHS) the British Nationality Act (1948) was introduced to permit residents of British Colonies to become British Citizens, and work in unskilled jobs. My parents arrived in England 1961, the last flurry of migrants to enter the country in anticipation of the 1962 Commonwealth and Immigration Act. The Act aimed to restrict the number of migrants coming to Britain as there were by then sufficient numbers to address the labour shortage. Additionally, the visual presence of black people in England was upsetting the equilibrium and racially motivated violence had started to occur (Pilkington, 1988). It is no coincidence that Jamaica also gained its' independence in 1962, uncoupling Britain from any responsibility to the Jamaican nationals who were experiencing high unemployment. These events from slavery through to colonisation demonstrate the differential power relations between black and white people and the embedded systemic racism that has continued to pervade throughout British society.

Postcolonial Theory – The Legacy

Postcolonial Theory reminds us that the ramifications of colonialism can remain inherent in a country in terms of economic stability, culture and national identity and continue to experience the reverberations in the postcolonial age (Walker, 2017). Hall (1996) posits how Postcolonial theory provides an understanding of culture and identity as fluid, contested, deconstructed and reconstructed. The theory suggests Postcolonial structures become reproduced in everyday life (Routledge 2016). Fernando (1991) argues how racism informed the diagnostic categories used by psychiatrists in America during the period of slavery sighting the example of proto-psychiatrist Cartwright (1851), who diagnosed the 'madness' of slaves who ran away from their owners. More recently, Metzl's (2009) identified African American protestors during the civil rights movement were diagnosed with schizophrenia. These are examples of how black people have been disempowered and socially abused when they exercise their right to be free from oppression. This brings me to the phenomena we are experiencing in Britain today. As I have argued, institutional racism is only a partial and inadequate explanation of the phenomena experienced by black men in Britain.

Systemic Racism Explanations

I have identified examples from England of the historical systemic racism Feagin (2001, 2006) suggests is steeped in America's history. I suggest England has a parallel legacy that has emerged from an oppressive, colonial mindset, passed through generations, institutions, organisations, legislation via a combination of racial bias, stereotyping, dysconscious racism, overt racism, omission of equity resulting in the maintenance and has been maintained in England. Firstly, colonisation and slavery have provided Britain with a culture of ownership of 'other'. The relationship between the England and the colonised country and the relationship between the people is immediately one exemplified by the dualisms of power/powerless, oppressor/oppressed, privilege/disadvantage. From a systemic perspective, the equilibrium has been established by these dichotomies which continue to reproduce themselves centuries after the abolition of slavery and decades after a country ceases to be colonised. The threat to this balance would be complete equality between the countries and the people who inhabit them. I have noted examples of where a diagnosis of mental health has been applied to run away slaves and civil rights protestors. These black people have challenged the status quo and attempted to re-balance the existing equilibrium where black people are disadvantaged or oppressed. The mental health diagnosis serves to punish and discredit the behaviour undesired by the privileged white community and prevent the punished black people from influencing the wider black community. It also serves to generate fear in the wider community that this will be the consequences for contesting oppression.

The over representation of black men in both the criminal justice and mental health systems also serve to maintain the equilibrium of oppressor/oppressed, privilege/disadvantage. When a black man is dehumanised in the construction of the big, bad and dangerous stereotype, there is a reticence by those in power to address his misdiagnosis or killing. Being perceived as superhuman and dangerous, the justification for being restrained and/or killed is to preserve the safety of others. As such, the risk to others is perceived as too great to implement recommendations that might change the status quo. Although the overt rational may be related to safety, the covert and underlying reason for the disproportionate imprisonment, restraint and death is a demonstration of white power and the devaluing of black lives. It shows that white power pervades throughout society and black people should fear the extent of this power. The unlawful killing as a result of restraint may just as well be seen as the modern version of lynching.

I struggled for weeks to draw this chapter to a close. It was a difficult chapter to write from the outset, yet somehow, I could not find the words to bring it to an end. That is until I was confronted with a situation similar to what I have been writing about. I was teaching a class of social work students, I had been teaching them all day so by the afternoon I was relaxed, I had kicked off my shoes and enjoying the interaction with them when a white man appeared at the door. He entered without knocking and was followed by two other white men. The class I was teaching were 95% black students; the presence of three white men standing in the room was domineering. The first white man spoke and said he did not want to disturb the class, but there had been an altercation, he was head of security and he was looking for the student involved. Rather than speak to me privately, this was said as an announcement to the class. I was stunned. I scanned the room puzzled thinking who would have had an altercation – and *when*? He walked over to a black, male student at the back of the room and said come with me; the doorway now flanked by the other two white men. I ran out after them in my stockinged feet, fearful of what was happening to my student. Surrounded by these three white men, my student was accused of being threatening and aggressive to a female student. He looked as shocked as I was at the allegations. Immediately I thought of Orville Blackwood, Rocky Bennett and the others that were killed. I could see the scene being replayed in front of me; a black man has an 'altercation' with someone white, the black man is reprimanded, in the process of defending himself he is accused of being aggressive, he is restrained and killed.

My student was trying to explain what had taken place, the white man was insisting he needed to listen. I heard words such as 'aggressive', 'threatening' and 'investigation'. I knew what the student or I said in the next few minutes could mean the difference between life or death – literally. I touched my student's arm and told him not to speak; for the moment just listen. I said we needed to move this out of the corridor into a private space. Still without my shoes, I led my student and the white man into a nearby office. I tried to put the 'altercation' into context. The situation began to defuse to whereby the white man concluded there was in fact no threat and he would draw the matter to a close. As soon as he left I burst into tears. I was so angry I could not speak. I had been scared for my students' life. That might seem an over-reaction to anyone unaware that black men in similar situations have ended up being restrained and killed. On one hand I felt guilty for silencing my student – who is an adult, a father and husband – but I was *afraid* the situation could escalate to where the police were called and I would have a dead student stereotyped as big, bad and dangerous. I felt I had compromised myself and my student rights by advising him to wait before speaking. Yet, this is what I believed I had to do for him to stay safe. In terms of the university hierarchy, I was absolutely higher ranked than this white man but my power was precarious and changeable depending on the situation (Hill-Collins, 1990). If the police were called my power would be completely diminished. This is the legacy of colonialism, oppression, disadvantage and being viewed as other. Knowing that black men are disproportionately imprisoned, sectioned under the Mental Health Act or killed made me fearful. I was scared for my students' life. Yet, this is the *purpose* for these disproportionalities; it sends a clear warning and a sense of fear to those in the black community that are aware of these 'dirty secrets' not challenge those in power. This is how the duality of oppressor/oppressed and privileged/disadvantage remains.

Understanding systemic racism is not enough to change it, however, it is a start to have this awareness. Also to recognise it is futile to expect those that benefit from the power imbalance to be the ones to implement recommendations that would diminish the power they have. Therefore, change will only happen when the black community becomes mobilised and united to overcome individual fears and begin to influence the institutional culture across the institutions where systemic racism has been reinforced.

References

Alarcon, R. D. (2009). Culture, cultural factors and psychiatric diagnosis: Review and projections. *World Psychiatry, 8*(3), 131–139.

Angiolini, E. (2017). Report of the independent review of deaths and serious incidents in police custody. Retrieved from https://www.gov.uk/government/uploads/system/uploads/attachment_data/file/655401/Report_of_Angiolini_Review_ISBN_Accessible.pdf

Bhugra, D., Hilwig, M., Hossein, B., (1996). First-contact incidence rates of schizophrenia in Trinidad and one-year follow-up. *British Journal of Psychiatry, 169*, 587–592.

Bhui, K., Stansfeld, S., McKenzie, K., Karlsen, S., Nazroo, J., & Weich, S. (2005). Racial/ethnic discrimination and common mental disorders among workers: Findings from the EMPIRIC Study of Ethnic Minority Groups in the United Kingdom. *American Journal of Public Health, 95*(3), 496–501. http://doi.org/10.2105/AJPH.2003.033274

Bourne, S. (2014). *Black Poppies: Britain's black community and the great war*. London: The History Press.

Bradley. (2009). *Lord Bradley's review of people with mental health problems or learning disabilities in the criminal justice system*. London: House of Lords.

Cabinet Office. (2017). Race disparity audit. Retrieved from https://www.gov.uk/government/uploads/system/uploads/attachment_data/file/650723/RDAweb.pdf

Campbell, D. (2000). *The socially constructed organisation*. London: Karnac.

Care Quality Commission. (2011). Count me in census. Retrieved from http://www.cqc.org.uk/news/releases/care-quality-commission-looks-ahead-last-count-me-census-published. Accessed on March 9, 2017.

Crichton, J. (1994). Comments on the blackwood inquiry. *Psychiatric Bulletin, 18*, 236–237. doi:10.1192/pb.18.4.236.

Crichton, J., & Sheppard, D. (1996). Psychiatric inquiries: Learning the lessons. In J. Peay (Ed.), *Inquiries after homicide* (pp. 65–78). London: Duckworth.

Cummins, I. D. (2015). Discussing race, racism and mental health: Two mental health inquiries reconsidered. Retrieved from http://usir.salford.ac.uk/35493/

Deloria, V. (1982). Institutional racism. *Explorations in Ethnic Studies, 5*(1), 40–51.

Department of Health. (2005). Delivering race equality in mental health care: An action plan for reform inside and outside services and the government's response to the independent inquiry into the death of David Bennett. Retrieved from http://webarchive.nationalarchives.gov.uk/20130123204153/http://www.dh.gov.uk/en/Publicationsandstatistics/Publications/PublicationsPolicyAndGuidance/DH_4100773. Accessed on October 14, 2017.

Downham, G., & Lingham, L. (2009). Learning lessons: Using inquiries for change. *Journal of Mental Health Law*, 57–69. Retrieved from www.northumbriajournals.co.uk/index.php/IJMHMCL/article/download/281/275

Dyer, J. (2017). Jacqui Dyer: Talking about race and mental health is everyone's business. Retrieved from https://www.theguardian.com/society/2017/nov/08/jacqui-dyer-race-mental-health-act-black-people-detentions-inequality

European Commission against Racism and Intolerance Report. (2016). ECRI. Retrieved from https://www.coe.int/t/dghl/monitoring/ecri/Country-by-country/United_Kingdom/GBR-CbC-V-2016-038-ENG.pdf

Feagin, J. R. (2001). *Racist America: Roots, current realities, and future reparations*. New York: Routledge.

Feagin, J. R. (2006). *Systemic racism: A theory of oppression*. Routledge/Taylor & Francis Group.

Fearon, P., Kirkbride J. B., Morgan, C., Dazzan, P., Morgan, K., Lloyd, T., ... & AESOP Study Group. (2006). Incidence of schizophrenia and other psychoses in ethnic minority groups: Results from the MRC ÆSOP Study. *Psychology Medicine, 36*(11), 1541–1550.

Fernando, S. (1991). *Mental health, race and culture*. Basingstoke: Macmillan/Mind.
Fitzpatrick, R., Kumar, S., Nkansa-Dwamena, O., & Thorne, L. (2014). Ethnic inequalities in mental health: Promoting lasting positive change report of findings to LankellyChase Foundation. Retrieved from https://lankellychase.org.uk/wp-content/uploads/2015/07/Ethnic-Inequality-in-Mental-Health-Confluence-Full-Report-March2014.pdf
Fung, W. L. A., Jones, P. B., & Bhugra, D. (2009). Ethnicity and mental health: The example of schizophrenia and related psychoses in migrant populations in the Western world. *Psychiatry, 8*(9), 335–341. doi:10.1016/j.mppsy.2009.06.002
Hall, S. (1996). Introduction: Who needs identity? In S. Hall & P. Du Gay (Eds.), *Questions of cultural identity* (pp. 1–17). London: SAGE Publications.
Hickling, F. W. (2005). The epidemiology of schizophrenia and other common mental health disorders in the English-speaking Caribbean. *Pan American Journal of Public Health, 18*(4–5), 256–262.
Hickling, F. W., McKenzie, K., Mullen, R., & Murray, R. (1999). A Jamaican psychiatrist evaluates diagnosis at a London psychiatric hospital. *British Journal of Psychiatry, 175*, 283–285.
Hickling, F. W., & Rodgers-Johnson, P. (1995). The incidence of first contact schizophrenia in Jamaica. *British Journal of Psychiatry, 167*, 193–196.
Hill-Collins, P. (1990). *Black feminist thought: Knowledge, consciousness and the politics of empowerment*. Boston, MA: Unwin Hyman.
Home Office. (1999). *The Stephen Lawrence inquiry. Report of an Inquiry by Sir William Macpherson of Cluny*. London: Stationery Office. Retrieved from https://www.gov.uk/government/uploads/system/uploads/attachment_data/file/277111/4262.pdf
INQUEST. (2015). Deaths in mental health detention Feb 2015. Retrieved from http://inquest.org.uk/pdf/INQUEST_deaths_in_mental_health_detention_Feb_2015.pdf
INQUEST. (2017). BAME Deaths in police custody, Retrieved from https://www.inquest.org.uk/bame-deaths-in-police-custody
Institute of Race Relations. (2004). Rocky Bennet: Killed by institutional racism? Retrieved from http://www.irr.org.uk/news/rocky-bennett-killed-by-institutional-racism/
Lambeth Black Health and Wellbeing Commission. (2014). From surviving to thriving. Retrieved from http://lambethcollaborative.org.uk/wp-content/uploads/2014/08/ENC-4.4-BHWB-Commission-Final-Report2-PDF-June-2014.pdf
Mahy, G. E., Mallett, R., Leff, J., & Bhugra, D. (1999). First-contact incidence rate of schizophrenia on Barbados. *British Journal of Psychiatry, 175*, 28–33.
Mental Health Task force. (2015). Terms of reference. Retrieved from https://www.england.nhs.uk/mentalhealth/wp-content/uploads/sites/29/2015/10/mh-tor-fin.pdf
Metzl, J. (2009). *The protest psychosis: How schizophrenia became a black disease*. Boston, MA: Beacon Press.
MIND. (2013, June). Mental health crisis care: Physical restraint in crisis. A report on physical restraint in hospital settings in England. Retrieved from https://www.mind.org.uk/media/197120/physical_restraint_final_web_version.pdf
Ministerial Advisory Group. (2017). Ministerial advisory group on mental health strategy. Retrieved from https://www.gov.uk/government/groups/ministerial-advisory-group-on-mental-health-strategy#terms-of-reference
Ministry of Justice. (2015). Statistics on race and the criminal justice system 2014: A Ministry of Justice publication under Section 95 of the Criminal Justice Act 1991. Retrieved from https://www.gov.uk/government/uploads/system/uploads/attachment_data/file/480250/bulletin.pdf
National Humanities Centre. (n.d.). Retrieved from http://nationalhumanitiescenter.org/pds/amerbegin/power/text1/SpanishEnglishRivalry.pdf. Accessed on November 15, 2015.

Norfolk, S., & Cambridgeshire Strategic Health Authority. (2003, December). *Independent inquiry into the death of David Bennett*. Cambridge. Retrieved from https://www.blink.org.uk/docs/David_Bennett_report.pdf

Paradies, Y., Bastos, J., & Priest, N. (2016). Prejudice, stigma, bias, discrimination, and health. In C. Sibley & F. Barlow (Eds.), *The Cambridge handbook of the psychology of prejudice* (Cambridge Handbooks in Psychology, pp. 559–581). Cambridge: Cambridge University Press. doi:10.1017/9781316161579.025

Peatfield, L. (n.d.). The story of the British West Indies regiment in the First World War. Retrieved from http://www.iwm.org.uk/history/the-story-of-the-british-west-indies-regiment-in-the-first-world-war

Pilkington, E. (1988). *Beyond the mother country: West Indians and the Notting Hill white riots*. London: Tauris.

Pinto, R., Ashworth, M., & Jones, R. (2008). Schizophrenia in black Caribbean's living in the UK: An exploration of underlying causes of the high incidence rate. *The British Journal of General Practice, 58*(551), 429–434. http://doi.org/10.3399/bjgp08X299254

Rajkumar, F. (2013). The Chinese in the Caribbean during the colonial era. In R. Cruse & K. Rhiney (Eds.), *Caribbean atlas*. Retrieved from http://www.caribbean-atlas.com/en/themes/waves-of-colonization-and-control-in-the-caribbean/daily-lives-of-caribbean-people-under-colonialism/the-chinese-in-the-caribbean-during-the-colonial-era.html

Routledge. (2016). Critical race and postcolonial theory. Social theory re-wired. Retrieved from http://routledgesoc.com/profile/critical-race-and-postcolonial-theory

Sharpley, M., Hutchinson, G., McKenzie, K., & Murray R. (2001). Understanding the excess of psychosis among the African-Caribbean population in England: Review of the current hypothesis. *British Journal of Psychiatry, 178*(Supplement 40), 60–68.

Singh, S., Burns, T., Tyrer, P., Islam, Z., Parsons, H., & Crawford, M. (2014). Ethnicity as a predictor of detention under the Mental Health Act. *Psychological Medicine, 44*(5), 997–1004.

Souhami, A. (2012). Institutional racism and police reform: An empirical critique. *Policing and Society, 24*(1), 1–21.

Special Hospitals Service Authority (SHSA). (1993). *Report of the Committee of Inquiry into the death in Broadmoor Hospital of Orville Blackwood and a Review of the deaths of Two other African- Caribbean patients, Big, Black and Dangerous*. London: SHSA (Chairman Professor H. Prins).

Stevenson, J., & Rao, M. (2014). *Explaining levels of wellbeing in Black and Minority Ethnic populations in England*. London: University of East London, Institute of Health and Human Development. Retrieved from http://hdl.handle.net/10552/3867. Accessed on August 30, 2017.

Stokely, C., & Hamilton, C. V. (1967). *Black power: The politics of liberation in America*. New York, NY: Vintage Books.

The Black Manifesto. (2010). The price of race inequality. Retrieved from http://www.oneeastmidlands.org.uk/sites/default/files/library/black_manifesto_race_inequality.pdf

The Guardian. (2017, September 3). Four black men die. Did police actions play a part? Retrieved from https://www.theguardian.com/uk-news/2017/sep/03/four-black-men-die-police-restraint-no-officers-suspended-bryant-cumberbatch-charles-da-costa

Thornicroft, G. (2006). *Ethinicity of patients in high security psychiatric hospitals in England. Delivering Race Equality in Mental Health Care*. London: Institute of Psychiatry, Kings College London.

Tortelli, A., Errazuriz, A., Croudace, T., Morgan, C., Murray, R. M., Jones, P. B., ... & Kirkbride, J. B. (2015). Schizophrenia and other psychotic disorders in

Caribbean-born migrants and their descendants in England: Systematic review and meta-analysis of incidence rates, 1950–2013. *Social Psychiatry and Psychiatric Epidemiology, 50*(7), 1039–1055. Retrieved from http://doi.org/10.1007/s00127-015-1021-6

Walker, S. (2017). Relationship based teaching with (social work) students affected by globalism and the politics of location. *Educational Alternatives, 15*, 48–55. Retrieved from https://www.scientific-publications.net/en/article/1001561/

Walker, S. (2020). Racism in Academia: (How to) Stay Black, Sane and Proud as the Doctoral Supervisory Relationship Implodes. In R. Majors, K. Carberry, T. Ransaw (Eds.), *The International Handbook of Black Community Mental Health* (pp. 89–107). Bingley: Emerald Publishing.

Xanthos, C. (2008). Racializing mental illness: Understanding African-Caribbean Schizophrenia in the UK. *Critical Social Work, Archive Volumes, 9*(1). Retrieved from http://www1.uwindsor.ca/criticalsocialwork/racializing-mental-illness-understanding-african-caribbean-schizophrenia-in-the-ukIndex

Chapter 2

In the Name of Our Humanity: Challenging Academic Racism and its Effects on the Emotional Wellbeing of Women of Colour Professors

Philomena Essed and Karen Carberry

Introduction

This chapter emerges from unconventional author collaboration. The work is largely based on an earlier article published by the first author originally called 'Dilemmas in leadership: Women of colour in the academy' (Essed, 2000). Intrigued by the theme, the second author (Karen Carberry) immediately recognised the connection to health challenges as a result of racism in the academy. Emotional wellbeing had hardly been touched upon in the original article. Race critical studies often shun the psychological ramifications of exhaustion due to constant racism stress and struggle, probably for fear of pathologising. At the same time, denial reinforces the myth of the 'strong' black woman, the family and community caretaker who can handle everything, thus implicitly dehumanising women of colour. The research findings discussed in Essed's original publication seem – sadly – still as relevant today. This can be inferred from public and campus debates invoked by the 'Black Lives Matter' movement and more recent publications focussing on 'being-a-scholar-while-black' including among others Alexander-Floyd's (2015) research, who applied Puwar's (2004) notion of 'space invaders' to the political sciences, and Essed (2013) who looked at women of colour social justice scholars. In light of this, we kept most of the original text of the original article, though written in the first author's voice, as a basis of this joint venture. Carberry, family therapist and researcher in the area of mental health, interjects at relevant moments to accentuate the mental health implications of professional stress and everyday racism in the lives of women of colour in Academia.

Thus with the embedded commentary folded into the (revised and updated) original the new text evolved into a research based conversation type of article.

Essed: In many ethnic communities, the norm prevails that those who have reached higher grounds support other group members. Coaching younger generations and witnessing their intellectual growth can be a rich and rewarding experience. At the same time, when support is taken for granted in the name of culture or solidarity, that claim can become a burden. A troublesome experience in this respect involves a black woman, a nurse by profession and university student, whom I had met a couple of times in the context of the Women's Movement. In my mailbox a draft paper on 'Women and Anti-Colonialism', with a little note from her attached saying: 'I have recently presented this paper at a workshop. I'd appreciate if you would give me credit points for this'. I replied that she was welcome to take a course with me and write a paper for that, but that it was not acceptable to demand credits out of the blue without having agreed with me in advance. Furious, she accused me of abusing my position of power. Yet, I suspected that she would never have approached a white professor, male or female, with the same request.

A more positive note, there is this high-school girl, an immigrant from Suriname, who telephones me on a Sunday afternoon in order to discuss with me, at length, her literature list for a paper on racism. How could I not be a one-time-mentor to this adolescent girl bravely challenging the racial prejudice she experiences in school.

Events like the above are not uncommon in the lives of the exceptional, visible, sometimes token, often solitary position of women of colour in university departments. As scholars, we operate in a competitive world, where we are constantly asked to adapt to norms largely made to fit, preferably, white, male profiles and career paths (Essed, 2004). At the same time, it is often the case that we engage in activities to promote social justice, above and beyond office hours, without any acknowledgement within the university system. In doing so, we constantly redefine the meaning of being a university professor. This process has its own consequences.

Carberry: This balancing act can affect mental and emotional wellbeing raising levels of stress which can covertly hijack the zeal for the profession. Thus, this important aspect will also overlay the chapter drawing on data and additional voices to illustrate the impact and pattern of surviving in the UK's academic institutions, the location where I am based as a professional.

In the UK, the swelling of white academics in higher education continues unabated. Although the Higher Education Staff Statistics (HESA) cite that in '2016/2017 15% of academic staff with known ethnicity were Black and Ethnic (BME)', a featured article by Black British Academics drew on 2014/2015 figures extracted from the HEDI database at Bournmouth University to present HESA statistics of professors by race and gender. At that time, the number of professors in the UK was numbered 19,630, but from this number less than 1%, 110, were from the black African/Caribbean communities, of which 80 were male and 30 female. Conversely, 16,350 were identified as white, of which 12,455 were male and 3,895 were female respectively. Recent 2016/2017 figures from HESA (2018) illustrate that figures for white professors had increased to 20,550, of which 15,500 were male and 5,050 where female. The dearth of promotion of UK black academics to leadership positions in higher education thus remains a source of tension and concern with promotion boards which are 'overwhelmingly white' (Khan, 2017).

Essed: But we have made some progress, be it slow and little. Against the background of many years of affirmative action in the US, changing demographics of the student body, the era of multi-cultural education programmes, and increasingly assertive strategic politics from communities of colour, the presence of people of colour at universities that used to be exclusively white challenges the face of education and questions the assumptions of previously taken for granted rules and expectations about the teaching profession (Mckay, 1997). Towards the end of the twentieth century there were the first signs of an emerging body of research about everyday oppositional and transformative potential among women of colour in white dominated colleges (Romero, 1997), followed up in the new millennium (Essed, 2013; Mirza & Joseph, 2013). The experiences of women of colour scholars are largely documented in autobiographies and other biographical materials. There are oral narratives of African-American women, who went to college in the period before World War II (Etter-lewis, 1993). Other women have utilised their own experiences as teachers in the academy, in critical essays about racism and the pedagogy of social change (Bannerji, 1995; Carty, 1991; hooks, 1984, 1989; Ng, Staton, & Scane, 1995; Tate, 2017; Williams, 1991).

Clearly, oppositional and solidarity work in the face of systemic marginalisation would be a challenge, not without risks, as Ruth Farmer (1993) points out referring to women of colour professors:

> Often she is said to be incompetent if she cannot or will not juggle all the responsibilities thrust upon her. She may feel guilty that she cannot help all who need her. Yet if she does all that is required of her as a person of color (…) for example, integrating all-White committees and functions and acting as unofficial, uncompensated and often unacknowledged counselor to students of color – she will not be viable in her own job and may bring emotional stress upon herself. (p. 204)

Ever since I (first author) first started to teach, this was in the Netherlands, the late 1980s, I have wondered whether other women of colour are also confronted with contradictory demands. There are the demands of scholarship, requiring solitude at times, individualism, discipline and self-assertion. On the other hand, there are pressures to participate in community events, requests to represent 'colour' at forums and other formal events, and last but not least, a commitment to supporting students of colour – and race/gender critical students in general – requiring among other things understanding, availability, sharing and giving. In the 1980s, there was no other person in a position similar to mine, to whom I could turn in The Netherlands. By the new millennium, the number of Dutch women of colour professors could still be counted on one hand (Essed, 1999; Wekker, 2016).

Reflecting on the contradictory demands of scholarship and justice work, in particular, with respect to teacher–student relations this chapter also draws from interviews with women professors of colour, six in all, conducted between the late 1980s and early 1990s in the context of a long-term cross-national endeavour where I (first author) collected (auto) biographical stories on the theme of gender, ethnicity and leadership. The professors, five African-American and one Caribbean Dutch, represent different fields in the humanities and the social sciences: arts, history, anthropology, sociology, psychology and educational sciences, but all engage in race and gender critical scholarship. 'What makes critical social theory "critical" is its commitment to justice, for one's own group and/or for other groups' (Collins, 1998, p. xiv). In addition, there are secondary materials, personal experiences to which women of colour refer in monographs and articles, for the purpose of this chapter predominantly from the US and Canada, countries with a larger representation of women of colour professors than Europe (Bannerji, 1995; Benjamin, 1997; Collins, 1998; James, 1993; Ng et al., 1995; Razack, 1998, and others).

Carberry: Our concern in this chapter is not with blue-prints, but with exploring modes for inclusion of diverse life experiences in the way that we relate as teachers to students (of colour), paying attention to the importance of maintaining wellbeing during periods of feeling stretched. Our mental health, wellbeing and physical health are inextricably linked in combatting work-related stress, in order to strengthen our general health. Work-related stress is defined as 'The adverse reaction people have to excessive pressures or other types of demand placed on them at work' (Health and Safety Executive, HSE, 2011, p. 3). It is one of the most commonly reported health problems, and academics with hidden and high stress levels have had long hours and a culture of intense workload, across universities in the UK (Kinman & Wray, 2013).

Leadership: Challenging Traditions and Setting another Example

Essed: Leadership qualities include the courage to challenge situations taken for granted, while identifying contingent and strategic possibilities, regardless of institutional constraints (Astin & Leland, 1991; Handy, 1992; James & Farmer, 1993; Sinclair, 2007). More than any other attributes, the capacity to move people to action, to strengthen confidence is at the heart of the notion of leadership (Gardner, 1990). This view is echoed in real life experiences:

> I encourage students to see the possibilities of their making fundamental decisions for the direction of this nation, and to use their know-ledge, training, creativity, and skills in the interest of the oppressed people of the United States (…). I encourage them (…) [to make] the first step in their own transformation, and perhaps, intellectual and spiritual liberation. (Coleman-Burns, 1993, p. 141)

In her reflections on her career as a black woman law professor Taunya Lovell Banks asserted that the academy needs black women as mentors to bring multiple life experiences to the classroom (Banks & Peller, 1995). The academy needs women of colour intellectuals to challenge unicultural perspectives in predominantly white colleges and universities. To use the words of Linda Carty (1991):

> As a Black woman now teaching university in a society where this is extremely rare, I am aware, like the few other 'non-White' women in a similar position, of the unique opportunity I now have to redress some of the historical inaccuracies perpetrated by Eurocentric scholars, including feminists, who refuse to recognize the changing nature of the social world. (p. 40)

Women of colour in the academy have contributed to the development and articulation of new epistemologies (Collins, 1998) in spite of the antagonistic conditions under which critical research and teaching often takes place (Carby, 1982; Collins, 1990, 1994; Mohanty, 1993; Moses, 1989; Ng et al., 1995, Parmar, 1982; Puwar, 2004; Tobin, 1983;). Critical writings of women of colour have shifted frameworks, while generating self-reflection on the part of white feminist scholars (Caraway, 1991; Chaudhuri & Strobel, 1992; Cock, 1992; Frankenberg, 1993; Ware, 1992; Ware & Back, 2002).

Race critical theory is not the prerogative of women of colour, but the conditions under which women of colour engage in critical work are particularly challenging, where neither race, ethnicity, gender nor class worlds can be taken for granted. Taunya Banks put it like this:

> We are misfits, not fully accepted by the black or white community; and as women, we still are not full members of the feminist community. (...) I am constantly asked to fit within one paradigm at a time. I am categorized as being part of a black world, or of a white world, or a world of poverty and cultural deprivation. Being so variously categorized often causes me to think about all of these worlds collectively when viewing common life experiences. (Banks, 1995, pp. 330–331)

All teachers operate in a changing world, but the majority are not experts in change processes. Moreover, as Fullan (1995) points out, teachers and educational systems are known more for their capacity to resist change than for their roles as agents of reform. Graduate schools do not only (re)produce standard models of professional identity that are exclusive of women of colour, but simultaneously perpetuate gender, race, ethnic, class and other forms of inequality (Margolis & Romero, 1998; Romero, 1997). This is not meant to suggest that women of colour are powerless:

> (...) we have tremendous power as teachers (...) to help students rethink and challenge their own socialization with respect to racism, sexism, heterosexism, to name only a few 'isms' that hurt all of us. (Guy-Sheftall, 1997, p. 121)

Much of the literature on women and leadership rejects a top-down conception of leadership as the process by which a group follows the objectives that a leader induces them to adopt (Gardner, 1990; Sinclair, 2007). Furthermore, rather than focussing on leadership as control, due emphasis is put on the leader's ability to mobilise talent, motivate others and support their 'empowerment' (Astin & Leland, 1991; Hall & Grey, 1988; King, 1988). Leadership in education means encouraging and assisting students in discovering their own interests and challenging their implicit theories of the way the world works and how it can be changed. An illustration of this is expressed in the following quote:

> A teacher gives to the students to the point they begin to question what they are doing. And begin to try to find answers from inside themselves or researching from outside themselves too. So that is what ideally I would like to do because I think that if I hide behind this authoritarian way of thinking, then what happens is I create students that don't ever get to the point where they realize that they have a certain power within themselves to make decisions and if they don't ever realize that then what happens is you do have authoritarian governments. [Professor of Film-Arts, interview first author]

Understanding and Solidarity

In his contribution to the volume *Educating Teachers for Leadership and Change* (O'Hair and Odell, eds), Michael Fullan (1995) points out that the knowledge base for being an effective teacher has changed dramatically over the past decade to include, among other things, an understanding of how diverse, multi-ethnic students learn and develop, as well as strategies to meet a wide range of individual needs. Drawing from their own experiences as minorities in graduate school, most women of colour are likely to have an understanding of the situation of students of colour. They are sensitive to the fact that life on a predominantly white campus can be hard on students of colour, many of whom come from low income families. The environment of white universities is different from their home and previous school experience. It has been pointed out that these and other factors add to the fact that black students, for instance, are often academically and psychologically ill-prepared for the fierce competitiveness and the 'survival of the fittest' mentality that they often encounter in predominantly white universities (Hall & Allen, 1989).

Graduate status in white institutions means operating in an environment which, if not hostile, is cool and chilly (Henry & Tator, 2009; Wilkerson, 1986). Pressures are high and many students develop hardly any other interest than in 'what is going to be the exam', or 'what do I have to do to pass in this course' [Professor of Psychology, interview first author]. There are students of colour who dissociate themselves from campus race politics and others who recognise when, for instance, black faculty contribute, on a structural (material) level, to improving facilities for black students. One professor explains:

> We provide fellowships for graduate students, research support and money to do their dissertation studies. They are closer to being professionals and I think they are better able to empathize with the situation of black academics, black administrators. [Professor of Psychology, interview first author]

Apart from grants and fellowships, other resources can be mobilised as well:

> Most of the time I really work hard to be supportive. I have been involved in committees in terms of working to find ways to get black students in and keeping black students in. I give support when I hear about job openings or when I hear about conferences or places where they can network, meet other people (...) I try to work alongside, get exposure for many when I can. [Professor of Film-Arts, interview first author]

There is also a downside to racial or ethnic solidarity. Some students make unrealistic claims, assuming that they can afford to perform poorly, because the professor will pass them on racial grounds:

> We have this expression, to 'cop a plea'. You have not worked during the course and so you come in at the last moment and say, 'But sister you know how it is with us, we are all poor, I need this grade to stay', this kind of solidarity thing. [Professor of English Literature, interview first author]

Another variant of disrespectful appeal to solidarity has to do with the hiring of staff. One professor recalls this enormous grant that she was getting for a project. Word got around and she had this Black male student who had heard about it yelling across the hallway area to me in my office saying, 'I heard you got the grant, I want to come talk to you, I think we need to talk about these things so we can talk about staffing'. Her explicit reference to the gender of the student suggests that the professor experienced this event as mediated through gender as well:

> He would have approached a white male very differently than saying I'm going to have to talk to you. There is a level of respect that is absent, and there is a refusal to acknowledge authority. [Professor of Psychology, interview first author]

There are also other indications that students' attitudes towards faculty have ethnicized and gendered dimensions. In her research among Chicana faculty, Mary Romero (1997) has found that they were expected to work with all the Chicano students, as well as other students of colour. As a result, all the women in her sample reported spending additional hours working with students of colour. Not surprisingly, white faculty are not expected to be working with every white student.

Carberry: This level of pressure and stress women of colour faculty are exposed to is indicative of the impact of the organisation's 'poor work design and lack of control over work processes' (Lekha, Griffiths, & Cox, 2004): engaging within a bi- or multiple-cultural life style with the trappings of upward mobility without a level playing field for the woman of colour. This adds pressure to living in a 'White' world while the teacher has to metaphorically work with her 'hands tied behind her back' (Boyd-Franklin, 1989, p. 207).

Advocacy in Case of Discrimination

Essed: (Gendered) racial stereotypes create barriers for students of colour aspiring to share with the college community an atmosphere of creativity and a mutual exchange of ideas and work. One professor, affiliated to a Center for Black Studies, has seen it happening many times: 'Students will contact a black faculty when an incident occurs on campus that has racist overtones. And that person will become a kind of an advocate for the student' [Professor of Sociology, interview first author].

Although there is an ombud office on campus, 'a lot of the black students tend not to trust that route at all' [Professor of Sociology]. Evidence of racism is often denied by the majority group, which makes it hard to deal with actual occurrences of discrimination (Essed, 1991; Feagin, 1992; Henry & Tator, 2009; Piliawsky, 1982; Wekker, 2016). Fearing that white faculty trivialises their experiences, students who are discriminated against rather approach one of the black teachers for obtaining advice and support:

> One black student here was telling me how one professor in the department has made racial jokes. And I am working with her on that. You have to deal with it all the time. And the person that she is dealing with, he is one of the most liberal ones in the department. But still I am not surprised that this kind of thing happens. It is like always having a guard up, but still operating as if nothing happens. It is hard, time consuming. It keeps you active. [Professor of Film-Arts, interview first author]

Another case involves a student of cultural anthropology, the only black student in class. An anthropology teacher had referred to Africa as a 'series of backward nations with no technical history and primitive characteristics, loosely translated' [Professor of Sociology]. Upset about the event, the student turned to the African-American professor, who recalls:

> I tell them to confront as long as they have the facts to do it. And apparently she did go up to the instructor after class and take issue with what he said. Of course, he claimed he didn't mean it that way and she goes on 'I can only take it the way you said it and your

information is very wrong'. She said, 'I resent it because you have a class full of students here who don't know any better than what you tell them and you're perpetuating myths and stereotypes'. Misinformation. Now, it is risk-taking, you see. Because if she is going to put herself in the position of constantly confronting the professor on the content of the lectures she may get penalized for that, and she recognizes that but, as she said she cannot sit there and allow it to happen. [Professor of Sociology, interview first author]

Orchestrating Multi-dimensional Identities

Cecile Wright asserted that the ability to play simultaneously on more than one dimension of identity, in this case race-ethnicity as well as identifying with teaching, can open up possibilities unique to women of colour. She acted effectively as an intermediary between students and staff, even when an intermediary role also gives rise to a dilemma.

> (...) I inevitably came to be 'caught in the crossfire' of relations between teachers and black students. (...) [Many] of the African Caribbean students would identify with me as a black woman and would look to me for support during conflicts with their teachers within the classroom. However, on the other hand, the teachers would see me as an adult and an ally within the classroom during these times of conflict, with my black identity offering a further resource that they would expect me to use to relate to, and help them control, the black students. (Wright, 1998, pp. 67–68)

Women of colour engaged in critical studies are and have been pioneers in making explicit the different, sometimes overlapping, dimensions of personal and political identities, including finding unique safe spaces for free expression via the internet, challenging racial and gendered identities portrayed in the media through blogs (Collins, 1998; Crenshaw, 1991; Gabriel, 2016, 2018).

A case in point concerns gender identity and specific roles or expectations attached to that. The normative (white male) standard of professional identity requires disconnection between private and public dimensions of our gender identities. Understanding and support for students of colour appeal to qualities of caring, in Western societies (including ethnic minority cultures) statistically a disposition more common or more extensively developed among women than among men, as daughters, partners and mothers.

Arguably, academic professionalism is not about caring as a sister, or as a mother, but one can also argue for another understanding of professionalism, where different layers of identity are not rigidly disconnected but remain linked and can be activated when relevant. I (first author) found one example where care for students of colour was expressed in a private form resembling a way of mothering, in this context meaning a,

> socially constructed set of activities and relationships involved in nurturing and caring for people (...) (at the heart of which is) an ethic of caring – knowing, feeling and acting in the interests of others. (Forcey, 1994, p. 357)

The event is about an immigrant student in need of a relationship to compensate for her lack of family relations in the US. The professor recalled:

> There is one woman, we don't know how to classify her, the computer has no place to put her. She is from the Dominican Republic and I see her as black. Last night she came to me and she said I need to go home with you, I am missing my mother. So she was obviously feeling that she is black and I am black and she wanted to be mothered by me. It is a very close kind of relationship, but our program is very close anyway. [Teacher, Education]

There is a hazard to racialised mothering as a mode for student support, particularly when it may invoke stereotyped images of black women. It seems to be hard, sometimes, to escape the pattern where, according to Patricia Hill Collins (1998) even

> Black women professionals find ourselves doing 'mammy work' in our jobs, work in which we care for everyone else, often at the expense of our own careers or personal well-being. (p. 49)

Arguably, without a sense of care one cannot be a good teacher (O'Hair & Odell, 1995). But care can have different meanings at different times. As younger women of colour increasingly enter the academy there may occur a shift designating generational differences in style and political engagement. Those who went to school during the highdays of the Civil Rights movement and the Black Power era may feel politically more engaged with a sense of community and the ideal of 'lifting the race' than younger scholars who grew up in times of individualism, diversity and politics of multi-culturalism in colleges and universities (Goldberg, 1994).

Carberry: The everyday life for black professors is like tightrope they walk in maintaining their level of integrity in their bi- or multiple-cultural experience and expectations of them by their white peers and black students (Essed, 2004). The 'fishbowl' experience illuminates the importance of striving for wellness, and emulating a pattern for the young black scholars to follow. There seem to be several levels in shifts in terms of social consciousness. The recent black male 'Black Excellence movement' led by Terry and Terrence Everett, Jonathan Brooks and Schyler Landrum rippling across campuses in the US and UK, juxtaposed with pride in the 'Black Child in Education Awards' led by Diane Abbott MP in the UK is heralding a Civil Rights movement where the slogan 'Black Lives Matter' is breathed into the atmosphere. Yet, there are conflicting nuances of internalised and external racism, and lack of awareness regarding white privilege, and lack of solidarity (Gabriel, 2017). Nick Pendry (2011), a black/Asian academic recounts a painful episode of attempting to create a safe space for conversations.

> I remember clearly the experience of co-facilitating a Black only group in a training context. My teaching colleagues and I were aware from the student body that our plans to separate the racially mixed group of students had become an emotive issue. Indeed, a number of students, Black and White, had expressed their considerable discomfort with this exercise. It would seem that this discomfort would be easily understandable, given the apparent emphasis on our separateness as people rather than our togetherness, which would seem to bring to mind stories of racial superiority and inferiority contained within this forced separation. I think I was prepared for this strength of feeling, but I wasn't certainly prepared for was a number of White students claiming places in the Black-only group. I felt my 'Blackness' being challenged … my strong Black Identity crumbling before me and was powerless to act … I was silenced by the act of challenge to this exercise, and couldn't imagine the Black students posing a challenge to the White group in quite the same way … I realised, not for the first time, that my Black voice was only heard if the White dominant group let it. (p. 11)

This 'silencing' has been one that many academics have voiced through working in what can often be the toxic environment of academia and white power. Shirley Ann Tate (2017) expands upon this descriptions of

> feelings of shame … and the unvoiceability of negative feelings through institutional silencing and finally the impact of deracination on black women academics 'well-being' from the standpoint of having liveable lives at work. (p. 55)

A person's emotional wellbeing is their ability to be able to function in society and meet the demands of everyday life. The opposite of high emotional wellbeing is severe psychological stress and all universities have a duty of care to both the employee and the student. Staff wellbeing is one of the keys to raising student satisfaction and emotional health.

Essed: Being a mentor to students is part of formal education, but in some of the examples caring is linked with or mediated through informal responsibilities that black women professors may feel for the wellbeing and the political 'conscientising' of their students (of colour). The latter speaks to social, political identities and to skills developed in the framework of gender identities. The following experience of mentorship, taken from an interview with a teacher and mother of a son in his early twenties, suggests the activation of gender dimensions of identity (appeal to a sense of mothering) intertwined with dimensions of identity as a teacher (appeal to intellectual coaching):

> This one young guy. (...) started coming up to my office after about the third week of school and he asked me if he could come and take a look at my bookshelf, and that is a real clue, and I said yes. (...) He will select a book off the shelf and he will look through it and then he will start writing down names. Then he begins to talk about some experiences that he had in high school. He is a neat young man, about 19. He said he never learned anything about himself in high school, (...) but he knew that there were some things he needed to know and tried to start reading on his own. Which a lot of them do. Not enough of them. (...) He is a very serious person, but he is wrestling with being Black. He is reading all about Malcolm X which he started reading on his own. [Professor of Sociology, interview first author]

Whereas extracurricular support to students of colour can be gratifying for personal and political reasons, it is not duly credited when it comes to faculty evaluations. Mary Romero (1997) interviewed a Chicana professor who, the focal point for all the students of colour on campus, reports:

> I was working with many Black students as well as Puerto Rican students and a handful of Chicanos (...) [It] was work I enjoyed doing, that I felt was important, and I felt committed to doing. But, at the same time, I always knew this was going to be working against me [in the tenure decision]. (p. 162)

In this case, the professor transcends ethnic and racial borders in solidarity with all (marginalised) students of colour. Racial and ethnic inclusion in catering to students has become increasingly accepted as normative practice among women of colour engaged in critical social sciences (Essed, 2013; Razack, 1998). Feminists, black and white, have been in the forefront of breaking through ethnic barriers in working together in pursuit of common goals, in particular in Western European countries (Afshar & Maynard, 1994; Anthias & Yuval-Davis, 1992; Essed, 1996; Kraft & Ashraf-Khan, 1994; Yuval-davis, 1998). Developments in the US are to a larger extent marked by (the history of) racial segregation. There is a tendency towards racial exclusiveness and US-centrism in representations of black feminism in publications of African-American spokeswomen like bell hooks, Joy James, and Patricia Hill Collins (Collins, 1990; James, 1999). The same holds for situations where African-American women professors in interviews with the first author, referred almost exclusively to *black* students in discussing issues of justice, and not to students of colour in general. This is a point of concern, but it would not do justice to African-American women to generalise. Patricia Hill Collins' (1998) most recent work is more inclusive, and there are some African-American women, Angela Davis and Andrée Nicola McLaughlin to mention but two, who have been consistent from an early stage in including in their academic and political orientation cross-national and cross-ethnic interests and experiences of women (Davis, 1988; James, 1998; McLaughlin, 1990).

Recognising multi-identities and speaking to students across marginalised borders poses its own problems as well. Sherene Razack courageously analyses a situation where it went 'wrong' in her own class. She recalls an incident from the summer college in human rights at the University of Ottawa, which brought together members of a range of marginalised groups, from women with disabilities to anti-racist groups. As the instructor and a woman of colour, she had purposefully chosen storytelling in her course as a pedagogical tool to make space for different voices and to forge a politics of alliances based on this mutual engagement in listening to and trying to understand one another's daily experiences.

> One participant in my group, a white disabled woman, frustrated by the silence of a Black woman from South Africa during a discussion about South Africa, directly confronted her with a firm 'Why don't you tell us your experiences?' Realizing the harshness of what was said, another participant also disabled but male, repeated the request more gently. The trust and sharing of the class, built over five days, instantly dissolved. The Black participant, confronted with a request to tell her story, defended her right to silence and then left the room in tears. (...) [The request] (...) recalled for every person of colour in the room (seven out of twenty and myself, the instructor) that this was not in fact a safe learning environment. (Razack, 1998, p. 48)

In many instances life stories are one of the best rhetorical tools because they connect the story teller and the message with the audience. Stories help to show the listener how to identify with a topic because of the detailed manner in which the stories are contextualised.

Accounts are useful in revealing the emotional toll of constant exposure to discrimination (Williams & Yu, 1997). In this particular case Razack, as she recalled, was amazed to find herself so immediately identifying, through 'race', with the South African woman in feeling hurt and indignant, that it took a conscious effort for her to maintain her composure as a teacher. Razack concluded that in the particular event they got carried away by the promises of the pedagogy of storytelling, while failing to consider how social hierarchies operate among subordinate groups, thereby influencing the way storytelling serves different groups. In other words, the initial intention that in a multi-layered society multi-dimensional identities of all the participants (national background, gender, colour and physical abilities) can be shared with equal care and understanding did not materialise. At the end of the day, race and ethnicity came to be the overriding dimension of group divide and experience. Race, the power relation setting white apart from non-white, clouded other markers of identity, including gender, class differences, national backgrounds, physical abilities, teacher–student distinction and other professional affiliations. This event probably also shows that even when we engage in sophisticated theory depicting experiences and identities as multi-dimensional, in practice it is hard to avoid trodden paths where identities are reduced to one single dimension of our existence, in this case, racial.

What goes into creating a 'safe' learning environment in a mixed class-room? One can agree with Razack that storytelling as a way of sharing daily experiences is a risky business. Advocating mutual openness (i.e. tolerance or even acceptance of difference) as a pedagogical tool is likely to create either a blind eye for privileges or over-emphasis on group disadvantages (Essed, 1996).

In *Diversity: Gender, Color and Culture* (Essed, 1996) I have discussed classroom dynamics when teaching about sensitive topics like gender, ethnicity, racism. I have suggested, among other things, that it is important to guide students in identifying and mutually acknowledging their individual strengths; to identify patterns of exclusion while discussing personal experiences of discrimination only against the background of structural relations of dominance; to protect, as a teacher, the principle of respect which means creating space for inclusive (critical) engagement of all participants in dialogue (better: multi-logue) where there is no tolerance for personal attacks or accusations. I have pleaded for the principle of reason over tradition, implying critical scrutinising of dominant traditions as well as traditions among ethnic groups. Last but not least, I have argued against the idea that one group claims its heroes only for itself. The transcultural and transnational adoption of inspiring examples can be instrumental in facilitating the abandonment of taken for granted (traditional) allegiances.

Critical Knowledge in a Multi-layered Society

One of the most challenging aspects of teaching in a multi-layered society has to do with questions of race identity and the transmission of knowledge of racism. Because they teach predominantly white classes all of the professors also have to deal with the race identity of white students and their political awareness, or the lack of it. Himani Bannerji (1995) comments about her course on 'Gender, Race, and Class'.

> [...] some white women students cringed every time I mentioned slavery, racism and colonialism. They were affronted by the possibility of their consciousness being constructed through a white, male, middle-class culture. They could not or would not see that they had to question their common sense, knowledge apparatuses and politics. (p. 117)

Formal education usually fails to expose students to critical views on race issues. Shocked to find that, in 1993, white students '[didn't] know who Angela Davis was', that they 'had heard about Malcolm X, but did not know who he was, that they hadn't got a clue about stuff we have grown up with', one professor decided to introduce the students to topics and to literature that had been absent from their previous education:

> I liked very much the power that it gives and the way you can influence class dynamics also by just choosing a particular kind of literature, how you can force students to think about issues. [Professor of Anthropology, interview first author]

Another woman, a professor of education, encouraged her (predominantly white) students to develop a 'healthy concern' for disadvantaged children, the majority of which are black:

> I scream and yell and jump up and down to make sure that we send our students (of education) to Black schools. (...) I am not saying that we need to handcuff students and send them down by force to where they don't want to be, because they do more damage than good if they were forced to be where they don't want to go, but if the philosophy of the program really is that we're set up here to change what is going on, quote 'down there', then we will do those supportive things so that the students won't feel punished being sent down there. They won't feel like they have some choices, they will want to go down there. [Teacher, Education, interview first author]

Women professors who seek to share responsibility and commitment in the struggle for racial, ethnic and gender justice explained how they are using education as a tool (Kershaw, 1992), sometimes specifically to affirm black culture:

> I want to make a clear and direct contribution to black women's lives. (...) All of my work, as diverse as it is, whether it is on subjectivity or sexuality or literature, language or poetry, it is all the time within one grand project: validating and describing black culture. [Professor of Anthropology]

Finally, some women emphasised the need to explore more extensively the transforming potential of Ethnic Studies. As an interdisciplinary field, Ethnic Studies is committed not only to criticise institutional operations, policies and laws and other social practices of domination informed by racial, ethnic, gender and class formations (San Juan, 1992), but also to explore the conditions for alternative models of social formation that advance the cause of justice in society. It seems therefore proper to highlight the following quote from the professor who had the most extensive teaching experience in the field of Ethnic Studies:

> A lot of the students that I get in my classes are going to be teachers, they are going to be counselors, they are going to have children, they are going into professions where if they didn't take some of our courses, they would have no perspective at all from the multiethnic point of view. They go into the classroom and they go into a counseling session, setting, or wherever they go without much knowledge about culturally diverse populations and that is a tragedy because they are the ones that are going to be responsible for changing some attitudes and they can't do it because their attitudes are limited. I feel very, very strongly about Ethnic Studies. I think it is probably one of the most critical disciplines that could be offered right now in institutions because of the diverse society that we live in. [Professor of Sociology, interview first author]

Conclusions

The redefining of educational leadership among women of colour as presented in this chapter has primarily dealt with leadership in teacher–student relations. Some women professors intentionally choose to develop and use certain leadership qualities in the pursuit of justice. They motivate students of colour to develop critical understanding of race and other systems of domination, they develop facilities to strengthen competitive skills, they offer understanding and support in the case of discrimination. In doing so the women include and speak to different dimensions of their identity and those of the students: including race, gender, national background, class and physical ability. There is a price tag to racial solidarity in the sense that extra activities involved are seldom acknowledged in evaluations and career paths. Until recently, the health consequences of racism have largely been ignored or underestimated in the social and educational sciences (Hansen, 2013). Racism can indeed have long-term effects on health (Paradies et al., 2013). At the same time, a range of factors can work to ameliorate the impact. Paradies, one of the most prolific interdisciplinary researchers in this field emphasised the health benefits of critical awareness and the positive impact of parents who educate their children about racism. Essed (1991) found the same in terms of the confidence young people feel about challenging racism when they have been socialised to understand that the injustices involved are not their personal fault. Paradies (2006) further found a range of empowering factors in facing and challenging racism, including, the strong sense of racial or ethnic identity, access to religious and social support systems and on a more personal level character traits such as hardiness.

With their inclusive interpretations of leadership, women of colour provide specific support that the university system fails to offer sufficiently to students of colour. We do not mean to suggest that women of colour are the only ones responsible to bridge this gap. Leadership inclusive of diverse experiences should be taken up by the university at large. In the meantime, rather than suggesting that women of colour should not use their critical knowledge and supportive skills on behalf of (racially) marginalised students, their understanding of leadership as teachers at institutions of higher education can be an example to others, which deserves to be acknowledged and credited accordingly. That is to say, teachers in privileged institutions *should* take up a specific role, which is precisely that of scrutinising practices of exclusion, and defining the conceptual frameworks for alternatives, which will do more justice to the diverse worlds and complex identities of students and the quality of student–teacher relationships.

Carberry: I hope that this chapter contributes to acknowledging in communities of colour, the psychological and emotional toll of the pressures of everyday racism. In doing critical work women of colour need to be able to draw on and develop emotional resilience. They often have come a long way.

Making the transition into university life as a black student is certainly not without its challenges and stress in moving back and forth between different levels of racial awareness. University policy, informal practices and institutional racism can add to the pressure of family expectations of perhaps being the first one in generations to achieve educational success. Teachers from black and some minority ethnic families are aware that there is an unspoken expectation that students seek positive role models within the extended community system including the education, church and wider community networks (Boyd-Franklin, 1989, p. 45). These role models are seen as key to building self-esteem and positive racial identity from teachers who seem to have made the bi-cultural and educational transition to an elite position within the educational system (Boyd-Franklin, 1989, p. 30). What does this mean for teachers or colour? Due to their university experience, teachers, through increased empathy, confidence in mentorship, over-identification of the black and minority student's experience, coupled with an over-arching workload, could find their wellbeing affected by being emotionally and physically over-extended. When it comes to dealing with a particular stress or strain in life, we are normally faced with a choice. We can either attempt to change the situation which is causing us difficulty, or we can do something about our capacity to deal with it. If we do not, the wrong type of pressure turns to stress and anxiety, and cumulative stress invariably results in trauma. Trauma has the capacity to make some people feel overwhelmed, while others appear to be able to cope. Whatever our response, traumatic events have a significant impact on our lives and invariably reduce our capacity for emotional resilience.

Affected by day to day racism, there are many teachers who are jaded, 'walking wounded' but without the right type of support. The symptoms of stress which include headaches, stomach upsets, high blood pressure, even a stroke or heart disease can escalate. It can also cause feelings of distrust, anger, anxiety and fear which in turn can destroy relationships at home and at work (Lekha et al., 2004). Developing a peer network of support is key to alleviate pressure and loneliness in academia. Creating fluid boundaries is key with the option of developing a capacity to look at evasive action for most of life's challenges. A good healthy diet, coupled with regular exercise is also an important strategy in maintaining wellbeing.

Many universities, and organisations, engage employment assistance providers (EAPs), who can help with free counselling, employment advice, family care and debt advice. Black and minority families have a healthy cultural suspicion regarding the discussion of their private matters, however, a confidential talk with a professional will help to reduce stress and enhance the capacity for personal wellbeing. At any sign of stress one should speak with their family doctor. Check your employment contract and/or ask human resources for your EAP. There are also several confidential self-help sites listed below:

http://www.moodjuice.scot.nhs.uk/
http://www.acas.org.uk
https://www.psychotherapy.org.uk
https://www.bacp.co.uk/
https://www.baatn.org.uk

We all develop different levels of resilience as we grow up and you might be afraid that you are not a naturally resilient person. However, resilience can definitely be developed, and there are many small changes that you can draw on, which can dramatically boost your capacity to cope. Women of colour professors can thrive against the odds, providing a healthy example to the students of critical awareness and action against institutionalised racism without compromising the community love and personal care it takes to sustain stamina in the struggle for racial and other social justice.

References

Afshar, H., & Maynard, M. (Eds.). (1994). *The dynamics of race and gender: Some feminist interventions*. London: Taylor & Francis.
Alexander-Floyd, N. G. (2015). Women of color, space invaders, and political science: Practical strategies for transforming institutional practices. *PS: Political Science & Politics, 48*(3), 464–468.
Anthias, F., & Yuval-Davis, N. (1992). *Racialized boundaries: Race, nation, gender, colour and class and the anti-racist struggle*. London: Routledge.
Astin, H. S., & Leland, C. (1991). *Women of influence, women of vision: A cross-cultural study of leaders and social change*. San Francisco, CA: Jossey-Bass.
Banks, T. L., (1995). Two life stories: Reflections of one Black woman law professor. In K. Crenshaw, N. Gotanda, G. Peller, & K. Thomas (Eds.), *Critical race theory* (pp. 329–336). New York, NY: The New Press.
Bannerji, H. (1995). *Thinking through. Essays on feminism, Marxism, and anti-racism*. Toronto: Women's Press.
Benjamin, L. (1997). *Black women in the academy*. Gainesville, FL: University Press of Florida.
Boyd-Franklin, N. (1989). *Black families in therapy: A multisystems approach*. New York, NY: Guilford Press.
Caraway, N. (1991). *Segregated sisterhood: Racism and the politics of American feminism*. Knoxville, TN: University of Tennessee Press.
Carby, H. (1982). White Woman Listen! The Boundaries of Sisterhood. In Centre for Contemporary Cultural Studies (Ed.), *The Empire Strikes Back: Race and Racism in 70s Britain* (pp. 212–235). London: Hutchinson & Co.
Carty, L. (1991). Black women in academia: A statement from the periphery. In H. Bannerji, L. Carty, K. Dehli, S. Heald, & K. McKenna (Eds.), *Unsettling Relations: The University as a Site of Feminist Struggles*, (pp. 13–44). Toronto: Women's Press.
Chaudhuri, N., & Strobel, M. (Eds.). (1992). *Western women and imperialism*. Bloomington, IN: Indiana University Press.
Cock, J. (1992). *Women and war in South Africa*. London: Open Letters.
Coleman-Burns, P. (1993). The revolution within: Transforming ourselves. In J. James & R. Farmer (Eds.), *Spirit, space and survival: African American women in (White) academe* (pp. 139–157). London: Routledge.
Collins, P. H. (1990). *Black feminist thought*. Boston, MA: Unwin Hyman.
Collins, P. H. (1994). Shifting the center: Race, class, and feminist theorizing about motherhood. In E. N. Glenn, G. Chang, & L. R. Forcey (Eds.), *Mothering: Ideology, experience and agency* (pp. 45–65). New York, NY: Routledge.
Collins, P. H. (1998). *Fighting words: Black women and the search for justice*. Minneapolis, MN: University of Minnesota Press.

Crenshaw, K. (1991). Mapping the margins: Intersectionality, identity politics, and violence against women of color. *Stanford Law Review*, *43*(6), 1241–1299.
Davis, A. (1988). *Women, culture and politics*. New York, NY: Random House.
Essed, P. (1991). *Understanding everyday racism: An interdisciplinary theory*. Newbury Park: Sage.
Essed, P. (1996). *Diversity: Gender, color and culture*. Amherst, MA: University of Massachusetts Press.
Essed, P. (1999). Ethnicity and diversity in Dutch academia. *Social Identities*, *5*(2), 211–225.
Essed, P. (2000). Dilemmas in leadership: Women of colour in the academy. *Ethnic and Racial Studies*, *23*(5), 888–904.
Essed, P. (2004). Cloning amongst professors: Normativities and imagined homogeneities. *Nora: Nordic Journal of Femininst and Gender Research*, *12*(2), 113–122.
Essed, P. (2013). Women social justice scholars: Risks and rewards of committing to anti-racism. *Ethnic and Racial Studies, 36*(9), 1393–1410.
Etter-lewis, G. (1993). *My soul is my own: Oral narratives of African American women in the profession*. New York, NY: Routledge.
Farmer, R. (1993). Place but not importance: The race for inclusion in Academe. In J. James & R. Farmer (Eds.), *Spirit, space and survival: African American women in (white) academe* (pp. 196–217). New York, NY: Routledge.
Feagin, J. (1992). The continuing significance of racism: Discrimination against Black students in White colleges. *Journal of Black Studies*, *22*(4), 546–578.
Forcey, L. R. (1994). Feminist perspectives on mothering and peace. In E. N. Glenn, G. Chang, & L. R. Forcey (Eds.), *Mothering: Ideology, experience and agency* (pp. 355–375). New York, NY: Routledge.
Frankenberg, R. (1993). *White women, race matters: The social construction of whiteness*. London: Routledge.
Fullan, M. (1995). Contexts: Overview and frameworks. In M. J. O'Hair & S. J. Odell (Eds.), *Educating teachers for leadership and change* (pp. 1–10). Thousand Oaks, CA: Corwin Press.
Gabriel, D. (2016). Blogging while Black, British and female: Critical study of discursive activism. *Journal of Information, Communication and Society*, *19*(11), 1622–1635.
Gabriel, D. (2017). White privilege exposes how Eurocentricity undermines the mission for race equality. Black British Academics. United Kingdom. Retrieved from http://blackbritishacademics.co.uk/2017/10/28/subu-event-on-white-privilege-exposes-how-eurocentricity-undermines-the-misson-for-race-equality/. Accessed on June 6, 2018.
Gabriel, D. (2018). Addressing anti-Black gendered racism requires critical leaders. Black British Academics. United Kingdom. Retrieved from http://blackbritishacademics.co.uk/2018/05/17/addressing-anti-black-gendered-racism-requires-critical-leaders/. Accessed on June 6, 2018.
Gardner, J. W. (1990). *On leadership*. New York, NY: The Free Press.
Goldberg, D. T. (Ed.). (1994). *Multiculturalism: A critical reader*. Oxford: Basil Blackwell.
Guy-Sheftall, B. (1997). Transforming the academy: A Black feminist perspective. In L. Benjamin (Ed.), *Black women in the academy* (pp. 115–123). Gainesville, FL: University Press of Florida.
Hall, M. L., & Allen, W. R. (1989). Race consciousness among African-American college students. In G. L. V. Berry & J. K. Asamen (Eds.), *Black students* (pp. 172–197). Newbury Park, CA: Sage.
Hall, N., & Grey, K. (1988). Leadership for Black women: Strategies for the future. *Sage*, *5*(2), 53–55.
Handy, C. (1992). The language of leadership. In M. Syrett & C. Hogg (Eds.), *Frontiers of leadership* (pp. 7–12). Oxford: Basil Blackwell.

Hansen, D. (2013). An apple a day keeps the doctor away ... but so does white privilege: everyday racism, perceived discrimination and the health costs of social exclusion for black people in Europe. *ENAR visible invisible minorities: Confronting afrophobia and advancing equality for people of African descent and Black Europeans in Europe* (pp. 206–235). Brussels: ENAR.

Health and Safety Executive (HSE). (2011). *Work related stress*. United Kingdom: Human Factors Ergonomics and Psychology Unit.

Henry, F., & Tator, C. (Eds.). (2009). *Racism in the Canadian university: Demanding social justice, inclusion, and equity*. Toronto: University of Toronto Press.

HESA. (2018). 2016/2017 Higher Education Staff Statistics (HESA) UK. Retrieved from https://www.hesa.ac.uk/news/18-01-2018/sfr248-higher-education-staff-statistics. Accessed on June 6, 2018.

hooks, b. (1984). *Feminist theory: From margin to center*. Boston, MA: South End Press.

hooks, b. (1989). *Talking back: Thinks feminist – Thinking black*, London: Sheba Feminist Publishers.

James, J. (1993). Teaching theory, talking community. In J. James & R. Farmer (Eds.), *Spirit, space and survival: African American women in (White) Academe* (pp. 199–235). London: Routlegde.

James, J. (1999). *Shadowboxing: Representations of black feminist thought*. New York, NY: St. Martin's Press.

James, J. (Ed.). (1998). *The Angela Y. Davis Reader*. Malden, MA: Blackwell.

James, J., & Farmer, R. (Eds.). (1993). *Spirit, space and survival*. London: Routledge.

Kershaw, T. (1992). The effects of educational tracking on the social mobility of African Americans. *Journal of Black Studies*, 23(1), 152–169.

Khan, C. (2017). Do universities have problem with promoting their BME staff. *Guardian Newspaper*. Retrieved from https://www.theguardian.com/higher-education-network/2017/nov/16/do-universities-have-a-problem-with-promoting-their-bame-staff. Accessed on June 6, 2018.

King, J. E. (1988). A Black woman speaks on leadership. *Sage*, 5(2), 49–52.

Kinman, G., & Wray, S. (2013). *Higher stress. A survey of stress and well-being among staff in higher education* (p. 6). London: University and College Union.

Kraft, M., & Ashraf-Khan, R. (Eds.). (1994). *Schwarze Frauen der Welt: Europa und Migration [Black women of the world: Europe and migration]*. Berlin: Orlands Frauenverlag.

Lekha, S., Griffiths, A., & Cox, T. (2004). *Protecting workers' health series 3*. United Kingdom: Institute of Work, Health & Organisation, Nottingham: University of Nottingham. Retrieved from http://www.who.int/occupational_health/topics/stressatwp/en/

Margolis, E., & Romero, M. (1998). The department is very male, very white, very old, and very conservative: The functioning of the hidden curriculum in graduate sociology departments. *Harvard Educational Review*, 68(1), 1–32.

Mckay, N. Y. (1997). A troubled peace: Black women in the halls of the white academy. In L. Benjamin (Ed.), *Black women in the academy* (pp. 11–22). Gainesville, FL: University Press of Florida.

McLaughlin, A. N. (1990). Black women, identity, and the quest for humanhood and wholeness: Wild women in the whirlwind. In J. M. Braxton & A. N. McLaughlin (Eds.), *Wild women in the whirlwind* (pp. 147–180). London: Serpents' Tail.

Mirza, H. S., & Joseph, C. (Eds.). (2013). *Black and postcolonial feminisms in new times: Researching educational inequalities*. London: Routledge.

Mohanty, C. (1993). On race and voice: Challenges for liberal education in the 1990s. In B. Thompson & S. Tyagi (Eds.), *Beyond a dream deferred: Multicultural education and the politics of excellence* (pp. 41–65). Minneapolis, MN: University of Minnesota Press.

Moses, Y. T. (1989). *Black women in academe: Issues and strategies*. Washington, DC: Project on the Status and Education of Women, Association of American Colleges.

Ng, R., Staton, P., & Scane, J. (Eds.). (1995). *Anti-racism, feminism, and critical approaches to education*. Westport, CT: Bergin & Garvey.

O'Hair, M. J., & Odell, S. J. (Eds.). (1995). *Educating teachers for lendership and change*. Thousand Oaks, CA: Corwin Press.

Paradies, Y. (2006). A systematic review of empirical research on self-reported racism and health. *International Journal of Epidemiology*, *35*(4), 888–901. Retrieved from http://journals.plos.org/plosone/article?id=10.1371/journal.pone.0138511. Accessed on June 24, 2018.

Paradies, Y., Priest, N., Ben, J., Truong, M., Gupta, A., Pieterse, A., & Gee, G. (2013). Racism as a determinant of health: a protocol for conducting a systematic review and meta-analysis. *Systematic Reviews*, *2*(1), 85.

Parmar, P. (1982). Gender, race and class. Asian women in resistance. In *Centre for contemporary cultural studies* (Ed.), *The Empire Strikes Back. Race and Racism in 70s Britain* (pp. 236–275). London: Hutchinson & Co.

Pendry, N. (2011). The construction of my Black voice. *Black voices. Context*, *117*, 10–12.

Piliawsky, M. (1982). *Exit 13: Oppression and racism in academia*. Boston, MA: South End Press.

Puwar, N. (2004). *Space invaders: Race, gender and bodies out of place*. Oxford: Berg.

Razack, S. (1998). *Looking White people in the eye: Gender, race, and culture in court-rooms and classrooms*. Toronto: University of Toronto Press.

Romero, M. (1997). Class-based, gendered and racialized institutions in higher education: Everyday life of academia from the view of Chicana faculty. *Race, Gender & Class*, *4*(2), 151–173.

San Juan, E. (1992). *Articulations of power in ethnic and racial studies in the United States*. Atlantic Highlands, NJ: Humanities Press.

Sinclair, A. (2007). Leadership for the disillusioned. *Melbourne Review: A Journal of Business and Public Policy*, *3*(1), 65.

Tate, S. A. (2017). How do you feel? Well-being as a deracinated strategic goal in UK universities'. In D. Gabriel & S. A. Tate (Eds.), *Inside the Ivory Tower. Narratives of women of colour surviving and thriving in British Academia* (pp. 54–66). London: UCL IOE Press.

Tobin, M. (1983). *The Black female Ph.D.: Education and career development*. Boston, MA: University Press of America.

Ware, V. (1992). *Beyond the pale*. London: Verso.

Ware, V., & Back, L. (2002). *Out of whiteness: Color, politics, and culture*. Chicago, IL: University of Chicago Press.

Wekker, G. (2016). *White innocence: Paradoxes of colonialism and race*. Duke University Press.

Wilkerson, M. B. (1986). A report on the educational status of Black women during the UN decade of women, 1976-85. In M. Simms & J. Malveaux (Eds.), *Slipping through the cracks* (p. 8536). New Brunswick: Transaction Books.

Williams, D. R., Yu, Y., & Jackson, J. S. (1997). Racial differences in physical and mental health: Socio-economic status, stress and discrimination. *Journal of Health Psychology*, *2*(3), 335–351.

Williams, P. (1991). *The alchemy of race and rights: Diary of a law professor*. Cambridge, MA: Harvard University Press.

Wright, C. (1998). Caught in the crossfire: Reflections of a black female ethnographer. In P. Connolly & B. Troyna (Eds.), *Researching racism in education. Politics, theory and practice* (pp. 67–78). Buckingham: Open University Press.

Yuval-davis, N. (1998). Beyond differences: Women, empowerment and coalition politics. In N. Charles & H. Hintjes (Eds.), *Gender, ethnicity and political ideologies* (pp. 168–189). London: Routledge.

Chapter 3

Racial Battle Fatigue: The Long-Term Effects of Racial Microaggressions on African American Boys and Men

William A. Smith, Rodalyn David and Glory S. Stanton

Introduction

One of the most significant and persistent concerns for African Americans is the effect of racism. African Americans are constantly stressed by the burdens of defending their humanity and existence. Rarely are the diversities and intersectionalities of their humanness considered, as they are forced to respond to how dominant white society sees and treats them: primarily as an inferior racial group. For example, a socially identified African American man might see himself not only at the intersections of race and gender but also at intersections of class, physical impairment, sexuality, phenotype, ethnicity, religion, geographic location, and heritage. Yet, dominant society forces him "back" into a more "simplified" racialized or racialized-gendered identity. Subjectification streamlines the process for classifying African American boys and men as racial/ethnic stereotypes, reinforcing discriminatory practices, and reducing the process to race, the easiest and most common group denominator. The stereotypes of blacks are the most significant global stereotypes there are of any racial/ethnic group. Historically, these global anti-black stereotypes have taken on a unique form in the USA that makes them stand out for various forms of racial antipathy, attacks, subjugation, and even genocide. Additionally, such reductionism activates and strengthens most whites' abilities to acquire psychological, emotional, physiological, economic, cultural, and residential wealth while reinforcing longstanding anti-black stereotypes despite reality. This white racial wealth is cumulative, reusable, and transferable to other whites, much like equity in a home or interest on stocks. According to Harvard psychologists Dr. Chester Pierce (1995), racism (including sexism and gendered racism) disadvantages blacks and other people of color because it adds additional burdens to their STEM: (1) *S*pace or the ability to control the environment in which a racially subjugated group lives, works, learns, and congregates; (2) *T*ime, which is the significant amount of time needed to address or seek redress from racism; (3) *E*nergy, which is the constant redirection of energy to deal with racism; and (4) *M*otion, the inability to move freely throughout society without the fear of danger, discrimination, or death simply because you are black. In the end, much of the conscious activity of targets of racism is spent explaining and utilizing resilient adaptive coping strategies dealing with racism and racial microaggressions/macroaggressions.

My research with my colleagues has focused primarily on racial microaggressions and gendered racism. According to Dr. Derald Wing Sue, a professor of counseling psychology,

> microaggressions are the everyday verbal, nonverbal, and environmental slights, snubs, or insults, whether intentional or unintentional, that communicate hostile, derogatory, or negative messages to target persons based solely upon their marginalized group membership. In many cases, these hidden messages may invalidate the group identity or experiential reality of target persons, demean them on a personal or group level, communicate they are lesser human beings, suggest they do not belong with the majority group, threaten and intimidate, or relegate them to inferior status and treatment. (Sue et al., 2007)

An example of gender microaggressions can be found in my own life experiences. Shortly after arriving in Utah, a state with only a 1.8% African American population, I was constantly followed by the police while driving and pulled over several times. On one occasion, this occurred after a breakfast meeting with a white female colleague. We both were doctoral students in the same program at the University of Illinois at Urbana-Champaign. She had arrived, as a professor, at the University of Utah several years before me, and she wanted to make sure my transition was going well. She met me at a local restaurant. We had a very good conversation about what I should expect in my new department, where we were professors. After our breakfast meeting, as we got up to leave, I asked her whether she had driven to the restaurant. She told me "no" and that she was going to walk back to her house. I offered her a ride home, she accepted and put on her hoodie, covered her head, and we left the restaurant. As we drove the short distance to her house, I noticed a police car with two officers following us. My colleague continued talking, unaware of what was happening behind us. I made sure to drive slower than the maximum speed limit while keeping both of my hands on the steering wheel. Keeping both of your hands on the steering wheel is not just for safety – as a black male, you are taught this strategy so that the police will always see your hands and feel less threatened in case you are stopped. The hope is that by having your hands visible at all times it will lower the police officer's suspicions, and you will not be "accidentally" shot.

As I pulled over to my colleague's house, the police car pulled up behind me. This was when I let my colleague know that we were followed and that the police officer on my side was approaching the car with his gun unholstered at his side, and the police officer on her side had his gun holstered, but with his hand on his gun. As a white woman who had never been stopped for "driving while black," my colleague thought that she could use her "whiteness" to defuse the situation. Without telling me, she jumped out of the car to approach the officers. At that point, I thought they were going to shoot me. She took her hoodie off of her head and asked the officers, "What is the problem?" The police officer on her side said, "Ma'am, are you all right?" Three more times they repeated those words. Finally, my colleague identified both of us as University of Utah professors and said that I was dropping her home. The police officer then said, "Sorry, we noticed that he parked a little far from the curb." My colleague looked down and saw that I was no more than 15 inches from the street curb. We both knew this was a bogus racial stop. It was something for which many years of personal experiences and those of my family and black friends had prepared me.

When we combine lived experiences with additional statistics regarding anti-black forms of discrimination and hatred, we become more aware of how many African American men and boys experience gendered racism, and how often. Gender and implicit bias, discrimination, and microaggressions are the poisons that are being added to the soup of human progress. The artist Joel Parés brilliantly captured in two contrasting photographs of Jefferson Moon, an African American male Harvard graduate,[1] the implicit biases held toward African American men by "some" well-meaning people. These implicit biases can range from the trivial and comical to the viciously criminal. Rarely are African American boys and men seen in the same way that they see themselves and their loved ones know them. Despite our accomplishments, regardless of the schools we attend, even with the income we make, irrespective of how large our house, we are seen and treated as criminals. Out of place. Ignorant. Violent. Lazy. Like a *beast* that must be controlled. Regardless of overwhelming evidence to the contrary, these perceptions have not been abandoned since they were created and justified in the late 1800s. This must be understood as acts of violence.

We have to consider what kind of environment we have created and continue to support when African American boys and men have to use as much, or more, energy fighting racial discrimination and assaults than they do in being intellectually creative in their school work or occupations. African American boys and men experience acute and chronic forms of stress from discriminatory treatment and racial microaggressions in what can be considered hyper-toxic environments. These hyper-toxic environments breed racist pathogens and an increased allostatic load that decrease their biopsychosocial health. Racial microaggressions include a range of racist behaviors impacting people of color on an individual or micro-level. For instance, some racial microaggressions are merciless and mundane exclusionary messages that are meant to make someone uncomfortable in a shared environment, such as a workplace or on a university campus. Other types are meant to "put you in your place," such as being treated as less than fully human to civil and human rights violations. This is why racial microaggressions are crucial to understanding

---

[1] See Joel Parés' photo of Jefferson Moon, Harvard Graduate in the series "Judging America" for visual background (http://www.joelpares.com/judging-america-1).

increases in racial battle fatigue (Smith, 2004). Racial battle fatigue results from the psychological and physiological stress that racially marginalized individuals/groups experience in response to specific race-related interactions between them and the surrounding dominant environment. Racial microaggressions/macroaggressions are those actions that produce race-related stress. These additional and often unanticipated race-related stressors tax and exceed available resilient coping resources that people of color (i.e., African Americans, Asian Americans, Latinas/Latinos/Latinx, Native Americans, Pacific Islanders, and bi- and multiracial people) have available to use and draw upon. Meanwhile, and as a consequence of not having to deal with the cost of racial discrimination, many whites easily build additional or stronger sociocultural and economic environments and resources that shield them from race-based stressors and threats to their unearned racial entitlements. These unearned racial entitlements are produced through a system of racial control based upon an internal colonial structure that keeps people of color in "their place." For African American boys and men and other oppressed people of color, we must understand this race-based internal colonial structure as psychological, social, and emotional environments of violence and control.

What is at stake, here, is the quest for racial equilibrium versus racial disequilibrium in a society that marginalizes human beings into substandard racial groups. Identifying and counteracting the biopsychosocial and behavioral consequences of actual or perceived racism, gendered racism, and racial battle fatigue will continue to be one of the most significant challenges of the twenty-first century. As a term, "racial microaggressions" was introduced in the 1970s to help psychiatrists and psychologists understand the nefariousness and impediments of the understated but constant racial attacks that African Americans face on a daily basis. More than four decades have passed since racial microaggressions were introduced to the academic community. Unfortunately, while more people are beginning to understand what they are, very few understand their impact. The remaining parts of this chapter will focus on the definition, identification, and long-term effects of racial microaggressions and the resultant racial battle fatigue within US environments.

Dr. Chester M. Pierce was a psychiatrist and education professor emeritus at Harvard Medical School. In 1970, he coined the term "racial microaggressions" to help psychiatrists and psychologists understand the enormity and complications of what he classified as racism's "subtle blows," which are "delivered incessantly" at blacks (p. 267). He subcategorized racial microaggressions as part of offensive mechanisms, "which assure that the person in the inferior status is ignored, tyrannized, terrorized, and minimized" (p. 267). Racial microaggressions, then, are subtle attacks or invalidations against individuals because of race or ethnic group membership. Let me pause for a moment to reassure you that the "micro" in racial microaggressions does not mean mini, small, insignificant, or trivial. As in microsociology, microeconomics, microbiology, or microorganisms, racial microaggressions are the microlevel racial pathogens responsible for much health-related sickness and disease in people of color, and as such, should be the target for elimination (Profit, Mino, & Pierce, 2000). Racial microaggressions are those stereotypes and institutionalized "threats in the air" as psychologist

Dr. Claude Steele (1997) describes to the direct individual-level attacks on a racially marginalized person of color.

My colleagues and I (Smith, Yosso, & Solórzano, 2006, 2007) have defined racial microaggressions as (1) subtle verbal and nonverbal insults directed at people of color, often automatically or unconsciously; (2) layered insults, based on one's race, gender, class, sexuality, language, immigration status, phenotype, accent, or surname; and (3) cumulative insults, which cause unnecessary stress to people of color while privileging whites. Sue and his colleagues (Sue et al., 2007; Sue, 2010) have expanded upon our understanding of racial microaggressions to include (1) microinsult, (2) microassault, (3) microinvalidation, and (4) environmental:

- *Microinsult (often unconscious)*: "behavioral/verbal remarks or comments that convey rudeness, insensitivity, and demean a person's racial heritage or identity."
- *Microassault (often conscious)*: "explicit racial derogations characterized primarily by a violent verbal or nonverbal attack meant to hurt the intended victim through name-calling, avoidant behavior or purposeful discriminatory actions."
- *Microinvalidation (often unconscious)*: "verbal comments or behaviors that exclude, negate, or nullify the psychological thoughts, feelings of a person of color."
- *Environmental*: "racial assaults/insults, and invalidations which are manifested on systemic and environmental levels."

Examples of racial microaggressions are racial slights, unfair treatment, hypersurveillance, and personal threats.

Racial microaggressions are all a part of the offensive racist mechanisms. Offensive racist mechanisms ensure African Americans are consistently kept in unbalanced positions, responding to micro- and macrolevel attacks. Racial microoffenses or microaggressions help explain how racism shortens life expectancy in targeted populations. We must understand that the body codes racism as a violent attack. For the targets of racial microaggressions, both stress and violence are noxious stimuli, conditions, or people. As a result, racism can be experienced as both a macrolevel (social) and microlevel (individual) stressor that negatively impacts the psychological, emotional, and physiological health of people of color in the USA (Anderson, 1989; Brondolo, Brady ver Halen, Pencille, Beatty, & Contrada, 2009; Carter & Forsyth, 2010; Pierce, 1970, 1974, 1975a, 1975b, 1988, 1995; Ramos, Jaccard, & Guilamo-Ramos, 2003; Smith, 2004, 2008a, 2008b).

Racial battle fatigue is caused by the constant redirection of energy needed for emergency situations, mainly for psychosocial reasons, to deal with race-related stress. This also compromises resilient coping resources when used for responding to mundane forms of racism. Energy redirection and loss deplete psychological and physiological resources needed for important, creative, and productive areas of life (Smith, 2008b). The cost of racism for African American men must be minimally acknowledged as the deterioration in their quality of life, stunted personal achievements, reduced interpersonal emotional effectiveness, and shortened life spans. These conditions occur from exposure to chronic and pathogenic forms of everyday and generational gendered racism.

Discussion

The cumulative effects of racial microaggressions can be linked to illnesses, shortened life spans, lack of self-confidence, lowered motivation, trouble concentrating, excessive worrying, avoidance, hyper-vigilance, irritability, headaches, diabetes, fatigue, weight gain or loss, rashes, and muscle tension (Anderson, 1989; Smith, 2004, 2008a, 2008b). Microaggressions affect most racially marginalized and oppressed people in the USA and cause stress hormones, designed to deal with acute danger, to operate as if they were in a chronic state of guardedness and threat. The threat can be at racial/ethnic group or racial-gender group levels. Disturbingly, the effects of real and anticipated racial microaggressions are supported within the larger societal structure, particularly in terms of anti-black racial misogyny and anti-black racial misandry.

Racial misogyny justifies and reinforces the subordination and oppression of black women. Offensive anti-black racial misogynistic mechanisms operate to specifically target and marginalize black women (Smith, 2010; Smith, Allen, & Danley, 2007). Again, a classic example of the social structure supporting anti-black racial misogyny and racial battle fatigue is the hyper-policing of black women. Sandra "Sandy" Bland's frustration at what many blacks perceived as an unwarranted police stop and arrest was highlighted in a police video recording in July 2015 in Waller County, Texas. Within days of her arrest, Bland was found hanged in her jail cell. Her death was ruled a suicide, despite public outcries of police-led racial violence against her. Bland had lived in towns in Texas and her home state of Illinois where blacks are up to four and a half times more likely to be stopped for traffic violations than white drivers and more than four times more likely to be searched (Nathan, 2016). This, and many other examples, causes African American women to have increased levels of racial battle fatigue that jeopardize their ability to live healthy and peaceful lives as partners, mothers, sisters, and friends.

Anti-black racial misandry refers to exaggerated pathological aversions toward racially marginalized black boys and men that are reinforced in societal, institutional, and individual ideologies, practices, and behaviors (Smith, 2010; Smith, Yosso, et al., 2007). For instance, despite video evidence, most police officers are acquitted or never charged for the unarmed killing of hundreds of African American men and boys (Hall, Hall, & Perry, 2016). African American boys must learn very early to negotiate a society that devalues their existence regardless of their innocence, age, education, or social-economic standing. Like racial misogyny, racially misandric environments cause African American boys and men to negotiate hostile and often caustic conditions at the expense of unimpeded growth and development. This places them in jeopardy of racial battle fatigue. Obviously, these environmental racial microaggressions impact not only the quality of life for African American men but also their ability to benefit from human capital development through hard work and education. At both the micro- and the macro-level, offensive racist mechanisms – experienced as continuous racial attacks – can lead to racial battle fatigue. There is not enough research on how racial microaggressions operate among oppressed racial groups.

This cannot continue. Available evidence shows that US classrooms from primary school years to graduate school are replete with race-related stress. Work-life and community life are not benign racial environments. Where can African American men, women, and children go where anti-black stereotypes and racism are not omnipresent?

A full understanding of the cost of racism and how it impacts African American boys and men in their pursuit of a healthy and productive life is needed. There are too many health disparities between whites and African Americans. Once offensive racist mechanisms are understood, successful strategies can be developed for reducing racial battle fatigue and promoting a healthier and successful life for African American men and *all* oppressed racial/ethnic groups. Dr. David Williams, a Harvard University social psychologist, has spent his career studying racial disparities and the health of African Americans in the USA (Williams, 1997, 2005; Williams & Collins, 1995, 2001; Williams & Mohammed, 2009, 2013; Williams & Neighbors, 2001; Williams, Neighbors, & Jackson, 2003). His research, among that of many other scholars, has led the discussion to locate the overall research conversation on personal or microlevel forms of discrimination inside the larger research on racism and health (Williams & Mohammed, 2009). Key points by Williams and his colleagues are outlined in the two lists below.

Racism and Health: Mechanisms

- Institutional discrimination can restrict socioeconomic attainment and group differences in social-economic status and health.
- Segregation can create pathogenic residential conditions.
- Discrimination can lead to reduced access to desirable goods and services.
- Internalized racism (acceptance of society's negative characterization) can adversely affect health.
- Racism can create conditions that increase exposure to traditional stressors (e.g., unemployment).
- Experiences of discrimination may be a neglected psychosocial stressor.

Sources: Williams and Mohammed (2009, 2013).

Racial Disparities in Health

- African Americans have higher death rates than whites for 12 of the 15 leading causes of death.
- Blacks and American Indians have higher age-specific death rates than whites from birth through the retirement years.
- People of color get sick sooner, have more severe illness, and die sooner than whites.
- Latinos have higher death rates than whites for diabetes, hypertension, liver cirrhosis, and homicide.

Sources: Williams and Mohammed (2009, 2013).

The takeaway from this research is that almost 100,000 US blacks die prematurely every year, unnecessarily, due to some unaddressed racial disparities in health, and that "there is also the need to more seriously begin to provide targeted relief to individuals suffering from exposure to discrimination" (Williams & Mohammed, 2009, p. 21). We agree with Williams and his colleagues. There is much more progress that needs to be made for all marginalized identity groups regarding health, oppression, and discrimination, in its micro-level and macro-level forms.

For African American boys and men, however, there remains a huge hole and lack of understanding of their unique positionalities, despite the great contributions by scholars such as Chester M. Pierce, Phillip J. Bowman, Walter R. Allen, Claude M. Steele, Norman Anderson, Na'im Akbar, Jim Sidanius, Joe R. Feagin, Lance Williams, Gloria Ladson-Billings, Eduardo Bonilla-Silva, Richard Majors, Fred A. Bonner II, Pedro Noguera, T. Hasan Johnson, J. Luke Wood, Tyrone C. Howard, Tommy J. Curry, Frank Harris III, James L. Moore III, Chance W. Lewis, Ivory Toldson, Shaun R. Harper, Jerlando Jackson, Jeremy D. Franklin, and Brian Burt, to name just a few of the important contributors to this topic. Black males in the USA are a social group that is distinctly different from white males. Therefore, their life experiences in a racist system position them away from the social-economic benefits and privileges that white men and white women receive (Smith, Mustaffa, Jones, Curry, & Allen, 2016). Being a black male means that you will always have to deal with discrimination in your everyday circumstances and your health will become compromised. As a result, we will continue to see reports stating that black men are much more likely to be targets of discrimination than black women. The image of the black male brute, thug, criminal, rapist, and murderer is burned into the American and global psyche. While black men tend to report higher levels of discrimination than black women (Carter, 2007), black women tend to use proactive and resilient coping efforts more often and more effectively than black men (Swim, Hyers, Cohen, Fitzgerald, & Bylsma, 2003). In short, there is much more work that needs to be done in the field of US black male studies, and likewise for black males outside of the USA, so that we can better develop an understanding of the links between race, racism, racial micro-level aggressions, racial macro-level aggressions, and racial battle fatigue for all black boys and men.

Conclusion

Racism does not appear that it will be eliminated within the next half of a century. Researchers must begin more complete investigations concerning how gendered racism, sexual assault, discrimination, systemic racism, institutionalized oppression, poverty, isolation, segregation, and racial microaggressions cause racial battle fatigue in the lives of people of color. These investigations must be undertaken at the racial/ethnic and racial/ethnic/gender levels, inclusive of multiple identities (e.g., age, social-economic class, education, phenotype, urbanicity, sexuality, ability, and language). We must understand commonalities across groups, but also more nuanced ways an oppressive system attacks specific marginalized identities within racialized structures. This represents the most significant gap in our understanding and in our ability to develop effective race-specific defensive mechanisms.

References

Anderson, N. B. (1989). Racial differences in stress-induced cardiovascular reactivity and hypertension: Current status and substantive issues. *Psychological Bulletin, 105*(1), 89–105.

Brondolo, E., Brady ver Halen, N., Pencille, M., Beatty, D., & Contrada, R. (2009). Coping with racism: A selective review of the literature and a theoretical and methodological critique. *Journal of Behavioral Medicine, 32*(1), 64–88.

Carter, R. T. (2007). Racism and psychological and emotional injury: Recognizing and assessing race-based traumatic stress. *The Counseling Psychologist, 35*(1), 13–105.

Carter, R. T., & Forsyth, J. (2010). Reactions to racial discrimination: Emotional stress and help-seeking behaviors. *Psychological Trauma: Theory, Research, Practice, and Policy, 2*(3), 183–191.

Hall, A. V., Hall, E. V., & Perry, J. L. (2016). Black and blue: Exploring racial bias and law enforcement in the killings of unarmed black male civilians. *American Psychologist, 71*(3), 175–186.

Nathan, D. (2016). What happened to Sandra Bland? Retrieved from http://www.thenation.com/article/what-happened-to-sandra-bland/. Accessed on April 28.

Pierce, C. M. (1970). Offensive mechanisms. In F. Barbour (Ed.), *The Black seventies* (pp. 265–282). Boston, MA: Porter Sargent.

Pierce, C. M. (1974). Psychiatric problems of the Black minority. In G. Caplan & S. Arieti (Eds.), *American handbook of psychiatry* (pp. 512–523). New York, NY: Basic Books.

Pierce, C. M. (1975a). The mundane extreme environment and its effect on learning. In S. G. Brainard (Ed.), *Learning disabilities: Issues and recommendations for research* (pp. 111–119). Washington, DC: National Institute of Education, Department of Health, Education, and Welfare.

Pierce, C. M. (1975b). Poverty and racism as they affect children. In I. Berlin (Ed.), *Advocacy for child mental health* (pp. 92–109). New York, NY: Brunner/Mazel.

Pierce, C. M. (1988). Stress in the workplace. In A. F. Coner-Edwards & J. Spurlock (Eds.), *Black families in crisis: The middle class* (pp. 27–35). New York, NY: Brunner/Mazel.

Pierce, C. M. (1995). Stress analogs of racism and sexism: Terrorism, torture, and disaster. In C. Willie, P. Rieker, B. Kramer, & B. Brown (Eds.), *Mental health, racism and sexism* (pp. 277–293). Pittsburgh, PA: University of Pittsburg Press.

Profit, W. E., Mino, I., & Pierce, C. M. (2000). Stress in Blacks. In G. Fink (Ed.), *Encyclopedia of stress* (pp. 324–330). London: Academic Press.

Ramos, B., Jaccard, J., & Guilamo-Ramos, V. (2003). Dual ethnicity and depressive symptoms: Implications of being Black and Latino in the United States. *Hispanic Journal of Behavioral Sciences, 25*(2), 147–173.

Smith, W. A. (2004). Black faculty coping with racial battle fatigue: The campus racial climate in a post-civil rights era. In D. Cleveland (Ed.), *A long way to go: Conversations about race by African American faculty and graduate students* (pp. 171–190). New York, NY: Peter Lang.

Smith, W. A. (2008a). Campus wide climate: Implications for African American students. In L. Tillman (Ed.), *A handbook of African American education* (pp. 297–309). Thousand Oaks, CA: Sage Publications.

Smith, W. A. (2008b). Higher education: Racial battle fatigue. In R. T. Schaefer (Ed.), *Encyclopedia of race, ethnicity, and society* (pp. 615–618). Thousand Oaks, CA: Sage Publications.

Smith, W. A. (2010). Toward an understanding of Black misandric microaggressions and racial battle fatigue in historically White institutions. In V. C. Polite (Ed.), *The state of the African American male in Michigan: A courageous conversation* (pp. 265–277). East Lansing, MI: Michigan State University Press.

Smith, W. A., Allen, W. R., & Danley, L. L. (2007, December). "Assume the position … you fit the description": Campus racial climate and the psychoeducational experiences and racial battle fatigue among African American male college students. *American Behavioral Scientist, 51*(4), 551–578.

Smith, W. A., Mustaffa, J. B., Jones, C., Curry, T. J., & Allen, W. R. (2016, September). 'You make me wanna holler and throw up both my hands!': Campus culture, black misandric microaggressions, and racial battle fatigue. *International Journal of Qualitative Studies in Education, 29*(9), 1189–1209.

Smith, W. A., Yosso, T. J., & Solórzano, D. G. (2006). Challenging racial battle fatigue on historically white campuses: A critical race examination of race-related stress. In C. A. Stanley (Ed.), *Faculty of color teaching in predominantly white colleges and universities* (pp. 299–327). Bolton, MA: Anker Publishing Company, Inc.

Smith, W. A., Yosso, T. J., & Solórzano, D. G. (2007). Racial primes and black misandry on historically white campuses: Toward a critical race accountability in educational administration. *Educational Administration Quarterly, 43*(5), 559–585.

Steele, C. M. (1997). A threat in the air: How stereotypes shape intellectual identity and performance. *American Psychologist, 52*(6), 613.

Sue, D. W. (2010). *Microaggressions in everyday life: Race, gender, and sexual orientation.* Hoboken, NJ: John Wiley & Sons.

Sue, D. W., Capodilupo, C. M., Torino, G. C., Bucceri, J. M., Holder, A. M. B., Nadal, K. L., & Esquilin, M. (2007). Racial microaggressions in everyday life: Implications for clinical practice. *American Psychologist, 62*(4), 271–286.

Swim, J. K., Hyers, L. L., Cohen, L. L., Fitzgerald, D. C., & Bylsma, W. H. (2003). African American college students' experiences with everyday racism: Characteristics of and responses to these incidents. *Journal of Black Psychology, 29*(1), 38–67.

Williams, D. R. (1997). Race and health: Basic questions, emerging directions. *Annals of Epidemiology, 7*(5), 322–333.

Williams, D. R. (2005). The health of U.S. racial and ethnic populations. *Journals of Gerontology: Series B, 60B*(Special Issue II), 53–62.

Williams, D. R., & Collins, C. (1995). U.S. socioeconomic and racial differences in health: Patterns and explanations. *Annual Review of Sociology, 21,* 349–386.

Williams, D. R., & Collins, C. (2001). Racial residential segregation: A fundamental cause of racial disparities in health. *Public Health Reports, 116*(5), 404–416.

Williams, D. R., & Mohammed, S. A. (2009). Discrimination and racial disparities in health: Evidence and needed research. *Journal of Behavioral Medicine, 32*(1), 20.

Williams, D. R., & Mohammed, S. A. (2013). Racism and health I: Pathways and scientific evidence. *American Behavioral Scientist, 57*(8), 1152–1173.

Williams, D. R., & Neighbors, H. (2001). Racism, discrimination and hypertension: Evidence and needed research. *Ethnicity & Disease, 11*(4), 800–816.

Williams, D. R., Neighbors, H. W., & Jackson, J. S. (2003). Racial/ethnic discrimination and health: Findings from community studies. *American Journal of Public Health, 93*(2), 200–208.

Chapter 4

Racism in Academia: (How to) Stay Black, Sane and Proud as the Doctoral Supervisory Relationship Implodes

Sharon Walker

Introduction

This chapter intends to provide a reflexive discussion of the experience I loosely refer to as the 'supervisory relationship breakdown', which led me to withdraw from a Professional Doctorate in the penultimate year of completion. The event left an indelible impact upon me; a reminder of my blackness, the contrast between that and the "ivory tower" of academia. I recount the emotional toil I endured as each incident unfolded, ultimately leading to my exit from the doctorate and the shattering of my mental wellness. The term 'supervisory relationship breakdown' is a superficial reference to my situation that disguises the hidden and complex entanglement of what I deemed to be dysconscious racism and attempts to control the access black people have to academia. I will explore how as a black woman in academia I believe I can be perceived through a dysconscious racial lens, a lens shaped by a dysconscious intention to maintain white privilege. I posit how a misalignment existed between who I am and who I was perceived to be by my doctoral supervisor. The space between this misalignment became filled with inequity, tension and oppression, culminating in the relationship breakdown and the emotional breakdown that I consequently endured. I present an 'implosion' of the relationship as a metaphor for the embodied affect having to withdraw from the doctorate had on me; it felt as though my 'self' – body, mind and spirit – were broken, in a state of collapse which I did not know how I would recover from. However, this is more than an autobiographical account; I am not unique in my experience. In order to set a context for this phenomenon, I discuss the concept of the ivory tower, present statistics on numbers of black people in academia in the UK, the number of PhD non-completers and those with related mental ill health. I explore some of the reasons which researchers have provided for PhD non-completion before discussing the role of the relationship breakdown. I will share the stories of two others, 'Rosie' and 'Peter' whose supervisory relationship led to the non-completion of their PhD. I finish by exploring how we each experienced these events and the coping mechanisms initiated to maintain our mental wellbeing.

The Conceptualisation of the 'Ivory Tower' of Academia

Although the disproportionately high number of black people experiencing mental ill health in the UK general population is well known (Care Quality Commission, 2011), there is less known about the emerging trend of mental ill health amongst black academics. Yet, there have been growing reports into the increase of mental ill health amidst the academic population, particularly students undertaking PhD's (Levecque, Anseel, Beuckelaer, Van der Heyden, & Gisle, 2017). My focus is on the mental health of black people in the ivory tower of academia.

Gullo, Li Volti, and Ristagno (2013) explain the term 'ivory tower' originated from the Bible and later used as a metaphor for institutions where intellectuals, often disconnected from the realities of life, gathered in order to pursue further knowledge. More recently, the ivory tower has been conceptualised as a privileged, closed and protected space. Broadfoot and Munshi (2007) argue that the exclusivity of who enters the ivory tower has resulted in a knowledge base developed from a dominance of rigid structures of exclusivity and superiority which colonises the world of lived experience. Gullo et al. (2013) posits that the 'Ivory Tower can be dangerous in its inherent privatization of knowledge and intellect' (p. 49). The word 'ivory' is itself associated with whiteness; for me this all equates to knowledge developed from a world view of privileged, white, male, middle class, intellectuals – a world view very different to the experiences of those who are often the subjects of research and are not privileged, not white or male; they are 'other' distinct and separate from those who conduct research about them.

There are people from these backgrounds with the intellectual capacity to contribute to knowledge from their *own* world view. One way of contributing to or contesting the knowledge emergent from the ivory tower is to enter it and develop a knowledge base conducted as a doctoral programme of research. Peelo (2011) notes:

> The PhD remains a key credential for an academic career and, as such, the demographics of who is successful in this degree becomes an equal-opportunities issue as it dictates the profile of the future academe. (p. 3)

Yet, there are (visible/invisible) processes designed to select in and out those deemed to be at doctoral standards, these processes serve to maintain the exclusivity within the ivory tower. Broadfoot, Munshi, and Nelson-Marsh (2010) suggests 'scholars also need to question who determines such standards and practices and how these can act as gate-keeping and "othering" practices designed to protect the walls of ivory towers' (p. 7). I am particularly concerned about the experience of black people being exited out of the ivory tower for a number of reasons.

Firstly, I am a black, female academic who has encountered this experience and understand the profound impact it can have, secondly, black people are the most under-represented racial group in academia and most likely to not complete their PhD, thirdly black people suffering with mental ill health are disproportionately represented in the UK community. There is now an emerging trend of black people in academia experiencing mental ill health and not completing their PhD. I refer to 'black people' as those who would identify their origins as black British, black Caribbean or black African as oppose to using the term black minority ethnic (BME) which would include people from Asian backgrounds. Gillborn (2008) notes some scholars use the term 'Black' to include all minority groups subject to white racism. Yet, he contends that this collectivism in research 'can obscure important social, historical, cultural and economic differences between groups' (Gillborn, 2008, p. 2). This is reflected in academic related statistics that identify different levels of attainment and experiences between black and Asian people.

The Under Representation of Black People on the Journey to the Ivory Tower

Prior to achieving the level of academic attainment to commence a PhD, there is an educational journey to navigate through higher education, which black people are disadvantaged on. Noden, Shiner, and Tariq Modood (2014) note that although black people attend university in reasonable numbers, they are disadvantaged by being concentrated in lower status universities. Noden et al. (2014) found black Caribbean and black other candidates were significantly less likely to apply to lower ranking institutions than elite institutions compared with white British candidates. Yet, black candidates were 'significantly less likely to result in an offer than applications from the white British group' (Noden et al., 2014, p. 4).

The UPP Foundation (2017) found that once in university, the drop-out rate was higher for black students, that is, 10.3%, whereas for the English students, the average was 6.9%. They associated this attrition rate to universities with high numbers of black students and black students with parents in lower level occupations. Conversely, the Race Equality Survey (Gabriel, 2014) identified that 20% of black students found the most pressing issue for them was a lack of diverse staff, followed by 16% who said the lack of diversity in the curriculum. Gabriel (2014) posits that even when diverse staff are in post, as a result of internalised racism, there are

> staff of colour who may promote Eurocentric knowledge and culture and place a lesser value on research that explores the experiences of Black, Asian and Oriental peoples and that draws on alternative epistemologies. (p. 13)

Jones (2000) defines internalised racism as 'characterised by their not believing in others who look like them and not believing in themselves' (p. 1213).

Bhopal and Jackson (2013) offer an alternative perspective and argue that staff from BME backgrounds feel the need to develop styles of interacting in culturally specific ways in order to progress. This suggests that some BME staff are taking an assimilationist position whereby they forgo their cultural identity in an attempt to integrate. As such, some black academics may feel the need to re-position who they are and what they teach, 'whitewashing' their own cultural lens. Dillard (2006) discusses the multiple identities black women academics have that help to define who we are. She asserts:

> Like many women scholars of colour, finding balance between, within and among our multiple identity positions in the varying global and local contexts and spheres where we work is a long-standing challenge in our academic lives. (Dillard, 2006, p. x)

To tip this balance by foregrounding a Eurocentric perspective whilst denying ones' own culture does not guarantee inclusion or equality in the ivory tower.

Outsiders in the Ivory Tower

Research in the education sector has ranged from the under representation of BME staff in further education colleges (Commission for Black Staff in Further Education, 2002), the disparity in pay between BME and white staff (Deem & Morley, 2006) to BME staff being overlooked for promotions or not encouraged to apply to posts for progression (The Equality Challenge Unit, 2011). These inequalities have resulted in significantly low numbers of black people represented in academic positions and when they are, it is usually those of lower ranking, sessional or part time work. The Equality Challenge Unit (2015) found BME staff comprised 3.9% of senior managers in UK academia and of those only 0.5% were black (p. 180). When the intersectionality of gender is introduced, they found 7.1% of BME men and 1.8% BME women were professors whilst 7.9% of BME men and 5.9% of BME women were non-professors (Equality Challenge Unit, 2015, p. 278). With such low representations of black staff, it may not be surprising to learn that Bhopal and Jackson (2013) found many BME academics felt like 'outsiders' in their own university ... this feeling of being an outsider resulted in part, experiences of subtle exclusion' (p. ii). Wright, Thompson, and Channer (2007) continued the use of Puwars' terminology referring to black women academics as 'space invaders' and 'out of place' in higher education. Mirza (2006) suggests that feelings of isolation can have negative emotional effects on BME teaching staff. Jones (2006) further states that feelings of isolation not only 'breeds insecurity' but results in BME staff unable to challenge racist experiences and 'militates against the formation of supportive and mentoring networks' amongst BME academics (p. 152). Therefore, the isolation of black staff becomes multi-purposeful in undermining confidence, reducing the ability to challenge racism and increasing the reluctance to join a network that could potentially counteract the isolation.

These feelings are also experienced by black PhD students, often compounded by the challenge of working and studying simultaneously in institutions that have these negative characteristics and have a low representation of other black academics or networks that they may be able to gain support from.

Mental Health within the Ivory Tower

The ivory tower in the UK is becoming a more stressful environment for academics and students of all colours. Cleary (2018) found that while universities compete to attract students to ensure profit margins are gained, academics are forced to work long hours due to increased student cohorts and decreases in the size of teams. Cleary identified academics who reported having more demands on them in terms of teaching, research and income-generating projects, which resulted in their becoming exhausted. For black academics, already on the 'outside', the reluctance to report overwork, stress, or exhaustion is likely to be compounded by existing feelings of isolation and insecurity from being positioned as an outsider by colleagues.

The Higher Education Statistics Agency (HESA, 2017) identified 1,180 students who experienced mental health problems left university early in 2014–2015. HESA highlight this as a 210% increase from 380 students in 2009–2010. There was also a 39% rise in students seeking counselling for depression over the same period. Although it is not known what percentage of these students was black, we do know that there is a higher attrition rate for black students in general. Therefore, it is possible, with the additional pressures that black students' experience, that the attrition rate due to mental health issues may be higher for black students than for students of other ethnicities. Part time doctoral students who are also employed in academia have the combined pressures of the academic work environments and the demands of conducting research whilst producing publications and conference presentations (Goh, Pfeffer, & Zenios, 2015). Levecque et al. (2017) found organisational factors in relation to the job demand and job role, decision-making culture, leadership style and perceptions of a career beyond academia were significantly related to the prevalence of mental ill health amongst PhD students culminating in non-completion of their research (p. 868). The relational aspect identified by Levecque et al. in terms of the leadership style which will impact on the student/supervisor relationship has been noted by others as potentially problematic. Etherington (2004) discusses the PhD supervisor relationship and notes 'the quality of this relationship has been found to be fundamental to completion rates for PhD students more generally across the social sciences (p. 165). This view is supported by evidence from research (Heath, 2002; Ives & Rowley, 2005; Marsh, Rowe, & Martin, 2002; McAlpine & Norton, 2006).

Budd (cited by Etherington, 2004) states 'the {supervisory} relationship remains perhaps the most fraught aspect of post-graduate life' (p. 165). It can become exceptionally fraught if the relationship is built on inaccurate perceptions of each other, particularly if the supervisor is inexperienced, has inadequate or no training and lacks self-awareness. I suggest the relationship is made more complex when the black student has a white supervisor who sees through a lens of dysconscious racism in attempt to maintain the privilege of the ivory tower.

Dysconscious Racism

King (2004) defines dysconscious racism as

> a form of racism that tactically accepts dominant white norms and privileges. It is not the absence of consciousness (i.e. unconscious) but an impaired consciousness or distorted way of thinking about race, as compared to, for example, critical consciousness. (p. 73)

This is different to being perceived through a lens of unconscious or implicit bias whereby the person is unaware of and has no control over their actions or thoughts. Although the Equality Challenge unit (2013) use the term "unconscious bias" to explain inequity in higher education, I am deferring to the dysconscious lens position as this appears to relate most closely to the experiences Rosie, Peter and I had. The consequence of us as black people not completing our doctorate serves to protect the dominant, white privilege of the ivory tower. My concern is that a dysconscious lens results in a misalliance, incongruity and discrepancy between the supervisor and student. This could lend itself to superficial or contentious relationships personified by subtle or overt misunderstandings and miscommunication as the perceiver is thinking, speaking and responding to the dysconscious racial lens rather than the person in front of them. I suggest these were all underlying features in the breakdown of the supervisory relationships, which the three of us had with our supervisors.

As I recount my experience, I need to be clear with the reader that this is *my* perception of events; it is likely that my ex-supervisor will have another. Young (2011) could argue that the misconception of self by the supervisor could prevent her from acknowledging how her power and position is being used to perpetuate the systemic racism in education. Young (2011) identified four categories of racism: the conscious perpetrators, the unconscious perpetrators, the deceived perpetrators/activists and the enlightened perpetrators/activists. Young found that the participants were largely deceived by their social activism and failed to recognise their perpetuation of racism through their practice. As such, some supervisors who perceived themselves to be enlightened activists – as I think my ex-supervisor would – were unconscious perpetuators of racism which could result in their detrimental perception of students through a dysconscious lens. It is also important for me to consider the issue of relational ethics (Ellis, 2007).

This means, keeping in mind as I tell our stories, those who were involved in the events may be identifiable particularly as Peter and I shared the same supervisor and the time, place and circumstances are unique and could only have involved a specific group of people.

Our Stories

Peter and I were on the same programme and had the same supervisor whilst Rosie was a year ahead of us on a different taught doctorate. At the start, I was worried that I did not know as much as the other students about the theoretical approach that underpinned the PhD. Importantly, I did not know that I was creating a narrative about myself as someone uncertain and insecure in my knowledge and my place in academia. I had located myself in the group in a position that reflected where black women invariably find themselves when in the ivory tower; as 'space invaders' and 'out of place'. *I* was saying that *I* did not have a right to occupy the space on the doctoral programme. Perhaps I had dysconsciously taken this stance to recreate the normative hierarchy of privilege in Western Society and the ivory tower. Hill-Collins (1990, p. 77) notes 'African-American women's status as outsiders becomes the point from which other groups define their normality'. This is also true for British black women whether at the bottom of the ivory tower or in the margins of Western society, the position of those at the top or centre becomes normalised and might only change after being continuously challenged and contested – which I clearly was not doing.

When Rosie started her doctoral programme, she stated 'I felt like I was in the out … I don't think they knew how to take me'. Peter recalls when a Scandinavian member of our cohort had a verbal exchange with him:

> *Peter*: 'she took it upon herself to say to me, "Peter, we love you in this group, you are part of the group" and I said "What gives you permission to think you can say that to me? I'm British, you're not, it's me who should be welcoming you"'.

There was a sense that we did not have a right to be present; we had to be *invited* in and given permission to remain. As Puwar, (2004) argued 'While they now exist on the inside, they still do not have an undisputed right to occupy the space'.

Black: The Lens We are Seen Through

Although I had just ended a long career in the Prison Service as a senior manager where I was in the minority as a black woman, I never *felt* my blackness or experienced it in the same way that I did in academia. In academia, my colour was what others seemed to define me by as though no other aspect of myself existed. Peter experienced a similar phenomenon:

> *Peter*: For me, one of the things that I was very much aware of was how race and ethnicity, my race and ethnicity would be referred to and it would be, Well, how do you see things from your perspective as a black person?, and I'm thinking, Why do you have to frame it for me? How do you know what vantage point I might be seeing things from?… I don't want you to be an expert on me. By all means share your formulation of me if you want but when it comes to defining me, I'm quite capable of doing that.

It seems there were assumptions made that the lens Peter and I saw through was a black lens first and foremost. Yet, we were undertaking a professional doctorate;

therefore, it could be assumed that we would see things through the lens of our practice or area of research. Peter went on to say how his supervisor once commented:

> 'It's hardly surprising is it, given what you've been through?' and I thought, 'What are you talking about?'. I'm not being positioned', so I thought, you know, 'I will contest the way you're positioning me but the way I'm gonna contest it is by not engaging with it, I am not going to give it any length, ... I'm thinking 'these are your projections, you are presuming to know what my experience has been like and therefore, you're then using that as if it's a fact'.

T. C. King (1995) identified the distorted lens that she categorised into four projective patterns whereby students perceive black, female academic staff. She suggests that these projections were based on a form of self-deception in the perceiver. These misalignments between the reality of who the black female academic is and what the students perceive her to be, personifies the potential historical, stereotypical and colonial projections that can occur from a dysconscious lens of a supervisors' perception of a supervisee. These projective patterns potentially fed by dysconscious racism may have been at the root of the comments said to Peter. This type of projection becomes dangerous and detrimental to the person perceived, particularly when the perceiver is the supervisor with the power to influence the doctoral journey.

I was unclear how our supervisor perceived me and Peter but I noted a dynamic between them which was tacit, subtle and difficult for me to name, yet I felt race was enshrined in the dynamic:

> *Me speaking to Peter*: There was lots of things that I feel I observed during that time and I think it was these things that kept reminding me, 'you're black', 'you're black', 'you're as black as Peter'! So where does that leave me, Sharon, where does that leave me? Because yeah, what's the difference, if this is what you're seeing {our supervisor} then apart from the gender, what's the difference between us {Peter and I}? There is none.

The Shift in Supervisory Relationships

A range of differences did develop between Peter and I during the first two years of the doctoral programme. I gained a job as a senior lecturer which meant that completing the doctorate had become a condition of my employment. I had also begun to publish articles, another expectation in my role as an academic. One of my supervisors left and I was allocated a woman of dual heritage in her place. Peter and I continued to share the same first supervisor, however our relationship had become particularly fractious:

> *Peter*: I think she got very frustrated because I was saying to her, 'I need more guidance in terms of how to actually write this' and

> I don't think she knew how to offer me guidance, she sent me loads of papers from other people .so I read this stuff and I said to her, 'I still don't quite understand this, can I have some time with you?', she never offered it because I think she actually didn't know how to do it.

There was a shift in my relationship with this supervisor after I secured the job as a senior lecturer in the same department; we were not only supervisor and supervisee but also colleagues. Reamer (2009) notes 'Supervisors should avoid dual relationships that have the potential to interfere with the quality and objectivity of their supervision' (p. 1). My employment in the same department also blurred hierarchical boundaries.

Hill-Collins (1990) suggests 'those individuals who stand on the margins of society clarify its boundaries' (p. 77). Yet, I had moved myself from the bottom/margins of the group and re-positioned myself more centrally and visibly. My transformation from not knowing to knowing, student to teacher, supervisee to colleague, reader to read (in terms of publications) contested the opposing nature of these dualisms. This blurred a range of boundaries that are often purposefully constructed to enable the privileged to feel secure and maintain their positions.

Having a supervisor of dual heritage did not cushion the growing discomfort between me and my first supervisor. We had yet to develop a relationship with each other to build trust, she had never supervised anyone before and had little knowledge of the theory that underpinned the doctorate. Her lack of knowledge and experience worried me; who would hear her voice if she disagreed with my first supervisor?

Questioning the Others' Competence

Peter noted what he perceived to be our supervisor's lack of knowledge and how that might have fed into feelings of insecurity about her position:

> *Peter:* I never took her seriously, I didn't think she knew what she was talking about, I thought I knew more {theoretical} stuff than she did ...
>
> *Me*: You did, you absolutely did ... I tried to hide, the fact that I'd cottoned on that you knew more than she did! Maybe that was part of my downfall as well, {I could not hide it} it's like {the supervisor thought} 'I can't have these people round me that I know that I don't know'... and then my first publication was in the journal she had published in'.
>
> *Peter*: I think that was too much of a threat because for her, there was space only for her.

Litalien and Guay (2015) suggest the level of competence the supervisor perceives the doctoral student to have is the cornerstone of doctoral studies persistence, determining the completion of the PhD. Yet, if the student is perceived as competent and the competence is experienced by the supervisor as a threat, then it can have negative impact on the relationship. Conversely, if the student is perceived as lacking in competence, when there is improvement, the supervisor may have reservations about the authenticity of the work. Rosie experienced this with her first supervisor when she re-submitted a piece of work:

> *Rosie:* She asked 'Is this your work?' ...
>
> *Me:* so basically, she was saying is, 'You can't write, full stop, so if this is a better draft, you didn't write it?'
>
> *Rosie*: Yeah. That's what I felt, yeah, that's what she was saying. I mean I was so humiliated.

This type of mistrust is not unusual, Puwar (2004) argued that when BME academics enter the ivory tower, they are responded to by their white counterparts with suspicion about the authenticity of their credentials. In addition to experiencing this type of scepticism about ones' work, Litalien and Guay (2015) state how the student perceives the supervisors support may be a determining factor of success or failure completing the PhD. Rosie felt unsupported by her supervisor from their very first contact:

> *Rosie:* I wanted her to have something to base the supervision on. So I thought, 'Let me send it to her' {a draft paper} and I sent it and then it came back with like red marks all the way through and then she said, 'Let's meet, this is not on' .... it was like she was writing in gobbledygook, so I thought, 'Let me meet with her' and so we met and went through it and we seemed to be on the same page – but we weren't.

In addition to not receiving the guidance on writing the thesis, Peter also felt that there was a lack of support during a period when a significant incident at his place of work had taken place. In fact, this was when our supervisor referred him to an academic progress panel.

Peter reflected on his feelings at the time:

> *Peter:* 'I really don't need to go through this, it's not being supportive, there is no compassion, there is this punitive stuff and it's almost like my ethnicity is being used, my race is being used to justify why I'm having these difficulties when I know it's got nothing to do with that, what it has to do with is the pressures I'm under {at work} and also I don't want to do what you're asking me to do.'

Changing Research Topic: For Whose Benefit

Peelo (2011) posits how PhD students can be persuaded to change their topic in the interest of the supervisor. Peter's comment that 'I don't want to do what you're asking me to do' is in relation to this:

> *Peter:* I had been misled or I had allowed myself to be misled by {the supervisor} who had said to me, what I was doing was fine and all of a sudden I was being referred {to the academic progress panel} and I'm thinking 'so I'm going to have to start something afresh?' ... She said that my insistence that I wanted to work with kids meant I wasn't ever going to get to where I wanted to get to, that she had advised me to work with the professionals.

In Peter's case, over a year had elapsed before he felt pressured into changing his topic; hence his feeling of being misled. However, Rosie was told to change her topic twice in her first year. The first time was during her initial meeting with her supervisor after receiving negative feedback on her draft paper:

> *Rosie:* 'she dismissed my idea, like "that doesn't exist" ... I let go of that, I said I wanted to talk about sexual exploitation, peer on peer. She dismissed that the peer on peer sexual exploitation was a thing, dismissed it. There was no nurturing of my idea ... I always say, if I'd have published that work, I'd been ahead of my time.

I was at the start of my fourth year when my supervisor suggested I collected new data. I had analysed the data using one method, which was unsuccessful therefore I was looking for an alternative method of analysis. Having new data would not have helped this process; what I needed was a new method. However, when I declined to collect new data, this felt like a defining moment where the relationship with both supervisors was under threat. I felt oppressed and under pressure to agree; the suggestion felt like an instruction that I had refused but purely because it was inherently unsound. Not only was I told to collect new data, I was instructed to stop writing for publication as it was 'distracting me' from writing the thesis. This was incomprehensible for two reasons: firstly, the publications were all intended to contribute to the thesis and secondly, she was aware that as a senior lecturer, there was an expectation that I would publish. These were Peter's observations of that period:

> *Peter:* you were basically doing what needed to be done and you were producing the work, and you were being told not to do that, 'slow down, slow down' and you weren't slowing down and I think that left her feeling like you had almost stolen her thunder, you weren't listening to what she was saying.

Misunderstandings

My supervisor would interchangeably refer to my research as 'reflexivity', 'responsivity' or 'relational'. Perhaps it was her ambiguity about the research focus that lead us to have dialogues that were interlaced with misunderstandings.

Peelo (2011) notes 'Staff–student relations can appear to sit on a continuum of misunderstandings and no matter how well the relationships appear to work they seem rooted in tacit expectations on both sides' (pp. 90–91).

These misunderstandings will be compounded in relationships that are not working well, especially if the student is being viewed through a dysconscious lens. Peter explained how his second supervisor often had to 'act as an interpreter' to clarify what was being said:

> *Peter*: I remember on one occasion, he was quite ... shocked with her because she was saying something different and he said, 'that's not what Peter is saying, Peter is saying this ...'

Peter's relationship with his second supervisor, an Asian man, was much more supportive and clear in their communication. As well as attempting to provide clarification, Peter felt he was like a big brother, cheering him on:

> *Peter*: he would say to me, 'Peter, you can do this' and I'm saying, 'Well, the way she and I don't seem to be connecting makes things difficult' but by then, she had reported me to the academic progress panel ... I think there was something about my disagreeing with her being seen as I was not understanding something".
>
> *Me:* 'I had also got to a point {with that supervisor} where I felt like, 'Okay, one of us is speaking Spanish and one of us is speaking English because there is nothing now that we are talking about where we even understand each other, nothing, there is nothing'.

Rosie also talked about never being 'on the same page' as either of her supervisors:

> *Rosie:* Because every time I tried to clarify, it's like saying to you, 'So what is it you would like?', I wasn't getting a straightforward answer ... I didn't know, I don't know, I just don't know, I just don't know, to this day I don't know what was wrong with it.

The Endings

Rosie's Ending

The end of the doctoral programme for Rosie came at the closing of her first academic year. After being asked to change research topic twice and then having a change of supervisor to someone with no previous experience of supervising a PhD student, Rosie failed an assessed paper:

> *Rosie:* I sent a draft in June which she rubbished and I had to submit it in September, which I did and it failed and it came back with loads of stuff. At that point, we changed supervisor because

she was sick ... I met {the new supervisor} twice, she seemed nicer, I was like 'oh thank God', but she turned out to be a complete bitch. {When I failed I felt} devastated, humiliated, they told me, asked me if I had a learning need because I couldn't write and this is after doing a degree in nursing, a diploma in counselling ... an MSc in CBT and the only thing that saved me is a postgraduate certificate in Leadership that I was doing and at the same time .... If it wasn't for the fact that I had that course, I probably would have, lost all confidence in my ability.

I asked Rosie how the experience made her feel:

Rosie: It made me ashamed. It's not something that I repeat to people, I tell people 'oh I didn't finish, I finished the first year, I didn't go on', I felt ashamed, I felt that somehow it gave a message that I wasn't good enough and I think that fed into a narrative already that I have, when working within a white dominated environment, that you're always fighting. I felt like I didn't know what the obstacles were and they weren't showing me or telling me ... I could have fought it but the reason that I left was I don't know how much of me it would have destroyed. So, I cut my losses and walked away.

Me: you've gone on to do other courses that involve high levels of academic writing, so what is it specifically about a PhD, why you wouldn't go back?

Rosie: The supervisor.

Me: That relationship?

Rosie: Yeah, because that relationship, now I know the importance and also I know that you have to be vulnerable and there was no way I am going to be vulnerable and I'll tell you this now, for me to show vulnerability to anyone they would have to reflect who I am, full stop and none of them do.

Peter's Ending

Peter was at the end of his second academic year feeling misled by his supervisor, who had initially supported his research ideas but then stated he needed to change topic because she thought he would not get ethical approval. Peter was asked to attend a meeting and only subsequently realised it was an academic progress panel, which had the power to decide if you should be withdrawn from the programme. Peter recalled the panel experience:

Peter: 'The supervisor said Peter doesn't seem to be doing the things that I've asked him to do' and this woman said to me, 'What's your response?' and I said 'I'm surprised to be here because I hadn't realised that there were these difficulties but I'm quite happy to hear from you, what you think as the university, given what I'm being accused of'. And then they came up with some points that required some action, I was supposed to produce this, produce that and produce everything else and I thought, 'I know a lot of people who are way behind me ... why am I being persecuted here?'

A review academic progress panel meeting was scheduled to take place some weeks later.

> *Peter:* That's when I dropped out ..., I was then given some tasks to do. My second supervisor then said he would take over {as the first supervisor} and said this is what needs to be done, he is more than happy to help me, so they just swapped roles. I just thought, 'No, I'm not going to bother doing this', so that's why I dropped out ....

Peter was unprepared to continue on the doctoral programme if after two years he would have to change to a research topic he did not want to do. I asked how he felt about having to make this decision:

> *Peter:* I actually thought to myself, 'Why am I putting myself through this?', 'this is becoming too painful, I'm being directed to do things I don't want to do because this isn't something I want to do ... I wasn't as angry because I just thought to myself, I saw this coming'.

I asked Peter how he was able to not feel angry.

Peter went on to explain the learning he took from a black academic who had become angry about his experiences of racism:

> *Peter:* Sometimes when you read some of his stuff, it was like he was being driven crazy. I was always determined that I would not allow any experience to drive me crazy, I was very clear about that, I was thinking, I don't know, nothing is going to drive me crazy whereas for him ... and it's painful, but I could identify with that pain as well. Now, when I experience some racist incidents, I know how to manage them but I don't allow them to affect me, I just see them like you often see the clouds in the sky, I don't confuse the clouds with the sky, I know that it might be cloudy but there is the blue sky beyond the clouds, therefore for me when I experience racism, I just see it as the clouds, I know who I am, I'm not going to allow someone else's opinion of me to influence the way I see myself.

My Ending

When Peter did not return at the start of the third academic year I was devastated. He had become my mentor, my confidant and my support. His leaving shattered my confidence; if someone with his level of knowledge and self-assurance could leave the doctoral programme, then I felt my position was untenable. It was already feeling contested since I began working in the same department as my supervisors. I had the oppressive supervision session with both supervisors where I felt I was instructed to collect new data. I then agreed to send a draft chapter of the thesis to them. The feedback I received was incomprehensible; it exemplified the gravity of misunderstanding between us. About a month later, I received an email from my first supervisor casually asking if I would be on campus to have supervision. Within three email exchanges of trying to arrange a date, my supervisor informed me she was worried about my progress and would be referring me to the academic progress panel. I was horrified. She had not asked me for an update of my progress, which I would have provided. I emailed and said as much. No response. I had no information about the panel or their remit. It was only when I researched into their role, I realised it was the same panel Peter had been referred to. Peter and I were the only two students from our cohort to ever be referred to the panel, despite by that stage others had yet to collect any data or start writing. I wrote a letter to the chair of the panel and my supervisors explaining my shock at the referral, the lack of transparency and the unjust, repressive nature in how the referral was made. I requested a change in supervisory team, which was my entitlement to do. No-one responded. I felt disempowered and oppressed. I attended the panel where my request for a new supervisory team was ignored. I had no voice. In fact, I was instructed to send the same supervisors something explaining my chosen methodology. The panel never specified what format they wanted me to explain my new methodology in. I spent the following weekend at home. I did not get dressed, I hardly ate or slept. I was frantically trying to find a format by which to present my methods. I was terrified that whatever I presented would not be good enough and would be reason for them to withdraw me from the doctoral programme.

The stress so was immense that I went to my doctor and was I signed off sick with depression and anxiety. Still, I organised myself to find black academic support networks to engage with. Hearing stories from other black academics made me determined to fight the system.

I gathered the courage to write a methodology chapter discussing the rationale for the methodology I had chosen and summarised it within a PowerPoint presentation. I sent these to my supervisors and received devastating feedback a few days before the review academic progress panel.

Not only was the feedback condemning but inaccurate; stating that it was only a few paragraphs that told them nothing about the methodology; it was ten thousand-word chapter! They were still commenting on the age of the data; my supervisor evidently continued to be aggrieved that I had not changed the data. I felt physically sick. I knew I would not survive the panel in light of those comments. I could not change the age of the data so I decided to change research focus altogether.

Driven by adrenalin and a high level of anxiety, I spent the next two days and nights before the panel meeting writing a new research proposal and ethical application. I attended the panel whilst signed off sick, sleep deprived with only adrenalin to keep me from falling. My supervisor said that my new area of research did not fit the theoretical underpinning which was central to the doctoral programme. This unilateral decision meant that I would need to move to another department to conduct the research. She added, in light of my referral to the academic progress panel, it was unlikely that any other academic would choose to supervise me. I then reneged and said I would continue with the original research. My supervisor said this was not possible; not only was my data 'old' but my writing was 'barely at Masters' degree level'. I was speechless. I had four Masters' degrees, was at the start of my fourth year of the PhD, with several publications and being told I could not write. I looked up at the ceiling and asked aloud 'how did it come to this?'

I formally withdrew myself from the doctoral programme and resigned from my job. What followed was a period of depression where I mourned the loss of the doctorate, the loss of my voice and the loss of my academic autonomy.

A New Beginning

Unexpectedly, I received an email from a publisher advising me a paper I had submitted some time ago had just been published. I read it with pride. It affirmed that I was capable of writing. It motivated me to secure another job as a senior lecturer with a manager I had previously work with. I also enrolled to complete the PhD by publication with my former manager as my supervisor. With hindsight I realise this was not the best decision considering Reamer (2009) warned against these dual relationships. At the time I believed the history with my manager/supervisor meant he would be supportive of me. However, race and gender issues began to emerge very quickly. He ensured my workload became increasingly demanding whereby it was impossible for me to focus on the doctorate. I became aware that as my manager and supervisor his power to sabotage the PhD was twofold. Once again I had to resign in order to protect my chance to complete the doctorate. Rosie had said she would not engage in a doctoral programme again unless the supervisor reflected who she was. I had to agree.

Ways Forward

In the absence of finding a supervisor where trust has already been established, it is helpful to start with a supervisor who not only has expertise in your area of research but also reflects you, minimising the potential for dysconscious racism which might add to the complexity of the relationship. Students also need to be mindful of the issues of internalised racism, inexperience and power dynamics which can also undermine the relationship. However, often, the student has little choice in whom they are given to supervise them. A supervisory contract could be useful in establishing some expectations and setting boundaries. The relationship should be one of mutual respect for the others experience, knowledge and ability with the supervisor as a supportive guide. There should also be clarity on the role of the second supervisor and to what extent they will be involved. The student should seek support networks both inside the university and externally. Have an understanding of the university systems and regulations in order to avoid having to learn to navigate them during a time of potential stress and worry. Ensure there is a ready established network of support.

Post Script

Despite many challenges, I gained my PhD by publication. The next task was to find a job. My PhD was meant to give me currency, promote my career and secure myself in an established position in the Ivory Tower. I applied for three jobs as a senior lecturer – none were promotions – and each time the job went to a white woman with less experience than me, fewer qualifications and no PhD. This is not unusual as Rollock (2019) noted black female professors experienced 'being over taken by less qualified and less experienced white female colleagues in appointments to new posts and in the promotion process' (p:4). One respondent from Rollock's research argued 'it's not always the person who is the most qualified (...) who is either shortlisted or appointed', that sometimes it is a question of who is perceived to best "fit" in the Department', (p:20). Coincidently, the feedback I received from Human Resources on the third post I was turned down for was that the other candidate was a better "fit". In the meantime, I became an associate lecturer. In doing so, I also became a personification of the inequalities in academia which result in black people gaining jobs of lower ranking, sessional or part time work.

One aspect of the recruitment process which there appears to be little research on is the role that references or recommendations play in influencing prospective employers. If black academics are to request a reference from a manager who perceives them through a dysconcious lens and deems them unworthy of progression, the reference or recommendation will be written with this racialised bias, consequently producing a "racialised reference" (Major, 2020). When I was unsuccessful in my applications, I decided to apply for a job at Cambridge University, one of the most prestigious in England. When my referee received a reference request, she contacted me to ask if it was a hoax. Such was her disbelief that I dared to apply to a high-ranking university or that they would consider employing me. She "joked" and said she should sabotage the reference so that I would continue to do sessional work for her. I did not get the job. I have no idea how influential her reference was in the decision not to pursue my application. However, references are requested because they are a persuasive tool and a racialised reference has the power to persuade employers to keep the doors to the ivory tower shut to anyone unable to maintain its ivoryness.

References

Bhopal, K., & Jackson, J. (2013). *The experiences of black and minority ethnic academics: Multiple identities and career progression.* Southampton: University of Southampton.

Broadfoot, K. J., & Munshi, D. (2007). Diverse voices and alternative rationalities: Imagining forms of postcolonial organizational communication. *Management Communication Quarterly, 21*(2), 249–267.

Broadfoot, K. J., Munshi, D., & Nelson-Marsh, N. (2010). COMMUNEcation: A rhizomatic tale of participatory technology, postcoloniality and professional community. *New Media & Society, 12*(5), 797–812. doi:10.1177/1461444809348880

Care Quality Commission. (2011). Count me in census. Retrieved from http://www.cqc.org.uk/news/releases/care-quality-commission-looks-ahead-last-count-me-census-published. Accessed on March 9, 2017.

Cleary, T. (2018). Social work education and the marketisation of UK universities. *The British Journal of Social Work, 48*(8), 2253–2271. Retrieved from https://doi.org/10.1093/bjsw/bcx158. Assessed on April 8, 2018.

Commission for Black Staff in Further Education. (2002). Challenging racism: Further education leading the way. Retrieved from http://consortium.hud.ac.uk/media/consortiumwebsite/content/documents/projects/equalitydiversity/BlackStaffinFEreport_000.pdf. Accessed on August 30, 2017.

Deem, R., & Morley, L. (2006). Diversity in the academy? Staff perceptions of equality policies in six contemporary higher education institutions. *Policy Futures, 4*(2), 185–202. doi:10.2304/pfie.2006.4.2.185

Dillard, C. B. (2006). *On spiritual strivings: Transforming an African American woman's academic life*. New York, NY: State University of New York Press.

Ellis, C. (2007). Telling secrets, revealing lives relational ethics in research with intimate others. *Qualitative Inquiry, 13*(1), 3–29.

Equality Challenge Unit. (2011). *The experience of black and minority ethnic staff in higher education in England*. London: ECU. Retrieved from http://www.ecu.ac.uk/wp-content/uploads/external/experience-of-bme-staff-in-he-final-report.pdf. Accessed on August 30, 2017.

Equality Challenge Unit. (2013). Unconscious bias and higher education: Literature review. Equality Challenge Unit. Retrieved from http://www.ecu.ac.uk/publications/unconscious-bias-in-higher-education/. Accessed on August 30, 2017.

Equality Challenge Unit. (2015). Equality in higher education: Statistical report 2015, Part 1 staff. Retrieved from http://www.ecu.ac.uk/wp-content/uploads/2015/11/Equality-in-HE-statistical-report-2015-part-1-staff.pdf. Accessed on August 30, 2017.

Etherington, K. (2004). *Becoming a reflexive researcher: Using our selves in research*. London: Jessica Kingsley Publishers.

Gabriel, D. (2014). *Race equality survey*. London: Black British Academics CIC.

Gillborn, D. (2008). *Conspiracy? Racism and education. Understanding race inequality in education*. London: Routledge.

Goh, J., Pfeffer, J., & Zenios, S. (2015). Workplace stressors and health outcomes: Health policy for the workplace. *Behavioural Science Policy, 1*, 43–52.

Gullo, A., Li Volti, G., & Ristagno, G. (2013). New burns and trauma journal celebrating translational research. *Burns & Trauma, 1*(2), 47–50. http://doi.org/10.4103/2321-3868.118922

Heath, T. (2002). A quantitative analysis of PhD students' views of supervision. *Higher Education Research & Development, 21*(1), 41–53.

Higher Education Statistics Agency. (2017). Students and qualifiers. Free Online Statistics. Retrieved from https://www.hesa.ac.uk/stats. Accessed on August 30, 2017.

Hill-Collins, P. (1990). *Black feminist thought: Knowledge, consciousness and the politics of empowerment*. Boston: Unwin Hyman.

Ives, G., & Rowley, G. (2005). Supervisor selection or allocation and continuity of supervision: PhD students' progress and outcomes. *Studies in Higher Education, 30*(5), 535–555.

Jones, C. P. (2000). Levels of racism: A theoretical framework and gardener's tale. *American Journal of Public Health, 90*(8), 1212–1515.
Jones, C. (2006). Falling between the Cracks: What diversity means for black women in higher education. *Policy Futures in Education, 4*(2), 2006.
King, J. (2004). Dysconscious racism, ideology, identity and the miseducation of teachers. In G. Ladson-Billings & D. Gillborn (Eds.), *The Routledge Falmer reader in multicultural education* (pp. 71–83). Abingdon: Routledge Falmer.
King, T. C. (1995). "Witness us in our battles": Four student projections of black female academics. *Journal of Organizational Change Management, 8*(6), 16–25. https://doi.org/10.1108/09534819510100536
Levecque, K., Anseel, F., Beuckelaer, A., Van der Heyden, J., & Gisle, L. (2017). Work organization and mental health problems in PhD students. *Research Policy, 46*(4), 868–879. doi:10.1016/j.respol.2017.02.008
Litalien, D., & Guay, F. (2015). Dropout intentions in PhD studies: A comprehensive model based on interpersonal relationships and motivational resources. *Contemporary Educational Psychology, 41*, 218–231.
Major, R. (2020). "Racialised References" a phrase created in conversation on 17th March 2020.
Marsh, H. W., Rowe, K. J., & Martin, A. (2002). PhD students' evaluations of research supervision. *The Journal of Higher Education, 73*(3), 313–348.
McAlpine, L., & Norton, J. (2006). Reframing out approach to doctoral programs: An integrative framework for action and research. *Higher Education Research & Development, 25*(1), 3–17.
Mirza, H. S. (2006). Transcendence over diversity: Black women in the academy. *Policy Futures in Education, 4*(2), 101–113.
Noden, P., Shiner, M., & Tariq Modood, T. (2014). *Black and minority ethnic access to higher education: A reassessment.* London: School of Economics & Nuffield Foundation. Retrieved from http://www.nuffieldfoundation.org/sites/default/files/files/BMEaccessHE_FINAL.pdf. Accessed on August 30, 2017.
Peelo, M. (2011). *Understanding supervision and the PhD continuum.* London: International Publishing group.
Puwar, N. (2004). Thinking about making a difference. *The British Journal of Politics and International Relations, 6*, 65–80. doi:10.1111/j.1467-856X.2004.00127.x
Puwar, N. (2004). *Space invaders: race, gender and bodies out of place.* New York, NY: Berg Publishers.
Reamer F. G. (2009). Boundaries in supervision. *Social Work Today, 9*(1), 1.
Rollock, N. (2019). Staying Power *The career experiences and strategies of UK Black female professors.* University and College Union: London.
UPP Foundation. (2017). Students from lower socio-economic groups. Retrieved from http://upp-foundation.org/wp-content/uploads/2017/07/1743-SMF-Foundation-Booklet-Digital.pdf. Accessed on May 30, 2017.
Wright, C., Thompson, S., & Channer, Y. (2007). Out of place: Black women academics in British universities. *Women's History Review, 16*(2), 145–167.
Young. (2011). The four personae of racism educators' (mis)understanding of individual vs. systemic racism. Retrieved from https://www.researchgate.net/publication/258198491_The_Four_Personae_of_Racism_Educators'_MisUnderstanding_of_Individual_Vs_Systemic_Racism. Accessed on August 30, 2017.

Chapter 5

Implicit Provider Bias and its Implications for Black/African American Mental Health

Andra D. Rivers Johnson

Introduction

Mental health is a public health issue that warrants special consideration, particularly among Blacks/African Americans who tend to suffer from mental health issues and disorders at the same rates as compared to their white counterparts, but whose mental health disparity outpaces their counterparts. According to the research, millions of Americans are affected by the health gap (Spencer et al., 2018). Issues associated with this mental health gap problem include lack of affordability related to insurance premiums, copayments, coinsurance, medications, provider service delivery, lack of quality health care, lack of advocacy, and lack of access to specialty care services, which include mental health (Spencer et al., 2018).

Lack of insurance coverage for mental health services has been an issue of concern in the Black/African American community. Many in this community are unemployed, underemployed, or intermittently employed and usually, their employers do not offer healthcare insurance. Also, insurance alone does not eliminate the disparity related to mental health care access by Black/African Americans (U.S. Department of Health & Human Services, 2001). As a fact, despite millions of previously uninsured Black/African Americans gaining access to health coverage under the Affordable Care Act 2010, millions of Black/African Americans continue to lack health insurance or adequate coverage for mental health care (Rhett-Mariscal, 2008).

According to Mental Health America (2013), Black/African Americans tend to experience more severe forms of mental health conditions due to unmet needs related to barriers such as institutional racism. The research indicates that Black/African Americans are 20% more likely to experience serious mental health problems than the general population (U.S. Department of Health & Human Services, 2001). Commonly experienced mental health issues and disorders in the Black/African American community include major depression, attention deficit-hyperactivity disorder, Black/African American male suicide, and posttraumatic stress disorder related to being victims of crime (Mental Health America, 2013). This writer believes that Black/African Americans also suffer from posttraumatic stress disorder related to the history, legacies, institutional racism, slavery, and domestic terrorism that have adversely impacted the Black/African American community.

Implicit Provider Bias and Black/African American Mental Health

The role of implicit provider bias is crucial to consider in the mental health gap, mental health disparities, and inequity in mental health care that Black/African Americans with mental health issues and disorders experience. Researchers are mindful that provider bias among mental health professionals exists, whether it is conscious or unconscious bias from providers toward Blacks/African Americans (Clark, 2003; Devine, Forscher, Austin, & Cox, 2012; FitzGerald & Hurst, 2017; Mental Health America, 2013; Rice et al., 1982; Snowden, 2003; Storrs, 2016; The Joint Commission, 2016; van Ryn et al., 2011; White, 2011). The research also highlights the fact that Blacks/African Americans and Black/African American women are more likely to complain of somatic symptoms related to depression, while Black/African American men are disproportionately misdiagnosed as schizophrenic when they are complaining of somatic symptoms related to posttraumatic stress disorder (Brown et al., 2000; Mental Health America, 2013).

Implicit provider bias has adverse implications on practice. It affects the quality of mental health care, including the formation, coordination, and completion of assessments and evaluations with Blacks/African Americans who have mental health concerns and disorders (American Psychological Association, 2016; Breathett, 2018; Hairston, Gibbs, Wong, & Jordan, 2019). Treatment plans that do not consider cultural, individual, and group experiences may not accurately reflect the needs and goals of Black/African American clients due to the underlying issues related to implicit provider bias, namely problems related to racism, prejudicial attitudes, and negative stereotypes about Blacks/African Americans that are learned, misinformed, and harmful to Black/African American clients.

The correlation between implicit provider bias and the lack of mental health service and quality care continues to be prevalent for Black/African Americans who need mental health intervention. The mental health disparity experienced by Black/African Americans is pervasive and illustrated by the lack of access to mental health services, identification, diagnosis of mental health concerns, lack of quality of care, lack of education about risk and management of mental health disorders, and stigma associated with mental illness. Implicit provider bias influences whether to make a clinical decision to engage with a prospective Black/African American client, and it impacts on the provider's choice of which assessment, evaluation, and testing instruments to use, and questions that are asked during clinical encounters with Black/African American clients (American Psychological Association, 2016; FitzGerald & Hurst, 2017; Hairston et al., 2019; Kugelmass, 2016).

Implicit provider bias with Black/African American clients is underlined with racial beliefs, negative attitudes, stereotypical language, and stigma during the clinical interview, evaluation, and ongoing encounters that are harmful to Black/African American clients (Brown et al., 2000; Johnson, 2017; Taylor, 2019; Washington, 2006). It affects the quality of assessment, can lead to misdiagnosis, development of a poorly constructed treatment plan, inadequate case coordination, inappropriate management of medication, and inadequate discharge planning (Cannon & Locke, 1977; Phelan, Atunah-Jay, & van Ryn, 2019; Sacks, 2017, 2019; Snowden, 2003; Taylor, 2019; Wolsiefer & Stone, 2019). The Joint Commission (2016) defines implicit provider bias as mental residue and purports that once providers align with racial distortions, discrimination, and/or prejudicial attitudes about Black/African Americans it is usually challenging to unlearn or to change even when there is contradictory evidence to implicit bias. By not being aware of one's own unconscious bias, the provider runs the risk of ethically harming Black/African American clients, engaging in medical malpractice, and misalignment with best practices or the Hippocratic Oath (The Joint Commission, 2016).

Implicit provider bias in mental health with the Black/African American community is prevalent (American Psychological Association, 2016; Clark, 2003; Dana, 2002; FitzGerald & Hurst, 2017; White, 2011; Snowden, 2003; The Joint Commission, 2016; Washington, 2006; Williams & Williams-Morris, 2000). This phenomenon is considered normative behavior with Black/African Americans who have mental health issues and disorders but who lacks access to care due to implicit provider bias. Implicit provider bias adversely influences the mental health gap, mental health disparity, and produces poor mental health outcomes among Blacks/African Americans as members of this community receive less patient-centered care when mental health professionals with implicit bias implications do not accept Black/African American clients and turn them away when they present with mental health symptoms, misdiagnose them, or unconsciously blame Blacks/African Americans for their socio-economic condition, and believe that Black/African American emotional pain differs from that of their white counterparts (Brown et al., 2000).

Implicit provider bias toward Blacks/African Americans exists in mental health as Blacks/African Americans lack access to mental health services and support (Clark et al., 1994). Normative implicit provider bias toward Blacks/African Americans stems from racism and the legacies of slavery and segregation. Washington (2006) points out that white supremacy in the form of institutional racism allows for Blacks/African Americans to receive more inferior treatment than their white counterparts and that this disparity dates to the days of slavery with a continuation into the twenty-first century American health care. The researcher argues that the legacy of American slavery has contributed to the perception that implicit provider bias among healthcare professionals toward Blacks/African Americans is the norm in the American healthcare industry (Washington, 2006). Provider bias is embedded in the historical and contemporary American psyche and rooted in racism (Washington, 2006).

Washington (2006) recounts that during the time of slavery, enslaved African Americans were not seen as human, were forced to have unnecessary surgeries at the requests of slave owners and in the name of medical advancement as African Americans were treated inhumanely and tortured. The reporting shows how enslaved African Americans were used as guinea pigs in medical experiments abused and systematically sterilized through forced surgeries that were for the benefit of slave owners. She concludes that the legacy of slavery has influenced implicit provider bias decisions which lead to providing African Americans with lower quality of care (Washington, 2006). The researcher also points out that at the end of slavery, African Americans were exposed to over 100 years of de jure segregation and de facto laws that were enacted to promote white supremacy and relegate African Americans to second class citizenship and inadequate or nonexistent health care (Edupedia, 2018; Washington, 2006).

Social Determinants of Health and Black/African American Mental Health

The overall health gap creates disparities in mental health treatment opportunities. Kohn, Levav, Saraceno, Saxena, and Kohn (2004), suggest that many have psychiatric disorders that continue to remain untreated despite the existence of effective treatments that are now available. In their examination of the community-based psychiatric epidemiology studies, Kohn et al. (2004) reviewed the use of standardized diagnostic instruments and related data on the percentage of individuals receiving care for mental health issues to understand the phenomenon related to mental health gaps in service.

The Institute of Medicine (2003) defines health disparities as solely racial and ethnic and not due to access to care issues, clinical considerations, or clinical preferences. Social determinants of health must be considered to gain more understanding of the root causes of the mental health gap that is experienced by Black/African Americans. Social determinants of health which determines who gets health care and what type of health care include criteria, such as race, ethnicity, gender, employment, income, education, neighborhood, zip code, food, water, language, immigration status, religion, biology, risk for disease and disability, and health care (Gracia, 2015; Johnson, 2017; Marmot, 2017).

According to Marmot (2017), social determinants of health are a reflection of social and economic injustice. Social determinants of health create health disparities, influence health inequity, and widen the mental health gap between rich and poor Americans based on race. The underlying principle of social determinants of health is health inequity, suggesting that there is a need to eradicate the social determinants of health while simultaneously advocating for health equity and for the fundamental human right for all to have health care, including that of marginalized, low-income, at risk, and communities of color who have the fundamental right to health care (Braveman & Gottlieb, 2014; Marmot, 2017).

Social determinants of health also play a role in the prevalence and practice of implicit provider bias with Blacks/African Americans who have mental health issues and disorders. The research highlights how implicit provider bias adversely impacts the quality of assessment, supports the use of culturally insensitive diagnostic tools, employs poor intervention strategies, enables the development of inadequate treatment plans, suggests difficulty with case coordination and poor referrals, disrupts the course of treatment with premature discharge planning, and results in poor mental health outcomes with Black/African American clients (Braveman & Gottlieb, 2014; Garcia, 2015; Hairston et al., 2019; Johnson, 2017; Neighbors, 1990; Sacks, 2019).

The high incidence of poverty among American Black/African Americans is apparent. According to the American Psychological Association (2016), 22% out of 34 million people who identify as Black/African American or African American live in poverty and are at risk for mental health issues and disorders, as well as for receiving substantially less treatment than their white counterparts. Given the phenomenon, it is, therefore, reasonable to assume that racial disparities continue to be evident in lack of access, identification, diagnosis, testing, education, and treatment of mental illness in the Black/African American community. The argument for mental health equity is therefore made and must be grounded in eradicating the underlying causes of health disparities and health inequity.

Barriers to Mental Health in the Black/African American Community

There is general agreement that the health gap exists in both urban and rural communities, and this is also true for mental health as well (Gabow, 2016). For this chapter, the barrier that is related to implicit provider bias perpetuates the gap that exists for Black/African Americans with mental health issues and disorders and adversely affects the Black/African American community as it responds to systemic racism and discrimination. According to the American Psychiatric Association (2013), Black/African Americans experience rates of mental illness that are like that of the general population. The difference is the disparities related to mental healthcare services to Blacks/African Americans, and the role of provider bias as gatekeepers to poor quality of mental healthcare services and care is generally not culturally competent (American Psychiatric Association, 2013).

Access to mental health services by Blacks/African Americans is limited and implicit provider bias serves as an institutional barrier to mental health and quality care for Black/African Americans who have mental health issues and disorders. Additional obstacles to psychiatric health care for Black/African Americans include distrust of the healthcare system, lack of mental health providers from diverse racial and ethnic backgrounds, lack of culturally competent mental health providers, and the stigma that is associated with mental illness (American Psychiatric Association, 2013; American Psychological Association, 2016; Cannon & Locke, 1977; Kugelmass, 2016; Mental Health America, 2013; Starfield, 2011; Taylor, 2019). Further, the lack of access to mental health care can be seen by the low numbers of Blacks/African Americans who receive mental health care. For instance, the research finds that only one in three Black/African Americans who need mental health services receive care and that Blacks/African Americans have lower rates of mental health services and medication intervention, but the highest rates of admission to inpatient psychiatric services (American Psychiatric Association, 2013).

Review of the Literature

The American Psychiatric Association (2013) reports that compared with their white counterparts, barriers to mental health care and mental health disparity occur when Black/African Americans are less likely to be offered evidence-based medication therapy or psychotherapy. Instead, the research argues that Black/African Americans are more likely to be incarcerated for mental health conditions such as schizophrenia and bipolar disorder, among other chronic mental illnesses than their white counterparts. Also, differences exist in how Black/African Americans' specific symptoms of emotional distress and how this difference contribute to provider misdiagnosis (American Psychiatric Association, 2013). In another study, the research highlights differences in the communication styles and language used by Black/African Americans and whites during clinical encounters, where physicians were 23% more verbally dominant and engaged in 33% less patient-centered communication with Black/African American patients than with white patients who present with the same symptoms (American Psychiatric Association, 2013).

According to Snowden (2003), there are differences between implicit and explicit bias due to the way these biases manifest in providers. Implicit bias is unique because it presents itself on an unconscious level and can go undetected and unchecked among practitioners at all levels of health care. Addressing implicit provider bias is essential, he argues, because it is particularly harmful and can have devastating effects on Black/African American mental health and related health outcomes. Snowden (2003) believes that implicit provider bias plays an essential role in the decision-making process that affects whether to identify, assess, intervene, and treat the mental health needs of the Black/African American community.

As a result, Snowden (2003) concludes that mental health administrators and providers make unwarranted judgments about people based on race and ethnicity. However, at the same time, the researcher pushes back on critics while contending that considering racial and ethnic differences does not in itself count as provider bias. There is agreement that appropriate mental health treatment includes considering cultural beliefs and sensitivities to customize one's treatment (Snowden, 2003). The researcher maintains that it is necessary to be aware of critical differences such as race and ethnicity when providing care because to ignore these vital factors reflects a kind of bias (Snowden, 2003).

The Joint Commission (2016) maintains that implicit bias is rooted in unconscious awareness that leads to the negative evaluation of a person based on race and gender. In their study about implicit bias, The Joint Commission (2016) reviewed 27 studies that examined racial/ethnic preferences. They found that 35 articles showed evidence of implicit bias in healthcare professionals, noting that there was a significant positive relationship between the level of implicit bias and lower quality of care (The Joint Commission, 2016). Understanding that implicit provider bias is a learned behavior at an early age is gaining more traction in the research.

According to The Joint Commission (2016), children chronically and systematically confront racial stereotypes and prejudices about Blacks/African Americans that reinforce throughout every aspect of society and promote ethnocentrism and inequity. It is argued that a predictable outcome of early instruction about Blacks/African Americans and race is the activation of implicit pro-white bias which occurs among children starting between the ages of three and five who learn, through repeated reinforcement of stereotypes associated with Blacks/African Americans, to perceive and to judge Blacks/African Americans solely by the values and standards of the white culture (The Joint Commission, 2016).

To drive this point home, The Joint Commission (2016) found that between October 1998 and October 2006, more than 4.5 million people completed a computerized Implicit Association Test which found that implicit bias is pervasive, although people may differ in their level of implicit bias. This instrument testing bias has also been administered in many healthcare organizations and has significant pro-white bias findings among physicians (The Joint Commission, 2016).

Provider bias has implications for the type of care that Blacks/African Americans receive compared to whites. According to van Ryn et al. (2011), Black/African Americans receive lower quality medical care than whites related to a phenomenon that is independent of disease status, setting, insurance, and other clinically relevant factors. Since little progress toward eradicating mental healthcare inequities are experienced by Black/African Americans, investigators developed a conceptual model which identifies mechanisms through which the provider's cognition, behavior, and decision-making are influenced by racial biases and stereotypes (van Ryn et al., 2011). The findings indicate that biases of white providers persist both independently of and in contrast to their explicitly conscious racial attitudes and that their implicit bias influences and adversely impacts their clinical decision-making and behavior during encounters with Black/African American clients (van Ryn et al., 2011).

In another study, FitzGerald and Hurst (2017) examined implicit bias toward Black/African American patients and found that there is a significant provider bias among healthcare professionals that exhibit at the same levels as the general population. The research team reviewed published peer-reviewed articles and papers and found that 25 articles that focused on a subject design using vignettes show the influence of the patient's physical characteristics on the healthcare professional's attitudes, diagnoses, and treatment decisions. They also found that 27 studies out of 42 items reviewed examined racial evidence of implicit racial bias in healthcare professionals and that 35 articles had a significant positive relationship between the level of implicit bias and lower quality of care (FitzGerald & Hurst, 2017). Besides highlighting the need for more research in actual care settings, the investigators recommend that healthcare professionals address the role of implicit bias in healthcare disparities (FitzGerald & Hurst, 2017).

Storrs (2016) reports that approximately 30% of middle-class Black/African American women and 60% of Black/African American men are less likely than their white counterparts to hear back from a therapist agreeing to see them. In her story for CNN, Storrs 2016) observes that Black/African American and working class people are less likely to find mental health therapists who will see them. The researcher cites a New York study where hired actors were portrayed to record 640 voice messages to therapists who never returned their calls for an appointment and who said they had no openings when they did return the calls (Storrs, 2016).

During this study, the actors read scripts where they said they had symptoms of depression, reported that they had health insurance, inquired about making an appointment for mental health, and asked for a return call to schedule an initial meeting (Kugelmass, 2016; Storrs, 2016). Therapists did not return the calls from Black/African Americans who sounded like working class people (Kugelmass, 2016; Storrs, 2016). According to the research, the return call rate among the therapists was in general low at 44%, and only 15% of those returned calls resulted in a mental health therapist offering an appointment time (Storrs, 2016). At the same time, findings indicate that overall, only 28% of the middle-class whites seeking mental health care were offered an appointment as compared with just 17% of the middle-class Black/African American prospective clients and 8% of the working class Black/African American and potential white clients (Storrs, 2016). These findings suggest for more exploration about the correlation between the effect of racial stereotypes, implicit provider bias, and their willingness to see Black/African American patients.

Fadus, Odunsi, and Squeglia (2019) studied the response of medical residents when presenting cases to emergency room doctors for patients who arrived at the hospital by ambulance due to symptoms of psychosis. The investigators found that when the medical residents showed the cases, they identified one of the patients as a 32-year-old and the other patient as a 25-year-old Black/African American male (Fadus et al., 2019). Racial identifiers are not attached to the case presentation of the non-Black/African American patient and the belief that racial differences in case presentation of psychiatric patients influenced the course of treatment (Fadus et al., 2019).

Neighbors (1990) takes the position that Blacks/African Americans are the casualties of mental health disparity. He argues that there is a need to take the mental health concerns and disorders in the Black/African American community seriously due to the high incidence of professional intervention that is warranted, as Blacks/African Americans are not being assessed, evaluated, nor given treatment due to the mental health disparity related to implicit provider bias (Neighbors, 1990). Furthermore, the researcher focuses on implications related to new provider bias that speak specifically to prior Black/African American experiences with historical misdiagnoses, inadequate treatment, and a lack of cultural understanding when working with Blacks/African Americans who have mental health concerns and disorders (Neighbors, 1990).

Some reports indicate that Blacks/African Americans are more likely to live with mental health problems, experiencing depression, anxiety, and high levels of stress for which they delay or decide not to seek treatment. Hamm (2014) exposes the high rates of depression among Black/African American women but low rates of mental health treatment, suggesting that when using services, it is inadequate in meeting their needs. The Center for Disease Control finds that 7.6% of Black/African Americans sought treatment for depression compared to 13.6% of the general population (Hamm, 2014). Accordingly, Blacks/African Americans experience major depression at a higher rate compared to the general population, yet Black/African American women are underrepresented in mental health care (Hamm, 2014).

To determine if particular sensitivity exists for Black/African American women suffering from depression, Barbee (1992) reviewed the literature on Black/

African American women and depression. The review critiqued major scales that were used to assess depression (Barbee, 1992). An interactive approach to risk factors for depression in Black/African American women provides a better basis for psychiatric nursing practice with this population (Barbee, 1992).

Brewer et al. (2013) present findings related to lack of patient-centered care with Blacks/African Americans. The research indicates that Blacks/African Americans tend to receive shorter visits, less psychosocial, and rapport building with providers and as a result, they receive neither adequate mental health counseling nor education about their illness or mental health management options and strategies (Brewer et al., 2013). The investigators conclude that Blacks/African Americans leave encounters without a full understanding of the need to continue with their mental health care.

Black/African Americans with mental health issues and disorders tend to display symptoms that are either underlying a specific mental disease or another health problem. For example, the U.S. Department of Health and Human Services (2001) suggests that symptoms of depression among Blacks/African Americans associated with increased risk of hypertension and that the prevalence of somatization appears high with this population. Reports of somatization occur at a rate of 15% among Blacks/African Americans and only 9% among whites, and that somatization symptoms may serve as the vehicle or segue by which they express psychiatric symptoms (U.S. Department of Health & Human Services, 2001). Studies show rates of suicide have increased in the Black/African American community, as during the last 15 years, suicide rates have increased 233% among Blacks/African Americans ages 10–14 compared to 120% among white in the same age group across the same span of time (National Association on Mental Illness, 2011; U.S. Department of Health and Human Services, 2001; Office of the Surgeon General. 2001).

Based on the Black/African American experience in America, there is a long-standing debate about whether being Black/African American in America is detrimental to one's mental health. Cannon (1977) argues that it is not the color of the skin, but the stressful social situations that come with being Black/African American. Finally, the researcher concludes that other effects of racism also contribute to the high prevalence of mental illness in the Black/African American community.

Helman (2007) believes that culture is the primary influence on people's lives, including their beliefs, behaviors, perceptions, and attitudes to mental health. In alignment with this perspective for closing the mental health gap involves breaking down barriers between mental health providers and the communities in which they serve (Helman, 2007). Also, Helman (2007) suggests that it is essential for providers to understand the heterogeneity within the culture they help to gain insight to get to know who they serve and gain cultural proficiency with that community. By engaging in this cross-cultural process, providers are taking a vital step toward identifying and confronting their own provider bias related to serving Blacks/African Americans with mental health issues. The need for this cross-cultural process and cultural proficiency development is critical to working effectively with this specific population, given that 55% of people who identified themselves as Black/African American living in the South, 18% in the Midwest, 17% in the Northeast, and 10% in the West (Black/African Americandemographics.com, 2017; U.S. Census Bureau, 2019).

Despite the growth in research about Black/African American mental health, there continues to be limited data on how racism affects Black/African American mental health in the United States. Researchers Williams and Williams-Morris (2000) assert that racism can lead to impairment in functioning on the part of some Blacks/African Americans who might accept the stigma of inferiority. It has been suggested that negative racial stereotypes and beliefs are incorporated into societal policies and institutions and can adversely affect Black/African American mental health (Williams & Williams-Morris, 2000). The researchers emphasize that mental health stressors experienced by Blacks/African Americans directly impacted by experiences with discrimination that activate physiological and psychological reactions. Finally, they illustrate how the scientific evidence shows that racism in societal institutions can lead to adverse outcomes for Black/African Americans, including truncated socioeconomic mobility, differential access to community and financial resources, and poor living conditions that can adversely affect Black/African American mental health.

Clark et al. (1994) suggest that there continues to be resistance to full equality of Blacks/African Americans by whites, although some improvements since the 1960s. The researchers provide a more in-depth analysis of the beliefs, attitudes, arrangements, and acts of how racism is manifested by those held by members of the same ethnic intergroup and those members of intragroup dynamics (Clark et al., 1994). The researchers support the notion that racism is a stressor for Blacks/African Americans, concluding that both intergroup and intragroup racism permeate the Black/African American psyche (Clark et al., 1994).

The Epidemiologic Catchment Area Study, a longitudinal study considered to be the most extensive mental health study with over 20,000 adults participating, interviewed these subjects from five research sites and used the Diagnostic Interview Schedule (Belle, 1990). Psychiatric epidemiology tends to center on the relationship between poverty and mental health. Belle (1990) contends that psychopathology is at least two and a half times and more prevalent in the lowest social class than in the highest. Her review of the positive association between poverty and mental health ties together the consistent documentation on the association between low-income and low-socioeconomic and mental health risks. She concludes that it is vital to pay attention to the mental health risks that accompany poverty because those from minority groups who are experiencing hardship are at high risk for mental health issues (Belle, 1990).

Psychosocial Issues Affecting Black/African American Mental Health

As resilient members of society, Blacks/African Americans have psychosocial issues and needs that require particular sensitivity from culturally competent providers of mental health services. Without knowledge and understanding of the Black/African American experience, providers cannot appreciate the mental health issues of Black/African American resilience in the face of institutionalized racism. From a strengths-based perspective, the legacy of slavery, institutional racism, and discrimination, along with collective group support, has influenced the resilience and survival of many Blacks/African Americans and despite the insurmountable odds; many have been able to do well (U.S. Department of Health and Human Services, 2001), Office of the Surgeon General (2001).

Institutional racism is systemic, impacts on the mental health of the Black/African American community (Williams & Williams-Morris, 2000). The systemic conditions related to institutional racism creates problems that leave Blacks/African Americans feeling personally vulnerable with little to no control over their environment. Some Blacks/African Americans struggle with issues related to racial identity, group pride, self-perception, and self-esteem (American Psychological Association, 2016; Assari et al., 2017; Breathett, 2018; Cannon, 2004; Clark, 2003; Johnson, 2017; Sacks, 2017, 2019; Washington, 2006; Williams & Williams-Morris, 2000; Wolsiefer & Stone, 2019). Black/African American racial identity, including self-perception and self-esteem, is one of the unique needs that require provider sensitivity and cultural competence when working with Blacks/African Americans who have mental health issues and disorders.

Blacks/African Americans have been the scapegoat of institutional racism, oppression, and discrimination as they have had to regularly and chronically engage in the rejection of negative messages, images, stereotypes, discrimination, and attacks on their Black/African American identities and self-concepts (Williams & Williams-Morris, 2000). It stands to reason that this constant and chronic engagement to reject the negative messages and stereotypes about Black/African Americanness is a lifelong process. The investigators suggest that for some, the stress can hurt their mental health (Johnson, 2017; Sacks, 2017; Whatley, 2010; William & Williams-Morris, 2000).

Psychosocial issues that affect Blacks/African Americans and that increase their risk for mental health issues include poverty, homelessness, housing discrimination, and exposure to violence and incarceration (National Alliance to End Homelessness, 2019). The risk factors for developing mental health issues in the Black/African American community increase as Blacks/African Americans make up to 40% of the homeless population in the United States despite being 14% of the overall population (Mental Health America, 2013; National Alliance to End Homelessness, 2019). According to both National Alliance to End Homelessness (2019) and the U.S. Department of Health and Human Services (2001), evidence of historical and institutional racism in housing is prevalent as the majority of Blacks/African Americans reside in segregated, low-income, and low-resource neighborhoods. Many are more likely to live in households with incomes below poverty levels. Upon review of these findings, the U.S. Department of Health and Human Services (2001) acknowledges that many of the same socioeconomic conditions exist for Blacks/African Americans today, as indicated in the twentieth century.

The research indicates that there is a correlation between high exposure of violence and mental health (American Psychiatric Association, 2013; American Psychological Association, 2016; Mental Health America, 2013; National Alliance to End Homelessness, 2019; National Association of Black Social Workers, 1998; National Alliance on Mental Illness Fact Sheet, 2011). Investigators have found that high exposure to violence in the Black/African American community increases the risk of developing depression, anxiety, and posttraumatic stress disorder, and that 25% of Black/African American children are especially at risk when compared with other children in the country as they meet the criteria for posttraumatic stress disorder (National Alliance on Mental Illness Fact Sheet, 2011).

Cultural Responses to Implicit Provider Bias

While implicit provider bias is problematic for Black/African Americans, an overview of the cultural responses to implicit provider bias is warranted. Implicit provider bias serves as a barrier to Black/African Americans receiving quality care services for mental health issues and disorders. As a result of implicit provider bias, there is a tendency to respond by having feelings of mistrust among Black/African Americans toward white providers (Cannon & Locke, 1977; Clark, Anderson, Clark, & Williams, 1999; Corrigan, 2004; Dana, 2002; Diala et al., 2001; Hamm, 2014; Parker & McDavis, 1983; Neighbors, 1988; Sacks, 2017, 2019; Shim et al., 2009; U.S. Department of Health & Human Services, 2001; Whatley, 2010). In its attempt to understand the differences between Black/African American and white utilization of mental health services, federal researchers acknowledge that some Blacks/African Americans automatically assume that racial bias exists from the provider; as a result, they view these services with distrust, believing that they might be victims of adverse treatment because they are Black/African American (U.S. Department of Health & Human Services, 2001).

Krieger, Sidney, and Coakley (1998) suggest that the perceived racism by Blacks/African Americans adversely impact on Black/African American mental health-seeking behaviors. Another investigation focused on a separate 13-year study where Krieger et al. (1998) examined the psychosocial stressors and cultural responses to institutional racism and discrimination from 1979 to 1992. The researcher found that perceptions and experiences with racism had adverse effects on the physical and mental well-being of Black/African Americans. These adverse effects found to be affecting the Black/African American community were mainly psychological distress along with a perception that whites want to keep Black/African Americans down (Krieger et al., 1998).

Another cultural response by Black/African Americans who encounter implicit provider bias in mental health is the stigma related to racism and stereotypes. For example, shame can serve as a barrier by Black/African Americans who refuse to access care out of fear of being crazy and due to lack of family or community support to seek help for mental health issues or disorders. The research indicates that Black/African Americans who perceive mental illness as a stigma are at high risk to terminate treatment prematurely and lack support to follow through with services (Barbee, 1992; Corrigan, 2004; U.S. Department of Health & Human Services, 2001). Another study cited by U.S. Department of Health and Human Services (2001) found that Black/African Americans were 2.5 times fearful of mental health treatment, and yet in the third study, Black/African American parents were less likely to describe their children's attention deficit-hyperactivity disorder symptoms using medical terminology and expected a shorter course of treatment.

Community Engagement with the Black/African American Community

As an institutional leader that addresses implicit bias at all levels of health care, The Joint Commission (2016) supports the position that all implicit bias should be reduced to ensure the best mental health outcomes, resulting in zero harm to all patients. They argue that racial diversity at all levels of mental health agencies, clinics, organizations, and hospitals must be the goal in health care. Leveraging both best practices in mental health and the adherence to the Hippocratic Oath is essential when working with Black/African Americans who have mental health issues and disorders. The Joint Commission (2016) emphasizes that stakeholders such as hospital administrations, mental health providers, medical educators, and policy-makers should understand that implicit bias and racial discrimination will not be tolerated and must be corrected. The Commission further emphasizes that the step of promoting racial diversity at all levels begins the process of addressing the impact of implicit bias on clinical care decisions with Black/African Americans (The Joint Commission, 2016).

Working with the Black/African American community requires a non-traditional level of engagement from mental health providers and organizations that provide mental health services. Reaching out to the Black/African American community is essential to develop partnerships and building trust with Black/African American clients. Outreach efforts by mental health professionals and organizations help to show their priority about and commitment to Black/African American mental health. The Joint Commission (2016) suggests that community engagement helps to spread the message that mental health services and Black/African American psychological wellness are benefits to the Black/African American community and that culturally appropriate mental health services provided are available to them. Therefore, connecting and partnering with the Black/African American community is a sign that a conscious decision has been made by the provider to engage in outreach activities that will show the community that the system of mental health care is an honest broker in the Black/African American healthcare continuum (The Joint Commission, 2016).

Before developing partnerships with this population, it is critical that mental health providers and organizations first gain the trust of the Black/African American community. To obtain the confidence of the Black/African American community, mental health providers and organizations that are willing to use community outreach and market innovative engagement strategies and that take extra, non-traditional steps might prove to be more successful at reducing implicit provider bias and thereby increasing the Black/African American community's access to mental health services and adequate care (The Joint Commission, 2016). Developing partnerships between mental health organizations, providers, indigenous residents, grassroots organizations, and other local stakeholders helps to convey to the Black/African American community that their mental health is essential and that everyone is on the same team working toward the mutual goal of Black/African American wellness (The Joint Commission, 2016).

To this extent, racial diversity among mental health agencies, clinics, organizations, and hospitals is a crucial component to demonstrating that the mental health needs of the Black/African American community are a priority to close the mental health gap. According to The Joint Commission (2016), this intentional investment includes the recruitment of racially diverse mental health providers that can be done by making a concerted effort to actively recruit racially and culturally diverse mental health staff and providers. Besides, a racially diverse mental health staff can help to evaluate the racial climate of the organization on an ongoing basis, and they can help by assessing their shared perceptions of policies and practices of the organization (The Joint Commission, 2016).

The emphasis on community engagement is a viable strategy that can be used to overcome and eliminate implicit provider bias in mental health care and increase the Black/African American community's access to mental health services and care. Outreach activities that can be held at churches, community centers, and in schools can range from events such as health fairs, book fairs, and ongoing community education made up of guest speakers, educator panels, and mental health narratives shared by members of the Black/African American community (Black Mental Health Alliance, 2019). Further, it is noted that to have success with outreach and marketing mental health in the Black/African American community, all outreach, and marketing staff from private, for-profit, and non-profit organizations must resemble the community that it intends to serve (Black/African American Mental Health Alliance, 2019; Lamb et al., 2015; The Joint Commission, 2016).

Such outreach efforts and innovative marketing techniques are designed to show genuine concern about the mental health and wellness of Blacks/African Americans outside of the traditional office setting. The successful recruitment of racially diverse mental health providers and that portray a sense of commitment, priority, urgency, care, and organizations will have the opportunity for more success in reaching the Black/African American community. This perspective is in alignment with the belief that acceptance of the outreach and marketing efforts by Black/African Americans will not happen overnight due to the long history and legacies of institutional racism and discrimination, and those mental health providers and organizations will have to accept that gaining the trust of the Black/African American community will take time.

Culturally focused groups that involve selected participants who engage in planned discussions about eradicating the mental health gap experienced by Black/African Americans are another opportunity to build community stakeholders and partnerships with the Black/African American community (Black/African American Mental Health Alliance, 2019; Mantovani et al., 2017; The Joint Commission, 2016). The goal of the culturally focused groups is to elicit the perceptions of Blacks/African Americans about mental health and related stigma and can be held in a non-threatening supportive environment to, as in this case, generate special topics presentations about Black/African American Mental Health (Black/African American Mental Health Alliance, 2019; Lamb et al., 2015; Mantovani et al., 2015; The Joint Commission, 2016).

Building partnerships in the Black/African American community is considered a best practice strategy. Parillo et al. (2011) provide a viable blueprint for building partnerships for health in the Black/African American community by emphasizing that the use of culturally appropriate approaches that rely on the strengths and resources within the Black/African American community is by far the best practice for building partnerships that will work to eliminate health disparities and build trust in the process. Parrillo and Kennedy (2011) suggest the following strategies for best practices, including the involvement and recognition that the pastors from community churches are the entry into the Black/African American community, utilizing the community-based participatory research process as the collaborative process that recognizes the strengths that each partner brings and equitably involve all partners in the collaborative research process.

To help reduce mental health disparities in the rural southern Black/African American community, the development and implementation of faith-based stress management intervention programs offer another option for Black/African American mental health. Bryant et al. (2015) propose that developing a community-based research approach to implement stress intervention programs that incorporate biblical principles, provide information, and uses the stress–distress–depression continuum will help to reach underserved Blacks/African Americans and effectively increase their access to mental health care. The research team supports both the development and use of community action boards whose goal is to help develop and implement the faith-based stress management intervention programs (Bryant et al., 2015). Use of the community action boards as a platform for community-based research and the participatory research approach, adds value to the engagement strategy because these boards are comprised of stakeholders, such as key informants, focus groups, and an academic research team (Bryant et al., 2015).

It is imperative to focus on Black/African American psychological wellness when intervening on this community. The increased awareness for the need to fund research projects that promote wellness centers on Afrocentric psychology, a worldview which focuses on qualitative, contextual, and human science (Bryant, 2015; Grills, 2006). It is crucial to use the Afrocentric worldview as the main point of Black/African American mental health intervention; it is imperative to start with the recognition that culture is a top value that is highly relevant to the everyday behaviors of Black/African American people (Bryant, 2015, p. 6; Grills, 2006). Also, Grills (2006) emphasizes that values, shared history, group experience, and language all affect how Black/African American see things, how they feel, and what matters to them. By starting where the client is, culture-based mental health providers working with Black/African American clients will need to understand how the individual client perceives the world and how the individual client gives meaning to things that are important to them and start mental health intervention from that starting point (Goldstein, 1983). Equally as important, Grills (2006) believes that Black/African American culture is motivational because it affects the freedom to choose one's own goals and level of commitment to those goals.

According to the research, culture-based treatment is the preferred approach with Black/African American clients. This approach expands the treatment agenda to include discussion of social context, history, racism, and other group-relevant issues which the client deems relevant and should expect to be part of the assessment, evaluation, and treatment plan discussion (Grills, 2006). An example of a culture-based treatment approach concerns depression. A culture-based therapist is one who works with the Black/African American client to identify cultural and personal factors to help motivate compliance with assessment, evaluation, diagnosis, and treatment planning.

Additionally, Grills (2006) rejects Eurocentric or western psychology's emphasis on qualitative, empirical research, and natural science when she systematically critiques the shortcomings of this approach when working with Black/African Americans. She argues that use of the western emphasis on methods, samples that are used, choice of research problems, evaluation techniques, and its culturally myopic theories fall short of effectiveness with Black/African Americans (Grills, 2006). Using the Eurocentric worldview, which centers on western psychology and philosophy are not valid with Blacks/African Americans who need mental health services and care since it is harmful to the psyche and wellness of Black/African American clients (Grills, 2006).

Cultural Competence and Cultural Humility in Black/African American Mental Health

Understanding the relevance of culture is vital to improving the quality of mental health care with Black/African Americans. Mental health providers should remember that they are bringing their own cultures into the helping relationship with Black/African American clients and that they should also keep in mind that the cultural background of patients influences how, when, and where they present with illness and how they express it. According to the National Association of Social Workers (2017), providers seek to understand culture and its function in human behavior and society and recognize the strengths that exist in all cultures. Culturally competent healthcare providers who are successful with these tenets are the ones who can identify with, relate to, and accommodate the cultural background of the client (National Association of Social Workers, 2017). Given this stance, it is crucial for providers to align with the mandate to understand the culture and its function in human behavior and society, and to recognize the strengths that exist in all cultures National Association of Social Workers, 2017).

Mental health providers who practice cultural humility tend to focus on critical self-reflection, engaging in lifelong learning (National Association of Social Workers, 2017). Although providers can demonstrate a willingness to challenge power imbalances and hold institutions accountable, they must also be willing to acknowledge and accept that they do not have all the answers and that they come from a place of not knowing when working cross-culturally (Kuwada, 2017). By acknowledging their limitations, providers are allowing Black/African American clients to act in the role of an expert (Kuwada, 2017).

Strategies to Reduce Implicit Bias

Implicit provider bias can be successfully addressed using organization support, skills training, and cognitive resources (Breathett, 2018; Hairston et al., 2019;

Hernandez, 2018; Institute for Healthcare Improvement, 2017; Kugelmass, 2016; The Joint Commission, 2016). At least three effective strategies are identified that can help mental health providers to lower implicit bias. The first strategy is called perspective-taking, and it involves the cognitive and physical use of empathy and putting oneself in another person's shoes, which in turn inhibits unconscious stereotypes and prejudices (The Joint Commission, 2016). A strategy that positively connects with Black/African American clients who are evaluating the authenticity of the mental health services that are available, offered, marketed, and provided (The Joint Commission, 2016).

The second strategy for reducing implicit provider bias involves the use of provider emotional regulation skills and the provider seeing the Black/African American client as an individual and not as a stereotype (Breathett, 2018; Maina, Belton, Ginzberg, Singh, & Johnson, 2018; The Joint Commission, 2016). Use of emotional regulation skills signals providers to have positive emotions during clinical encounters with Black/African American clients because this might help providers to see the individual uniqueness and attributes of Black/African American clients (Maina et al., 2018; The Joint Commission, 2016). In using this strategy, providers will be less willing to view the client as the "other," begin to use more socially inclusive categories, and be more likely to act consciously to adjust and replace the stereotypes and prejudices that are recognized as implicit bias (Breathett, 2018; Maina et al., 2018; The Joint Commission, 2016).

The third strategy to reduce implicit provider bias is the use of partnership building skills (Breathett, 2018; Maina et al., 2018; The Joint Commission, 2016). The research supports the notion that providers create partnerships as collaborative equals with Black/African American clients to underscore that providers and Black/African American clients are on the same team working together toward common goals that close the mental health gap, and that includes Black/African American wellness (Breathett, 2018; Institute for Healthcare Improvement, 2017; Maina et al., 2018; The Joint Commission, 2016).

Effective evidence-based strategies to reduce provider bias also include increasing their personal and professional intergroup contact, increase their awareness of their bias through implicit association bias testing, raise their knowledge of individual patterns of micro-aggressions and practice micro-affirmations (Finnerty, 2015; Devine et al., 2012; Institute for Healthcare Improvement, 2017). Another strategy to reduce implicit provider bias is offered by White (2011) who advises that providers gain a basic understanding of the culture from which their Black/African American clients come, to be mindful to understand and respect the power of implicit boundaries and to be aware of situations that might trigger bias and stereotyping.

Summary

Implicit provider bias is a standalone issue in Black/African American mental health that is rooted in institutional racism and the social determinants of health, both of which are at the root cause of the mental health gap that is experienced by the Black/African American community in the United States. Providers find it challenging to recognize implicit bias because of its unconscious nature that is usually left unchecked. The research indicates that implicit provider bias toward Black/African American clients is difficult to unlearn because of the historical legacies of slavery, institutional racism and discrimination, prejudicial attitudes, and stereotypes about Black/African Americans that also affect mental health assessment, evaluation, diagnosis, inadequate treatment plans, inappropriate psychotropic medication management, and poor prognosis.

Implications for best practices in mental health with the Black/African American community suggest that providers need skill sets that include cultural competence, cultural humility, and starting where the client is to ensure their understanding of provider bias and institutional racism in Black/African American mental health. To demonstrate the link between institutional racism, implicit provider bias, and Black/African American cultural responses to implicit provider bias, a brief overview of the Black/African American experience in America provides context for increased understanding of the individual and group trauma experienced by heterogeneity and diversity in the Black/African American community. Evidenced-based strategies help to reduce implicit provider bias and are innovative and presented. These strategies have implications for best practices in mental health with the Black/African American community, including the use of non-traditional and innovative personal and professional community engagement strategies that work to build partnerships in the Black/African American community that show authenticity, concern, and teamwork with the Black/African American community and other stakeholders who have an investment in Black/African American psychological wellness.

References

American Psychiatric Association. (2013). *Diagnostic and statistical manual of mental disorders: DSM-5* (5th ed.). Arlington, VA: American Psychiatric Association.

American Psychological Association. (2016). African Americans have limited access to mental and behavioral health care. Retrieved from http://www.appa.org/advocacy/cvil-rights/diversity/african-american-health.aspx

Assari, S., Moazen-Zaden, E., Caldwell, C. H., & Zimmerman, M. A. (2017). Racial discrimination during adolescence predicts mental health deterioration in adulthood: Gender differences among Blacks. *Frontiers in Public Health, 5*, 104. http://doi.org/10.3389/fpub.2017.00104

Barbee, E. L. (1992). African American women and depression: A review and critique of the literature. *Archives of Psychiatric Nursing, 6*(5), 257–265. https://doi.org/10.1016/0883-9417(92)9003601

Belle, D. (1990). Poverty and women's mental health. *American Psychologist, 45*(3), 385–389. http://dx.doi.org/10.1037/0003-066X.45.3.385

Black/African Americandemographics.com. (2017). *African American Population Report* (1st ed.).

Black Mental Health Alliance. (2019). Retrieved from https://blackmentalhealth.com/

Braveman, P., & Gottlieb, L. (2014). The social determinants of health: It's time to consider the causes of the causes. *Public Health Reports, 129*(1_suppl2), 19–31.

Breathett, K. (2018). *Overcoming physician clinical bias of minority patients: A department spotlight*. Tucson, AZ: University of Arizona Department of Medicine. Retrieved from https://deptmedicine.arizona.edu/news/2018/overcoming-physician-clinical-bias-minority-patients

Brewer, L., Carson, K., Williams, D., Allen, A., Jones, C., & Cooper, L.. (2013). Association of Race Consciousness with the Patient-Physician Relationship, Medication Adherence, and Blood Pressure in Urban Primary Care Patients. *American Journal of Hypertension, 26*(11), 1346–1352. https://doi.org/10.1093/ajh/hpt116.

Brown, T., Williams, D., Jackson, J., Neighbors, H., Torres, M., Sellers, S., & Brown, K. (2000). "Being Black/African American and feeling blue": The mental health consequences of racial discrimination. *Race and Society, 2*(2), 117–131. https://doi.org/10.1016/S1090-9524(00)00010-3

Bryant, K., Moore, T., Willis, N., & Hadden, K. (2015). Development of a faith-based stress management intervention in a rural African American community. *Progress Community Health Partnership, 9*(3), 423-430. doi:10.1353/cpr.2015.0060

Cannon, M., & Locke, B. (1977). Being Black/African American is detrimental to one's mental health: Myth or reality? *Phylon, 38*, 408–428.

Clark, R., Anderson, N. B., Clark, V., & Williams, D. (1999). Racism as a stressor for African Americans: A biopsychosocial model. *American Psychologist, 54*(10), 805–816.

Clark, P. A. (2003). Prejudice and the medical profession: A five-year update. *Journal of Law Medical Ethic, 37*(1), 118–33. doi: 10.1111/j.1748-720X.2009.00356. x. PMID:19245608

Dana, R. H. (2002). Mental health services for African Americans: A cultural/racial perspective. *Cultural Diversity and Ethnic Minority Psychology, 8*(1), 3–18. http://dx.doi.org/10.1037/1099-9809.8.1.3

Devine, P., Forscher, P., Austin, A., & Cox, W. (2012). Long-term reduction in implicit race bias: A prejudice habit-breaking intervention. *Journal of Experimental Social Psychology, 48*(6), 1267–1278. https://doi.org/10.1016/j.jesp.2012.06.003

Diala, C. C., Muntaner, C., Walrath, C., Nickerson, K., LaVeist, T., & Leaf, P. (2001). Racial/ethnic differences in attitudes toward seeking professional mental health services. *American Journal of Public Health, 91*(5), 805–807.

Edupedia. (2018, June 13). What are de jure and de facto segregation? Retrieved from https://www.theedadvocate.org/edupedia/content/what-are-de-jure-and-de-facto-segregation/

Fadus, M., Odunsi, O., Squeglia, L., & Fadus, M. (2019). Race, Ethnicity, and Culture in the Medical Record: Implicit Bias or Patient Advocacy? *Academic Psychiatry: the Journal of the American Association of Directors of Psychiatric Residency Training and the Association for Academic Psychiatry, 43*(5), 532–536. https://doi.org/10.1007/s40596-019-01035-9

Finnerty, D. (2015). Evidenced-based strategies to overcome unconscious bias. *Developed for strategies to overcome unconscious bias workshop series, Fall 2013*. Retrieved from https://lawprofessors.typepad.com/files/interventions-evidencebased-11-22-13.pdf

FitzGerald, C., & Hurst, S. (2017). Implicit bias in healthcare professionals: A systemic review. *BMC Medical Ethics, 18*(1), 19. doi:10.1186/s12910-017-017-8

Gabow, P. A. (2016). Closing the health care gap in communities: A safety net system approach. *Academic Medicine, 91*(10), 1337–1340.

Goldstein, H. (1983). Starting where the client is. *Social Casework, 64*(5). Retrieved from http://search.proquest.com/docview/1305257171/

Gracia, N. (2015, August 25). Moment of opportunity: Reducing health disparities and advancing health equity. *National conference on health statistics*, U.S. Department of Health and Human Services, Office of Minority Health. Retrieved from www.minorityhealth.hhs.gov

Grills, C. T. (2006, 28 April). *Strategies for Psychological Survival & Wellness*, Microsoft PowerPoint – London Talk 2 REV DAY 2. Retrieved from https://baatn-org.wildapricot.org/.../Cheryl%20Grills%20Powerpoint%202%5B1%5D

Hairston, D. R., Gibbs, T. A., Wong, S. S., & Jordan, A. (2019). Clinician bias in diagnosis and treatment. In M. Medlock, D. Shtasel, N. H. Trinh, & D. Williams (Eds.), *Racism and psychiatry. Current clinical psychiatry*. Cham: Humana Press. https://doi.org/10.1007/978-3-319-90197-8_7

Hamm, N. (2014, September 25). High rates of depression among African American women, low rates of treatment. Retrieved from https://www.huffingtonpost.com/nia-hamm/depression-african-american-women_b5836320.html

Helman, C. (2007). *Culture, health, and illness* (5th ed.). London: Hodder Arnold.

Hernandez, R. (2018). Medical students' implicit bias and the communication of norms in medical education, teaching. *Learning in Medicine, 30*(1), 112–117. doi:10.1080/10401334.2017.1359610

Institute for Healthcare Improvement. (2017, September 28) How to reduce implicit bias. Retrieved from http://www.ihi.org/communities/blogs/how-to-reduce-implicit-bias

Institute of Medicine. (2003). *Unequal treatment: Confronting social and ethnic disparities in health care.* Washington, DC: National Academies Press.

Johnson, C. (2017). America is a world leader in health inequality. *The Washington Post*, June 5. Retrieved from https//www.washingtonpost.com/news/wonk/wp/2017/06/05/america-is-a-world-leader-in-health-inequality/?noredirect=on&utm_term=.d862968b9121

Kohn, R., Levav, I., Saraceno, B., Saxena, S., & Kohn, R. (2004). The treatment gap in mental health care. *Bulletin of the World Health Organization, 82*(11), 811–890. https://doi.org/10.1590/S0042-96862004001100011

Krieger, N., Sidney, S., & Coakley, E. (1998). Racism and the physical and mental health status of African Americans: A thirteen-year national panel study. *Journal of Public Health, 88*(9), 1308–1313. doi:10.2105/AJPH.88.9.1308

Kugelmass, H. (2016). "Sorry, I'm not accepting new patients," an audit study of access to mental health care. *Journal of Health and Social Behavior, 57*(2), 168–183.

Kuwada, B. (2017). Cultural humility, empathy, & compassion: Teaching & learning retreat powerpoint presentation [PowerPoint slides]. Retrieved from https://www.everettcc.edu/files/programs/arts/transformative-teaching/kuwada-cultural-humility-presentation.pdf

Lamb, J., Dowrick, C., Burroughs, H., Beatty, S., Edwards, S., Bristow, K., ... Gask, L. (2015). Community engagement in a complex intervention to improve access to primary mental health care for hard-to-reach groups. *Health Expect, 18*(6), 2865–2879. doi:10.1111/hex.12272

Maina, I., Belton, T., Ginzberg, S., Singh, A., & Johnson, T. (2018). A decade of studying implicit racial/ethnic bias in healthcare providers using the implicit association test. *Social Science & Medicine, 199*, 219–229. https://doi.org/10.1016/j.socscimed.2017.05.009

Mantovani, N., Pizzolati, M., & Gillard, S. (2017). Engaging communities to improve mental health in African and African Caribbean groups: A qualitative study evaluating the role of community well-being champions. *Health & Social Care in the Community, 25*(1), 167–176. https://doi.org/10.1111/hsc.12288

Marmot, M. (2017). Closing the health gap. *Scandinavian Journal of Public Health, 45*(7), 723–731. https://doi.org/10.1177/1403494817717433

Mental Health America. (2013, November 6). Black/African American & African American communities and mental health. Retrieved from http://www.mentalhealthamerica.net/african-american-mental-health

National Alliance on Mental Illness. (2011). African American Community Mental Health Fact Sheet. Retrieved from https://www.nami.org/

National Alliance to End Homeless. (2019). Homelessness in America. What causes homelessness: racial inequality. Retrieved from https://endhomelessness.org/homelessness-in-america/what-causes-homelessness/inequality/

National Association of Black/African American Social Workers. (1998). Harambee: 30 Years of unity. Our roots position statement. Retrieved from https://cdn.ymaws.com/www.nabsw.org/resource/collection/E1582D77-E4CD-4104-996A-D42D08F9CA7D/NABSW_30_Years_of_Unity_-_Our_Roots_Position_Statement_1968.pdf

National Association of Social Workers. (2017). *NASW Press, Item #X2B Pamphlet, Section 1.05(a)*. Washington, DC. Retrieved from socialworkers.org

Neighbors, H. W. (1988). The help-seeking behavior of Black Americans: A summary of findings from the National Survey of Black Americans. *Journal of National Medical Association, 80*(9), 1009–1012.

Neighbors, H. W. (1990). Clinical care update: Minorities the prevention of psychopathology in African Americans: An epidemiologic perspective. *Community Mental Health Journal, 26*(2), 167–179.

Office of the Surgeon General. (2001). Chapter 3: Center for Mental Health Services (US); National Institute of Mental Health (US). Chapter 3 Mental Health Care for African Americans Mental Health: Culture, Race, and Ethnicity: A Supplement to Mental Health: A Report of the Surgeon General. Rockville (MD): Substance Abuse and Mental Health Services Administration (US). Retrieved from https://www.ncbi.nlm.nih.gov/books/NBK44251/

Parker, W. M., & McDavis, R. J. (1983). Attitudes of Black/African Americans toward mental health agencies and counselors. *Journal of Non-White Concerns in Personnel and Guidance, 11*, 89–98. doi:10.1002/j.2164-4950.1983.tb00106.x

Parrillo, R., & Kennedy, B. R. (2011). Partnerships for health in the African American community: Moving toward community-based partnership. *Journal of Cultural Diversity, 19*(4), 150–154.

Phelan, S. M., Atunah-Jay, S., & van Ryn, M. (2019). The patient experience: Stereotype threat in medical care. In L. Barkley, M. Svetaz, & V. Chulani (Eds.), *Promoting health equity among racially and ethnically diverse adolescents* (pp. 139–148). Cham: Springer. https://doi.org/10.1007/978-3-319-97205-3_11

Phelan, S. M., Atunah-Jay, S., & van Ryn, M. (2019). The patient experience: Stereotype threat in medical care. In L. Barkley, M. Svetaz, & V. Chulani (Eds.), *Promoting health equity among racially and ethnically diverse adolescents*. Cham: Springer. https://doi.org/10.1007/978-3-319-97205-3_11

Rhett-Mariscal, William. (2008, November). Promotores in Mental Health in California and the Prevention and Early Intervention Component of the MHSA Policy Paper. The California Endowment and the Center for Multicultural Development at the California Institute for Mental Health. Retrieved from https://www.cibhs.org/sites/main/files/file-attachments/promotores_policy_paper.pdf

Rice, M., & Jones, W. Jr. (1982). Black health inequities and the American health care system. *Health Policy and Education, 3*(3), 195–214

Sacks, T. (2019). Invisible visits: Black/African American middle-class women in the American healthcare system. In *Invisible visits*. Oxford: Oxford University Press. https://doi.org/10.1093/oso/9780190840204.003.0003

Sacks, T. K. (2017). Performing Black/African American womanhood: A qualitative study of stereotypes and the healthcare encounter. *Critical Public Health*. doi:10.1080/09581596.2017.1307323

Shim, R. S., Compton, M. T., Rust, G., Druss, B. G., & Kaslow, N. J. (2009). Race-Ethnicity as a predictor of attitudes toward mental health treatment seeking. *Psychiatric Services, 60*(10), 1336–1341. http://doi.org/10.1176/ps.2009.60.10.1336

Snowden, R. L. (2003). Bias in mental health assessment and intervention: Theory and evidence. *American Journal of Public Health, 93*(2), 239–243.

Spencer, M., Walters, K., Allen, H., Andrews, C., Begun, A., Browne, T., & Uehara, E. (2018). Close the health gap. In *Grand challenges for Washington (2006) social work and society*. Oxford: Oxford University Press. https://doi.org/10.1093/oso/9780190858988.003.0003

Starfield, B. (2011). The hidden inequity in health care. *International Journal for Equity in Health, 10*, 15. Retrieved from http://link.galegroup.com.libproxy2.usc.edu/apps/doc/A256366861/AONE?u=usocal_main&sid=AONE&xid=2ca0472

Storrs, C. (2016). Therapists often discriminate against Black/African American and poor patients, study finds. *CNN Wire*, June 1. Retrieved from http://amsterdamnews.com/news/2016/jun/01/therapists-discriminate-against-Black/AfricanAmerican-and-po/

Taylor, J. (2019, March 20). *Unconscious bias in health care setting preceptor conference 2019* [PowerPoint presentation]. University of Mississippi Medical Center Office of Diversity and Inclusion.

The Joint Commission, Division of Health Care Improvement. (2016). Implicit bias in health care. Quick Safety, Issue 23.

U.S. Census Bureau. (2019). News release. 2010 Census shows Black/African American population has highest concentration in the South: People who reported as Both Black/African American and white more than doubled. Retrieved from https://www.census.gov/newsroom/releases/archives/2010_census/cb11-cn185.html

U.S. Department of Health and Human Services. (2001). *Mental health: Culture, race, and ethnicity – A supplement to mental health: A report of the surgeon general*. Rockville, MD: U.S. Department of Health and Human Services, Substance Abuse and Mental Health Services Administration, Center for Mental Health Services.

van Ryn, M., Burgess, D. J., Dovidio, J. F., Phelan, S., Saha, S., Malat, J., & Perry, S. P. (2011). The impact of racism on clinician cognition, behavior, and clinical decision-making. *Du Bois Review: Social Science Research on Race, 8*(1), 199–218.

Washington, H. (2006). *Medical Apartheid: the dark history of medical experimentation on Black/African American Americans from colonial times to the present* (1st ed.). New York, NY: Doubleday.

White, A. (2011). *Unconscious bias in health care*. Cambridge, MA: Harvard University.

Williams, D. R., & Williams-Morris, R. (2000). Racism and mental health: The African American experience. *Ethnicity and Health, 5*(3–4), 243–268. https://doi.org/10.1080/713667453

Wolsiefer, K, & Stone, J. (2019). Addressing bias in healthcare: Confrontation as a tool for bias reduction and patient and provider self-advocacy. In R. K. Mallett & M. J. Monteith (Eds.), *Confronting prejudice and discrimination: The science of changing minds and behaviors* (pp. 275–297). Cambridge, MA: Academic Press. https://doi.org/10.1016/B978-0-12-814715-3.00013-8

Part II
Policy

Chapter 6

Thirty Years of Black History Month and Thirty Years of Overrepresentation in the Mental Health System

Patrick Vernon

Why Black Mental Health Matters

> The present state of Black Britain is a grim and unpleasant one, but an understanding of the issues, coupled with commitment to effect a fundamental change in policy directions on the part of both white institutions and black organisations, could substantially improve the quality of life in Britain and lead to a more integrated and equal society. (Haynes, 1983)

Although there has been a black presence in Britain since the time of the Roman Empire, it has been since the Windrush era and the subsequent generations that we have established a critical mass in the British population. Over the past 60 years, research evidence, government reports, and lived experiences highlight that black people are still on the extreme margins of mainstream society despite individual achievements and success. The familiar story of overrepresentation reflects state of the black experience in Britain from school exclusions, mental health institutions, the criminal justice system, children in care, gun violence fatalities, living in the most deprived neighborhoods, poor access to health care, and widening health inequalities. It is not surprising that all these factors have an impact on our self-esteem, identity, and mental wellbeing.

Often the relationship between identity, culture, and mental wellbeing, as well as the legacy of empire, is overlooked in the development of social policy and service delivery, especially when you look at the development of public health and health inequalities policy at the national level from the Black Report in the 1960s, the Acheson Report in the 1980s, the Wanless Review in the 1990s, and the Marmot Report (2010).

The 2015 Care Quality Commission (CQC) annual monitoring report of the 2007 Mental Health Act (MHA) provided additional commentary highlighting the overrepresentation of African and Caribbean men and women who have been sectioned in secure wards or on Community Treatment Orders (CTOs) in the psychiatric system over the past 30 years, recognizing that no fundamental shift has taken place. The CQC has subsequently revised the MHA code of practice to further recognize issues around race equality as part of wider perspectives and principles of human rights.

Since there is no consensus on or collective approach to tackling racial inequalities in mental health services, this has resulted in politicians and policymakers being dependent on the medical model and thus deferring to the influence of clinicians and mainstream charities in seeking solutions and answers. Every so often there is a media story or news report that jolts a degree of consciousness which reminds the National Health Service (NHS) leaders, the politicians, and the community why black mental wellbeing still matters. The following stark statistics remind us that sadly this is one of the biggest travesties of human rights and system failure in health and social policy since the closure of asylums in the 1980s:

- Research shows that black people are overrepresented by three times at the acute end of services and six times more likely to suffer from death under restraint in police custody.
- Black people are less likely to receive preventative services and talking therapies.
- Detention rates under the MHA are 44% higher among black patients.
- Young men are three times more likely to have been in contact with mental health services in the year before they committed suicide than their white counterparts, and their suicides are more likely to be considered preventable.
- As psychiatric inpatients, they are twice as likely to commit suicide as white psychiatric inpatients.
- Current services are Eurocentric and not culturally sensitive, which has an impact on patient outcomes.
- In any given year, 20% of children and young people are said to have a mental health problem, but there is no data available about how many are from black and minority ethnic (BME) backgrounds.
- Young black people are disproportionately overrepresented in the youth justice system, social services and looked-after provision, exclusion from school, and educational underachievement.
- Research indicates that older people may experience dementia and depression at a higher rate than among indigenous older people.
- Depression among BME older people from several different groups is known to be associated with a range of disadvantageous conditions, including chronic health problems, stroke, poor housing, low family support, and poor socioeconomic status.

The current mainstream discourse presented by psychiatrists and academics suggests that you cannot blame mental health services or psychiatry for the overrepresentation of black people, as they are simply responding to issues of societal problems rather than racial inequality. This view is clearly articulated in the AESOP research project looking at mental illness within the Caribbean community (Morgan et al., 2006). Although this is a crucial point, just like the lack of senior representation in the civil service, Parliament, the judiciary, and the board room, we cannot pretend that institutionalized racism does not exist. However, such claims have produced tensions between psychiatrists, academics, activists, service users, and carers from the black community around approaches to mental illness. Over the past 30 years, organizations such as Afiya Trust, National Survivor User Network, Mental Health Foundation, Mind, and Centre for Mental Health, and Black Mental Health UK have campaigned and advocated on the experiences and concerns of the black community. In addition, there have been several campaigns established by the families of those who died under the care of the mental health services, such as Orville Blackwood, Rocky Bennett, Sean Rigg, Christopher Alder, Olaseni Lewis, and Sarah Reed, which are now part of the wider international campaign around Black Lives Matter.

The impact of overrepresentation of black people in mental health services for the past 30 years, as reflected in the last "Count me in" survey (Care Quality Commission, 2011), has consequences for policymakers, politicians, NHS and social care providers, and the black community:

- Many black communities have lost trust in services due to experiences of racism and cultural differences, as highlighted in the 2002 report "Breaking the circles of fear" (Sainsbury Centre for Mental Health, 2002).
- Stigma around mental health still exists, making it difficult to talk about problems and to seek early help for fear of being given a diagnosis.
- The ingrained prejudice and stigma of the notion of "big, black, and dangerous" presents a massive challenge to the black community involved in the mental health system and the engagement of frontline staff.
- Inequality and discrimination of black communities can lead to increased risk of psychosis.
- There is a lack of black representation in decision making within the NHS, as well as among mental health services employees.
- There is a lack of capacity in communities to deliver mental health interventions.
- Most health spending is tied up in acute rather than preventative services.
- There is difficulty in addressing causal factors for poor mental health, such as deprivation and social exclusion, which are disproportionately present in poorer and black communities.

What is clear reflecting on issues around policy development and commissioning of mental health services is that there is collective system failure, plus a lack of leadership, at all levels. Sadly, the current models of service development and thinking are not working and there is no space to develop a black perspective on solutions and new models of care.

From Uprising and Riots in the 1980s to the Millennials

> Some authors have suggested that people of Afro-Caribbean descent are liable to a form of reaction which is seldom seen elsewhere, and the name "West Indian Psychosis" has even been coined for it. The characteristics of the syndrome are said to be excitement and over-activity, with pressure of thought and speech, sometimes accompanied by cognitive confusion with subsequent loss of memory. Bizarre behaviour may occur (e.g. removal of clothes in public) and violence is common, especially if attempts are made forcibly to restrain the patient. Talk is often fragmented or incoherent, and there often seems to be some paranoid ideation, which stops short of systematized or complex delusions. (Rack, 1982)

Britain was in turmoil in the Thatcher era with the after-effects of the riots in Brixton, Tottenham, and Toxteth. Black Britons were fighting for tolerance and acceptance, and against marginalization and racism, and trying to define a sense of identity and purpose. For instance, during the 1980s the concept of "ganja psychosis" was adopted within the community and by many psychiatrists to explain the growing phenomenon of young black men being sectioned, especially under section 136 of the 1959 (subsequently 1983) MHA. The issue revolved around whether weed was the cause or just the symptom of psychosis. The label "ganja psychosis" for several years replaced the typical diagnosis of schizophrenia, which meant black men with this label still received significant levels of medication and more physical restraint. One of the recommendations from the report of the inquiry into the care and treatment of Christopher Clunis in 1994 (Ritchie, Dick, & Lingham, 1994) was the introduction of advanced directives, and for psychiatrists to adopt higher levels of risk assessment for black men, which often put pressure on bed occupancy and increased out areas placements as local health budgets were squeezed.

It was during this period that we see a growing trend of black men going to the special hospitals such as Broadmoor, Ashworth, and Rampton, plus several medium-secure units, at alarming rates, often via the criminal justice system. The concept of "mentally ordered offenders" was the standard norm, especially for black men, to be escalated through the prison system and the special hospitals.

For many, the MHA was another form of state repression, a powerful narrative which sadly was still strong in 2017.

> One modest estimate has it that black men are twice as likely to be "caught" by this section (section 136 of the 1959 Mental Health Act). It has thus earned itself the nickname of the "mental health sus law." In other words, to understand how racism has been institutionalised in patterns of police use of this power (and bearing in mind that up till now no serious and detailed study has been carried out on this issue) we need to set the issue in the context of the scapegoating of (especially young) black people for the economic and social crises of the 1970s. (Mercer, 1983)

The death of Orville Blackwood at Broadmoor in 1991, which led to an inquiry and two inquests, again highlighted the injustice and the narrative of treatment of black people in one of the most secure mental health hospitals in the country (Special Hospitals Service Authority, 1993). The title of the inquiry report into Orville Blackwood's death, "Big, black, and dangerous," reflects past and current stereotypes of black men's relationship with the police and mental health services.

However, in response to the experiences of black men and women, a growing network of black-led community and grassroots organizations began to emerge around the country, delivering an alternative response to mainstream services in health, social care, housing, employment, and criminal justice. One such organization grew out of the concerns and experiences of black men, particularly of Rastafarian faith, who were overrepresented in the psychiatric wards at New Cross Hospital in Wolverhampton. During the 1980s, the notion of "ganja psychosis" was of concern to the Wolverhampton Rastafarian Progressive Association, which laid the initial ground work for the African Caribbean Community Initiative (ACCI) to be established in 1987 to provide a range of preventative, educational, housing, and support services. ACCI is one of the longest-running black self-help organizations in Wolverhampton, and is at the heart of the community, where it plays a key role in promoting mental health awareness and breaking the stigma. The year 2017 was the 30th anniversary of ACCI, which is now an important landmark in the black mental health history of the UK as one of the few organizations still in existence – the clear majority of black service providers around mental health, housing, employment, and criminal justice have disappeared. Sadly, there has been very little research on the growth and demise of funded voluntary sector and grassroots organizations which played an important role as a buffer and alternative cultural perspective. Also, these organizations created and established a new class of community activists, academics, service users, and professionals, many of whom would run and commission mainstream services targeting the black community from the 1990s.

It was also in this context of the 1980s that Black History Month was adopted in the UK in 1987. In that year, the concept of black history was developed by Akyaaba Addai-Sebo, a special project officer at the Greater London Council, and later at the London Strategic Policy Unit. It was also the year that African Jubilee Year Declaration was launched, which called on local and national government to recognize African contributions to the cultural, economic, and political life of London and the UK.

The declaration also called on authorities to implement their duties under the Race Relations Act 1976 and to intensify their support against apartheid. It required authorities to support and continue the process of naming monuments, parks, and buildings to reflect the contributions of historical and contemporary heroes of African descent, thus giving positive affirmation to children and giving young people identity and self-worth. The above activities created the catalyst for many local authorities in the UK to formally institute October as Black History Month, which was subsequently adopted by the NHS and other public bodies. The role of Black History Month is not to be underestimated as it provides the platform to raise issues around black identity and the need for culturally relevant and sensitive services across a range of social policy issues, especially in the NHS and local government, and greater visibility of black representation at the senior level in public life.

After the 1990s, there was already a decline in and decommissioning of cultural sensitive led projects in NHS trusts and black-led mental health charities, even though the NHS and local government received significant funding during this period under New Labour. With the introduction of the National Service Framework from 1998, this led to a growing approach around standardization of services and commissioning. However, it was the murder of Stephen Lawrence in 1993 and the Macpherson inquiry in 1999 (Home Office, 1999) which led to the Race Relations Amendment Act 2001 and the recognition of institutionalized racism and how BME communities were systematically discriminated against.

This led to major reforms in policing and the criminal justice system, but it did not trickle down to mental health policy and services. Even with the death of Rocky Bennett in 1998, which led to an inquiry in 2001 (Norfolk, Suffolk & Cambridgeshire Strategic Health Authority, 2003) and the 2003 "Inside out" report by Professor S. P. Sashidharan to the Department of Health with recommendations on tackling racism (National Institute of Mental Health, 2003), these were not taken on board. Instead, the Delivering Race Equality (DRE) program, a five-year strategy with a £300 million budget and a delivery agency and high-profile advisory board, was established to improve services and better engagement between BME communities and the NHS (Department of Health, 2005). The program generated a range of feelings, especially as the government decided not to follow the Macpherson approach in recognizing mental health services as institutionalized racism because of the growing backlash from the police, politicians, and several commentators who felt that the line around race equality had gone too far (McKenzie, 2007). Others saw the DRE as a once-in-a-lifetime opportunity to tackle the wrongs of the last 25 years of black overrepresentation in the system (RAWOrg, 2011). The government funded the DRE for less than five years; it introduced a new mental health strategy, called "New Horizons," in 2009, which had a weak focus on race equality and lasted for less than six months. When the Coalition government came into power in 2010, "New Horizons" became redundant with the introduction in 2011 of "No Health Without Mental Health," but despite undertaking an equality impact assessment, the final strategy had no recommendations or plans to tackle black mental health.

MHA and CTOs

The issues were compounded with the New Labour government's plans to update the 1983 MHA with the introduction of CTOs as a way of extending powers into the community for mental health services to provide treatment and medication against patients' will. This was the result of the Christopher Clunis case in 1994 where a young black man killed a member of the public, Jonathan Zito, in an unprovoked attack in North London. This was a high-profile case, with lots of media attention, where the label "big, black, and dangerous" was again introduced to the public. This led to new guidance and executive powers around risk assessment and advance directives to ensure mental health trusts and providers could intervene on grounds of public safety. Ongoing lobbying by medical professional bodies and charities representing victims and families also had a major impact, influencing Conservative and New Labour government for stronger enforcement and greater risk assessment. CTOs were seen as a way of reassuring the public and mental health professionals that the MHA could be extended in the community in managing risk of potentially violent mental health service users. The debate around violent crime was part of a wider conversation around gun crime and "black on black" violence, which was also a major issue during the 1990s.

Several organizations and campaigners had bitter battles with the government, outlining that this would have a disproportionate impact on black communities and would further undermine the relationship with mental health services (Fernando, 2017). The Act was passed in 2007, but over the last several years there has been increasing evidence that CTOs have no impact on clinical outcomes, while at the same time increasing the overrepresentation of black people in mental health services (Burns et al., 2013).

From Striving to Thriving

Since the demise of the Delivering Race Equality strategy in 2010 under the last Labour government (1997–2010), the government at times has adopted a "colorblind" approach to race and health. One of the only exceptions has been the introduction of the Workforce Race Equality Standard in 2015, which was in response to "Snowy White Peaks," a report by Middlesex University looking at poor levels of black senior management on NHS boards and the evidence that black staff in the NHS were being bullied and discriminated against in their career development, which has an impact on patient experience.

The United Nations (UN) report on the August 2016 meeting of the Committee on the Elimination of Racial Discrimination (CERD), which every five years reviews the UK government record on race equality, criticized the government for not tackling issues of overrepresentation of African and Caribbean people in the mental health system.

The 2016 Equality and Human Rights Commission report "Fairer Britain" further highlighted mental health inequalities facing the black community. In response, Prime Minister Theresa May launched the Race Disparity Audit across all government departments. In October 2017, the government launched a comprehensive analysis on a dedicated website highlighting the nature of structural racism in Britain.

Nevertheless, over the last few years there has been a growing consensus among mainstream political parties and philanthropists and think tanks as to how to tackle the issue of neglected mental health services and the poor health outcomes experienced by many service users, and their carers, from health and social care services. The concern has been ongoing, and of great significance, for BME communities. This challenge was reflected in NHS England's Independent Mental Health Taskforce, established in 2015, which brought together health and care leaders, people who use services, and experts in the field to create a "Five Year Forward View for Mental Health" for the NHS in England. The taskforce launched its report in February 2016 (NHS England Mental Health Taskforce, 2016).

The taskforce concluded that the best way to revolutionize care is to treat people's minds and bodies equally, and so by hardwiring mental health into the NHS once and for all, this vision will be attained. This means greater transparency in spend and outcomes, and a relentless focus on inequalities. The report's recommendations for the NHS have been adopted, with a target that by 2020/2021 at least one million people with mental health problems will be accessing high-quality care that they are not getting today. This is further backed by £1 billion in new investment by the year 2021. The report also challenges the government for stronger leadership because a mentally healthy society – and one which cares well for people with mental health problems – involves social care, housing, employment, education, and schools. The issues and experiences of African and Caribbean service users, carers, and frontline staff were not overlooked in the taskforce's considerations. There were a number of community dialogue events and informal conversations – direct and honest conversations – with black service users and professionals who shared their positive but also negative experiences of the mental health services. The conversations also raised issues of stigma and discrimination, not only across services but in how the black community views mental health and the stigma it holds against people with mental health challenges.

The Royal College of Psychiatrists in 2015 established an independent commission, chaired by Lord Nigel Crisp, to review the provision of acute inpatient psychiatric care for adults. The commission launched its report in 2016, recognizing the issue of black people's overrepresentation in detained services, with a clear recommendation for a Race Equality Patient Charter. The government was due to respond to this report in 2017.

We have had more than 30 years of race equality training, strategies, pledges, and measurement tools which have failed to shift the agenda, much to the dismay of many service users, frontline staff, senior system leaders, activists, and politicians. This further adds to the malaise and the perception that "black mental health" is an intractable issue that is impossible to address.

Thus, we need to create a new agenda by exploring structural racism in society and its impact on mental health services alongside the impact of the legacy of enslavement to unpack new models or solutions for tackling racial mental health inequalities. A new initiative, Black Thrive, was established in June 2017 to tackle the issue of metal health in the London borough of Lambeth, which has one of the largest black populations in Britain and is often seen as the center of black cultural expression and the home of black Britons as a result of the Windrush migration from 1948. Black Thrive came out of the 40 recommendations from Lambeth Council establishing an independent commission called the Black Health and Wellbeing Commission, which looked at the implications of the death of Sean Rigg, a young man with mental health problems who died in police custody in Brixton in 2008. Black Thrive is working with the black community and statutory services to look at how mental health services and the public health agenda could be improved to support the African and Caribbean community.

In October 2017, the government established an independent review of the 2007 MHA as a way of providing more safeguards for patients and service users. The review, under the leadership of Sir Simon Wessely, is due to report to the government in 2018 and provides an opportunity for an informed public debate on the historical and contemporary roles of psychiatry and the experiences of mental health in Britain's African and Caribbean communities. The review examined community anxieties about the proportionally larger numbers of black ethnic minorities receiving inpatient care and CTOs, or in the criminal justice system. The review was launched in December 2018 with a series of recommendations. This was followed up in June 2019 with a summit held by the outgoing Prime Minster, Theresa May that a White Paper will be produced by the end of the year which to respond to the review. However, the following priorities were agreed as immediate action:

- The first ever Race Equality Framework will ensure NHS mental healthcare providers work with their local communities to improve the ways in which patients' access and experience treatment, and ensure data on equality of access is monitored at board level and acted on.
- Working with Black African and Caribbean community groups alongside others to develop a White Paper formally setting out a response to Sir Simon's review.
- Further work toward eradicating the use of police cells as a place to detain people experiencing mental illness ahead of banning it in law, building on the Prime Minister's work to end this practice for under-18s.
- Launching a pilot program of culturally sensitive advocates in partnership with local authorities and others, to identify how best to represent the mental health needs of ethnic minority groups.
- A partnership between the CQC and Equality and Human Rights Commission to review how they can use their regulatory powers to better support equality of access to mental health services.
- An open call for research into how different ethnic minority groups experience mental health treatment and how this can be improved – to be launched later this year by the National Institute for Health Research.

However, there has been criticism around the process of the review and recommendations in not addressing the key issues of structural racism and the rights of service users particularly with the continued use of CTOs (Fernando, 2018; Nazroo, 2018).

Another recent change in 2018 was the passing of the Mental Health Use of Force Act (Seni's Law) was inspired by Olaseni Lewis who died in 2010 soon after being restrained by 11 police officers in Bethlem Royal Hospital, Beckenham. The Act which was led by Steve Reed MP for Croydon North aims to ensure the use of force against patients in mental health units is better governed and requires police to wear body cameras while carrying out restraint unless there are legitimate operational reasons for not doing so. The Act requires NHS providers and others to provide regular data and information on the use of restraints. This is another milestone in making the system more accountable.

Thus, after 30 years of Black History Month in the UK, we can ask: Are those of African descent overrepresented in the systems are still being left behind? If so, is serious mental illness over diagnosed among these groups due to the persistence of stereotypes rooted in the experiences of enslavement, or do they in fact experience distinctive patterns of mental health and illness, perhaps due to the wider fallout of historical enslavement around structural racism? Or perhaps the experience is located only in modern inequalities such as family breakdown, social capital, education, and housing?

As we move forward toward the next decade we need more research and analysis to see the issues and challenges facing black communities around mental health:

- The impact of Children and Adolescent Mental Health Services and "looked after children."
- Gangs, gun, and knife crimes.
- LGBTQ.
- Gender and domestic violence.
- Migrants and refugees/asylum seekers living in the shadows.
- Dementia.
- The impact of austerity.
- Windrush scandal and the impact of hostile environment.

Maybe we should also be putting pressure on the government to adopt two of the key recommendations below from the UN CERD report in 2016 especially if there will be a future White Paper and follow strategies and action plans:

> The State party should take effective measures to ensure the accessibility, availability and quality of health care services to persons belonging to ethnic minorities throughout its jurisdiction. The Committee stresses the particular importance of adopting measures to effectively address the overrepresentation of persons of African Caribbean descent treated in psychiatric institutions and the disproportionate use of restraint, seclusion and medication.
>
> Recalling its general recommendation No. 34 (2011) on racial discrimination against people of African descent, the Committee recommends that the State party consider adopting a national action plan to combat discrimination against persons of African descent, in partnership and consultation with communities of African descent, with concrete targets, implementation mechanisms and adequate resources. The Committee also encourages the State party to prepare and implement a suitable programme of measures and policies for the implementation of the International Decade for People of African Descent, proclaimed by the General Assembly in its resolution 68/237, considering General Assembly resolution 69/16 on the programme of activities. (UN Committee on the Elimination of Racial Discrimination, 2016)

This could contribute to thinking around issues of Afriphobia, which the UN International Decade for People of African Descent has recognized, to counter the stigma, stereotypes, and misunderstanding which present black people as big, black, and dangerous something with politicians, clinicians, senior leaders in health and social care are still not engaged or open to a way new way of looking at racism and over representation.

References

Burns, T., Rugkåsa, J., Molodynski, A., Dawson, J., Yeeles, K., Vazquez-Montes, M., ... Priebe, S. (2013). Community treatment orders for patients with psychosis (OCTET): A randomised controlled trial. *Lancet, 381*(9878), 1627–1633.

Care Quality Commission. (2011). *Count me in 2010: Results of the 2010 national census of inpatients and patients on supervised community treatment in mental health and learning disability services in England and Wales.* London: Care Quality Commission.

Department of Health. (2005). *Delivering race equality in mental health care: An action plan for reform inside and outside services, and the government's response to the independent inquiry into the death of David Bennett.* London: Department of Health.

Department of Health and Social Care. (2018). *Modernising the Mental Health Act – Final report from the independent review.* London: Palgrave Macmillan. Available at https://www.gov.uk/government/publications/modernising-the-mental-health-act-final-report-from-the-independent-review.

Fernando, S. (2017). *Institutional racism in psychiatry and clinical psychology: Race matters in mental health* (Contemporary Black History Series). Chippenham: Palgrave Macmillan.

Fernando, S (2018). Blog for ROTA. Retrieved from https://www.rota.org.uk/content/review-mental-health-act-fails-put-%E2%80%98race%E2%80%99-its-agenda-change-acknowledges-reality

Haynes, A. (1983). *The state of black Britain.* London: Root Publishing.

Home Office. (1999). *The Stephen Lawrence inquiry.* Report of an inquiry by Sir William Macpherson of Cluny, Stationery Office, London.

McKenzie, K. (2007). Institutional racism in mental health care. *The British Medical Journal, 334*(7595), 649–650. Retrieved from http://www.bmj.com/content/334/7595/649

Mercer, K. (1983). Black communities' experiences of psychiatric services. Paper presented at the Transcultural Psychiatry Society, London.

Morgan, C., Dazzan, P., Morgan, K., Jones, P., Harrison, G., Leff, J., ... Fearon, P. (2006). First episode psychosis and ethnicity: Initial findings from the AESOP study. *World Psychiatry, 5*(1), 40–46.

National Archives. (2018). *Mental Health Units (Use of Force) Act 2018.* Parliament UK.

National Institute of Mental Health. (2003). *Inside out: Improving mental health services for black and minority ethnic communities in England.* London: NIMH.

Nazroo, J. (2018). Blog Mental Health Today. Retrieved from https://www.mentalhealthtoday.co.uk/innovations/modernising-the-mental-health-act-a-missed-opportunity-to-address-ethnic-inequalities

NHS England Mental Health Taskforce. (2016). Retrieved from https://www.england.nhs.uk/wp-content/uploads/2016/02/Mental-Health-Taskforce-FYFV-final.pdf

Norfolk, Suffolk & Cambridgeshire Strategic Health Authority. (2003). *Independent inquiry into the death of David Bennett: An independent inquiry set up under HSG(94)27.* Norfolk, Suffolk and Cambridgeshire Strategic Health Authority, Cambridge.

Prime Minister's Office. (2019, June). *10 Downing Street*. Retrieved from https://www.gov.uk/government/news/measures-to-end-unequal-mental-health-treatment-kickstarted-by-pm

Rack, P. (1982). *Race, culture and mental disorder*. London: Tavistock Publications.

RAWOrg. (2011). *The end of delivering race equality: Perspectives of frontline workers and service users from racialised groups*. London: RAWOrg.

Ritchie, J. H., Dick, D., & Lingham, R. (1994). *The report of the inquiry into the care and treatment of Christopher Clunis*. Norwich: HMSO.

Sainsbury Centre for Mental Health. (2002). *Breaking the circles of fear: A review of the relationship between mental health services and African and Caribbean communities*. London: SCMH.

Special Hospitals Service Authority. (1993). *Report of the committee of inquiry into the death in Broadmoor Hospital of Orville Blackwood and a review of the deaths of two other Afro-Caribbean patients: 'Big, black and dangerous?'* London: SHSA.

UN Committee on the Elimination of Racial Discrimination. (2016). Retrieved from http://tbinternet.ohchr.org/_layouts/treatybodyexternal/Download.aspx?symbolno=CERD%2fC%2fGBR%2fCO%2f21-23&Lang=en

Chapter 7

Race and Risk – Exploring UK Social Policy and the Development of Modern Mental Health Services

Patricia Clarke

Safety and its pursuit are integral to health care. Within mental health care, an inability to manage risks within agreed parameters, including risk to self or others, may result in an adult or child being compelled by law to receive it. The Mental Health Act 1983 (Jones, 2018), together with its various "sections," is one of the key legal instruments used to detain adults at risk within mental health hospitals and also to manage people in the community.

Improving safety for all, including black communities, will result in universal safety improvements for users and staff. The idea of sanctuary, safety, and security is an important one within mental health care.

Concerns remain regarding the excessive use of restraint, deaths in custody, and the convergence of factors affecting access to preventative health care for African-Caribbean men and women, and other diverse communities.

In 2017, headlines such as "Grenfell Tower fire: death toll may have been covered up to prevent a riot" were widespread following the West London fire (Oppenheim, 2017). Politicians including David Lammy and Diane Abbott – two of the most high-profile black MPs – continue to play a key role in trying to establish the root cause of the deaths of more than 70 London residents who lived in social housing at Grenfell Towers. Arguments continue about the care of the most vulnerable and the impending inquiry is tasked with trying to identify key lessons. The safety of the most vulnerable remains paramount; exceptions to this may result in loss of life.

For the purpose of this chapter, I will attempt to summarize the emergence of modern mental health services and will conclude with opportunities and potential for improving services and, ultimately, for service users. I am particularly concerned about the experience of the black, Asian, and minority ethnic (BAME) men, women, and children who use mental health provision.

From Asylums to Community Care

Addressing mental health care, particularly when considering the mental health journey within the UK, has an interesting trajectory.

The Bethlem Royal Hospital, based in South London, is widely considered to be one of the earliest examples of state care for men and women with mental health problems. The hospital was built in 1247 and has evolved from the once feted "asylum" model, which was hospital based, to offering inpatient and community services models of care in which children, men, and women can also be cared for at home.

By 1774, the Madhouse Act enabled the "insane" to be treated by non-licensed practitioners, and in 1808, the County Asylum Act gave counties the power to levy a rate to build asylums. The apparent intention was to remove the "insane" from the workhouses to offer more care, according to the Royal College of Psychiatrists (Bewley, 2008). William Tuke, a Quaker, is largely credited with injecting a more caring approach into the care of people with mental health problems, including recreational activities in the nineteenth century (Bewley, 2008).

The evolution of services from charitable organizations to the involvement of the state, plus the interface of the religious values within the culture of modern mental health care, is evident.

The professionalization of the workforce, along with the development of more person-centred terminology regarding the care of adults with mental health problems, has been an impact of social policy too.

With regard to language, professionals speak much more about "wellbeing," and offensive colloquialisms relating to mental health are considered to be discriminatory. Language and the way in which professionals interact with the users of their services are key ways in which alliances can be improved.

Even for the purposes of this chapter, using the in-vogue BAME term is problematic. With regard to men and women of African origin, there is a distinction between the experiences of different ethnic groups in terms of mental health care. It is therefore important to make clear that with regard to diversity, an acronym does not accurately convey the distinctions and experience within the social group. Current parlance no longer allows individuals with mental health problems to be described as "insane," thankfully, and the evolution of language within the wider culture is inherent within considerations of social policy.

The complexities of diversity are such that it is appropriate to consider how minorities manage within the wider organization – while ensuring the workforce is reflective of the community it serves, there are nuances that need consideration.

I was recently involved in a statutory Mental Health Act assessment on an acute ward in London. The entire inpatient nursing team could be described as BAME, largely female.

I observed an acutely ill, young African-Caribbean male approach staff in a courteous manner and request leave. As an inpatient, acquiring leave is essential to wellbeing – inpatients can be bored and feel "trapped" without access to leave, though depending on levels of risk, staff may need to escort the individual.

There is no question that wards are under-resourced and the National Health Service (NHS) is subject to record pressures; however, there were six staff members who were able to assist by speaking with this young man to respond to his needs.

Unknown to the service user, I could hear the staff communicating with each other about not being able to take him out. Unfortunately, no staff member had told him. The matter escalated. The young man became more aggressive and in my view, a fairly pedestrian matter of communication resulted in a man being nursed intensively because he was so distressed.

I chose to speak to the nurse in charge and escalated matters further. Young black men are particularly at risk with regard to control and restraint, and in my mind, he wasn't treated with dignity. The white female independent doctor, who had observed the matter, discreetly thanked me for escalating the matter. The doctor later said that she had felt uncomfortable challenging the staff because of the "power dynamics."

On this occasion, the presence of largely African staff did not contribute to safe care and reinforced the need to ensure that organizations are aware of the nuances within staffing and care. There are sometimes distinctions of manner, approaches to care, and how groups work together in the delivery of health and social care. Diversity continues to require difficult conversations in the quest to improve.

A key part of the debate about race and mental health centers upon "labeling," which is in direct contrast to the newer philosophies of "person-centered care" and strengths-based approaches, which are an attempt to mitigate against the damaging impacts of stereotyping individuals and their difficulties.

The high rates of labeling black people of African descent with a diagnosis of psychosis are no real finding, but rather an indication of bias in diagnostic practice – this is what urgently demands scrutiny and reform.

Prime Minister Theresa May has commissioned a review into mental health law – specific attention to race is inherent. The Independent Review of the Mental Health Act has a specific African and Caribbean group. Professor Simon Wessely is yet to report back to the government, but there are different ways in which social policy initiatives interact within the provision of mental health policy.

Staffing the NHS

The contributions of young men and women from the Commonwealth who dedicated their professional and personal lives within the NHS are inextricably linked. It is no coincidence that the arrival of the SS Windrush and the NHS are celebrating 70 years in 2018.

Keeping people with mental health problems from "view" and the arrival of visible minorities because of the postwar effort, particularly around the provision of health care, has resulted in change. Nurses, porters, doctors, and bus drivers who arrived as part of mass migration ensured that the social transformation in the UK was under way.

At the time of the introduction of the NHS in 1948 (see England, 2013), Aneurin Bevan, the minister for health, made clear that the NHS had the following core principles:

- It meets the needs of everyone.
- It is free at the point of delivery.
- It is based upon clinical need, not on the ability to pay.

The ideological shift toward care within the community continued. Enoch Powell (1961), the controversial former minister for health, made clear that his intention was to eliminate the greater part of the country's mental hospitals:

> We have to get the idea into our heads that a hospital is a shell, a framework, however complex, to contain certain processes, and when the processes change or are superseded, then the shell must probably be scrapped.

Financial considerations were undoubtedly a catalyst for ideological change. New practices, including the introduction of medication no longer requiring long inpatient stays, contributed.

While modern mental health care is increasingly delivered at home, an inability to treat people based on clinical need and failing to meet their needs is unsafe.

Debating Poor Outcomes

As an experienced mental health professional, I feel that services could benefit from viewing diversity/race not within a silo but largely within the interrelationship with risk and safety.

Mental health problems can be an incredibly frightening experience for service users and carers; however, there is now more "health promotional" work to help allay wider fears. Despite reports of violence and aggressive behavior at the hands of people with mental health problems, fortunately the risks posed to the public are fairly low. Nevertheless, fear of using services is stigmatizing. A more helpful approach would be to be more emphatic about BAME as victims, not simply perpetrators, who needed help and attention, and therefore to be more vocal about experiences of poor care and risk. It is my view that there are parallels with the increasing incidence of knife crime. Safety and its perceptions will be central to any resolution of the problem and will include collaboration between the most affected communities and partners. Improvements within mental health are therefore no different.

One in Four

One in four of the population will suffer from a mental health problem; disorders include depression or a psychotic illness. The incidence of mental health problems is common, costly to the nation, and a contributory factor to social exclusion.

Almost 10% of mental health patients are identified as black or mixed race. However, these groups make up just 3% of the UK population. Fears about the disproportionate and adverse experiences remain, and agencies are engaged in trying to respond in different ways. Ethnic monitoring has been mandatory within health services since 1995, although more than 20 years later, progress is still required.

The Mental Health Foundation (2017) wrote about the different ways in which the black and minority ethnic community accessed health services. The Foundation was particularly concerned that this distinct group is more likely to:

- be diagnosed with mental health problems;
- be diagnosed and admitted to hospital;
- experience a poor outcome from treatment; and
- disengage from mainstream mental health services, leading to social exclusion and a deterioration in their mental health.

Discriminatory practices and a failure to meet the needs of the entire community which the organizations should serve fail to address core business, are unsafe, and lead to poor outcomes.

Tolerating poor outcomes within organizations, and failing to maintain focus on publicly stated aims, can be usefully challenged by broadening the discourse; in practice, forcing agencies to ensure that staff are properly trained and identify particular risks. Compassion and kindness are an integral part of health and social care.

Viewing substandard care within a context of safety and quality is particularly helpful when you consider the impact of communities mobilizing themselves into direct action. The Stafford Hospital is an excellent model to consider.

The Stafford Hospital – Campaigning for Quality Care

Staffordshire is in the Midlands, north of the comparatively more diverse city of Birmingham, which is the UK's second city.

Bella Bailey was admitted to the Stafford Hospital for eight weeks in 2007 and died. Lovingly supported by her family, who were shocked and appalled at the care delivered by the hospital, Julie, her daughter, initially raised her concerns with the hospital.

Julie's account notes that she did not receive an acknowledgement to her concerns. She reports that she eventually received a lawyer's letter explaining that it wasn't "the local authority's role to listen to complaints about the hospital." Complaints included:

- Patients were left in excrement in soiled bed clothes for lengthy periods.
- There was no assistance with feeding for patients who could not eat without help.
- Water was left out of reach.
- In spite of persistent requests for help, patients were not assisted in their toileting.

- Wards and toilet facilities were left in a filthy condition.
- Privacy and dignity, even in death, were denied.
- Triage in A&E was undertaken by untrained staff.
- Staff treated patients and those close to them with what appeared to be callous indifference.

The observations from family and carers dated back to 2007 and were particularly appalling considering that they applied to a hospital. While the population served there was largely white, there are useful parallels. Poor care would have continued had it not been for the efforts of a local carer, who established an incredibly influential pressure group rejecting this version of care.

One of the consequences of Julie's campaign, which was supported by politicians and the media, is that the relatively new culture of listening to service users and carers appears to have improved. However, Julie was met with an inadequate response from the hospital and enlisted the help of her local newspaper to appeal to the locality to hear their experiences. Julie describes being "flooded" by letters and what began as a single issue emerged into a pressure group entitled "Cure the NHS."

Despite openness and collaboration being encouraged as part of foundation trust status, Julie's frustrations and her work with users and carers shamed the authorities – calling into question the usefulness of adhering to a "tick box culture."

The group moved from impromptu meetings in a local cafe to finally forcing the government to hold an independent inquiry into the Stafford Hospital's failings. Nevertheless, the route to this was controversial and dogged – members of Cure the NHS worked with the then regulator, the Health Complaint Commission (HCC). The HCC, along with the hospital itself, was aware of the uncharacteristically high mortality rates (for a hospital of its size) and the documented issues of poor care. It is estimated that approximately 400–1200 people lost their lives at the hospital "unnecessarily" over 50 months.

Lord Francis, chair of the inquiry, made clear that there should be zero tolerance of any service that does not comply with fundamental standards. Recommendation 12 of the report makes explicit that standards should be subject to regular review, with a defined set of duties to maintain and operate them.

Within mental health services it is possible to observe a tragic narrative involving African-Caribbean men and women while in need of care. The case of Sarah Read is recent and worthy of consideration.

Too Late to Receive Care?

Sarah Read had a long history of mental health problems and took her life while in HMP Holloway in 2016. Sarah's case became public following the inquest into her death and the matter of care failings arose again. The inquest heard that despite waiting at the top of the list for a transfer for urgent health care, prison officers had found her to be "low risk" (see Gentleman & Gayle, 2017).

It is reported that Sarah's family are distressed that she did not receive the care that she required to keep her safe. INQUEST (2017), a UK-based charity reporting state deaths, stated in its July newsletter that despite the matter of death now being closed, the question remains: why was Sarah ever sent to prison, particularly given her long and documented risk history and need for treatment.

Learning lessons from inquiries or serious case reviews is incumbent upon agencies, particularly with the growing numbers of offenders with a mental disorder within prisons and cuts to preventative mental health care.

While I am not in possession of the full facts of Sarah's case, that an individual with her risk history could ever be deemed low risk is a concern and gives further weight to my view that diversity discussions need to be more emphatic about links to safety.

In 2010, an independent inquiry began, leading to a comprehensive report being published in 2013. The report's chair, Lord Francis (2013, p. 7), made 290 recommendations:

> Healthcare is not an activity short of systems intended to maintain and improve standards, regulate the conduct of staff, and report and scrutinise performance. Continuous efforts have been made to refine and improve the way these work. Yet none of them appreciated the scale and deficiencies at Stafford and, therefore, over a period of years did anything effective to stop them.

Lessons from the Staffordshire hospital interface with the experience of bereaved families. Francis (2013) asks a vital question within the inquiry report:

> Why did it have to take a determined group of families to expose those failings and campaign tirelessly for answers? I pay tribute again to the Work of Julie Bailey and Cure the NHS.

The independent organization Cure the NHS, which continues its work today, has not only achieved its aim to force state agencies to examine themselves more rigorously – the irony that the most vulnerable people were subject to "unnecessary harm" cannot be diminished – but has also forced complaints processes and obliged state agencies to respond to the recommendations of the report.

Social policy can therefore result from the "rule of law," but increasingly in response to direct action from families and loved ones, who can have an impact on a safer context. Public agencies are required to consider the impact of the report upon their business, largely due to the actions of a campaigning family member, that is, the efforts of Julie Bailey and the recommendations of Lord Francis in his report.

The adoption of a shared culture in which the patient is the priority in everything is the second recommendation. Lord Francis made clear that there should be zero tolerance of any service that does not comply with fundamental standards.

There is a more strengthened regulatory framework and a dynamic policy context to ensure that state agencies are much more vigilant about delivering safe and compassionate care.

Working with the Mental Health Act – Responsibilities and Rights for Relatives

The disproportionate numbers of largely black service users subject to compulsory treatment remains a very real fear for families. Not only is a mental health problem common, the black experience is often reported with a view to adverse health benefits.

At the time of writing there is a workforce review under way, which has yet to report to the Department of Health and Social Care (DHSC), although at a National Approved Mental Health Professional Conference, held in London in June 2018, Claire Barcham's work with the DHSC indicated that initial findings are that black people access crises services at a comparatively higher rate and subject to a greater degree of compulsion.

It is a serious concern that certain parts of the community do not appear able to be involved in key aspects of decision-making without the force of the law. This is particularly so when considering the coercive aspects of welfare, such as compulsory treatment to manage risk and health which feature heavily within the BAME experience of receiving vital care. In practice, more intelligence around reasons why informal admissions to hospitals appear less likely within BAME communities is needed.

Mental health law makes clear that informal admissions are a vital option to consider. The use of the more controlling aspects, that is, detentions under the Mental Health Act 1983, is likely to be multi-causal. Gould's (2012) work, which focused upon the lived experience within the application of the Care Program Approach (CPA), is relevant in terms of the BAME patient experience.

Gould found that with regard to ethnicity, African-Caribbean men and women were particularly dissatisfied with services. In addition, there were a significant number of respondents who were not sure that they had received identification of risk.

Risk assessment remains an integral part of the CPA process – which is a government attempt to coordinate health and social care for people with mental health problems. The process was introduced 20 years ago and has been subject to reform.

Dissatisfaction may lead to disengagement with care, which has implications in the way therapeutic alliance can be achieved for those in need. While compulsion has its place, I hope that the independent review which is under way can make useful recommendations that can achieve real change.

However, within the busy inner-city London borough in which I work as an approved mental health professional (AMHP), it increasingly feels as if the opportunities for informal admissions continues to diminish.

An AMHP is a social worker who undertakes specialist training and is authorized to be involved in the detention of a child or adult. A Mental Health Act assessment usually involves two doctors and an AMHP, who consider risk and the least restrictive place for a mentally incapacitated person to receive care. An informal admission is a legal consideration at all times, but not always possible. Decision-making is also supported by the Mental Capacity Act 2005 in the undertaking of a Mental Health Act. If a formal detention is required, a "section" of the Mental Health Act will be used to enable compulsory treatment to be provided.

While making an application under the Mental Health Act 1983 is a huge responsibility, there are safeguards, and it is important that all service users and their families are sufficiently empowered.

Staying Involved

Following a Mental Health Act assessment in which I was minded to make an application for Section 3 of the Mental Health Act 1983, I was unable to do so after being informed about her mother who had objected to her daughter receiving compulsory treatment.

In the presence of two doctors, I interviewed a young African-Caribbean woman who was detained in a London mental health hospital after her family raised concerns following an acute period of bizarre behavior. A detention for an assessment under Section 2 had taken place 28 days previously, which the law allows. However, her bizarre and increasingly aggressive behavior, along with an inability to look after herself and keep safe, led to a medical recommendation from the ward consultant, which resulted in a coordinated assessment.

One of the most important legal safeguards of the longer-term Section 3 (which lasts for up to six months) is that the AMHP must identify and consult with the nearest relative. A mother, partner, or sibling could be considered, although on this occasion, I identified her mother as the nearest relative. While the inpatient's mother (Mrs B) was fully versed with risk and her daughter's deteriorating mental state, she continued to object, and there is provision to go to court to displace a nearest relative if they are perceived to be acting unreasonably.

After detailed discussion, it became apparent that the objection was based upon her fears of "letting her daughter down" because "hospitals are racist" and "terrible things happen to black people in hospital."

I acknowledged her fears and supported both the clinical team and the nearest relative to speak about treatment, the processes, and care plans. In addition, we spoke at length about ensuring that she remained close to her daughter's care and not on the perimeters of it should a court displacement of her role be agreed.

I spoke to Mrs B about the hospital system and trying to get the most out of it for her daughter and herself. While lengthy and difficult, I found that acknowledging the parent's fear – being transparent – avoided a situation in which the more controlling aspects of law superseded the caring function.

Mrs B was also made aware that while I was of a similar ethnic background, the pursuit of health care and safety is critical, problematic, and all communities have a right to access it and exercise stated rights.

The nearest relative role has essential rights relating to applying for discharge if appropriate. This is a powerful right, which is to be respected. Time pressures and the demands of work priorities could have resulted in a swift hearing at court and would have been hugely impactful for a family embarking on a frightening and distressing episode in their lives.

Following the interventions of listening and getting senior leaders to speak with Mrs B and make clear their treatment plans, Mrs B removed her objection and the application was made. This was an incredibly difficult decision – but Mrs B told me that she appreciated the time, effort, and understanding given. One of the implications being, that a court order to displace a mother from her nearest relative role may have resulted in her not exercising influence in the care of her daughter. It was so important to try to avoid isolating her family – on this occasion; her mother was her key advocate and it is essential that professionals support carers wherever possible.

While I heard Mrs B's fears, I am also a parent, as well as a professional. There is much to do in terms of engagement with primary care to ensure that at the time of crisis, formal, statutory detentions are the most likely options.

The Rise of Safeguarding and New Opportunities

So far, I have considered the impact of social policy in its widest sense – through laws, "people power," and policy relating to the welfare of the black community in the UK. It does not appear that black communities are currently well served or safe.

However, while there is an argument that lessons are not learned in the vigorously pursued inquiries and ensuing publicity about poor standards and risk management with regard to the black community, it is also important to realize that agencies can be confronted with clear facts and be encouraged to change their culture. Equality impact statements, scrutiny by politicians, increased accountability, and the introduction of the new Speak Up Champions – which the NHS is now required to employ to bolster whistle-blowing activities – are modern tools to combat inequalities.

Agencies are increasingly required to listen to their stakeholders like never before. The Care Act (2014), which repealed the postwar welfare state laws, ensures that adults and autonomy are central to new, mental health care arrangements.

Safeguarding Is Personal

Legal obligations regarding safeguarding are enshrined in the Care Act. At its heart is the idea that safeguarding is *personal*. As the Act is new, there is a dearth of research documenting the interrelationship between race and safeguarding. There is some potential for the development of high-quality, personalized, and accessible services.

An emphasis on "personal" and a shift from a service-led philosophy offers opportunities for individual care, which reflects a person's needs. While the local authority is the lead agent with regard to adults at risk within its borough of responsibility, adults with care and support needs who appear to be at risk are required to be assessed.

Black communities engage with services in specific ways and access primary care much later than their white counterparts (discussed in Gould, 2012) and have an impact upon the management of risk.

It is my view that there is now an opportunity to review the impact upon BAME communities with regard to safeguarding and their risks.

Adults at risk with care and support needs are the very focus of safeguarding, and the pursuit of enquiries and safeguarding planning may result in greater numbers of BAME considered within the safeguarding adults' statistics.

In short, if there is a disproportionate number of BAME using mental health services, there is a greater likelihood of BAME men and women meeting the eligibility criteria.

It is therefore possible that the safeguarding arena could also helpfully contribute to renewing the focus on safety for the most at-risk members of the community.

There is the wider social context of the impact of economic austerity, political change, along with tightening service thresholds. The Care Act (2014) provides a greater focus upon the assessment and management of risks for the most vulnerable within our community. It is also opportune for increased research into the interrelationship between safeguarding and the impact of care planning and ways in which state agencies support adults at risk to ensure that safeguarding is truly personal.

There is a real opportunity to be empowered by pursuing requests for statutory, community care assessments, especially if certain adults are at risk of harm.

There is a new legal impetus created by the emphasis on safeguarding to ensure that vulnerable people can approach statutory services for assessment if they are at risk of abuse. This is a new lever to compel agencies to collaborate with service users, and it offers opportunities. While safeguarding formalities do not apply within prisons, users and families who believe that their loved ones are being neglected or abused have a right to have their circumstances reviewed and the adult at risk is to be consulted about their view and aspirations for the management of risk.

Categories of Abuse

The Care Act (2014) broadened the category of risks to be considered, with regard to adult safeguarding.

In addition to the categories of physical, emotional, and sexual abuse to consider within the undertaking of safeguarding enquiries, consideration must now be given to adults at risk of domestic violence, modern slavery, and neglect.

Individuals with care and support needs (which includes' the presence of mental health issues) who appear to be at risk are entitled to have a statutory assessment. This is new legislation and something that marginalized communities are able to utilize. There is an opportunity to work closely with the agencies that are designed to offer care and support and not to be "written off."

Diversity is an inherent part of mental health provision. Poor care, in my view, is also a manifestation of poor assessment and management of risk. Assessments of care and risk are the lifeblood of health care, so greater attention to improving

162 Patricia Clarke

Funding shortages, poor training, increased demand, and expectation are a real challenge for the future. Highlighting the ways to challenge quality, by asserting legal rights, formally pursuing complaints processes, and the unique advantages of the independent sector that marginalized communities, can challenge an anachronistic and unsatisfactory status quo.

It is compelling that services lead a new debate, which broadens the professional understanding of safety, risk, and diversity.

References

Bewley, T. (2008). *Madness to illness: A history of the Royal College of Psychiatrists.* Cambridge: RCPsych Publications by Cambridge University Press.

Care Act. (2014). Retrieved from http://www.legislation.gov.uk/ukpga/2014/23/contents/enacted

England, N. (2013). *The NHS Constitution for England*. London: Department of Health.

Francis, R. (2013). *Report of the Mid Staffordshire NHS Foundation Trust public inquiry: Executive summary*. London: The Stationery Office.

Gentleman, A., & Gayle, D. (2017). Sarah Read's mother: "My daughter was failed by many and I was ignored". *The Guardian*, February 17. https://www.theguardian.com/society/2016/feb/17/sarah-reeds-mother-deaths-in-custody-holloway-prison-mental-health.

Gould, D. (2012). Service users' experience of recovery under the 2008 care programme approach.

INQUEST newsletter. (2017) Retrieved from https://www.inquest.org.uk. Accessed on July 2.

Jones, R. (2018). *The Mental Health Act manual* (21st ed.). London: Sweet & Maxwell/Thomson Reuters.

Mental Capacity Act. (2005). Mental Capacity Act. http://www.legislation.gov.uk/ukpga/2005

Mental Health Foundation. (2017). Mental Health Crisis Care. Retrieved from https://www.mentalhealth.org.uk/a-to-z/b/black-asian-and-minority-ethnic-bame-communities. Accessed on July 1.

Oppenheim, M. (2017). Grenfell Tower fire: "Death toll may have been covered up to prevent a riot", says David Lammy MP. *The Independent*, June 27.

Powell, E. (1961). The Water Tower speech; Speeches 1957–65. Retrieved from https://enochpowell.info/resource

Chapter 8

Remaining Mindful about Children and Young People

Mhemooda Malek and Simon Newitt

My culture and identity are understood and respected when I am in contact with services and professionals. I am not stigmatised by services and professionals as a result of my health symptoms or my cultural or ethnic background. The strengths of my culture and identity are recognised as part of my recovery. My behaviour is seen in the light of communication and expression, not just as a clinical problem. (The Mental Health Taskforce, 2016, p. 43)

Mental health and wellbeing are an asset whatever an individual's age, race or ethnicity and mental health problems don't discriminate on the basis of these attributes. So do we give equal attention to planning and providing services that sustain good mental health and address mental health problems irrespective to people's age, race or ethnicity?

This question is explored here in relation to children and young people who are described, by themselves or society, as Black and minority ethnic (BME) or the range of related terminology in use. Inequalities in the provision of mental health care for BME communities have been noted for some time (National Institute for Mental Health in England, 2003; The Sainsbury Centre for Mental Health, 2002); however, children and young people have received relatively less focus than adults on this issue. Statutory Child and Adolescent Mental Health Services (CAMHS) in England generally cater for young people up to the age of 18 years, some voluntary and community sector provision offers services up to the age of 25 years.

The first part of this chapter considers the landscape of policy and strategy and the extent to which Black and minority children and young people have received due focus and attention. The second part presents a case study from a frontline Youth Information Advice and Counselling Service (YIACS). These perspectives are based on experience in England where mental health provision has experienced significant cuts in funding, increased demand and significant unmet need (Mental Health Foundation, 2017; NHS Providers, 2016; The Mental Health Taskforce, 2016). In this scenario, services in the voluntary and community sector such as YIACS are experiencing unprecedented demand and presentation of more complex needs than has previously been the case, including increased referrals from statutory sector services (Kenrick, 2013; Malek, 2016). The report of the House of Commons Health Committee published in 2014 notes:

> YIACS have always been vulnerable, largely because they sit between a wider system of young people's services and statutory mental health. A lack of ownership and ambivalence, despite often representing the most significant resource alongside CAMHS in meeting mental health needs, has allowed YIACS to be easy targets for cuts. Over the years, individual services have set up and closed, including some closures over the past four years. With national policy stressing the importance of mental health and better early intervention and prevention, these cuts make no sense at all. (House of Commons Health Committee, 2014, p. 24)

The supply chain to young people receiving relevant support is a long and complex one spanning a range of sectors, services and professionals including: service commissioning; education, health, social services and youth justice sectors; community provision such as youth groups and recreational facilities; primary care; and specialist community and inpatient mental health services. It is not within the scope of this chapter to examine the range of components in this chain, nevertheless it is essential to highlight the need for a holistic approach to identify and address issues that impact on BME children and young people receiving appropriate support.

Impact of Race and Ethnicity Terminology

The term 'Black and minority ethnic' or 'BME' is used with some caution because they raise a number of issues regarding the people they aim to describe and in the planning and provision of services, as well as related research and evaluation activity (Bhopal & Rankin, 1999; Malek & Joughin, 2004; Smaje, 1995; Street, Staplekamp, Taylor, Malek, & Kurtz, 2005). A range of other terms are also in current use in the UK to refer to people who are in a minority due to their race and ethnicity as compared to the majority White British population. However, while generic terms and categories are useful for identifying broad patterns and trends they do not provide sufficient detail about the full range of communities encompassed.

The search for accurate terminology regarding race and ethnicity in health provision is described as controversial (Bhopal & Rankin, 1999; Smaje, 1995) because, though in frequent use, the term 'race' lacks scientific validity and the term 'ethnicity' is a fluid concept that changes over time. This has implications for administrative and research activities that rely on accurate categories and for social reasons because people may not identify with the broad terminology created and imposed by others.

Intersectionality is also a key consideration regarding how aspects such as faith, sexuality and disability interact with race and ethnicity. BME communities are also at greater risk of exposure to social and economic disadvantage (Joseph

Rowntree Foundation, 2011; Office for National Statistics, 2014). A further consideration is that 'visible minorities' and 'people of colour', whose ethnicity is visible, can be subject to different or greater racism and discrimination. It is therefore imperative that mental health needs are considered in the context of broader inequalities experienced by individuals and their communities.

The national census (Office for National Statistics, 2014) is a relevant example in this respect because the categories used to collect data on race and ethnicity inform the planning and provision of services, as well as the collection of service user data and other activities including estimates regarding prevalence of mental health problems. However, census categories do not sufficiently distinguish between the range of people encompassed and can wrongly imply homogeneity between them. This scenario presents a number of challenges including (Bhopal & Rankin, 1999; Malek & Joughin, 2004; Smaje, 1995; Street et al., 2005):

- The need to balance simplicity in data collection and use against the dangers of stereotyping and inaccuracy. Generic terms such as 'BME' and categories such as 'African' do not indicate who the specific individuals and communities encompassed are, their needs, the extent to which they are reached by services and their needs addressed.
- Information generated by tick box categories alone is insufficient to usefully inform planning and provision of appropriate services and clinical interventions. For example, the concept of eating disorders may be understood differently across cultures and this will in turn impact on recognition of the issue as a problem, help seeking behaviour, diagnosis, treatment and aftercare that are culturally relevant and appropriate. Without this information, there is a real risk of commissioning services on the basis of incomplete information about local population groups. The extent to which additional data are generated and used to plan and commission local services for children and young people is unclear, the sparse published literature on this issue suggests that, some notable examples excepted, this is generally not the case.
- The level of international agreement on categories has implications for comparative research and other studies as well as interventions developed for particular groups. For example, the people encompassed in the term 'Asian' can differ between countries; in the UK it largely refers to people with origins in the Indian subcontinent, whereas in other countries it can include people of South East Asian origin.

These examples are intended to illustrate the potential wide ranging impact of terminology on planning and providing relevant services and the need for due vigilance regarding implications for service users.

Lack of Data

The scarcity of data on mental health and ethnicity is frequently highlighted and contributes to an incomplete overall picture of who is affected, how and where (Atkinson et al., 2001; Dogra, Singh, Svirydzenka, & Vostanis, 2012; Fitzpatrick, Kumar, Nkansa-Dwamena, & Thorne, 2014; Malek & Joughin, 2004;

Messent & Murrell, 2003; Minnis et al., 2003). A key area in which a lack of relevant data has a significant impact is in local and national initiatives such as service reviews. For example, an independent review of CAMHS (Department for Children, Schools and Families, 2008) found that data in relation to BME children and young people was inconsistent and at times contradictory. Site visits carried out by the review team indicated an under-representation in statutory CAMHS and the team conclude that these young people are more likely to reach a crisis point before coming into contact with services.

Lack of accurate, robust data further adds to the invisibility of BME children and young people in the context of their mental health. Consequently, many of the issues highlighted, including in this chapter, are informed by literature that covers a broader age range.

Why Focus on Children and Young People?

Mental health problems are said to have started to develop during childhood and adolescence (Department of Health, 2009b; Department of Health and NHS England, 2015). There is an overrepresentation of some BME people in adult in-patient services in the UK (Care Quality Commission, 2010) and an under-representation in CAMHS (Department for Children, Schools and Families, 2008; Street et al., 2005). This suggests a link between lack of effective interventions at an early age and becoming a mental health in-patient as an adult.

Furthermore, children and young people from some BME groups are overrepresented in the youth justice system, social services looked after provision, exclusion from school and educational under-achievement (Malek, 2011); situations which are described as having an adverse impact on young people and their mental health.

National initiatives with a focus on BME people's mental health have tended to subsume all age groups and paid insufficient attention to children and young people (Department of Health, 2005, 2011; National Institute for Mental Health in England, 2003). This is problematic because it contributes to a lack of visibility and profile; furthermore, the structure of provision for this age group is fundamentally different to that for adults, thereby meriting specific attention.

Similarly, a raft of programmes that focus on all children and young people tend to give insufficient, if any, attention to matters of race equality (Malek, 2011). This lack of focus serves to marginalise BME young people at multiple levels, as illustrated by looking at some key policy and strategic developments.

Policy and Strategic Landscape

Over the past two decades or so there have been a number of developments at the national level which have made specific references to the mental health of people from BME communities and some have specifically focussed on them. However, BME children and young people have received scant attention in these initiatives.

The National Service Framework 1999 (Department of Health, 1999) highlighted that BME people experienced particular difficulties in accessing services and some were diagnosed as having higher rates of disorder than the general population. It also acknowledged that mental health services were not adequately meeting the mental health needs of this population group. There is no specific reference to provision for BME children and young people.

The reports 'Breaking the Circles of Fear' (The Sainsbury Centre for Mental Health, 2002) and 'Inside Outside' (National Institute for Mental Health in England, 2003) published in 2003/2004 focussed specifically on mental health provision for BME communities and were significant to informing national policy (Department of Health, 2005). However, while some reference is made to the experiences of 'young people', including those aged over 18 years, there is no specific exploration regarding the context in CAMHS.

The National Service Framework for Children, Young People and Maternity Services (2004) (Department of Health, 2004) includes specific recommendations regarding the mental health needs of BME children and young people. A welcome inclusion but limited to a small section of the standard on mental health and in isolation, does not address the need to give due consideration to race equality in all aspects of provision and recommendations covered in this standard. Thereby presenting the risk that addressing the specific recommendations will be inappropriately seen as sufficient to addressing race equality in all aspects of service planning and delivery. Neither has there been any overall evaluation regarding the extent to which the specific recommendations for BME communities have been implemented across all CAMHS and what outcomes have been achieved.

The national government action plan 'Delivering Race Equality in Mental Health Care' published in 2005 (Department of Health, 2005) is applicable across all age groups; however, the extent of its implementation in CAMHS is unclear and said to be piecemeal. The review of this action plan (Department of Health, 2009a) highlights some good practice but there is no overview of its implementation in provision for children and young people and the nature of further developments needed.

The Count Me In Census (Care Quality Commission, 2010) introduced as part of the national action plan (Department of Health, 2005) concluded that the number of BME children and young people in inpatient settings was small for some groups and average for others as compared to their numbers in the national population. However, the census is limited to mental health inpatient providers registered with the Care Quality Commission and therefore does not include those cared for in other settings such as paediatric wards and social care provision. The shortage of inpatient facilities is likely to contribute to young people being cared for in a range of settings the conclusion of this census therefore needs to be treated with some caution.

The government strategy for all age groups 'No health without mental health' published in 2011 (Department of Health, 2011) has a section on 'race' which does not mention children and young people. Nor do the sections focussing on children and young people indicate how many of BME origin are affected by mental health problems, or how belonging to the high risk groups listed in the strategy interacts with race and ethnicity.

A range of other national policies and programmes follow similar patterns (Malek, 2011). This further contributes to invisibility of BME children and young people and their needs, making them vulnerable to oversight in key policy and strategic planning activities that inform the commissioning and delivery of services.

Commissioning Services

Commissioning appropriate and responsive services is dependent on a reliable overview of local population needs. In this respect, cultural awareness and competency is as important at the level of strategic planning and commissioning, as it is to the operational delivery of services and interventions (Bahl, 1998; Bhui, Christie, & Bhugra, 1995; Malek & Joughin, 2004; Rawaf, 1998; Street et al., 2005). The availability of training, resources and skills required for effective strategic planning and commissioning of services for diverse communities are in short supply, which compromises good practice in this respect.

Population needs assessments are a vital aspect of the commissioning process and regular updating would enable taking account of changes in local demographics as well as changes in population needs. The extent to which any such assessments routinely and effectively incorporate race and ethnicity is unclear and likely to require significant development (Malek & Joughin, 2004).

Setting quality standards and taking forward findings highlighted by regular reviews are essential to effective service commissioning and delivery. Standard setting and review can include mental health promotion, identification of mental health problems, assessment, diagnosis and clinical interventions. Furthermore, service commissioners can communicate local population needs to providers and specify requirements to meet the needs of specific local population groups. It is unclear to what extent reviews of service provision to BME children and young people are undertaken or what, if any, guidelines are given to service providers in relation to meeting their needs. Nor is there any overview regarding the extent to which requirements about providing culturally sensitive services are specified in service contracts and their implementation monitored.

The Voluntary and Community Sector

The voluntary and community sector is increasingly acknowledged as a key provider of essential mental health services and support, particularly where statutory services fail to address inequalities (Bahl, 1998; House of Commons Health Committee, 2014; Singh, 1998). Provision in this sector may be targeted at BME communities or be available as part of broader provision for all communities, some may be delivered in partnership with the statutory sector. Services in the voluntary and community sector can also struggle to effectively engage diverse ethnic communities and in this respect should be subject to the same level of scrutiny as other services. Nevertheless, there is wide acknowledgement that this sector tends to have significant knowledge about local communities, is able to engage people whom other provision fails to reach and can provide valuable training to other sectors. A wide range of support is provided from primary care to specialist interventions as well as acting as a filter to statutory specialist mental health and social care provision (Fitzpatrick et al., 2014; Kurtz, Thornes, & Wolkind, 1994).

A key feature highlighted for this sector is the provision of holistic support that ranges from counselling and therapy to support with wider issues such as housing, education, employment, advice and advocacy. However, a significant proportion of this sector works under constraints including insecure and inadequate funding combined with lack of capacity to effectively engage with strategic planning structures that would benefit from its participation. This has wide ranging impacts including on long-term planning and sustaining innovative approaches developed to meet local needs. Currently in the UK, this sector is increasingly competing for contracts with relatively better resourced statutory sector services; a situation that presents a number of challenges, especially for small community organisations that operate on minimal resources but can be a lifeline to local people. Some promising partnerships and consortium arrangements are emerging in the context of CAMHS provision, though there are also concerns about some contractual requirements that can be potentially damaging to voluntary and community sector approaches in engaging with and providing for communities (Malek, 2016).

Services such as YIACS, which mostly have charitable status, are acknowledged as having a key role in supporting young people's mental health. The provision of holistic support, under one roof, to young people up to the age of 25 years is noted as a valuable asset of YIACS which should be seen as a key part of local provision (Department of Health and NHS England, 2015).

> Provide a key role for the voluntary and community sector to encourage an increase in the number of one-stop shop services, based in the community. They should be a key part of any universal local offer, building on the existing network of YIACS (Youth Information, Advice, and Counselling Services). Building up such a network would be an excellent use of any identified early additional investment. There may also be a case in future for developing national quality standards for a comprehensive one-stop-shop service, to support a consistent approach to improving outcomes and joint working. (Department of Health and NHS England, 2015, p. 43)

The case study example which follows this section illustrates the work of a YIACS and its endeavour to focus on meeting the needs of BME children and young people.

What Young People have to Say

The sparse published information available about the views of BME young people (Malek, 2011; Street et al., 2005) highlights that they experience problems that impact on all young people as well as additional issues specific to their culture, race and ethnicity. These additional concerns are wide ranging depending on individual circumstances and include racism and discrimination, conflicting demands of family or community and wider society, stigma that is specific to their culture and community and encounters with services and professionals that lack sufficient knowledge and skills to provide them with culturally relevant support. The following are some of the features BME young people have highlighted as helpful:

- Relevant information that can be accessed through friendly outlets, explaining mental health services and what various mental health professionals can offer.
- A range of venues and opening times for accessing support.
- Friendly, approachable staff who show an appreciation of diverse religious and cultural values and awareness of factors that BME young people specifically encounter in society and in their daily lives.
- Suitable interpreters where needed and staff experienced in working with them.
- Support with onward referral so that young people do not move between services that demonstrate different levels of cultural sensitivity.
- Being listened to and given opportunities to be involved in making decisions.

Given the opportunity to express their views, ideas and concerns it is clear that young people have much to say and contribute. The co-production of services with services users and local communities is a key theme currently being promoted (The Mental Health Taskforce, 2016; NHS England, 2015). The extent to which this is occurring in a meaningful way for all young people is unclear; let alone BME young people. Nevertheless, co-production provides a valuable mechanism for developing community and service user engagement that goes beyond time limited and, at times, tokenistic approaches. The development of initiatives that facilitate co-production should ensure BME children and young people are sufficiently and appropriately engaged, their contributions valued and feedback provided regarding progress on implementation of relevant actions.

There are many issues that need to be addressed before we can say with some confidence that we give due and equal attention to the mental health of BME children and young people. The range of areas that require attention cut across policy, planning and service delivery spanning prevention and early intervention through to treatment and aftercare.

The needs of BME children and young people require consideration as a core aspect of service development and provision; not as an afterthought whereby consideration of their needs occurs at a later stage after key components of a policy, strategy or service are already in place.

Importantly, facilitating participation in the planning and provision of services, through the mechanism of co-production and in collaboration with community and faith groups, is an important cornerstone to future provision of equitable services.

> **Case Study: Project Zazi**
>
> *I think it's because of the stereotyping Black people. Say for example someone was driving a nice car, coming towards a group of Black kids, and you went; 'what person you think is driving that car?' They'll never say a Black man. If a Black man was driving that car, they'd be, like ... well you look twice. So their stereotype even stops them seeing the Black people who are doing like the right thing, like the positive stuff in the area. That's all they're focussed on now, their mindset, 'cos it's not normal to them and so they shoot that person down and cuss on them. It's not normal for them to be where they're wearing suits instead of wearing the baggy jeans and the latest name brands and stuff. So, it's not like they do it on purpose, but their mindset is so corrupted that they don't see it as normal. They try to diss the person, so then it kind of stops them from doing it too. I think that's what's happening here.* (Lawrence, 19 years)

Emerging out of a three-year participatory social research project with young men from the inner city neighbourhood of St Pauls in Bristol, Project Zazi[1] aims to engage BME young people aged 11–25 with support well-upstream of the over-representations and poorer outcomes that too frequently characterise the Black experience of adult mental health services and the criminal justice system. Funded by a progressive grant-making foundation, the project operates out of Off the Record (OTR), a third sector (non-profit) organisation working across the city of Bristol and its surrounding area.

Project Zazi has three broad, over-arching but interconnected outcomes:

- To improve the personal and collective resilience of young people and communities.
- To improve the mental health and wellbeing of young people.
- To improve access to mental health support for young people.

The project also has three goals that relate to how these outcomes will be realised:

- To be a consistent local presence well beyond three years and to evolve into a local movement.
- To embed economic opportunity and participation for young people in the project structure.
- To change policy responses to this population of young people.

Project Zazi uses youth work and community psychology to proactively target and offer support to individuals, but the team also co-designs group work and

---

[1] Zazi is a Zulu word that means 'know yourself, know your strength'.

participatory social action campaigns (Cahill, 2006) alongside young people. These are vehicles for the application of de-colonising approaches drawn from liberation psychology (Martín-Baró, 1994) and critical pedagogy (Freire, 1971). More generally, the project is conceptually underpinned by feminist, critical race and postcolonial critiques of Western psychological sciences and the social conditions they operate in. The specific goal of the team is to challenge and unpick the epidermalised inferiority (Fanon, 1967) and hidden injuries (Sennett & Cobb, 1972) inflicted by structural inequality on the structure of feeling (Williams, 1977), cultural politics and psychological landscape of young people positioned at an intersection of race, class, gender and history.

> Too much people have the story of failure round here … try and fail. Not much people can say they done this and it worked out. Once you get success you're gone, they have to leave here. No-one stays. (Jermaine, 16 years)

On this reading, the hypervigilance, anxiety and anger expressed by many local young people is adaptive not disordered; a normal, even healthy response to an environment of economic injustice, structural and actual violence. As well as working directly with young people and families, Project Zazi exists to influence the wider system of statutory and non-statutory services and professionals around young people from this conceptual position, challenging mainstream services to understand the experience behind the presentation; to not be complicit in oppression by misreading social conditions as personal problems, and so effect 'an ideologization of reality that winds up consecrating the existing order as natural' (Martín-Baró, 1994, p. 21).

> It's like this, if I'm hungry and I see fruit on a tree, but you tell me you own the tree and the fruit and the land around the tree, so I can't even get the old fruit that's fallen on the floor. If I'm hungry and got no money to buy your fruit, if I'm hungry and you tell me that; sorry, I'm just gonna take the fruit. (Marcel, 18 years)

The Zazi team work iteratively, through cycles of planning, participatory action and reflection to develop content for the project structure, some examples of which are included below:

- Girl Talk is a weekly group for young women aged 11–16 that uses participatory action learning to explore themes of gender and sexual politics, healthy relationships, stress, aspirations and female empowerment through the lens of race, faith and postcode. The group is delivered in collaboration with another non-statutory agency from a local community flat, and its action learning structure facilitates the production of small-scale social action projects, including film and photography.
- Real Talk is a weekly group for 11- to 19-year olds that uses group discussion to explore identity and culture, co-opting in external speakers and agencies

and putting on new activities that encourage participants to learn new skills. The sessions holistically promote good physical and mental health, relationships and lifestyles.
- Corner Man is a weekly session for boys and young men aged 11–15 based in a local boxing gym. Using detached, street-based youth work project staff engage young people who are in contact with the justice system, engaged in youth violence, and participating in gang activity. The collaboration with boxing coaches offers a structured programme of sport and life coaching that helps individuals manage and regulate their (often strong and problematic) feelings, control their aggression and develop their self-discipline. Alongside the training and (non-contact) boxing, Project Zazi staff use psychological tools to support young people to develop gang exit strategies and set personal goals, exploring masculinity and transitions to adulthood in the process (Sewell, 1997). Often this means finding routes back into education and/or employment, but it can also involve managing conflict at home. The gym is home to three world champion boxers, and their presence is a source of inspiration and guidance.
- Street 2 Boardroom is an eight-week programme of group work that supports young people 16–25 to develop the entrepreneurial skills they learn on the streets into lawful enterprises and small businesses. Alongside the group work, which pulls in external speakers and uses motivational and solution focussed techniques in one-to-one mentoring, the project staff support their alumni into mentoring relationships with business leaders and allied agencies working to encourage youth enterprise.

> We feel like we can talk to you about anything and that you listen to us and plan stuff around what we say, so we can talk about things that are happening and learn stuff. (Arafa, 16 years)

Project Zazi is in many ways an exploratory piece of work, testing ideas and approaches in an iterative structure but through a clearly articulated conceptual model. The outcomes so far are modest in the sense that it is too early to claim, given the systemic circumstances facing this population of young people, that any individual life trajectories have been irreversibly altered. That said, the signs are encouraging, with numerous case examples of re-integration to school, cessation of anti-social and self-injurious behaviour, and improved communication skills. Allied to this – and in the vernacular of mental health services – self-reported feelings of anxiety and low mood are also seemingly improved by the team's approach. Indeed, qualitative feedback is overwhelmingly positive in relation to the ability of the Project Zazi staff to engage marginalised young people in the work, and with ideas, concepts and activities that have in them at least *the potential* to be therapeutic and transformative. With mainstream NHS child and adolescent mental health services struggling (persistently and by design) to engage young people from some BME communities, this is, in itself, an encouraging sign.

> It's good to just chill and talk, it don't ever happen normally. I like it. (Tyreese, 15 years)

About Off the Record (Bristol)

Founded in 1965, OTR is one of the oldest YIACs in the UK, with a simple and unchanged offer of free, confidential, self-referral support unburdened by service thresholds and criteria. The organisation is thriving in an emerging landscape characterised by increasing marketisation of public service provision, austerity and the wider retrenchment of the welfare state, the blossoming of social enterprise, and a public health crisis (including concomitant moral panic) in young people's mental health that has seen demand and 'clinical complexity' escalate year-on-year. OTR has achieved operational growth of 1,600% in eight years and today employs over 100 staff drawn from a wide range of professional backgrounds. The agency supports several thousand young people each year across a diverse and heavily targeted portfolio of community-based mental health support and social action work.

Focussing on prevention and early intervention, OTR operates in a highly integrated and systemic way, delivering in formal collaborations and commissioned partnerships with other third sector agencies and the NHS. The mission of the charity is 'to support, promote and defend the mental health, rights and social position of young people' (LinkedIn: Off The Record, 2017), a statement that immediately reveals the psychocultural and psychopolitical (Sedgwick, 1982) character of its work and approach; features central to the inception and delivery of Project Zazi, and which are explored briefly below.

For OTR, one of the most enduring ways mental health services have historically served to recycle societal inequalities is by not being transparent (with themselves; let alone the people that might come to need them) about *what it is they believe about what it is they do*. At OTR, 'mental health' is shorthand for the ways human beings experience the world and each other in it. A consequence of this definition is that mental health is an important lens through which to peer at and understand society – not just the individual and their distress. More than this, being explicit about and engaging with the cultural assumptions underpinning the organisation's mission is key to the ongoing capability of OTR and its various project teams to work with culture and difference intelligently, reflexively, and, ultimately, inclusively. In all service design, recruitment, induction and training processes OTR underwrites it's work with the following seven core assumptions and beliefs:

1. Mental health is social and political as well as personal.
2. The work we do is a vocation and we are on the side of young people.
3. All theoretical models are wrong, but all of them are useful.
4. Relationships are what make the difference.
5. Social networks are more sustainable than individual solutions.

6. Building on strengths and capabilities is more powerful than meeting needs and vulnerabilities.
7. Participatory services are more transformative than transactional ones.

OTR believes that clinicians, researchers and government alike make a number of implicit assumptions about mental health that are ideological in character and thus possess the potential to control, dominate and oppress marginalised groups. In the commissioning, evaluation, design and delivery of public services, these assumptions latently express fundamental ideas about the world and what it means to be human. They include powerful ethno-centric and socio-economic beliefs about the role of the individual and society, happiness, the emotions, status, the nature and meaning of knowledge and time, and of course the relationship between our mind and body. They come underwritten by a medical language that veils them with an aura of objectivity and scientific validity. But for OTR they are little else than cultural constructs that mirror the prevailing socio-economic and political narrative of the time.

This matters because these assumptions frame what is meant in a body of research, a social policy response, or an individual clinical intervention by healthy and unhealthy, normal and abnormal. They draw a line between 'us' (healthy and normal) and 'them' (sick and abnormal) that serves to other and stigmatise the latter. And they persist because of the enduring belief that it is the individual (and their pursuit of happiness) that is the most meaningful unit of enquiry in mental health; an ideological perspective that actively strips our emotional landscape of context and locates the mental health problem and solution inside the individual or perhaps some other external (but nearby) trauma.

Western approaches to psychological health are steeped in socio-political beliefs (individualism, hedonism, positivism, ahistoricism and homeostasis) that dressed up by scientism, embed and naturalise themselves as unconscious bias in the everyday and conceptual lexicon of professionals and services. This is important for any analysis of Black mental health because, alongside more obvious and well-documented racialised discourses, these ideological beliefs prop up a socio-economic order predicated on the existence of winners (cultural insiders) and losers (cultural outsiders).

Instead, OTR works through an engaged political psychology, which is defined as:

> the psychological processes through which persons and groups shape, struggle over, and exercise the power needed for satisfying certain interests within a social formation, the way they are mediated through the individual psyche of the various actors, and

> the behaviour involved in shaping, struggling over, and wielding power. (Martín-Baró, 1994, p. 55)
>
> To exclude this 'bigger picture' from any analysis of human suffering is, for OTR, to be complicit in its continued existence. To include this context at the very least changes the role of mental health professionals – from neutral 'experts' to activists and advocates for social change (Watkins & Shulman, 2008).

References

Atkinson, M., Clark, M., Clay, D., Johnson, M., Owen, D., & Szczepura, A. (2001). *Systematic review of ethnicity and health service access for London.* Warwick: University of Warwick, Centre for Health Service Studies.

Bahl, V. (1998). Ethnic minority groups: National perspective. In S. Rawaf & V. Bahl (Eds.), *Assessing health needs of people from minority ethnic groups* (pp. 3–18). London: Royal College of Physicians.

Bhopal, R., & Rankin, J. (1999). Concepts and terminology in ethnicity, race and health: Be aware of the ongoing debate. *British Dental Journal, 186*(10), 483–484.

Bhui, K., Christie, Y., & Bhugra, D. (1995). The essential elements of culturally sensitive psychiatric services. *International Journal of Social Psychiatry, 41,* 242–256.

Cahill, C. (2006). The personal is political: Developing new subjectivities through participatory action research. *Gender, Place and Culture, 14*(3), 1–39.

Care Quality Commission. (2010). *Count me in: Results of the 2009 National Census of Inpatients and Patients on Community Treatment Orders in Mental Health and Learning Disability Services in England and Wales.* London: Care Quality Commission and National Mental Health Development Unit.

Department for Children, Schools and Families. (2008). *Children and young people in mind: The final report of the National CAMHS review.* London: Department for Children, Schools and Families.

Department of Health. (1999). *A National Service Framework for Mental Health: Modern Standards and Service Models.* London: Department of Health.

Department of Health. (2004). *National service framework for children, young people and maternity services: The mental health and psychological well-being of children and young people.* London: Department of Health.

Department of Health. (2005). *Delivering race equality in mental health care: An action plan for reform inside and outside services.* London: Department of Health.

Department of Health. (2009a). *Delivering race equality in mental health care: A review.* London: Department of Health.

Department of Health. (2009b). *New horizons: A shared vision of mental health.* London: Department of Health.

Department of Health. (2011). *No health without mental health: A cross-government mental health outcomes strategy for people of all ages.* London: Department of Health.

Department of Health and NHS England. (2015). *Future in mind: Protecting and improving our children and young people's mental health and wellbeing.* London: NHSE.

Dogra, N., Singh, S., Svirydzenka, N., & Vostanis, P. (2012). Prevalence of mental health problems in children and young people from ethnic minority groups. The need for targeted research. *British Journal of Psychiatry, 200*(4), 265–267.
Fanon, F. (1967). *Black skin, white masks*. New York, NY: Grove Press.
Fitzpatrick, R., Kumar, S., Nkansa-Dwamena, O., & Thorne, L. (2014). *Ethnic inequalities in mental health: Promoting lasting positive change*. London: LankellyChase Foundation. Retrieved from https://lankellychase.org.uk/wp-content/uploads/2015/07/Ethnic-Inequality-in-Mental-Health-Confluence-Full-Report-March2014.pdf
Freire, P. (1971). *Pedagogy of the oppressed*. Harmondsworth: Penguin.
House of Commons Health Committee. (2014). *Children's and adolescents' mental health and CAMHS: Third report of session 2014–15*. London: The Stationery Office.
Joseph Rowntree Foundation. (2011). *Poverty and ethnicity: A review of evidence*. London: Joseph Rowntree Foundation.
Kenrick, J. (2013). *Picking up the pieces: Results of a survey on the state of young people's advice, counselling and support services*. London: Youth Access.
Kurtz, Z., Thornes, R., & Wolkind, S. (1994). *Services for the mental health of children and young people in England: A national review*. London: South West Thames Regional Health Authority and Department of Health.
LinkedIn: Off The Record. (2017). Off The Record. Retrieved from https://uk.linkedin.com/company/off-the-record-bristol-
Malek, M. (2011). *Enjoy, achieve and be healthy*. London: Afiya Trust. Retrieved from http://www.stbasils.org.uk/files/2014-07-30/Enjoy-achieve-and-be-healthy.pdf
Malek, M. (2016). *Young people in mind: Transforming service delivery*. London: Youth Access. Retrieved from http://www.youthaccess.org.uk/downloads/ypimtransformingservicedelivery.pdf
Malek, M., & Joughin, C. (Eds.). (2004). *Mental health services for minority ethnic children and adolescents, chapters 1 and 4*. London: Jessica Kingsley Publishers.
Martín-Baró, I. (1994). *Writings for a liberation psychology*. Cambridge, MA: Harvard University Press.
Mental Health Foundation. (2017). *Surviving or thriving: The state of the UK's mental health*. London: Mental Health Foundation.
Messent, P., & Murrell, M. (2003). Research leading to action: A study of accessibility of a CAMH service to ethnic minority families. *Child and Adolescent Mental Health, 8*(3), 118–124.
Minnis, H., Kelly, E., Bradby, H., Oglethorpe, R., Raine, W., & Cockburn, D. (2003). Cultural and language mismatch: Clinical complications. *Clinical Child Psychology and Psychiatry, 8*(2), 1791–1186.
National Institute for Mental Health in England. (2003). *Inside outside: improving mental health services for Black and minority ethnic communities in England*. London: Department of Health.
NHS England. (2015). *Local transformation plans for children and young people's mental health and wellbeing: Guidance and support for local areas*. London: NHS England.
NHS Providers. (2016). *Funding mental health at local level: Unpicking the variation*. London: Foundation Trust Network.
Office for National Statistics. (2014). *2011 Census: Key statistics for England and Wales, March 2011*. London: Office for National Statistics.
Rawaf, S. (1998). Theoretical framework. In S. Rawaf & V. Bahl (Eds.), *Assessing health needs of people from minority ethnic groups*. London: Royal College of Physicians.
Sedgwick, P. (1982). *Psychopolitics*. London: Pluto Press.
Sennett, R., & Cobb, J. (1972). *The hidden injuries of class*. London: Cambridge University Press.
Sewell, T. (1997). *Black masculinities and schooling*. Stoke-On-Trent: Trentham.

Singh, J. (1998). *Developing the role of the black and minority ethnic voluntary sector in a changing NHS*. London: Department of Health.
Smaje, C. (1995). *Health, race and ethnicity: Making sense of the evidence*. London: King's Fund Institute.
Street, C., Staplekamp, C., Taylor, E., Malek, M., & Kurtz, Z. (2005). *Minority voices: Research into the access and acceptability of services for the mental health of young people from Black and minority ethnic groups*. London: Young Minds.
The Mental Health Taskforce. (2016). *The five year forward view for mental health*. London: NHS England. Retrieved from https://www.england.nhs.uk/wp-content/uploads/2016/02/Mental-Health-Taskforce-FYFV-final.pdf
The Sainsbury Centre for Mental Health. (2002). *Breaking the circles of fear*. London: Sainsbury Centre for Mental Health.
Watkins, M., & Shulman, H. (2008). *Toward psychologies of liberation*. New York, NY: Palgrave Macmillan.
Williams, R. (1977). *Marxism and literature*. Oxford: Oxford University Press.

Part III

Interventions

Chapter 9

Cultural Competencies in Delivering Counselling and Psychotherapy Services to a Black Multicultural Population: Time for Change and Action

Nicholas Banks

This chapter will consider the provision of counselling and associated mental health support services and the need for multicultural competencies (MCC) in delivering ethical and efficacious services to a black multicultural population with some emphasis on the UK. Notions of culture, important for the effective delivery of MCC will also be discussed.

Tao, Owen, Pace, and Imel (2015) report that MCC are generally seen as having the ability/skill set to work effectively across diverse cultural groups, together with the specific expertise to provide intervention to clients from culturally diverse groups, including minority and under-represented groups (Sue, Zane, Nagayana Hall, & Berger, 2009).

The 2011 Census of England and Wales (Office for National Statistics) identified black communities in general (those of African descent including African-Caribbean) as forming 3.4% of Britain's overall population. In 2011 those specifically identifying as black Caribbean were 1.1% of the total UK population. This does not include those who identified as 'black other' or 'mixed' at 0.05%. From these figures, it follows there is a substantial British population with potentially unmet counselling needs. This is in the context of research identifying that people of ethnic minority status, including African-Caribbean groups, are less likely than their white British counterparts to receive and request mental health support. Cooper et al. (2013) suggest this is due to African-Caribbeans being less likely to attend for mental health consultation with their GP. There have, however, been various explanations as to why this lack of service engagement may be, focussing on the suspicion by African-Caribbeans of what services may offer (Karlsen et al., 2005) and the concern of black clients that they may experience a racialised service with stigma (Marwaha & Livingstone, 2002). Different understandings and models of mental health may also exist (Brown, 2011; Marwaha & Livingstone, 2002).

The lack of engagement with mental health services and counselling is despite research identifying that minority groups as a whole, when compared to the white ethnic majority, report higher levels of psychological distress and a marked lack of social support (Erens et al., 2001). Earlier research (1994, British Fourth National Survey of Ethnic Minorities; Bhui, 1995), found that African-Caribbeans were less likely to make use of medication for depression than their white counterparts. Use of antidepressants also needs to be seen in the context of prescription of antidepressants, where black people may be prescribed fewer antidepressants (Cooper et al., 2010). For black people, medication may not be the treatment of choice (Brown, 2011; Marwaha & Livingstone, 2002). Little research exists about the possible reluctance by mental health professionals to identify the availability of alternatives to medication and refer for the relevant psychological therapy. The 'reluctance to engage' may be more based on pre-existing professionals' prejudice about what is of use for people of African-Caribbean origin. In addition, different perspectives and models of mental health may deter black people from making use of antidepressants (Brown, 2011). In the US, data suggests that medical professionals may prescribe antidepressants similarly to black patients as with white patients, with black patients much less likely to make use of these (Miranda & Cooper, 2004). For black people, spiritual values may feature more highly, focussing on the need for intervention more on social and psychological support than chemical support (Allen, Davey, & Davey, 2010; Brown, 2011; Dempsey, Butler, & Gaither, 2016). US data suggests that medical professionals may prescribe antidepressants similarly to black patients as with white patients, with black patients much less likely to make use of these (Miranda & Cooper, 2004). Different perspectives and models of mental health may deter black people from making use of antidepressants (Brown, 2011).

Notions of Culture

Understanding of the influence of culture in MCC is important as a conceptual base for MCC service delivery. Culture is a term that has broad meaning. Culture can be seen as a way of processing, understanding and responding to group derived expectations, through a process of inculturation and socialisation. This brings about shared expectations of behaviours that are seen to be meaningful, acceptable and/or unacceptable, passed through generations and becoming a collective experience over time. Gerstein, Rountree, and Ordonez (2007) believe that there are four basic components in the construction of culture:

> (1) it is socially transmitted through inculturation; (2) knowledge (people share enough knowledge that they can behave in ways that are acceptable and meaningful to others so that they do not constantly misunderstand one another; (3) there are shared behavioural regularities or patterns; and (4) there are shared collective experiences of a specific group. (p. 20)

From this perspective, if one ignores the separate components, misunderstandings of how to go about achieving MCC may come about; for example, a

Cultural Competencies in Delivering Counselling and Psychotherapy **183**

primary focus on courses on 'knowledge-building' that may be offered. With this focus alone, counsellors may set about learning specific aspects of culture that can be easily taught, for example, traditions around important ceremonies, dressing or food preparation. This is likely to miss the importance of building depth of cultural understanding, as shared understanding components of culture are not likely to be well taught or understood by those who attempt to learn culture from a distance in a classroom informed setting. Without meaningful social interaction with others from a different culture, over time in informal settings, the shared understandings, and expectations and ways of construing and responding to the world, are not likely to be well-understood.

The teaching of 'knowledge' may be likely to initiate 'othering', where one simply studies 'those who are different' as objects. What will be missing are key reflections on self and one's own cultural underpinnings as a way of seeing the interaction of those from a different culture, hidden assumptions and expectations of how those different groups may interact with one's own culture with all this creating an active dynamic in the delivery of counselling services. Without affiliation with other cultures, one may not begin to understand and respond to the complexities of the cultural dynamic that will exist between individuals and groups. This transcendence of the status quo is not as easy as one may initially envisage. There are also issues of economics, gender and social status that may form boundaries which are difficult to penetrate and interpret.

As Banks (1999) identified, theories of counselling tend to be composed of philosophical assumptions regarding the nature of 'man' (rarely women) and theories of personality. These characteristics are based on those observed with Western Europeans and, as such, are both ethnically and culturally bound. When not recognised by the counsellor, a misapplication of theory and/or practice may occur, with the result that service delivery becomes increasingly Eurocentric with a danger of becoming inappropriate for meeting the needs of black client groups.

Banks (1999) also identified that culturally biased stereotypes and negative perceptions of black people can be related to the conceptual framework internalised by counsellors who may unwittingly subscribe to the deficit hypothesis. This may mean that rather than searching for environmental and, importantly, in the provision of counselling services, issues of systemic inequality as causal explanations for non-engagement with services, explanations attributed to cultural and/or social pathology act to limit the potential to engage. Thus, the onus of difficulty is placed on the client with the institutional limitations and restrictions not sufficiently recognised and acknowledged.

With this in mind, how is MCC expected to come about? Early writers such as Ho (1995) argued that for successful counselling or mental health interventions, counsellors would need to transcend their own internalised culture through the process of 'inculturation' which is a process by which people are exposed and learn and are influenced by that culture. Ho (1995) argued that in any cross-cultural transaction, complications are likely to arise where there are rapid changes to a culture, where different cultures are coming into contact with an element of conflict or threat and where there exist individuals more enculturated to more than one culture. To better understand these issues, Ho (1995) used the construct of 'internalised culture'. Ho (1995) has raised the important point, from a psychological perspective, of distinguishing group cultural issues, looking at intercultural or between group differences, and that of intracultural or variation between individuals within that cultural group.

This variation between individuals in the same culture is an issue which appears to have been often neglected where culture is more often seen as a group phenomenon, with little attention paid to how individuals within that group may experience and express conflict about cultural expectations. Ho (1995) saw internalised culture as 'the cultural influences operating within the individual that shape (not determine) personality formation and various aspects of psychological functioning'. Ho (1995) made the further point that internalised culture should be separately conceived from cultural group membership. Cultural group membership is not, on its own, a psychological variable; however, internalised culture is. As Ho (1995) noted, there can be subcultural differences within a cultural group related to age, gender and social class and financial income differences. As Ho (1995) argued, there appears clear evidence that men and women in the same cultural group are differently socialised and thus, different internalised cultures exist within the same cultural group. This construct is related to that of 'subjective culture' as was argued by Triandis (1972). Subjective culture refers to the typical world view that people have within their culture related to ways of behaving and ways of construing the world, or their cultural cognitive map or world view. A demonstration of similar responses by individuals within a cultural group is a way of construing the subjective culture of a group. Such a construct, however, has limited benefit in understanding individuals. Knowing that individuals are from a particular culture, does not allow us to make predictions about their preferences, likes or dislikes or specific world view. Complicating the issue, there are major aspects of culture which have a shared, common understanding or world view. Thus cultural knowledge on its own for counsellors to achieve sufficient MCC is of limited use.

One may get stuck, if simply teaching knowledge, in thinking of culture in increasingly concrete, rigid and inflexible terms and be further in danger of allowing counsellors to activate automatic fixed and rigid notions about individuals from a particular cultural group. Thus, simplistic judgements about individuals may be made if one simply imbibes facts without understanding the dynamic interplay between an individual and their culture and, importantly, their individual experiences and way of processing information. Generalisations and stereotypes of over-simplified images and beliefs about what individuals are capable of, and how they should react and respond, may come about. There will be a danger of sweeping and inaccurate generalisations. In developing MCC, Ho's (1995) view was that one must have:

> [...] sensitivity to the discrepancies, tensions and conflicts which may exist side-by-side with conformities, between the client's beliefs and values and those shared by members of his or her cultural group ... These discrepancies, tensions and conflicts are not to be viewed necessarily in a negative light. They may be the driving forces for adaptation, creativity and change. (p. 4)

Ho (1995) also reminded us of the useful distinction between the concepts of over-generalisation and stereotyping, where a generalisation is formed by a level of observation of some members of a group, which is useful for hypothesis-generating and testing. However, difficulties will arise if from generalisations, unfounded assertions about a whole group are then made and acted upon. This then moves into the concept of stereotyping where there exists rigidity and inflexibility in construing the behaviours of individuals within a group and the likely 'group behaviours'. Stereotyping becomes a particularly extreme and rigid way of seeing the behaviours of individuals within a group and the group as a whole based simply on group membership. Awareness of individuals and individual differences is therefore negated.

Insightfully, Ho (1995), identified that when individuals are in contact and/or conflict and/or undergoing rapid changes, they may become increasingly bi-cultural which requires an enhanced dynamic understanding of cultural processes. Thus, culture is not necessarily a stable position, but is a construct where change may need to be factored in to understand the particular experiences of individuals. The present writer suggests integrated cultural identities tend to enable more adaptive coping patterns.

Earlier writers, Rohner (1984) argued the point that individual behaviours and personalities cannot be predicted from knowledge of a culture or a social system. Holding a view that individuals are the result of cultural determinates is related to the early notion of 'cultural determinism' (White, 1948), where this notion is one that human behaviour is solely the result of responses to cultural stimuli and therefore, that behaviour is determined by culture alone. This can lead to over-generalisation and rigid stereotyping. In construing these views, one also needs to take into account Bandura's (1978) early notion of reciprocal determinism, where the relationship between an individual and their behaviour and culture, should be seen as one of continuous interaction. Here, culture should not be seen as the cause and neither should individual behaviour be seen as the effect. People influence and create environments which, in turn, influence culture. As Ho (1995) noted, the rigid idea that culture determines behaviour does not take into account psychological universals in behaviours. As Ho (1995) argued, learning about differences between groups often negates understanding of similarities between groups and individual variation or differences within groups. Furthermore, MCC often suggests a social discontinuity or holding a construct of understanding others as distinct from understanding oneself.

Carter (1991) argued that a misunderstanding of cultural values/behaviours may produce ineffective mental health service delivery, as well as impact on the communication process and the interpersonal communication dynamic. Examples of how misunderstandings of behaviours may occur due to different world views was given by Carter (1991) where a white middle class mental health professional or counsellor, may perceive being late for an appointment as resistance and lack of commitment to the counselling session. On the other hand, the non-white middle class individual, may see their arrival and participation in the counselling process as a clear indication of the commitment criterion being met. The differences here relate to the white counsellor's Western notions of a time perspective and the cultural values associated with this. As Carter (1991) identified, in Western culture, time is perceived as linear and future-oriented, with time as a commodity, needing to be saved, potentially lost and wasted. Other cultures may have a tendency to live more in the present not be over-concerned about looking towards and planning for the future (Trimble, 1976). Thus, different cultural values may be misunderstood and clash in the counselling relationship. Carter (1991) argued that an important characteristic for a culturally competent counsellor would be the awareness of their own culturally based assumptions, values and biases.

The Evidence for MCC Efficacy

Regardless of the reasons for black people not featuring strongly in psychological support services, Arredondo and Toporek (2004) argued that to disregard MCC is a form of unethical practice. In the United States, there exists research criticising counselling practice for assuming that all therapy practice was effective independent of ethnicity and culture, with no evidence to support this (Miranda, Bernal, & Lau et al., 2005). Likewise, when Miranda et al. (2005) reviewed published data in counselling efficacy studies, it was discovered that only 6% of the samples were African-American, 1% Latino and 0.1% Asian, thus, it was argued that this limited the clinical application of findings with different ethnic groups.

Tao et al. (2015) note that the argument put forward by Kleinman and Benson (2006) requesting evidence that culture impacts on clinical efficacy. Research exists supporting the value of MCC efficacy. A review of 20 independent samples and 53 effects showed strong and positive effects of client perceptions of therapist MCC attributions on the clinical processes, with a moderate relationship between MCC and treatment outcomes. A recent meta-analysis in the United States (Nagayama et al., 2016) considered close to 14,000 participants, 95% of whom were non-European, in 78 studies evaluating culturally adapted therapy interventions. The meta-analysis findings supported the effectiveness of culturally adapted interventions with a medium effect size confirming the effectiveness of culturally adapted interventions over versions of the same non-adapted intervention. Culturally adapted interventions had significantly greater impact than other conditions to produce remission from psychological distress.

Confirming this view, meta-analysis by Chowdhary, Jotheeswaran, Nadkarni, and Hollon (2014) upheld the finding that cultural adaptations of evidence-based psychological treatments are required to make them universally applicable. The authors systematically reviewed the literature on psychologically adapted cultural interventions for depressive disorders for ethnic minorities in Western countries and for any population in non-Western countries to explore the treatments used and their effectiveness. Twenty studies met their search criteria with 16 included in the meta-analysis. Specific cultural adaptations were observed in the use of language, context and therapist administering the treatment. The meta-analysis revealed a statistically significant benefit for adapted cultural interventions involving the implementation of the treatment rather than its content for depressive disorders.

In addition, a UK randomised control trial (Afuwape et al., 2010) with 40 African-Caribbean patients with previously untreated mental health difficulties with a culturally sensitive intervention including ethnically matched therapists, using interventions which included mentoring and advocacy, obtained intervention results with significantly lower rates of depression after three months.

Importantly, Tao et al. (2015) in a meta-analysis found that client perceptions of MCC accounted for some 8.4% of the variance in therapy outcomes. As such, Tao et al. (2015) concluded that MCC should be seen as an evidence-based therapy relationship factor similar to the working alliance, empathy, genuineness and collaboration. Tao et al. (2015) explored the notion of the value of MCC through assessing the relationship between measures of MCC and treatment process and outcome. In doing so, it was said to be important to pay attention to the way that MCC have been measured and then to review studies testing the relationship between MCC and the psychotherapy process and outcome measures. Sue, Arredondo and McDavis's (1992) model, was argued to be the most influential model specifying the knowledge, skills, beliefs and attitudes that defined the MCC counsellor. Competent counsellors were said to be those who continually worked hard in expanding knowledge of their client's cultural background and world view, those who developed and used culturally relevant interventions and treatment strategies for diverse client groups, and counsellors who had an awareness of their own assumptions, beliefs, values and bias and how these may interact in the counselling process. Also important was the counsellor's skill in recognising how the interaction of their own culture and ethnicity impacted on their own behaviour and the client's response and behaviour to therapy.

The findings above identify a continuing need for adapted culturally specific service interventions. Importantly, in achieving MCC, counsellors and the services which provide counselling, may be better placed in working from a systemic position as one culturally adapted intervention. This adaptation arises from recognising that counsellors are not always dealing with an individual client, but one who may be part of an influential family and social system, with due emphasis on this needing to take place for successful therapeutic outcome. As such, there may be limitations on any individual therapy approach that does not sufficiently consider the person within a family system and also a larger social cultural and power matrix (Banks, 1999). Early writing, by Burke (1986), a black British psychiatrist, considering the mental health needs of African-Caribbean clients found that often family or group therapy could be a more appropriate form of intervention than the more common one-to-one counselling interactions used with indigenous British clients. In extending this notion, Burke (1980) found that with African-Caribbean clients diagnosed as mentally ill, family–patient interaction was one of the most important factors in influencing a positive outcome. As such, there is always a need to resist imposing techniques according to the need of theoretical orientation, rather than making use of approaches and techniques which are based on culturally different client needs and values.

The Need for Targeted Therapy Services and Training

Despite the evidence showing that African-Caribbean people significantly respond to targeted therapy services, a report by the UK Department of Health (2003) admitted that there was no national strategy or policy specifically targeting the particular mental health needs of black people or their care and treatment in mental health services. There was also an acknowledgement that historical approaches were fragmented and selective, making such interventions marginalised. The UK Department of Health further acknowledged that the experiences of black people in mental health care were that of 'an over-emphasis on institutional and coercive models of care: professional organisational requirements being given priority over (client) individual needs and rights, with institutional racism being prominent'. In particular, young men of African-Caribbean origin were over-represented in coercive care contexts (Sainsbury Centre for Mental Health, 2002). The Department of Health (2003) also recognised that there was a trend of ignoring cultural dimensions of service efficacy and outcome which resulted in less beneficial service delivery. This lack of targeted services can therefore be argued to severely disadvantage African-Caribbean people in their access to mental health services and suggests a poor quality of relevant service delivery if and when services are accessed.

In enabling services to African-Caribbeans, early UK research (Shaw, Creed, Tomenson, Riste, & Cruickshank, 1999) suggested that GPs had difficulties in recognising the mental health needs of people of African-Caribbean origin and making adequate services available. One important aspect recognised by the UK Department of Health (2003) was that of the need to develop a mental health workforce capable of providing efficacious mental health services to a multicultural population. Although there were stated strategic objectives, little appeared to exist to identify how to meet the stated objectives. This is still the case despite the context of research (Afuwape et al., 2010) showing that targeted service provision could show real benefit. Although the Department of Health (2003) did not see

> developing cultural capability (as) and end in itself; by making services more capable than they are at present, it is expected that there would be an enhancement of the overall quality of care received by people from minority ethnic groups. (p. 22)

Unfortunately, there was little guidance in how this important and practical piece of policy would be put into practice. As the document noted, the enhanced capability was not focussed on 'dealing adequately with cultural issues' but about improving the 'quality of assessment, care, support and treatment'. The Department of Health appeared to lose focus when considering the development of the workforce, as it targeted 'attitudes, behaviours, knowledge and skills necessary for the staff to work respectfully and effectively' with minority groups, but provided little detail of how to provide a culturally skilled and focussed service delivery. Although advice was offered where

> A culturally competent mental health service will be prepared to adapt the conventional ways of working to meet the needs of culturally diverse groups of people. Flexibility and adaptability in service provision, as well as an awareness of different cultural norms, are necessary to achieve this. (p. 23)

In the context of services struggling to deliver culturally competent services, little specific guidance on how this advice should be developed and practically implemented was provided. No specific guidelines on cultural competencies were offered. No means of monitoring and evaluating the beneficial effects of services was given. Cultural awareness training of GPs was suggested, although there was little evidence that this was likely to have any impact on service delivery. The Department of Health appeared to use the term 'cultural awareness' in a broad sense to include sensitivity, skills and competencies. The value of individual religious, cultural and spiritual beliefs was recognised where assessments were focussed on a care plan which acknowledged these issues. However, the care plan may require additional resources to meet the various needs, with little indication that extra resources would be available. The Department of Health Guidelines focussed on the need to change what it termed 'conventional practice', but was not specific in what this conventional practice might be, or even how this could improve services to ethnic minorities. There was discussion of cultural competencies without defining what these were or referencing publications where these would be identified and made use of. There was a rather vague suggestion that recent work had begun to occur, but no indication that this had been evaluated and shown to have value or impact.

Gomez (2015) in line with the view that direct clinical and social experience of other cultures is required to be able to work with an MCC ethos, cites critical race theory (Yosso, Smith, Ceja, & Solorzano, 2009), as stressing the importance of direct knowledge of different cultures, as a way of negating the privilege and legitimacy of narratives that support dominant racist ideology.

The additional need for personal reflexivity and a focus on the white counsellor's self and not 'the other' is underlined by the work around micro-aggressions perpetuated by those with the power to define and construct reality (Sue, 2010), which are imposed onto culturally devalued groups. Sue's notions of micro-aggressions include 'micro-assaults', 'micro-insults' and 'micro-invalidations'. Micro-assaults are covert and direct degradations. These micro-assaults resemble direct racist insults. Micro-insults and micro-invalidations are more subconscious with individuals unaware they are communicating offensively. Concerningly, micro-aggression can be processed through a guise of perceived compliments, for example, 'I don't see you as black'. Micro-invalidations are the hallmark of the power to define reality, for example, 'people are hired on their merit'. This appears to suggest that there is a meritocracy in operation rather than privilege. For this meritocracy to be in place there would need to be a level playing ground from the start.

Sue (2010) notes that micro-aggressions are typically beyond the conscious awareness of the perpetrator. These are ways in which unintended, but nonetheless damaging personal insults, reflecting racism, are displayed. Although overt racism may, for some, be taboo, the view may be that white society's collective unconscious continues to reflect racist assumptions. Micro-aggressions not only occur in wider society, but also in the counselling relationship (Constantine, 2007). Being politically correct is a form of micro-aggression, as it may involve micro-invalidation, where there is an avoidance of discussing cultural factors in counselling sessions or an accusation that the client is over-sensitive about racial issues. The impact of micro-aggressions in the counselling session is likely to effect a weaker therapeutic alliance (Constantine, 2007).

Colour-blind racial attitudes, where the social and political impact of colour is not discussed/acknowledged is seen by the current writer as 'colour muteness', and is likely to be experienced as micro-aggression. Higher levels of colour muteness and attitudes tend to correlate with less empathy and a blaming of black clients for institutionalised issues (Burkard & Knox, 2004). Micro-aggressions, even out of the counselling scenario, have been found to have significant impact (Sue et al., 2007), where these have been reported as resulting in feelings of powerlessness, a sense of invisibility, sacrificing personal integrity to meet white colleague's perceptions, and feeling forced to be a social representative of one's ethnic group (Sue et al., 2008).

In considering the efficacious delivery of MCC from a politicised perspective, Drinane, Owen, Adelson, and Rodolfa (2016) argue that factors of colour/race, sexual orientation, ethnicity and gender are also 'political factors'. This is in the context of decisions made of political service provision priorities, intersecting with psycho-socio factors which have been shown to impact on the therapeutic environment with therapists needing to engage with clients in a culturally competent manner. For example, the American Psychological Association's (APA) Code of Ethics (2010) explicitly states that psychologists need to be aware of, and demonstrate, respect clients' cultural identities (e.g. race, ethnicity, sexual orientation, socioeconomic status and gender). The APA's UK equivalent, the British Psychological Society (BPS) has no equivalent statement. Similarly, the British Association for Counselling and Psychotherapy (BACP) Ethical Framework for Counselling Professions Glossary appears weak in focussing on multicultural issues. The BACP tends to talk in terms of 'diversity and equality', which are general and vague terms. Diversity is interpreted as:

> variations and differences between people .... Equality is treating all people with equal fairness and impartiality, regardless of their differences .... The precise legal requirements vary between the different nations in the UK. Nonetheless, all practitioners in all nations and settings are ethically committed to respecting these characteristics.

There is no indication of the competencies in either of the UK organisations that should exist to determine whether the 'diversity and equality' service delivery requirements are met. There is no explicit, detailed discussion on culture or race or ethnicity as separate social and political concepts. The BACP discussion related to 'culture' asserts

> The provision of culturally sensitive and appropriate services is also a fundamental ethical concern. Cultural factors are often more easily understood and responded to in terms of values. Therefore, professional values are becoming an increasingly significant way of expressing ethnical commitment....

This appears to be a dilution of the importance of race, culture and ethnicity as feared by Quinn (2013) as it does not have a perspective located in social, political and historical issues. The BACP perspective can be argued to be avoidant of socio-political influences. The BACP however appears further ahead of its consideration of issues than the BPS. Without this consideration and clear policy and training statements being made, little progress may be made in meeting the specific needs of black client groups. With both the BPS and the BACP, difficulties may exist with conceptualising the issues as suggested by Quinn (2013). In reviewing the literature, Quinn (2013) cautioned against an ongoing conceptual struggle in the area of MCC with attempting to rank order oppressions and also that of attempting to establish an 'equality of oppressions' that may dilute the history and ongoing effects of racial oppression. Attempting to create an equality of oppressions was said to be likely to perpetuate a 'colour-blind' perspective, perpetuating notions of universal human experience which perpetuated oppression, particularly in counselling, where Quinn believed this notion of universal human experience would receive general acceptance in humanistic inspired settings.

Individual and Professional Practice Issues Effecting MCC

Banks (1999) found in a BACP survey that counsellors who did have specific training in the needs of black clients were much more open in their belief of the potential limitation of Eurocentric interventions in working with black clients. Self-directed reading was seen as a significant predictor of greater cultural awareness, where this may have been related to greater commitment and personal involvement in exploring the related issues of differing cultural need.

The MCC model adopted by the APA was one based on the work of Sue, Arredondo, and McDavis (1992). Importantly, Sue and Sue (2008) later went on to argue that therapists should demonstrate awareness and sensitivity to a client's cultural heritage and the awareness of therapist bias that may influence a client. This awareness is said to involve knowledge about wider diverse socio-political systems that clients live in and the social and political barriers that are experienced due to diverse client backgrounds. As in the UK, research (Afuwape et al., 2010) looking at client experiences with therapists with high levels of MCC, was said to show a positive correlation with therapy outcome and client satisfaction (Fuertes & Brobst, 2002; Owen, Leach, Wampold, & Rodolfa, 2011). In addition, clients' ratings of therapists' competence, empathy and credibility were also shown in these studies to be related to good levels of MCC. This was said to work through a process of the therapeutic working alliance and a congruent relationship (Owen, Tao, Leach, & Rodolfa, 2011). Other factors related to client satisfaction, and therefore efficacious therapy, were said to be those of cultural humility (Hook, Davis, Owen, Worthington, & Utsey, 2013) and an absence of racial micro-aggressions (Constantine, 2007).

Of interest is that client–therapist racial/ethnic matching has been found to be unrelated to MCC perception by clients (Owen et al., 2011) and also unrelated to client satisfaction with therapy (Fuertes et al., 2006). General counselling competence measures were seen to more impact on client perception of therapist competence, particularly those involving congruence and therapist relational skills (Zane et al., 2005). Importantly, empathy is seen as a particularly important factor (Elliott, Bohart, Watson, & Greenberg, 2011). This appears related to highly rated therapists perceived as more likely to engage with issues of cultural difference and to score more highly on tests of emotional intelligence (Miville, Carlozzi, Gushue, Schara, & Udea, 2006). Of further interest is that therapists who were found to be highly 'colour-blind' (ignoring cultural and ethnic difference) also received lower scores for empathy (Burkard & Knox, 2004). As Quinn (2013) argued, therapist empathy and its demonstration may be a major factor in multicultural counselling competence.

Tao et al. (2015) questioned whether the general counselling competence of the therapist, where this relates to the expertise of the therapist, involving their general skills and knowledge, genuineness and congruence, were distinct factors from MCC. They cited an early study (Coleman, 1998) where MCC and general counselling competence measures were explored with 112 clients involving predictors of satisfaction of therapy. As might be expected, the results confirmed that MCC and general counselling competence had a high positive correlation ($r = 0.78$). A later study (Fuertes & Brobst, 2002) confirmed the results of Coleman (1998). Other measures of MCC and general counselling competence have links with, what is termed, 'session impact', which refers to a client's evaluation of a counselling session, including the immediate effects and the client's post-session mood. This is said to be influenced by the working alliance effecting depth in treatment outcomes (Owen, Hilsenroth, & Rodolfa, 2013). Depth is said to be the degree to which a therapy session is considered powerful or valuable to a client. Treatment outcomes are those influences that have impact on the client with regard to both change and process.

The model developed by Sue et al. (1992) focussed on a counsellor's capacity to recognise their membership in a dominant group culture and to be able to recognise the impact of this membership on the minority membership client or their group. Quinn (2013) has argued that an obstacle in facilitating counsellors understanding the negative implications of bias is one of white culture being a dominant norm that presents an invisible veil preventing individuals from seeing counselling as a biased system. This is said to exist because there is little critical analysis in training by counsellors in understanding their own experiences and how these interact with the experiences of clients within a socio-political system which impact on client and counsellor both in different ways.

In focussing on counsellor personal and professional development, Ivers, Johnson, Clarke, Newsome, and Berry (2016) suggested a relationship between the construct of mindfulness and multicultural counselling competence. The concept of mindfulness was seen as related to 'acceptance and attentive observation of both intra and interpersonal experience'. Ivers et al. (2016) saw MCC as the 'effectiveness with which a counsellor provides counselling services to clients whose cultural world views and cultural group affiliations, differ from those of the counsellor' (p. 72). Empathy too was seen as related to MCC and mindfulness (Constantine, 2002; Fulton, 2012). Given the agreed significance of the process of empathy as universally agreed as important for effective counselling, Constantine (2002) emphasised that counsellors with higher levels of empathy would be able to more accurately conceptualise individuals from a multicultural perspective, due to an enhanced capacity to take the perspective of other people and develop an empathic focus. Constantine et al. (2008) found that levels of empathy in counselling students accounted for a higher degree of variance in MCC, beyond that explained by simple classroom instruction in multicultural counselling, and beyond that of theoretical orientation. This appears to confirm the earlier argument in this chapter that 'taught knowledge' of different cultures is not sufficient for MCC. Furthermore, Chao (2012) found that although multicultural training influenced counsellors' multicultural knowledge, it did not develop their multicultural awareness in service delivery with clients. Mindfulness is essentially an Eastern spiritual tradition (Shapiro, Brown, Thoresen, & Plante, 2011; Shapiro & Karlson, 2009) which has been incorporated into western psychological counselling approaches. It is seen as developing a unique form of attention to bring about a complete focus on the individual's present moment experiences in an accepting and judgement-free way (Kabat-Zinn, 2003). Mindfulness tends to be associated with an increased sense of wellbeing and empathy (Chiesa & Serretti, 2011). Importantly, it is also associated with positive outcomes for clients (Ryan, Safran, Doran, & Muran, 2012), and increased ratings of therapeutic alliance. In making the further connection with MCC, Niemiec et al. (2010) explored mindfulness and defensiveness and found that more mindful undergraduate students responded less defensively to culturally different viewpoints compared to those students who were less mindful.

Ivers et al. (2016) also found that multicultural awareness and empathy were related. Ivers et al. (2016) also found that mindfulness non-reactivity to inner experience and mindfulness describing, respectively, correlated with self-perceived multicultural awareness and multicultural knowledge. This appears to resonate with other findings (Sue et al., 1992), who argued that counsellors who were culturally aware tended to be in tune with their own internal reactions and have higher levels of comfort in working with diverse client groups. Ivers et al. (2016) believed that the connection between these positions was that counsellors who were mindful were likely to not let biased, stereotyped thoughts 'take root' and may more easily recognise negative automatic thoughts and more readily dispense with these through mindfulness processes. Ivers et al. (2016) also tentatively explored the possibility that mindfulness was a deeper and more internalised form of empathy, allowing counsellors to better understand the lived day-to-day reality of clients. Ivers et al. (2016) believe that the mindfulness constructs of non-reactivity and describing, were likely to interact with counsellors who struggled with MCC, due to the personal challenges required. It was suggested that defence mechanisms may come into play to protect the individuals from experiencing and processing issues of cultural difference which were, in turn, likely to limit counsellors' MCC development (Sue & Sue, 2008). Counsellors and mental health professionals who lack mindfulness characteristics are likely to struggle to accurately recognise and come to terms with the influence of culture, both that of their own and that of others' influences on their lives and the significance of cultural difference. Thus, the single action of completing a multicultural counselling course may do little to enhance multicultural awareness and skills. Cultural immersion activities and multicultural clinical experiences, may better help counsellors (Dickson & Jepsen, 2003; McDowell, Gosling, & Melendez, 2012).

In conclusion, Mele and Sanchez-Runde (2013) have insightfully argued that MCC may generate ethical dilemmas and conflicts. These may arise from different world views and the different lived experiences of white counsellors notions on MCC are not only about respect for others, but also likely to involve significant debate and challenge when one encounters a different perspective. MCC is not simply about reading and classroom-based learning, it is more likely to involve active and critical debate and a personal challenge with regard to ethics. As Mele et al. (2013) argue, there can be huge differences in outlook and social judgement between cultures, with this potentially creating a tension between moral or ethical universalism (universal ethical principles or standards) and moral cultural relativism (local or cultural ethnical norms) (Vendemiati, 2008).

An effective means of supporting the needs of counselling in delivering MCC may be through the training of MCC supervisors who are able to help counsellors develop their awareness and service delivery. At the time of the BACP survey, Banks (1999) found that only 61% of counsellors received supervision. This was in conflict with the BACP's counselling code of practice. It would therefore be important for more counsellors to receive supervision and, importantly, to ensure that notions of MCC are instilled in the various supervisor training programmes which are recently appearing.

Also, as Banks (1999) found in a BACP survey, the outcome did not suggest that white counsellors were unable to effectively counsel black clients, but were more likely to be effective if they sought out information to enable their cultural understanding of how cultural differences may affect the cross-cultural counselling encounter. The acknowledgement of difference, the recognition that this can influence the counselling process and outcome, together with active attempts to gain information about cultural differences, are likely to be good baseline indicators of potential for MCC.

References

Afuwape, S. A., Craig, T. K. J., Harris, T., Clarke, M., Flood, A., & Lajide, D. (2010). The cares of life project: An exploratory randomised controlled trial of a community-based intervention for black people with common mental disorder. *Journal of Affect Disorders*, *127*(1–3), 370–374.

Allen, A. J., Davey, M. P., & Davey, A. (2010). Being examples to the flock: The role of church leaders and African American families seeking mental health care services. *Contemporary Family Therapy*, *32*, 117–134.

American Psychological Association. (2010). Ethical principles of psychologists and code of conduct.

Arredondo, P., & Toporek, R. (2004). Multicultural counselling competencies equals ethical practice. *Journal of Mental Health Counselling*, *26*(1), 44–55.

Banks, N. (1999). *White counsellors, black clients: Theory, research and practice*. Aldershot: Ashgate.

Bhui, K., Christie, Y., & Bhugra, D. (1995). The essential elements of culturally sensitive psychiatric services. *International Journal of Social Psychiatry*, *41*(4), 242–256.

British Association for Counselling and Psychotherapy (BACP). Retrieved from www.bacp.co.uk/ethicalframework/glossary.phpaccess12122016

Brown, J. S. L. (2011). How black African and white British women perceive depression and help-seeking: A pilot vignette study. *International Journal of Social Psychiatry, 57*(4), 362–374.

Burkard, A. W., & Knox, S. (2004). Effect of therapists' colour-blindness on empathy and attributions in cross-cultural counselling. *Journal of Counselling Psychology, 51*, 387–397.

Burke, A. W. (1980). Aetiological aspects of depression: A community survey. Transcultural Psychiatry Workshop, Edinburgh. In R. Littlewood & M. Lipsedge (Eds.), *Aliens and alienists: Ethnic minorities and psychiatry*. London: Unwin & Hyman.

Burke, A. W. (1986). Racism and mental illness. In J. L. Cox (Ed.), *Transcultural psychiatry* (pp. 139–157). London: Croom Helm.

Carter, R.T. (1991). Cultural values: A review of empirical research and implications for counseling. *Journal of Counselling and Development, 70*(1), 164–173.

Chao, R. C. L. (2012). Racial/ethnic identity, gender-role attitudes, and multicultural counseling competence: The role of multicultural counseling training. *Journal of Counseling & Development, 90*(1), 35–44.

Chowdhary, N., Jotheeswaran, A., Nadkarni, A., Hollon, S., King, M., Jordans, M., Rahman, A., Verdeli, H., Araya, R., & Patel, V. (2014). The methods and outcomes of cultural adaptations of psychological treatments for depressive disorders: A systematic review. *Psychological Medicine, 44*, 1131–1146.

Constantine, M. G. (2002). Predictors of satisfaction with counseling: Racial and ethnic minority clients' attitudes toward counseling and ratings of their counselors' general and multicultural counseling competence. *Journal of Counseling Psychology, 49*(2), 255–263.

Constantine, M. G., Smith, L., Redington, R. M., & Owens, D. (2008). Racial microaggressions against black counseling and counseling psychology faculty: A central challenge in the multicultural counseling movement. *Journal of Counseling & Development, 86*, 348–355.

Coleman, H. L. K. (1998). General and multicultural counselling competencies: Apples and oranges? *Journal of Multicultural Counselling and Development, 26*, 147–156.

Constantine, M. G. (2007). Racial micro-aggressions against African American clients in cross-racial counselling relationships. *Journal of Counselling Psychology, 54*(1), 7–31.

Cooper, C., Bebbington, P., McManus, S., Meltzer, H., Stewart, R., & Farrell, M. (2010). Treatment of common mental disorders across age groups: Results from the 2007 Adult Psychiatric Morbidity Survey. *Journal of Affect Disorders, 127*(1–3), 96–101.

Cooper, C., Spiers, N., Livingstone, G., Jenkins, R., Meltzer, H., Brugha, T., ... Bebbington, P. (2013). Ethnic inequalities in the use of health services for common mental disorders in England. *Social Psychiatry and Epidemiology, 48*(5), 685–692.

Dempsey, K., Butler, K., & Gaither, L. (2016). Black churches and mental health professionals: Can this collaboration work? *Journal of Black Studies, 47*(1), 73–87.

Department of Health. (2003). *National Institute for Mental Health in England: Inside out: Improving mental health services for black and minority ethnic communities in England*. London: Department of Health.

Dickson, G. L., & Jepsen, D. A. (2011). Multicultural training experiences as predictors of multicultural competencies: Students' perspectives. *Counsellor Education and Supervision, 47*(2), 76–95.

Drinane, J. M., Owen, J., Adelson, J. L., & Rodolfa, E. (2016). Multicultural competencies: What are we measuring. *Psychotherapy Research, 26*(3), 342–351.

Elliott, R., Bohart, A. C., Watson, J. C., & Greenberg, L. S. (2011). Empathy. *Psychotherapy, 48*(1), 43–49.

Erens, B., Primatesta, P., & Prior, G. (2001). *Health Survey for England: The health of minority ethnic groups*. London: HMSO.

Fuertes, J. M., & Brobst, K. (2002). Clients' ratings of counsellor multicultural competency. *Cultural Diversity and Ethnic Minorities Psychology, 8*, 214–233.

Fuertes, J. N., Stracuzzi, T. I., Bennett, J., Scheinholtz, J., Mislowack, A, Hersh, M., & Cheng, D. (2006). Therapists' multicultural competency: A study of therapy dyads. *Psychotherapy: Theory, Research, Practice, Training, 43*, 480–490.

Gerstein, L., Rountree, C., & Ordonez, A. (2007). An anthropological perspective on multicultural counseling. *Counselling Psychology Quarterly, 20*, 375–400. doi:10.1080/09515070701567788.

Ho, D. Y. F. (1995). Internalized culture, culturocentrism, and transcendence. *The Counselling Psychologist, 23*(1), 4–24.

Hook, J. N., Davis, D. E., Owen, J., Worthington, E. L., & Utsey, S. O. (2013). Cultural humility: Measuring openness to culturally diverse clients. *Journal of Counselling Psychology, 60*, 353–366.

Ivers N. N., Johnson, D. A., Clarke, P. B., Newsome, D. W., & Berry, R. A. (2016).The relationship between mindfulness and multicultural counseling competence. *Journal of Counselling and Development, 94*(1), 72–82.

Kabat-Zinn, J. (2003). Mindfulness-based interventions in context past, present, and future. *Clinical Psychology Science and Practice, 10*, 144–156.

Karlsen, S., Mazroo, J. Y., McKenzie, K., Bhui, K., & Weich, S. (2005). Racism, psychosis and common mental disorder among ethnic minority groups in England. *Psychological Medicine, 35*(12), 1795–1803.

Kleinman, A., & Benson, P. (2006). Anthropology in the clinic: The problem of cultural competency and how to fix it. *Plos Medicine, 3*, E294.

Marwaha, S., & Livingstone, G. (2002). Stigma, racism or choice? Why do depressed ethnic elders avoid psychiatrists? *Journal of Affect Disorders, 72*(3), 257–265.

Mele, D., & Sanchez-Runde, C. (2013). Cultural diversity and universal ethics in a global world, *Journal of Business Ethics, 116*, 681–687.

Miranda, J., Bernal, G., Lau, A., Kohn, L., Hwang, W. C., & Lafromboise, T. (2005). State of the science on psychosocial interventions for ethnic minorities. *Annual Review of Clinical Psychology, 1*(1), 113–142.

Miranda, J., & Cooper, L. J. (2004). Disparities in care for depression among primary care patients. *The Journal of General International Medicine, 19*(2), 120–126.

Miville, M. L., Carlozzi, A. F., Gushue, J. V., Schara, S. L., & Udea, M. (2006). Mental health counsellor qualities for a diverse clientele: Linking empathy, universal-diverse orientation and emotional intelligence. *Journal of Mental Health Counselling, 28*, 151–165.

Nagayama, G. C., Hall, A. H., YeeIbaraki, E., Huang, C., Marti, N., & Eric Stice, E. (2016). A meta-analysis of cultural adaptations of psychological interventions. *Behavior Therapy, 47*(6), 993–1014.

Nemiec, C., Brown, K., Kashdan, T., Cozzolino, P., Breen, W., Levesque-Bristol, C. l., & Ryan, R. (2010). Being present in the face of existential threat: The role of trait mindfulness in reducing defensive responses to mortality salience. *Journal of Personality and Social Psychology, 99*, 344–65.

Office for National Statistics. (2011). Census: Ethnic groups in local authorities in England and Wales.

Owen, J., Hilsenroth, M. J., & Rodolfa, E. (2013). Interaction among alliance, psychodynamic-interpersonal and cognitive-behavioural techniques in the prediction of post-session change. *Clinical Psychology and Psychotherapy, 20*, 513–522.

Owen, J., Leach, M. M., Wampold, B., & Rodolfa, E. (2011). Client and therapist variability in clients' perceptions of their therapists' multicultural competencies. *Journal of Counselling Psychology, 58*(1), 1–9.

Owen, J., Tao, K., Leach, M., & Rodolfa, E. (2011). Clients' perceptions of their psychotherapists' multicultural orientation. *Psychotherapy, 48*, 274–282.

Quinn, A. (2013). A person-centred approach to multicultural counselling competence. *Journal of Humanistic Psychology, 53*(2), 202–251.

Rohner, P. (1984). Toward a conception of culture for cross-cultural psychology. *Journal of Cross Cultural Psychology, 15*(2), 111–138.
Sainsbury Centre for Mental Health. (2002). *Breaking the circles of fear: A review of the relationship between Mental Health Services and the African and Caribbean Communities*. London: Sainsbury Centre for Mental Health.
Shapiro, S. L., Brown, K. W., Thoresen, C., & Plante, T. G. (2011). The moderation of Mindfulness-based stress reduction effects by trait mindfulness: Results from a randomized controlled trial. *Journal of clinical Psychology, 67*(3), 267–277.
Shapiro, S. L., & Carlson, L. E. (2009). *The art and science of mindfulness: Integrating mindfulness into psychology and the helping professions*. American Psychological Association. https://doi.org/10.1037/11885-000
Shaw, C. M., Creed, F., Tomenson, B., Riste, L., & Cruickshank, J. K. (1999). Prevalence of anxiety and depressive illnesses and help-seeking behaviour in African Caribbean's and white Europeans: Two phase general population survey. *British Medical Journal, 318*, 302–306.
Sue, D., & Zane, N. S. (1987). The role of culture and cultural techniques in psychotherapy: A critique and reformulation. *American Psychologist, 42*, 37–45.
Sue, D. W. (2010). *Microaggressions in everyday life: Race, gender and sexual orientation*. Hoboken, NJ: Wiley.
Sue, D. W., Arredondo, P., & McDavis, R. J. (1992). Multicultural counselling competencies and standards: A call to the profession. *Journal of Counselling and Development, 70*, 477–486.
Sue, D. W., Capodilupo, C. M., & Holder, A. M. B. (2008). Racial microaggressions in the life experience of Black Americans. *Professional Psychology: Research and Practice American Psychological Association, 39*(3), 329–336.
Sue, D. W., Capodilupo, C. M., Torino, G. C., Bucceri, J. M., Holder, A. M. B., Nadal, K. L., & Esquilin, M. (2007). Racial microaggressions in everyday life: Implications for clinical practice. *American Psychologist, 62*, 271–286.
Sue, D. W., & Sue, D. (2008). *Counselling the culturally diverse: Theory and practice* (5th ed., p. 45). Hoboken, NJ: John Wiley & Sons.
Sue, S., Zane, N., Nagayana Hall, J. C., & Berger, L. K. (2009). The case for cultural competency in psychotherapeutic interventions. *Annual Review of Psychology, 60*, 525–548.
Tao, K. W., Owen, J., Pace, B. T., & Imel, Z. E. (2015). A meta-analysis of multicultural competencies in psychotherapy process and outcome. *Journal of Counselling Psychology, 62*(3), 337–350.
Triandis, H. (1995). The self and social behavior in differing cultural contexts. *Psychological Review, 96*(3), 506–520.
Vendemiati, A. (2008). *Universalism versus relativism and contemporary ethics*. Milano: Marietti.
Yosso, T., Smith, W., Ceja, M., & Solorzano, D. (2009). Critical race theory, racial microaggressions, and campus racial climate for Latina/o Undergraduates. *Harvard Educational Review, 79*, 659–691. 10.17763/haer.79.4.m6867014157m7071.
Zane, N., Sue, S., Cheng, J., Huang, L., Huang, J., Lowe, S., & Lee, W. (2005). Beyond ethnic match: Effects of client–therapist cognitive match in problem perception, coping orientation and therapy goals on treatment outcomes. *Journal of Community Psychology, 33*, 569–585.

Chapter 10

Social and Emotional Education and Emotional Wellness: A Cultural Competence Model for Black Boys and Teachers

Richard Majors, Llewellyn E. Simmons and Cornelius Ani

Young people who struggle in school often lack the social and emotional skills (or "soft skills") needed to succeed academically, deal with anger, make sound choices, handle challenging situations constructively, and manage behaviors in ways that prevent them from being suspended, excluded, or dropping out of school (Majors, 1994, 2001, 2006, 2010, Majors, Cook, & Read, 2011; Okonofua, Paunesku, & Walton, 2016). In educational settings, Black boys often suffer disproportionately from poor achievement, high exclusions, suspensions, and drop-out rates (Ransaw, Gause, & Majors, 2018; Ransaw & Majors, 2017). Although most of the evidence regarding the lack of soft skills among Black boys comes from studies in Europe and America, similar findings are emerging from low-income countries such as Nigeria (Abdulmalik, Ani, Ajuwon, & Omigbodun, 2016; Ani & Grantham-McGregor, 1998).

Some teachers see pupils' problems as lying inherently within the child (rather than considering possible external factors, such as poverty, family factors, and teachers' inability to communicate effectively with the young person) and readily fall back on punishments and sanctions to fix the "so-called problems," rather than analyzing and reflecting on their own reactions and/or considering other environmental or socio-cultural factors that could trigger or escalate undesirable behaviors. In such situations, it would also be beneficial for teachers to consider using appropriate communication and relationship styles to address and remediate problems. Sometimes, it is the teacher's own behavior that escalates classroom tension and conflict (for instance, what they say and how they say things), damaging the teacher–student relationship and contributing to the emotional and physical stress of both. At other times, however, the triggering stressors may relate to the physical and/or wider socio-cultural environment within which the students and teachers have to work.

Unfortunately, because of these challenges, Black boys are disproportionately placed in special education classes (Neal, McCray, Webb-Johnson, & Bridgest, 2003; Majors & Billson, 1992). Moreover, they are often raised in poverty and exposed to violence and toxic environments that create different levels of trauma and can cause social and emotional issues that lead to mental health problems. Therefore, it is crucial that not only pupils/students but also teachers should be emotionally literate to help diffuse and understand such problems.

The authors are particularly interested in Black boys in the middle school years because this is a critical and important time period due to puberty and it is a time Black males they are becoming more and more aware of how race impacts how both society and teachers treat them for being Black. Being privy too and/or aware of more negative experiences for being Black and male they began to stand up more and challenge injustices which in turn create more problems for them both in society and school. Therefore, these educational years can be a very difficult time developmentally for young people aged 9–13 generally (Ransaw & Majors, 2016), but when race is added to the mix, this period becomes still more complicated. During pre-adolescence/puberty, children may experience a range of physical, cognitive, social, and emotional challenges. As well as tending to become more aware of their appearance and taking on more responsibility for caring about their image, pre-adolescence is a period when children develop their self-identity and begin to assert their independence.

For many Black boys, then, pre-adolescent developmental/puberty changes occur within a broader racial and cultural context in which others may begin to view them stereotypically and potentially as troubled and deficient "Black men." During this period, Black boys who begin to have more conflict and misunderstandings with their teachers are punished more often and more harshly (Okonofua et al., 2016). Educational institutions tend to place too much emphasis on punishment and discipline to manage behaviors and raise academic performance (Majors, 2001). Although there can be a role for non-punitive sanctions in managing students' disruptive behavior, studies show that primary reliance on punishment is a less effective disciplinary strategy. The perceived wisdom, when looking for the causes of punishment, is to blame the student for his or her own difficulties (Majors, 2004). That is, the view that the pupil/student is "broken" and needs to be "fixed" ("internally focused solution") tends to be privileged over that of a breakdown in the communication ("externally focused solution"). If punishment is perceived as a power relationship and about "getting even with" or being "one up on" the other person or persons, pupils/students may feel that teachers do not like them, or are out of touch with their needs. It can therefore be more helpful to frame these challenges as a communication or relationship breakdown.

In a competition run by *The Guardian* in 2001, "What Makes the Perfect School," entries were received from 15,000 young people all over the UK. In the report, young people expressed a need for more democratic teachers and classrooms. For example, they wanted teachers to be fairer, show them more respect, listen more, and be more enthusiastic. Perhaps if we had league tables for relationships, instead of the current focus on academic achievement, which unwittingly drives exclusions and punishment, we would be more effective at raising academic attainment and reducing behavioral problems.

The pre-adolescent/puberty years of many young Black boys are often complicated by various forms of trauma, including poverty, family instability, community violence, and cultural misconceptions, which create additional burdens and challenges that limit their ability to succeed in school. By the time many Black boys reach fourth grade (in the USA), they may find themselves significantly behind their white peers (Majors, 2001). Research suggests that academic disidentification (Osborne, 2001) and the "burden of acting white" (Fordham & Ogbu, 1986) may also affect the academic outcomes of many Black boys as they mature. Therefore, the social and the academic needs of Black boys in middle school are complicated. At a time when children are experiencing major physical and emotional changes, many Black boys are not only dealing with these changes but are also struggling with "cultural", racial and masculine identity along with academic challenges both in and out of school which complicates their lives even further. Hence, we need a social and emotional curriculum that is sensitive to these issues and is culturally competent to help them negotiate school life and relationships successfully. Unfortunately, a cultural competence led Emotional Literacy (EL) programme added to the school's curriculum which is not a priority currently and is often lacking, could make a major difference to not only Black children but all children.

What is EMOTIONAL LITERACY?

Emotional Literacy, is a model that helps us to recognize, understand, interpret, and manage our own behaviors, as well as the behavior of others (Maurer & Brackett, 2004). EL is about using emotions effectively. It enables individuals to adapt techniques and skills to manage difficult situations. Emotional resilience helps teachers to engage young people "at risk" and develop the interpersonal and intrapersonal skills needed to connect, develop better relationships, and communicate more effectively with young people. This in turn reduces the need for punishment. EL also promotes teachers' interpersonal and intrapersonal skills and competencies that are needed to motivate young people. Heavily influenced by the field of positive psychology – which emphasizes happiness, optimism, caring, and relationships – EL proposes that all learning has an emotional base, and that there is a correlation between thinking, feeling, and behavior. People who are "emotionally literate" use their emotions more effectively to deal with day-to-day challenges. EL provides them with the resilience and capacity to gain control and persevere when faced with difficult situations, disappointments, or other challenges (Powell & Kusuma-Powell, 2013). Being emotionally literate does not mean you are an "emotional superhero," capable of keeping calm in all circumstances. In the school context, it might simply mean that you seek to understand other people as you communicate with them to solve a problem, or that you can model behaviors that may motivate someone who is facing barriers to success. It may also mean that you know when you need to hand over a situation to someone else, and when you are losing emotional control. In this context, there is no cause to feel guilty or embarrassed – we are all emotional beings, and we are all subject to negative emotional responses triggered by certain situations, words, or actions. Learning to acknowledge these triggers can help us greatly when working within a stressful situation – we learn not to conquer our emotions but to control them.

As human beings, it is nearly impossible for teachers to "get along" with every student they educate. However, in a school setting, it is vital that every student feels liked and valued. School staff therefore need to be able to handle their emotions well and remember to separate the behavior from the student. By recognizing which behaviors trigger a negative emotional response in us, we can prepare for those situations and find ways to handle them. Additionally, we must understand how a student might react to what we say and do, and try to find the best way to accomplish our objectives without creating unnecessary conflict. We may find their behavior infuriating, but we need to draw upon our EL skills to support them in a consistent and considerate manner at all times. Some days can be more difficult and stressful than others when one feels hopeless. However, an emotionally literate teacher knows how to marshal his or her emotions in the service of a goal, despite difficulties, frustrations, and challenges, in order to find the motivation necessary to persevere at a difficult task.

EL is also about being able to convey "forgiveness" (Majors, 2006; *see Teacher Emotional Literacy curriculum below*). For example, if a teacher loses the temper and shouts at a student during a confrontation in school, can he or she demonstrate that they can let go of the grudge and move toward reconciliation? After a period of calm, when both teacher and student show emotional intelligence, we would expect the teacher to feel comfortable by acknowledging their role in the confrontation by saying something like, "Your behaviour was not appropriate, but neither was mine. I am sorry I lost control and shouted at you. How can we now both move forward?" The teacher's acknowledgement has the potential to allow both the teacher and the student to learn from each other and transform the situation so that both can progress without any grudges being held. Being able to move on without blame or anger is something that most adults, let alone children, struggle with. However, it is just one social skill that can work to a teacher's advantage in the classroom. Being able to admit one is wrong is one of the most difficult things one can do, as is accepting an apology and then leaving the past in the past. The teacher shows respect for the student by engaging him or her as a partner to find the solution to the problem. The student may then feel inclined to respond in kind and show a willingness to improve their relationship. By using EL, the teacher is thus able to turn a profoundly negative interaction into a positive step forward.

One Cambridge study (Rodeiro, Bell, Emery, & Assessment, 2009) has found an association between EL and enhanced academic performance. Research has also shown that individuals with higher EL scores report better quality friendships and dating experiences and, as part of a married couple, have more satisfaction and happiness in their relationships. Additionally, people with higher EL scores seem to handle stress better, and demonstrate less problem behavior and more pro-social behavior. Meanwhile, students with lower EL scores report higher levels of drugs and alcohol consumption and more deviant acts, including stealing and fighting (Maurer & Brackett, 2004). Lower EL scores are also associated with higher levels of anxiety and depression. This trend has been shown in both in high- and low-income countries (Ani & Grantham-McGregor, 1998; Dodge, 1980). Because of these trends over a long period of time, the National Assessment of Educational Progress in the USA, often dubbed the "nation's report card," from 2017 began to include measures of non-cognitive factors in education because of the impact of social and emotional factors (Bertling, Marksteiner, & Kyllonen, 2016).

To maximize the benefits for Black boys, EL must work within an emotional wellness model. Emotional wellness is concerned with how organizational infrastructures create and promote their activities and policies to support healthy behaviors to improve health outcomes. EL and emotional wellness work on both the "micro" and "macro" levels of behavior, respectively. EL focuses on the "micro" behaviors of the individuals, while emotional wellness focuses on the "macro" structures, systems, and/or policies that improve the emotional wellbeing and lives of young Black boys. For Black boys to benefit from EL and emotional wellness, these must be presented within a cultural competence model to have an optimal effect on them.

Some of the areas that emotional wellness focuses on include:

- Health and risk factors in education.
- Medical screening.
- Behavior and lifestyle coaching.
- Stress management.
- On-site fitness programs/facilities and flex-time workouts.

Such activities and programs in the organizational setting encourage and support individuals to adhere to specific self-managed care protocols toward the goal of better long-term health and positive lifestyle choice.

With emotional wellness in mind, we propose a new framework for EL for Black boys – one that takes into consideration emotional wellness and cultural competence. Cultural competence can be described as understanding and appreciating the values, attitudes, traditions, customs, history, language, beliefs, and experiences of different groups of people one may choose to work with, in order to prevent one from becoming judgmental and using stereotypes. Being aware of the different ways some cultures display emotions and teaching young people how to code-switch, for example, altering the way one may speak or behave depending on the context can help prevent sending young people the wrong message that they are inferior to others and their culture is not valued (Andrews & Majors, 2004; Majors, 1991; Majors & Billson, 1992; Simmons, 2017). We must be willing to appreciate the world from the viewpoint of those who are different and avoid bringing our culture into discussion in our interactions with others with the intention of imposing our own views. Therefore, cultural competence is important for motivating Black boys to learn and enjoy learning.

Currently, the first two authors of this chapter are involved in one of the first pilot projects of its kind on emotional development/literacy and cultural competence for Black boys in Bermuda, which is also one of the first countries in the world in the process of developing a demonstration project on social and emotional education and cultural competence for its students. One of the major reasons Bermuda is developing this new curriculum is to take steps to more adequately support pre-adolescent boys in particular during the very difficult social and emotional middle school years. Students will be involved in various learning activities and programs in school that help them process, identify, recognize, and understand their emotions. Bermuda's public school system will partner with the Spirit of Bermuda to help students to become emotionally literate.

One of the activities in the new social and emotional curriculum to which pupils/students will get access in school is the Spirit of Bermuda high seas program, which is part of the Bermuda Sloop Foundation. The goal of the program is to build students' resilience and increase their long-term chances of success by providing character and educational development through experiential learning. In the process of undertaking sea voyages, Bermuda's middle school students will learn social and emotional skills. This is just one program where the pupils/students will be involved in to promote EL and learn new skills. In Bermuda, the cultural competence model will take into consideration how boys' masculine identities, female-dominated households and particular child-rearing styles, among other cultural factors, impact emotional development and positive outcomes in school. The aim of the program will be to determine whether EL and cultural competence used together can improve Black boys' academic performance, motivate and stimulate them to success, help them regulate and manage their behavior more effectively, reduce discipline, exclusions and drop-outs, and improve their overall quality of life.

Based on the well-established evidence of social information processing deficits seen in children with antisocial behaviors (Ani & Grantham-McGregor, 1998; Dodge, 1980), the third author of this chapter and his colleagues in Nigeria developed a group-based psychological intervention to support aggressive primary school children with social and emotional problems. This program was tested in a controlled trial in primary schools in Ibadan, Nigeria (Abdulmalik et al., 2016), which showed significant reductions in both teacher- and student-rated aggressive behaviors. This study suggests that impairments associated with poor emotional and social literacy are observed among children across cultures and in different countries with varying socio-economic profiles. Importantly, it also shows that interventions to improve these attributes are feasible and effective across cultures.

There is a cognitive/non-cognitive divide in education that limits the influence of social and emotional learning in our schools. Most of our schools tend to focus on cognitive aspects of education/learning (e.g., memory-based education) at the expense of non-cognitive aspects (e.g., "soft skills" and social and emotional learning factors). If our young people are to realize their full potential in our schools, it is crucial that we begin educating the "whole child." Accordingly, we must increase social and emotional provisions in our schools and in community organizations that work with Black boys. It is the cognitive and non-cognitive aspects of learning combined that make young people successful. We therefore need a new educational mind shift. After all, educating the whole child makes sense, since all learning has an emotional base.

In a meta-analysis of 213 social and emotional learning programs in US schools involving a broad representative group of 270,034 students from urban, suburban, and rural elementary and secondary schools, Durlak, Weissberg, Dymnicki, Taylor, and Schellinger (2011) found that when compared with students who do not experience social and emotional learning in their schools, they show significant improvement in a number of areas:

- Academic achievement and test scores (an 11 percentile point gain).
- Conduct problems such as classroom misbehavior and aggression.
- Emotional distress such as stress and depression.
- Attitudes about themselves, others and school, and more motivation to learn.

We now have the science and technology to help Black boys and others to choose their emotions. To facilitate success, motivation, and connectedness, our social and emotional development and emotional wellness program utilizes and incorporates a cultural competence model, whose framework is culturally competent for the purpose of contextualizing, validating, and optimizing our effectiveness with Black boys. In our pilot project, this framework considers how factors like authoritarian child-rearing and communication styles, fatherlessness, masculine identity (e.g., "Cool Pose"), traumatic experiences/environments, racial identity (e.g., "burden of acting white" theory) (Fordham & Ogbu, 1986), and academic misidentification (Osborne, 2001) impact social and emotional development and contribute to poor mental health.

Social and emotional development programs are important not just for pupils/students but also for teachers if we are to engage young people effectively. Teachers who are committed to teaching and making a difference with Black boys should not only use a cultural competence framework to motivate and inspire them, however; they themselves need to be emotionally literate. Teachers cannot expect their pupils to be emotionally literate unless they are emotionally literate themselves and capable of demonstrating emotional competence. Teachers often lack EL and understanding of how to develop relationships with young people, and this, along with their "default punitive mindset" versus "an empathetic mindset," leads to high rates of disaffection, drop-outs, and exclusions in our schools (Majors, 2001; Okonofua et al., 2016). However, there is a lack of literature on the role of emotions in teaching (Majors, 2000, 2002; Majors et al., 2011). Existing research focuses mostly on the role of emotions in learning among students and tends to overlook the importance of emotional education of teachers (Jennings & Greenberg, 2009; Madalinska-Michalak, 2015; Majors, 2000, 2006, 2010, 2011, 2012). Hence, if we are to engage and motivate students and teachers, and create better conditions for learning, we will need to radically shift our current focus on punitive strategies and engage young people in more programs like those above.

Because of historical concerns about teachers' difficulties in forming adequate relationships, and communicating with and engaging young people adequately, the first author developed an EL-friendly program/curriculum, "Teacher Empathy: How to Help to Make Our Teachers More Relationship Friendly and Communicate More Effectively with Young People" (Majors, 2000, 2002), aimed at developing more empathetic relationships, better communication, reducing punitive discipline/exclusions, and helping to make education more interactive/relational between Black boys and their teachers (see also Majors, 2001, 2004; Okonofua et al., 2016). The teacher empathy program, which has a culturally competent curriculum, has nine teacher EL competencies to help teachers develop better relationships with their students, and includes a toolkit, a Teacher Emotional Literacy Scale, an online computer teacher empathy interactive tool, and a variety of student–teacher group activities (e.g., "mini-communications" and "teaching moments") (see the addendum for samples of the *Teacher Empathy Curriculum*). This program/curriculum was first trialed in 2006 as a demonstration piloted in eight further education colleges in London for the Learning and Skills Council. It was then piloted in 2010 and 2012 respectively in two separate transfer of innovation-awarded projects from the European Union: *Teachers First-Using Emotional Literacy to Improve VET Teaching in the 21st Century* and *Emotional Literacy In Action*. The Teacher Empathy pilots involved eight countries: Austria, Switzerland, Poland, Malta, Cyprus, Bulgaria, the Czech Republic, and the UK.

Teacher empathy takes into consideration the student's and the teacher's values, beliefs, experiences, customs, languages, and traditions to relate to the pupils'/students' lives, and to motivate and inspire them. Teachers sometimes "fear" pupils/students who are different from them and do not know how to relate to students who look and behave differently than they do. They may also have difficulties unpacking the "cultural baggage" young people bring to the classroom. An empathetic approach also makes use of EL and relationship/communication strategies and approaches to engage young people. The goal of this empathic relationship program was aimed at identifying the interpersonal and intrapersonal skills teachers need to communicate, raise attainment, manage difficult behavior, and cultivate effective relationships with young people.

Building teacher–student relationships is also extremely important for creating an appropriate climate for motivation and learning. Research by the UK's National Association of Head Teachers (2001) found that the classroom climate is a powerful predictor of pupil learning, motivation, curiosity, and engagement, and that this climate can increase the "discretionary effort" of teachers by as much as 30% (the effort that individuals give to their job or task over and above the minimum required to complete it). The classroom climate also affects how hard students work and how inspired they feel. The teacher empathy curriculum involves nine teacher relational/emotional competencies to help teachers connect with young people (see addendum for the nine teacher emotional/relational competencies).

In our teacher empathy program, in order for teachers to earn course continuous professional development credits, teachers are required to go into the classroom and use strategies they have learned on the course and put into practice, to satisfy each competency area. Teachers have a choice of either assessing themselves or asking a peer to assess them in the classroom. They make use of pre- and post-test instruments to establish a baseline of knowledge and diaries to document individual experiences such as new insights. The workshops also focus on group work, exercises, and other tasks to familiarize participants with each area. The project showed that teacher empathy helps teachers to reconnect with many of their earlier passions and virtues that brought them into teaching (see the addendum for samples of the TE program/curriculum). These virtues and new skills should in turn help teachers develop more effective relationships with young people in democratic learning environments. Democratic learning environments and the promotion of positive relationships are more beneficial for managing behaviors than focusing on punitive strategies that do not work and can destroy children's futures (Majors, 2001).

High exclusion rates and punitive discipline affect the lifelong learning opportunities and job prospects of young people. In the UK, the number of school-leavers not in education, work, or training reached a record year-on-year high at the end of 2009. The number of 16–18 year olds who are not in education or training rose significantly over the last year by more than two percentage points to 15.5% in England (Pells, 2017).

The fact is that while many teachers have good relations with young people, some are not engaging young people, do not know how to develop relationships with them, or do not have the confidence to do so. Just as teachers need the appropriate skills and competences to be successful in the classroom, they also need to be aware of the importance of their own temperament. Being aware of what can trigger an undesirable response or calm down a student can be of great value. Are you a teacher who always has to be right at all costs? Are you able to say you are sorry when you have made a mistake? Do you motivate or demotivate pupils/students? Are you patient? Do you know what to say and when to say something to de-escalate a situation? Do you know how to lighten up and use humor when appropriate? Are you a teacher who holds grudges or are you able to let go of things? Are you able to forgive a student? Do you "personalize" things when a student acts out? Are you able to control your anger? As Aristotle said, "Anyone can become angry ... that is easy. But to be angry with the right person, to the right degree, at the right time, for the right purpose, and in the right way, that is not easy".

The current focus on punitive strategies in many of our schools dictates that we make a paradigm shift that addresses new ways of thinking. If this paradigm shift is to happen, we will need to help our teachers and educators to develop the appropriate interpersonal and intrapersonal skills needed to engage, motivate, raise attainment, and communicate more effectively with our young people (Corrie, 2003; Madalinska-Michalak, 2015; Majors, 2006, 2010, 2012; Majors et al., 2011). We often assume that our teaching staff have the capacity, knowledge, and appreciation of how to communicate/interact properly with young people (Mortiboys, 2005). While the self-confidence to engage, communicate, or develop relationships comfortably with young people is a communication skill that many teachers may not have, it can be learned. For example, in a study on communication skills among teachers, Rosemary Sage (2003), a researcher at Leicester University, found in her sample that half of the teachers and three quarters of the support staff reported that they lacked the confidence and communication skills to interact with young people and they especially did not enjoy interactive learning. Hence, teacher training should not only focus on teachers' specialist subjects but should also involve helping trainees learn how to teach the whole person and relate to their students.

Young people often say they would like their teachers to "lighten up," use humor, and be more approachable. Michael O'Connor (personal communication, March 1998) said that teachers often do not have "constructive conversations" with our young people. O'Connor suggests there are two kinds of dialogue between teachers and students: "constructive" and "non-constructive." "Nonconstructive" dialogue makes up 70% of the conversations that teachers have with young people (yelling, screaming, sarcasm, confronting, talking down to, being condescending and patronizing, etc.), with the remaining "constructive" 30% involving use of humor, positive feed-back, praising, etc. Additionally, Gottman, Gottman, and DeClaire (2007) reported that it takes five positive strokes to one negative stroke to feel good about yourself, but that the opposite happens where there are difficult relationships (one positive stroke to every five negative strokes). Some studies have even found a one to nine ratio. Thus, we need to spend more time on developing teachers' self-confidence, EL, communication skills, and social justice (e.g., fairness and respect issues) if improvements in relationships are going to be made to motivate them and raise academic performance.

As the educator Haim Ginott (1972) so eloquently stated:

> I have come to a frightening conclusion.
>
> I am the decisive element in the classroom.
>
> It is my personal approach that creates the climate.
>
> It is my daily mood that makes the weather.
>
> As a teacher I possess tremendous power to make a child's life miserable or joyous.
>
> I can be a tool of torture or an instrument of inspiration.
>
> I can humiliate or humor, hurt or heal.
>
> In all situations it is my response that decides whether a crisis will be escalated or de-escalated, and a child humanized or de-humanized.

General Overview: Comments and Recommendations

More time and resources need to be allocated in the future to teaching/training school staff for the development of empathetic communication/relationships, EL, and cultural competence to help Black boys to improve their success in school and overall life quality. These areas are not "add-ons" but are crucial competencies that help teaching staff to motivate their pupils/students, manage difficult behaviors, and raise academic attainment among both Black boys and people of color. Giving attention to the social emotional learning, EL and cultural competence of Black boys, and to youth culture, represents a paradigm shift from the more punitive practices administered by schools in many parts of the world. For a more significant and long-term impact, empathetic relationships, discipline strategies, culturally competent approaches, and EL and emotional wellness need to be incorporated into teacher training. Programs like the Spirit of Bermuda, the Teacher Eempathy project in Europe and the social–emotional problem-solving skills program in Nigeria can be scaled up for wider implementation to reach many more Black boys and other children to improve both their social and emotional development/learning and that of their teachers.

Note

For those schools/organizations seeking members from our team to conduct training, workshops or master classes on topics in this article and the *chapter addendum* below please contact the first author at the following email: rmajorsuk@yahoo.co.uk

References

Abdulmalik, J., Ani, C., Ajuwon, A., & Omigbodun, O. (2016). Effects of problem-solving skills for aggressive primary school children in Ibadan Nigeria. *Child and Adolescent Psychiatry and Mental Health*, *10*(1), 31. doi:10.1186/s13034-016-0116-5

Andrews, V. L., & Majors, R. (2004). African American nonverbal culture. In R. Jones (Ed.), *Black psychology* (pp. 313–352). Berkeley, CA: Cobb & Henry.

Ani, C., & Grantham-McGregor, S. (1998). Family and personal characteristics of aggressive Nigerian boys: Differences from and similarities with western findings. *Journal of Adolescent Health, 23*(5), 311–317.

Bertling, J. P., Marksteiner, T., & Kyllonen, P. C. (2016). General noncognitive outcomes. In S. Kuger, E. Klieme, N. Jude, & D. Kaplan (Eds.), *Assessing contexts of learning. Methodology of educational measurement and assessment*. Cham: Springer.

Corrie, C. (2003). *Becoming emotionally intelligent*. Stafford: Network Educational Press.

Dodge, K. A. (1980). Social cognition and children's aggressive behavior. *Child Development, 51*, 162–170.

Durlak, J. A., Weissberg, R. P., Dymnicki, A. B., Taylor, R. D., & Schellinger, K. B. (2011). The impact of enhancing students' social and emotional learning: A meta-analysis of school-based universal interventions. *Child Development, 82*(1), 405–432. doi:10.1111/j.1467-8624.2010.01564

Fordham, S., & Ogbu, J. U. (1986). Black students' school success: Coping with the 'burden of acting white'. *The Urban Review, 18*(3), 176–206.

Ginott, H. (1972). *Teacher and children: A book for parents and teachers*. New York, NY: Macmillan.

Gottman, J. M., Gottman, J. S., & DeClaire, J. (2007). *Ten lessons to transform your marriage: America's love lab experts share their strategies for strengthening your relationship*. New York, NY: Three Rivers Press.

Jennings, P. A., & Greenberg, M. T. (2009). The prosocial classroom: Teacher social and emotional competence in relation to student and classroom outcomes. *Review of Educational Research, 79*(1), 491–525. doi:10.3102/0034654308325693

Lloyd, S. C., & Harwin, A. (2016, December 30). Nation's schools get middling grade on quality counts report card. Retrieved from https://www.edweek.org/ew/articles/2017/01/04/nations-schools-get-middling-grade-on-quality.html

Madalinska-Michalak, J. (2015). Developing emotional competence for teaching. *Croatian Journal of Education, 17*(2), 71–97. doi:10.15516/cje.v17i0.1581

Majors, R. (1991). Nonverbal behaviors and communication styles among African Americans. In R. Jones (Ed.), *Black psychology* (3rd ed., pp. 269–294). Berkeley, CA: Cobb & Henry.

Majors, R. (1994). *The American black male: His present status and his future*. Chicago, IL: Nelson-Hall.

Majors, R. (2000). *Teacher empathy (TE) training curriculum: How to help to make our teachers more relationship friendly and communicate more effectively with young people*. Unpublished manuscript.

Majors, R. (2001). *Educating our black children: New directions and radical approaches*. London: Routledge/Falmer.

Majors, R. (2002). *Teacher empathy (TE) training curriculum: How to help to make our teachers more relationship friendly and communicate more effectively with young people* (2nd ed.). Unpublished manuscript.

Majors, R. (2004). Can we break the punishment cycle? Broadcast, Spring, 38–39.

Majors, R. (2006). *The teacher empathy project with the learning and skills council (LSC), emotional literacy and teacher's education*. Learning and Skills Council Final Report.

Majors, R. (2010). *Teachers first: Using emotional literacy to improve VET teaching (EL4VET)*. European Union, Transfer of Innovation, Leonardo Da Vinci, Education and Culture DG, Lifelong Learning Program, 2010–2011.

Majors, R. (2012). *Emotional literacy in action (ELIA)*. European Union, Transfer of Innovation, Leonardo Da Vinci, Education and Culture DG, Lifelong Learning Program, 2011–2012.

Majors, R., & Billson, J. M. (1992). *Cool pose: The dilemmas of black manhood in America*. New York, NY: Touchstone.

Majors, R., Cook, S., & Read, D. (2011). Applying emotional literacy to teaching assistants to improve classroom relationships. *Supporting Learning*, *19*, 20–27.

Maurer, M., & Brackett, M. A. (2004). *Emotional literacy in the middle school: A 6-step program to promote social, emotional, & academic learning*. Port Chester, NY: National Professional Resources.

Mortiboys, A. (2005). *Teaching with emotional intelligence: A step by step guide for higher and further education professionals*. London: Routledge.

National Association of Head Teachers (NAHT). (2001). *Primary leadership paper 3 (Summer)*. Haywards Heath: NAHT.

Neal, L. I., McCray, A. D., Webb-Johnson, G., & Bridgest, S. T. (2003). The effects of African American movement styles on teachers' perceptions and reactions. *The Journal of Special Education*, *37*(1), 49–57. doi:10.1177/00224669030370010050

Okonofua, J. A., Paunesku, D., & Walton, G. M. (2016). Brief intervention to encourage empathic discipline cuts suspension rates in half among adolescents. *Proceedings of the National Academy of Sciences*, *113*(19), 5221–5226. doi:10.1073/pnas.1523698113

Osborne, J. W. (2001). Academic disidentification: Unraveling underachievement among boys. In R. Majors (Ed.), *Educating our black children: New directions and radical approaches* (pp. 45–68). London: Taylor & Francis.

Pells, R. (2017, May 25). Significant increase in number of 16–18 year-olds not in work or school. Retrieved from http://www.independent.co.uk/news/education/education-news/teenagers-not-in-work-school-significant-increase-15-per-cent-rise-unemployment-youth-a7755321.html

Powell, W. R., & Kusuma-Powell, O. (2013). *Becoming an emotionally intelligent teacher*. New York, NY: Corwin.

Ransaw, T. S., Gause, C. P., & Majors, R. (2018). *The handbook of research on black males: Quantitative, qualitative and multidisciplinary themes*. East Lansing, MI: Michigan State University Press.

Ransaw, T. S., & Majors, R. (2016). *Closing the education achievement gaps for African American males*. East Lansing, MI: Michigan State University Press.

Ransaw, T. S., & Majors, R. (2017). *Emerging issues and trends in education*. East Lansing, MI: Michigan State University Press.

Rodeiro, C. V., Bell, J. F., Emery, J. L., & Assessment, C. (2009). Can emotional and social abilities predict differences in attainment at secondary school? *Research Matters*, *7*, 17–22.

Sage, R. (2003). Learn through talking. The ESCALATE Student Feedback Project, British Education Research Association (BERA), September.

Simmons, D. (2017, June 7). Is social-emotional learning really going to work for students of color? Retrieved from https://www.edweek.org/tm/articles/2017/06/07/we-need-to-redefine-social-emotional-learning-for.html

Addendum

Emotional Literacy

Social and emotional development programmes are important not just for students but also for teachers if we are to engage young people and connect with them more effectively. Teachers who are committed to teaching and making a difference with Black boys should not only use cultural competence to understand, motivate and inspire them, they themselves need to be emotionally literate too. Therefore, teachers must be capable of demonstrating emotional competence in their everyday interactions and communications with young people. Teachers who tend to be more emotionally literate are able to manage their anger, yell less in the classroom and know how to talk more appropriately with the young people they serve (see the concept of 'adultism', Creighton & Kivel, 1991).

The first author was fortunate to have received two European Union Transfer of Innovation (TOI) Awards (EL4VET and ELIA) in 2010 and 2012, for a curriculum on teacher empathy and emotional literacy/soft skills for teachers (Majors, 2000, 2002). Teacher Empathy is one of the first programmes of its kind ever to focus on teachers' emotional literacy. The Teacher Empathy curriculum/toolkit (Funge & Majors, 2011) focuses on helping teachers to develop the appropriate interpersonal and intrapersonal skills to connect, interact and communicate more effectively with young people to motivate and inspire them to excel in the classroom. There is an assumption that teachers know how to communicate with young people or feel comfortable doing so, yet the fact is that many do not know how to or do not feel it is important to communicate effectively outside of normal day-to-day classroom teaching obligations. The Teacher Empathy curriculum is designed to improve the daily experience of being in the classroom with young people and learning how to interact and communicate with them in positive ways that result in positive outcomes.

The curriculum is made up of a toolkit, a teacher's scale and a reflective interactive tool. The Emotional Literacy Toolkit is a 150-page document which includes emotional/relational competencies, assessment tools, exercises, case studies, strategies, suggested approaches and techniques to promote positive relationships between teachers and students. The Emotional Literacy Reflective Interactive Tool (ELRIT) allows teachers to evaluate critical events/incidents via a variety of prompted questions. This tool and the questions help teachers and others to identify, better understand, analyze and interpret not only their behaviours, feelings and emotions but the behaviours, actions and feelings of their students. The Teacher Emotional Literacy Scale (TELS), meanwhile, provides each teacher with a unique communication/interactive style profile – the underlying assumption is that particular communication/interactive styles are more conducive than others for connecting with and motivating students and raising academic performance. These emotional literacy technologies, tools and resource materials have been rolled out in nine countries, including the UK.

Because of limited space we can share with you only a very small sample of the Teacher Empathy curriculum materials (for information on the complete curriculum, contact the first author). If teachers follow this programme and develop the appropriate inter/intrapersonal skills, they are likely to find that the experience of teaching becomes less stressful and should offer greater job satisfaction. These relational competencies must be used within a culturally responsive framework.

The methodology

The nine Teacher Empathy emotional/relational competencies (see Funge & Majors, 2011 Teacher Empathy Toolkit) discussed here were developed by Dr Richard Majors. The methodology involves the format given below. Each emotional and relational competency section is formatted as follows.

Aim of the section

- To identify why each competency is important to both the teacher's and the student's emotional development.

Case study

- To help teachers recognize, understand and discuss the emotions/feelings experienced by the characters. The characters used are all based on the experiences of real people, although details and names have been altered to protect anonymity.

Points for discussion

- To encourage reflection and understanding of the consequences.
- To increase teachers' understanding, awareness and recognition of how their behaviours and emotions can impact their students' feelings/emotions, motivation, behaviour and attainment.

Role play

- To reinforce the need to recognize the emotions of oneself and others.
- To experience the feeling of dealing with issues and themes discussed here in an emotionally literate and culturally responsive way that will help them connect and become closer to their students in the classroom.

Activity sheet

- To highlight how students respond to various approaches, strategies and techniques learned here and adopted by the teacher.

Self-reflection

- To encourage teachers to become more self-aware and reflective.
- To help teachers deal with their emotions more productively in the future.
- To develop knowledge and strategies that benefit both the teacher and the students.

Final group discussion

- To offer a further opportunity to reflect on and summarize the key learning outcomes of each competency.

Teacher empathy emotional and relational competencies

'All learning has an emotional base.'

Plato

Attribute	Recognizing & understanding emotions in self (self-awareness)	Understanding & recognizing emotions in others (interpersonal)	Managing emotions in self & others (intrapersonal)	Emotional-relational approach	Cultural competency
Compassion	• Be attentive to emotional cues and listen well • Are you blaming the child/student for problems at home?	• Be able to sympathize with the suffering of others and be willing to help when necessary	• Show sensitivity towards others • What can I say/do at this moment in time that tells the child/student I care?	• Develop trusting relationships with young people	• Help out based on understanding other people's needs and feelings
Enthusiasm	• Have a passionate interest in sharing their knowledge of a subject • Does your tone of voice and body language show that you are enthusiastic and that you like the student(s)?	• Be eager to engage learners	• Deliver lessons with energy and interest • Be responsive to the needs of learners	• Be willing to consider different modes of delivery to excite learners • Encourage learners to want to find out more	• Be approachable and willing to listen to students' ideas and suggestions • Ensure that lesson plans and delivery relate to all students
Forgiveness	• Are you able to say you are 'sorry' for making a mistake and in front of the class? • Are you holding a grudge? Are you preventing a student from becoming successful because you are angry with them or do not like them?	• Help the person who upset them to see what they have done • Do you think a student knows when you do not like them? Why?	• Understand what hurt them in the first place • Address the problem appropriately	• 'Let go' of feelings of anger and move on	• Accept that they and others make mistakes but everyone can learn from them if they are dealt with effectively

Optimism	• Do you have a belief in a positive outcome for a student(s) and see setbacks as due to a manageable circumstance rather than a personal flaw?	• Belief in the capabilities of all students • Have a positive attitude and be enthusiastic	• Operate from hope of success rather than fear of failure • Hold high expectations of the students	• Persist in seeking goals, despite obstacles and setbacks • Read successful case stories of famous people and celebrities who made it 'in spite of'
Power	• Be aware of the potential for power to be misused • Lead by example • Challenge your 'punitive mind set/default position'	• Manage difficult situations with fairness and reasonable control • Use your skills as a communicator to defuse difficult situations • Be willing to listen and not teach in an authoritarian and overly 'strict' manner	• Acknowledge the contribution young people can make and that they should be heard and not just seen • Negotiate and agree consequences rather than punishing young people	• Manage their authority with respect to others and themselves • Be guided by a 'bottom up' rather than 'top down' approach to managing the school environment	• Reflect the values of a fair, open and trusting environment where power is not used to bully or intimidate

Attribute	Recognizing & understanding emotions in self (self-awareness)	Understanding & recognizing emotions in others (interpersonal)	Managing emotions in self & others (intrapersonal)	Emotional-relational approach	Cultural competency
Relational	• Be willing to seek out and talk with young people outside the classroom and enjoy interacting with them • Do you feel comfortable talking to young people? • Do you know what to say? • Do you tend to overreact too much to what young people say and do?	• Be able to empathize with young people • What was I like at their age? How did I dress? What was the latest fad/music of the time?	• Be approachable and offer time to listen • Recognize their issues, aspirations and problems and work with them to achieve a positive outcome	• Build appropriate relationships with young people and others	• Promote friendly relationships with young people and create a cooperative climate
Self-confidence/teacher efficacy	• Are you approachable – why or why not? • How can you be more confident about communicating with young people? • Do you believe in your abilities to connect with and make a difference with young people? Why or why not? • What is it about your past experiences or the way you were raised that makes you feel this way?	• Communicate effectively • Be a good listener • Adopt a positive body stance • Acknowledge and reward people's strengths, accomplishments and development	• Be open to candid feedback, new perspectives, continuous learning and self-development • Provide feedback and encouragement to young people	• Be able to show a sense of humour • Be comfortable interacting with young people • Be able to approach and talk to young people outside the classroom	• Be willing to admit mistakes and learn from them • Be willing to learn from young people and their families • Respond to the identified cultural norms of a young person

Social justice	• Are you fair in the actions you take towards young people (e.g. 'adultism')? • Do you appreciate how a student's behaviour in school may be impacted by gender, race, disability or gay right issues?	• Do you talk down to young people? • Are you able to relate and interact with others fairly and respectfully?	• Do you let go of any potential bias caused by staffroom gossip or other prejudgements of a young person's, his sister/brother's or his family's capabilities?	• Be fair and reasonable, especially in the way people are treated or decisions are made • Respect and relate well to people from varied backgrounds • Challenge bias and intolerance
Attribute	Recognizing and understanding emotions in self (self-awareness)	Understanding and recognizing emotions in others (interpersonal)	Managing emotions in self and others (intrapersonal)	Emotional-relational approach
Youth culture	• Recognize that young people are in a period of transition between childhood and maturity • Know that for young people this will be the most challenging and difficult time probably in their lives	• Recognize that part of youth culture is about defining and learning who they are and 'experimenting' • Know there is no need to fear young people	• Acknowledge young people are likely to be different from you – with different interests, clothes and music, etc. – but they are no less of a person or less intelligent • Be sensitive and caring	• Be yourself and try not to be fake – they will respect that, even if you think you are 'corny' • Do not mimic them or patronize young people • Know that with the right guidance they will come through this period of transition to become responsible, rounded adults

(Social justice row, 5th column):
• Understand diverse worldviews and be sensitive to group differences
• See diversity as an opportunity, creating an environment where diverse people can thrive

(Attribute row, 5th column): Cultural competency

(Youth culture row, 5th column):
• Have an appreciation of youth culture
• Accept that they are capable of learning despite these differences

School ethos

In order for these emotional/relational competencies and attributes to be effective it is essential that they are reflected throughout the school or learning institution. Once teachers have worked through the detailed sections for each competency, the final section of the curriculum will look at effective ways to develop a whole-school ethos where these values should permeate the entire learning environment.

Relational

Time	Activity	Resources
0.00	Introduction to the attribute of Relational – Consider behaviours associated with emotional-relational approaches as a group – Refer to Maslow's Hierarchy of Needs to consider how a young person will not be able to achieve if some of the lower level needs have not been met	Handout – Why this attribute is important & Maslow's Hierarchy of Needs Flipchart paper and pens or use of a SMART board
0.10	Case study – Read out the scenario and use handouts to discuss how the characters feel	Handouts – Scenario and Points for discussion Flipchart paper and pens or use of a SMART board
0.40	Role play – Volunteers act out characters in scenario to demonstrate how adopting a relational approach can make a difference to the outcome	
1.00	Activity sheet – An opportunity for participants to reinforce what they have learned from the role play	Activity sheet
1.10	Self-reflection – Individual teachers complete these sheets to consider how far they already display this attribute or what they might need to do to become a more emotionally-relational teacher	Self-reflection sheet
1.20	Final group discussion – A chance for the group to discuss how useful they have found this section and to identify what they have learned from the session	Flipchart paper and pens or use of a SMART board
1.30	End	

Relational

> 'Relational progress is impossible as long as blame is the focus because blame and progress are enemies ... we must take care that focusing on fault ... doesn't carry over into interpersonal relationships. The heart of loving communication is listening to understand.'
>
> Jeffrey Bryant

Why is this attribute important?

The relationship between teacher and student is built on the values of respect, trust, empathy, fairness, openness and a willingness to listen and learn. The teacher will be self-aware, with a clear understanding of their emotions, and have the self-confidence to interact with students in a caring and positive manner. The teacher will value different perspectives and be able to manage potentially difficult situations with relative ease. For example, using an emotional-relational approach, if a young person is upset the teacher will take time to talk with them to find out what has caused them to feel upset. They will use the skills similar to those of a mentor to develop trust and openness between the young person and themselves. They will use active listening skills, be aware of their non-verbal prompts as well as the words they use to encourage this relationship to work. By using skilful questioning, and a calm and open manner, the teacher can help the young person to express how they are feeling and help them to gain a greater understanding of what has upset them and to learn how to articulate this in a way that helps them to be heard.

By utilizing these skills a teacher is learning to respond rather than react to situations and this is more likely to lead to a positive outcome for everyone. Students can appreciate they are being respected and valued and they will be most likely to respond to the teacher in a similar way – with respect and appreciation for their teacher.

Behaviours associated with relational:

Expressing a relationship – Connection – Be in touch with someone – Rapport

Can you think of any others? Jot them down here

Case Study

Thomas is 15 and was adopted as a toddler along with his older sister, Katie. Their early years had been spent living with their biological mother who led a chaotic life. Social services removed them from the family home and sought permission to have them adopted. Thomas recalls less of these early years than his sister. Thomas and Katie seemed to settle into their adoptive family well and their new parents were loving and supportive. Sadly, Katie's behaviour has begun to escalate out of control since she was 14. Thomas is worried about her as their parents have now refused to have her home because she has stolen from them; she is taking drugs and she has also hinted that she might be pregnant by a young man who is in and out of prison.

This is affecting Thomas greatly and his behaviour has changed in school. He has become withdrawn and sullen and is lagging behind in all subjects. In the lunch break a boy teased Thomas about his sister and Thomas punched him and they began fighting. Thomas was taken to see the head teacher, along with the other boy, and the head teacher said they would both receive a two-day suspension for fighting as this could not be tolerated in school. Thomas accepted the punishment and waited to be told off by his parents when he got home. He didn't want to disappoint his parents, so he decided not to share with them what the fight had been about.

Points for discussion

1. Jot down what you think Thomas is feeling.

How Thomas is feeling

2. Consider what support Thomas needs to help him through this difficult time.

How can the school and teachers help Thomas?

Additional points

Young people such as Thomas have already had to cope with a great deal in their young lives. If a teacher had been more 'connected', utilizing an emotional-relational approach with Thomas, they would have been more likely to see the change in Thomas and realize something must be wrong. By taking the time to get to know young people individually, a teacher is more likely to develop a relationship with a young person that could make a difference. If the consequence of troubles leads to behaviour similar to Thomas's and they receive a punishment for it, then it is likely to lead to a further decline in the young person's sense of self-worth. If we recall Maslow's Hierarchy of Needs (see below), then it is clear it will be difficult for a young person to achieve the higher levels if, for example, they are having problems with their relationships.

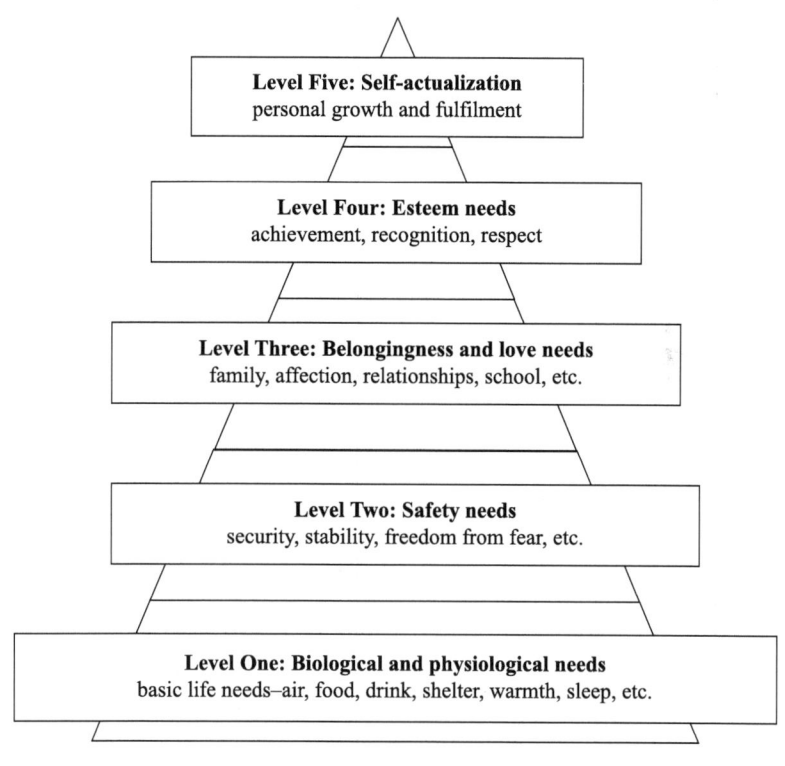

Level Five: Self-actualization
personal growth and fulfilment

Level Four: Esteem needs
achievement, recognition, respect

Level Three: Belongingness and love needs
family, affection, relationships, school, etc.

Level Two: Safety needs
security,stability, freedom from fear, etc.

Level One: Biological and physiological needs
basic life needs–air, food, drink, shelter, warmth, sleep, etc.

Maslow's Hierarchy of Needs

Role play

Discuss as a group how a teacher can develop their relationships with young people.

1. Select two participants to role play the head teacher and Thomas, utilizing an emotional-relational approach to demonstrate how the outcome might have been different.
2. The rest of the group can contribute ideas and suggestions to ensure that the head teacher is displaying an emotional-relational approach.
3. If agreed, alternative participant(s) can take over the role of the head teacher or Thomas to develop the scenario and practise these skills.
4. Check how the person playing Thomas is feeling – does he feel safe to share his true concerns? Does he feel he will be listened to and gain some support?
5. How does the head teacher feel? Does it seem that interacting using an emotional-relational approach is making a difference?

Activity Sheet

In observing the behaviours of a teacher who practises an emotional-relational approach through the role play, consider what behaviours they displayed for the young person to change their attitude and responses.

Behaviours of a teacher who practises an emotional-relational approach	How is this demonstrated?
Body stance	
Tone of voice	
Eye contact	
Facial expression	
Questioning skills	
Timing	
Environment	
What has worked particularly well in this interaction?	
Is there anything that could have improved the interaction further?	
Note some of the differences in the response from the student when a teacher interacts using an emotional-relational approach.	
How could a more culturally responsive approach make a difference?	

(See Majors, 1991 and Andrews & Majors, 2004 on nonverbal behaviour and culture)

Self-reflection

In your experience as a teacher, consider how far you already display the qualities of a teacher who practises an emotional-relational approach.
In what ways could you improve these skills?
What emotions might get in the way of you offering an emotional-relational approach towards young people?

How can you manage these emotions to develop the skills and practice of an emotional-relational approach?
Noting down reasons why an emotional-relational approach can make a difference can remind you of the benefits of adopting this method.
Are there any areas in which you feel you need more help to develop these skills?
Action points

Final Group Discussion

Finally, as a group, consider how this session has helped you in your role as a teacher.

Do you feel you can use an emotional-relational approach in your role as a teacher?

Do you feel that the key learning outcomes have provided you with the opportunity to:

- be willing to seek out young people outside the classroom and enjoy interacting with them
- balance a focus on task with attention to relationships
- empathize with young people
- collaborate with young people, sharing plans, information and resources
- be approachable and offer time to listen
- recognize their issues, aspirations and problems and work with them to achieve a positive outcome
- build appropriate relationships with young people and others
- promote a friendly, cooperative climate?

Crisis Time/Non-crisis Time Interactions and 'Mini-communications': How to Improve Behaviour and Communication with Young People

Adapted by Dr Richard Majors

Non-crisis communication is a period of time that is available to communicate/interact with a student to build up a relationship with them. It is this relationship that is the foundation for success, motivation and academic success. Tipping moments are a form of non-crisis interactions/mini-communications that teachers can have with their students. Tipping moments involve doing something different in the teacher–pupil relationship that is unique and out of the ordinary. These encounters can tip the balance in favour of a deeper and more empathetic relationship between the teacher and the student. These changes in relationships are not likely to be instigated by students, particularly boys; teachers need to take responsibility for seeking such opportunities and 'seizing the moment' when they arise. In these moments the teacher and student engage emotionally in a deeper personal way than in regular classroom activities, although the way into such 'tipping moments' could be through a cognitive challenge. The 'tipping student' could be the kind of key character whose relationship with the teacher can actually move the whole class forward. Tipping moments with such students are essential for the progress of not only the student but the whole class.

Learning outcomes

Understand the concepts and connections between tipping moments, praise and relationships.

Success criteria
Complete the 'Tipping moment exercise'.

Tipping moment exercise (in pairs)
Can you call to mind a time at work or in your private life where you experienced a 'tipping' moment where some small but significant interaction produced an unexpected positive change in your relationship with someone?

Note down:

- What were you pleased with? (three things)
- Which skills did you bring to this (three things)
- What have you learned from this that you can use again?

'Crisis time' vs. 'non-crisis time' interactions and 'mini-communications': how to improve behaviour and communication with young people

How many minutes are you spending with young people during 'crisis time' (e.g. when there is a problem) versus 'non-crisis time' (e.g. when there is not a problem)? Each day? Each week?
 List here how many crisis time minutes. (Each day? Each week?)
 List here how many non-crisis time minutes. (Each day? Each week?)
 What percentage of interaction each day or each week is crisis time versus non-crisis time with students?
 Consider how you can begin to create opportunities to have non-crisis time/ mini-communications interactions with your students both in and out of the classroom, e.g. coming into and leaving the classroom, in the hallway between classes,

during lunch, on your way to school, at the bus stop and in the community, e.g. at the shopping centre when you bump into one of your students. Non-crisis time/ mini-communications do not have to be long – they may be a few minutes or even only a few seconds. See below for the non-crisis time/mini-communications exercise – how many ideas can you come up with for each time interval?

Non-crisis Time Interaction Exercise

Adapted by Dr Richard Majors

'Non-crisis time' interactions Create opportunities for a positive encounter with a student in either the classroom or outside the classroom	
10-second interaction: What things can you do in **10 seconds** that may help you to develop a relationship with a particular student (e.g. greeting/trading of pleasantries)?	
20-second interaction: What things can you do in **20 seconds** that may help you to develop a relationship with a particular student (e.g. greeting/trading of pleasantries)?	
30-second interaction: What things can you do in **30 seconds** that may help you to develop a relationship with a particular student (e.g. greeting/trading of pleasantries)?	
45-second interaction: What things can you do in **45 seconds** that may help you to develop a relationship with a particular student (e.g. greeting/trading of pleasantries)?	
One-minute interaction: What other things can you do in **one minute** that may help you to develop a relationship with a particular student?	
Two/three-minute interaction: What other things can you do in **2–3 minutes** that may help you to develop a relationship with a particular student?	
Four/five-minute interaction: What other things can you do in **4–5 minutes** that may help you to develop a relationship with a particular student?	

The Emotional Literacy Reflective Interactive Tool

Adapted by Dr Richard Majors

The purpose of this tool (which was originally developed as a software package) is to help teachers develop understanding of their emotions to become more 'emotionally literate' and, in turn, enhance their effectiveness in the classroom/learning environment/workplace and in other areas of their professional practice.

Our emotions have a significant effect on our behaviours. Often we might find ourselves experiencing powerful emotions, though we may not always be aware of why we are feeling the way we are. These emotions can have a positive impact on others, but they can have a negative impact as well.

The Emotional Literacy Reflective Interactive Tool will help you precisely identify and communicate your feelings, work through your emotions, understand their causes and think about how you may change these to result in more effective behaviour for both yourself and others. This tool has been designed for you to use to contribute to your ongoing personal and professional development.

There are four broad stages to the process that the tool will take you through in a structured way:

Emotional Recognition: In this stage you will identify the specific emotions associated with the problem that you experienced.

Emotional Understanding: During this stage you will try to understand how your emotions affect your thinking and behaviour and how it impacts the behaviour of others. It is also important to understand how this knowledge helps you to improve relationships with others.

Emotional Analysis: This stage is about identifying the underlying messages embedded within your emotions in order to identify solutions to their causes for both you and others.

Emotional Regulation: This stage takes the emotions that you have identified, analyzed and interpreted in previous stages and gets you to formulate concrete strategies for how you can regulate your emotions to achieve a constructive solution to the problem. Furthermore, it will encourage you to consider ways to inspire and influence.

Exercise

Think of a difficult incident you have had with a student/trainee recently. This might be confrontation in or outside the classroom/learning environment. It could have happened because of what or how you said something. It might have resulted from the student/trainee being disruptive, rude or inconsiderate or them having an open and direct argument with you.

Try to be specific about the conflict you have selected:
Try to remember the setting, approximate time and date.

- What caused the conflict? What actually happened?
- What did the student/trainee say or do?

- How did you react/respond?
- Was the conflict resolved?

We will now try to re-live the incident with you using the four stages of the Emotional Literacy Reflective Interactive Tool and the questions and interactions outlined below.

We hope that the tool will help you better understand the incident. It will help you consider your emotions and thereby analyze the resulting reactions and behaviour.

I. Emotional Recognition

According to Mayer et al. (2000), the first branch of emotional intelligence is 'the capacity to perceive and express feelings'. This initial step therefore endeavours to identify and record the feelings experienced by both the teacher/trainer and student/trainee. It is the basic aspect of emotional intelligence as it will make further processing of emotional information possible.

The aim of this first step is to:

- identify emotions felt by the teacher/trainer during the difficult incident

  paying close attention to:

- identifying emotions in the student through their language, sound, appearance and behaviour
- what emotions were felt, expressed and observed
- discriminating between expressed and concealed/masked emotions, accurate/honest and inaccurate/dishonest expressions of feeling.

1. **What emotions did you feel?**

- User selects from a range of emotions.

2. **Which of these emotions did you express visibly and which might have been hidden to the student/pupil?**

    - (your expressed emotions/concealed or masked emotions).

3. **What emotions was the student/trainee displaying**

    - User selects from a range of emotions:

    a) What did he/she do?
    b) What kind of language did he/she use?
    c) What about his/her tone of voice, posture and demeanour?

4. Based on your answers above, what additional emotions might the student/pupil have felt that were underlying to the conflict and were not visibly expressed by him/her?

After submitting these four answers, the tool contrasts the feelings of both teacher and student.

II. Emotional Understanding

The next stage in the Emotional Literacy Reflective Interactive Tool will explore how the emotions perceived and expressed in step 1 are harnessed and tied together to facilitate cognitive functions such as thinking and problem solving. It will help the user to understand and manage the feelings they experienced in order to exploit emotions to improve performance.

The aim of this stage is to:

- discover how the emotions identified in the previous step have affected cognitive functions in both teacher/trainer and student/trainee
- explore how emotions are guiding and prioritizing the thinking of the teacher/trainer
- create awareness of factors that have influenced cognitive processing of emotion
- consider the impact of emotions on teacher/trainer decision making
- reflect on ways to capitalize on changing moods to empower the teacher/trainer
- facilitate self-management by controlling one's emotions and impulses to adapt to changing circumstances.

5. As a result of your feelings, what went through your mind during the confrontation?
6. How does your body respond to these situations/events (e.g. avoid, withdraw, run away)?
7. Which of these factors do you think influenced your mind during the confrontation?
    - User adjusts sliding scales from 'Big Influence' to 'No Influence' of: cultural/racial background, religious/spiritual beliefs, similar personal experiences, family upbringing, experience in childhood, social class, an unrelated current event in your life, prior learning, stereotypical beliefs about the student, previous experience with students, teacher's temperament, information shared by other staff member (negative or positive information sharing), fear of student/pupil.
8. As a result of their feelings, how did the student/trainee respond? What do you think was their reasoning?
9. How do you think you could capitalize on your mood and emotions to respond in a more effective manner in a similar situation?

III. Emotional Analysis

The third stage of this tool is about analyzing the emotional use. Emotions usually convey information that can give valuable indications in regard to the cause of the conflict and potential solutions. Emotions tend to express their own pattern of possible messages and potential actions. Anger, for example, could mean that someone feels treated unfairly. Possible actions might then include attacking, retribution, revenge-seeking or peacemaking.

Consequently, the aim of this stage is to:

- appreciate and understand the complicated relationship among emotions
- identify emotions that might be connected to the feelings recorded in the first stage

- become sensitive to slight variations between emotions
- recognize and describe how emotions evolve and change over time
- discover the messages and information conveyed by the emotions
- consider possible actions to resolve conflict and respond to the student.

10. Can you break the emotions listed in stage 1 into further more specific variations?
11. Create a mini-timeline of emotions experienced during this conflict and show how emotions have evolved during this confrontation.
12. How can you interpret the emotions you identified in step 1 in regards to:

    a) your underlying wants and needs in this situation?
    b) your relationship with this student?
    c) potential solutions to the problem?

13. What do you think the student/trainee is trying to display, tell you or express?

IV. Emotional Regulation

The final stage enables the user to combine everything considered and recorded within the first three stages. After emotions have been recognized, understood and interpreted, the user will reflect on strategies to regulate and manage emotions to achieve his/her goals. Remaining aware of our emotions as we go through this process will mean that we can also use these to monitor the effectiveness of any actions that we may take.

The last step aims to:

- regulate emotions in oneself and others by moderating negative emotions and enhancing pleasant ones without repressing or exaggerating information that these might convey
- harness and channel positive and negative emotions to achieve intended goals
- consider ways to inspire, influence and develop others while managing conflict
- remain open to both pleasant and unpleasant feelings
- influence and control emotions of both teacher/trainer and student/trainee
- reflectively engage with or detach from an emotion depending upon its judged informative value and utility.

14. How can you regulate your emotions during confrontation?
15. How can you influence the student's emotions during and after the event?
16. Can you channel the negative emotions to effect a change in the circumstances and variables surrounding the conflict?
17. Can you think of ways to inspire and develop the student as part of this conflict?
18. What strategies can you put in place to detach yourself from unhelpful emotions in order to make more objective and constructive decisions and responses?
19. How can you improve the classroom climate by regulating your emotions and becoming more emotionally literate?
20. In what ways can your school use and promote emotional literacy to improve the school ethos and atmosphere?

TELS Teacher Emotional Literacy Scale

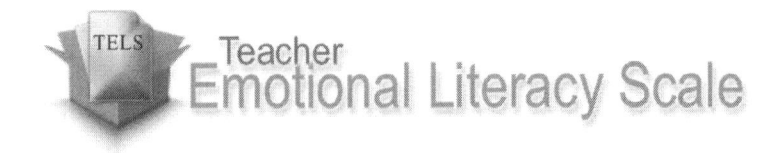

Adapted by Dr Richard Majors

1	2	3	4	5
Strongly Disagree	**Disagree**	**Neither Agree nor Disagree**	**Agree**	**Strongly Agree**

1	I wish I could be more demonstrative when I teach.	1	2	3	4	5
2	I believe that I am a highly effective staff member.	1	2	3	4	5
3	As a member of staff in this school/college/organization, I am involved in the community.	1	2	3	4	5
4	I have a significant positive impact on my students'/trainees' future.	1	2	3	4	5
5	With time, I am understanding the mistakes students/trainees make.	1	2	3	4	5
6	I am familiar with the places where my students/trainees spend their free time.	1	2	3	4	5
7	I am rarely sarcastic or patronizing to my students/trainees.	1	2	3	4	5
8	My students/trainees feel free to talk to me about non-academic matters.	1	2	3	4	5
9	My students/trainees trust me.	1	2	3	4	5
10	It is important for me to try to help fix a problem or assist one of my students/trainees when they have a problem or are in need.	1	2	3	4	5
11	Students/trainees seem enthused when I enter the classroom/learning environment.	1	2	3	4	5
12	Students/trainees do not seem at ease around me.	1	2	3	4	5
13	I feel like I am an important part of where I teach.	1	2	3	4	5
14	I believe that with the right teaching and mentoring, all students/trainees will be successful learners.	1	2	3	4	5

1	2	3	4	5
Strongly Disagree	**Disagree**	**Neither Agree nor Disagree**	**Agree**	**Strongly Agree**

15. I don't talk down to my students/trainees or patronize them.   1   2   3   4   5
16. When something goes wrong in my class, I can quickly stop dwelling on it and move on.   1   2   3   4   5
17. Though I may have many different values from my students/trainees, I still try to relate and get on with them.   1   2   3   4   5
18. I like teaching students/trainees from diverse backgrounds.   1   2   3   4   5
19. I find it difficult to approach and interact with my students/trainees.   1   2   3   4   5
20. I readily place trust in students/trainees when I first meet them.   1   2   3   4   5
21. I get upset when I see one of my students/trainees being treated unfairly.   1   2   3   4   5
22. I feel excited when I step into the school/college/organization.   1   2   3   4   5
23. I believe that other staff and students/trainees think that I make a valuable contribution to the educational environment.   1   2   3   4   5
24. School/college/organization policy supports the development of positive relationships with my students.   1   2   3   4   5
25. I believe that given the right approach to teaching my students/trainees will learn.   1   2   3   4   5
26. I consider the opinions of my students/trainees when making decisions but I don't feel I have to go along with their opinions.   1   2   3   4   5
27. If I make a mistake with my students/trainees, I feel bad at first but I do not keep feeling bad about it.   1   2   3   4   5
28. I dislike the types of clothes that my students/trainees are wearing these days.   1   2   3   4   5
29. Relationships are very important in raising academic performance.   1   2   3   4   5
30. I can count on my students/trainees to do their work to the best of their ability.   1   2   3   4   5

1	2	3	4	5
Strongly Disagree	Disagree	Neither Agree nor Disagree	Agree	Strongly Agree

31	If my students/trainees have any problems outside of school/college/organization that affect their learning, I want to show empathy.	1	2	3	4	5
32	My teaching stimulates me.	1	2	3	4	5
33	I believe that my students/trainees value my advice.	1	2	3	4	5
34	I believe that the staff in my school get along well together and like each other.	1	2	3	4	5
35	Teachers should direct the activities and decisions of their students/trainees through both reasoning and discipline.	1	2	3	4	5
36	I approve of the different forms of slang that my students/trainees use.	1	2	3	4	5
37	I believe my relationships with my students/trainees are overall very positive.	1	2	3	4	5
38	Generally, I trust all my students/trainees.	1	2	3	4	5
39	I worry about the feelings of my students/trainees when they are unhappy or upset.	1	2	3	4	5
40	I have learned a great deal from the differences I have seen between students/trainees.	1	2	3	4	5
41	I think that the school/college/organization's policy and schedule support my job role.	1	2	3	4	5
42	I feel confident approaching my students/trainees during non-class time.	1	2	3	4	5
43	My students/trainees would agree that I am enthusiastic.	1	2	3	4	5
44	Students think school/college/organization discipline policy overall is fair.	1	2	3	4	5
45	I like the types of music that my students/trainees listen to.	1	2	3	4	5
46	Before judging my students/trainees, I always try to hear their side of the story.	1	2	3	4	5
47	My students/trainees are reliable and will generally do what they say.	1	2	3	4	5
48	I feel good when I help one of my students/trainees who is in need.	1	2	3	4	5

1	2	3	4	5
Strongly Disagree	**Disagree**	**Neither Agree nor Disagree**	**Agree**	**Strongly Agree**

49	My students/trainees like me.	1	2	3	4	5
50	After one of my students/trainees has done something wrong, I do not hold it against them.	1	2	3	4	5
51	I can influence my students/trainees to learn.	1	2	3	4	5
52	I believe that I have the skills to do my job effectively.	1	2	3	4	5
53	I am always eager to help my students/trainees with their work.	1	2	3	4	5
54	My school/college/organization is an enjoyable place to work.	1	2	3	4	5
55	I try to incorporate some of my knowledge of youth culture in my work because it helps me to understand and relate to young people.	1	2	3	4	5
56	I am always fair to my students/trainees.	1	2	3	4	5
57	My students/trainees feel I am always approachable.	1	2	3	4	5
58	I am a good judge of students/trainees and have rarely been let down because of the trust I placed in them.	1	2	3	4	5
59	I am very aware of how my students/trainees are feeling when I interact with them.	1	2	3	4	5
60	I find it easy to forgive any mistakes students/trainees make.	1	2	3	4	5
61	What I do will in some way help my students/trainees to have successful lives in the future.	1	2	3	4	5
62	My school/college/organization has a friendly atmosphere.	1	2	3	4	5
63	I show passion when I teach.	1	2	3	4	5
64	Most students like this school/college/organization.	1	2	3	4	5
65	When one of my students/trainees disappoints me, I can eventually move past it.	1	2	3	4	5
66	I understand that the different backgrounds of my students/trainees may mean that they do not always see things in the same way as I do.	1	2	3	4	5

1	2	3	4	5
Strongly Disagree	Disagree	Neither Agree nor Disagree	Agree	Strongly Agree

67	Even when I am not present, I know my students/trainees will usually be working hard.	1	2	3	4	5
68	Relationships are important for motivating young people.	1	2	3	4	5
69	Teachers' opinions rather than students'/pupils' opinions should always be valued more.	1	2	3	4	5
70	The school's mission and vision statement needs to be more student-friendly.	1	2	3	4	5
71	I believe that I make a positive difference to the lives of my students/trainees.	1	2	3	4	5
72	In teaching, I have found the right career for me.	1	2	3	4	5
73	I understand how the school/college/organization's vision and mission underlie its most important decisions.	1	2	3	4	5
74	I do not know what to talk about when with my students/trainees.	1	2	3	4	5
75	I give clear directions about how my students/trainees should behave but am understanding when they disagree.	1	2	3	4	5
76	I respect my students/trainees.	1	2	3	4	5
77	Students/trainees feel free to talk to me about their work at school/college/organization.	1	2	3	4	5
78	My students/trainees appreciate the trust that I place in them.	1	2	3	4	5
79	I am put off by students/trainees with non-mainstream values or lifestyles.	1	2	3	4	5
80	Students'/trainees' rights should be respected always.	1	2	3	4	5
81	I feel confident approaching my students/trainees in class.	1	2	3	4	5
82	The school/college/organization's goals are consistent with the vision I have for it.	1	2	3	4	5
83	If I make a mistake, I'm willing to admit it to my students/trainees.	1	2	3	4	5
84	I believe that I make a positive difference to my school/college/organization.	1	2	3	4	5

1	2	3	4	5
Strongly Disagree	**Disagree**	**Neither Agree nor Disagree**	**Agree**	**Strongly Agree**

85	I often communicate with students/trainees outside the classroom/learning environment.	1	2	3	4	5
86	I can give my students/trainees a lot of freedom to learn without fear of this freedom being abused.	1	2	3	4	5
87	Relationships are important for managing behaviour.	1	2	3	4	5
88	My students/trainees can count on me to help them with a problem.	1	2	3	4	5

Scoring the TELS

After completing the 88 questions, a score can be calculated for each of the 11 constructs. If a person completes the online TELS, these scores will be calculated automatically; the paper version has to be scored manually.

What the TELS scores mean

The TELS will provide the user with a 10-point score for each of the 11 constructs (see screenshot below for an example submission on the online TELS).

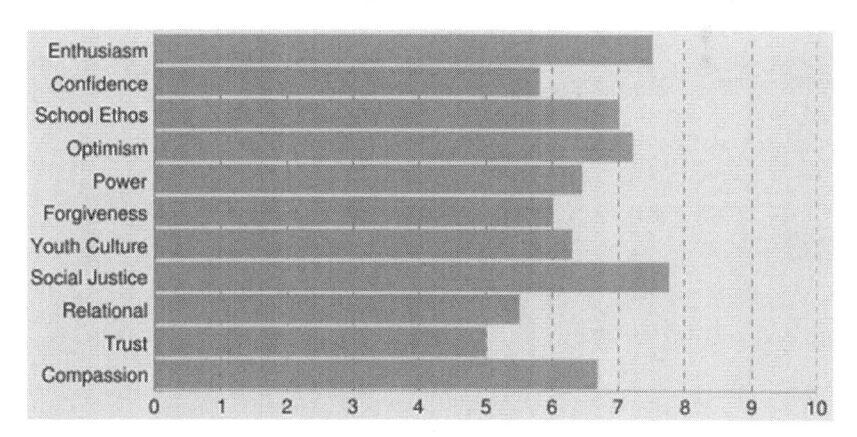

The score for each construct will indicate the emotional literacy strengths and weaknesses of the test user. Higher scores reflect higher self-reports on each construct. For example, a score of 7.6 for Confidence pre-intervention and a score of 8.8 for Confidence post-intervention shows that the user has increased in their level of teaching confidence.

As a further example, the screenshot above might indicate that the teacher's/trainer's emotional literacy strengths are both Enthusiasm and Social Justice while Confidence, Relational and Trust aspects of emotional literacy require further work through intervention coaching or training. In general, the user should aim to increase their scores for all constructs as this will have a positive impact on their effectiveness as a teacher/trainer.

Nevertheless, as with all self-report measures, the results should be treated as indicators only as the responses will depend on how a user has approached the questionnaire.

Scoring the paper-based version

The steps below describe the process of manually scoring the TELS, which might take 20–30 minutes. It is therefore recommended to use the computer tool instead as this will do the scoring automatically.

Enthusiasm:

1. Combine the scores for questions 22, 54, 11, 64, 44, 73, 33.
2. Add the reverse score for question 1.
3. Divide the resulting number by 40.

Confidence:

1. Combine the scores for questions 82, 43, 34, 53, 2, 72, 85, 23.
2. Add the reverse score for questions 1, 2 and 75.
3. Divide the resulting number by 50.

School Ethos:

1. Combine the scores for questions 83, 63, 13, 74, 42, 35, 3, 55, 45, 65, 24, 71.
2. Divide the resulting number by 60.

Optimism:

1. Combine the scores for questions 62, 14, 52, 4, 25.
2. Divide the resulting number by 25.

Power:

1. Combine the scores for questions 84, 26, 76, 15, 36, 81, 70.
2. Divide the resulting number by 35.

Forgiveness:

1. Combine the scores for questions 66, 16, 51, 27, 5, 61.
2. Divide the resulting number by 30.

Youth Culture:

1. Combine the scores for questions 56, 6, 37, 46, 17.
2. Add the reverse score for questions 28 and 80.
3. Divide the resulting number by 35.

Social Justice:

1. Combine the scores for questions 77, 47, 7, 41, 29, 57, 18, 67.
2. Divide the resulting number by 40.

Relational:

1. Combine the scores for questions 78, 8, 86, 50, 89, 38, 58, 30, 69, 88.
2. Add the reverse score for question 19.
3. Divide the resulting number by 55.

Trust:

1. Combine the scores for questions 87, 79, 20, 59, 48, 31, 68, 9, 39.
2. Divide the resulting number by 45.

Compassion:

1. Combine the scores for questions 21, 49, 32, 60, 40, 10.
2. Divide the resulting number by 30.

Chapter 11

ASD and Cultural Competence: An ASD Multicultural Treatment-Led Model

Mary Henderson and Richard Majors

Introduction

It became very clear from researching this chapter title that there is a real research gap around autism within a Black and Minority Ethnic (BME) population. Funding has been available for autism research in the mainstream populations but funds are very limited within a BME population.

Reports estimate that the prevalence of those on the autism spectrum disorder (ASD) is about 1% in the UK (Elsabbagh et al., 2012). It is also estimated that the occurrence was 157 per 10,000 (Baron-Cohen, Scott, Allison, & Williams, 2009). Based on these estimates, roughly 700,000 to a million people in the UK would appear to be autistic with a significant percentage arising from within a BME population (Nevison, 2019).

This chapter shall explore an ASD diagnosis and the crucial need for early diagnosis along with the need for cultural competence in the ASD diagnostic process especially with those from a BME population. Treatment options and support shall then be explored along with recommendations for essential improvements in patient diagnosis and treatment. First, let's try to understand what it might feel like to be on the autism spectrum in the eyes of a young man who is living with it.

An Example of How It May Feel to Be on the Autism Spectrum

"Prime numbers are what is left when you have taken all the patterns away. I think prime numbers are like life." *The Curious Incident of the Dog in the Night-time.*

The National Theatre recently staged a widely acclaimed play entitled *The Curious Incident of the Dog in the Night-time*, by Mark Haddon and adapted for theatre by Simon Stephens premiered in 2012. This was a superbly staged insight into how Christopher Boone, a young person on the autism spectrum, perceives the world.

The play tells the story of a boy with an outstanding gift for mathematics and science who, being on the autistic spectrum, also struggles to cope with everyday life. When Christopher accidentally finds the neighbor's dog dead, having been slain by a garden fork, this causes such revulsion within him that he determines to discover the killer. Whilst playing amateur detective, he learns his mother has not in fact died as his father informed him but is living safely in London after their separation. Christopher, in his role of sleuth, had discovered a bundle of unopened letters addressed to him from his mother. He then realizes that his father lied about his mother's death. At this point, the production highlights Christopher's utter vulnerability in the face of a newly destabilized world. He falls apart, with no inner reserves to sustain him post revelation. The production depicts his angst and confusion, with pained screaming culminating in collapse.

The drama emphasizes Christopher's rigidly literal view of the world, as well as his struggles to communicate effectively with others within the constraints of ASDs; he appears friendless and limited by his overly simplistic way of seeing the world. The stage set utilizes neat and ordered gridlines which represent the tight and safe boundaries in which Christopher has managed to construct his sense of the world, and thereby create a tenuous impression of safety and harmony. Conversely, when Christopher's world jars or refuses to make sense, the production makes use of screeching, discordant sounds to allow the listener to step into his agitated and confused world where disharmony seems to persist. The intensity of his emotions at these moments is reflected in his behaviors of heightened stammering, aggression, violence, and withdrawal.

The production manages to depict Christopher's typical time delay in understanding what is being said to him and, at other times, frantic processing of those words. It also dramatizes the ASD tendency to distill a waterfall of highly intense electronic emotion into comprehensible communication, facilitated often by using signs. When Christopher is trying to find his mother, the deafening sounds and train noises of a bustling town and city are all heightened to fever pitch, as externalizations of Christopher's inner turmoil and helplessness. The script depicts the natural buildup of strong emotions at various crisis points in the drama and beautifully draws out the overwhelming lack of containment which results in an emotional outburst, as well as collapse and regression into the fetal position.

When Christopher loses his pet rat in the London Underground and immediately, with no perceived sense of danger, begins searching on the rails, bystanders frantically try to "speak sense to him" regarding the dangers of an oncoming train. The passengers then feel compelled to put their own lives at risk by rescuing him. Christopher is so caught up in his obsession for the lost pet that he barely notices their dilemma and shows an acute lack of awareness of their plight in rescuing him. The production beautifully demonstrates his total focus on the potential loss of his pet, and his lack of awareness of any threat to himself or others.

The production depicts Christopher's mathematical giftedness as almost separate from other aspects of his world until near the end of the play when the beginning of an integration starts to emerge. The ASD support therapist is clearly most helpful in enabling Christopher to better understand himself and his world, and provides him with a repertoire of strategies to help him cope. The play closes with a far happier and empowered Christopher, who understands himself, is understood by others, and is accepted for both his giftedness and his difference. He inhabits and conceives a truer and more cohesive world, better able to manage rules and patterns as absolutes.

ASD's Definition and Diagnosis Criteria

ASD is a complex developmental condition that involves persistent challenges in social interaction, speech and nonverbal communication, and restricted/repetitive behaviors. "The effects of ASD and the severity of symptoms are different in each person" American Psychiatric Association (APA) (2013) (J. Nathan Copeland, 2018).

The *DSM-5* classifies ASD as persistent deficits in social communication and social interaction across multiple contexts, as manifested by the following, currently or by history:

(A) 1. Deficits in social–emotional reciprocity, ranging, for example, from abnormal social approach and failure of normal back-and-forth conversation; to reduced sharing of interests, emotions, or affect; to failure to initiate or respond to social interactions.
2. Deficits in nonverbal communicative behaviors used for social interaction, ranging, for example, from poorly integrated verbal and nonverbal communication; to abnormalities in eye contact and body language or deficits in understanding and use of gestures; to a total lack of facial expressions and nonverbal communication.
3. Deficits in developing, maintaining, and understanding relationships, ranging, for example, from difficulties adjusting behavior to suit various social contexts; to difficulties in sharing imaginative play or in making friends; to absence of interest in peers.

(B) Restricted, repetitive patterns of behavior, interests, or activities, as manifested by at least two of the following, currently or by history (examples are illustrative, not exhaustive:

1. Stereotyped or repetitive motor movements, use of objects, or speech (e.g., simple motor stereotypes, lining up toys or flipping objects, echolalia, or idiosyncratic phrases).
2. Insistence on sameness, inflexible adherence to routines, or ritualized patterns of verbal or nonverbal behavior (e.g., extreme distress at small changes, difficulties with transitions, rigid thinking patterns, greeting rituals, the need to take the same route, or eat the same food every day).
3. Highly restricted, fixated interests that are abnormal in intensity or focus (e.g., strong attachment to or preoccupation with unusual objects, excessively circumscribed or perseverative interests).
4. Hyper- or hypoactivity to sensory input or unusual interest in sensory aspects of the environment (e.g., apparent indifference to pain/temperature, adverse response to specific sounds or textures, excessive smelling or touching of objects, visual fascination with lights or movement).

In conclusion, the *DSM-5* classification states in its criteria C, D, and E that symptoms must be present in the early developmental period and cause clinically significant impairment in social, occupational, or other important areas of social functioning, and that these symptoms are not better explained by intellectual disability or global developmental delay.

Impact of Changes to the Diagnostic Criteria

Under the new stricter diagnostic criteria for ASD within the *DSM-5*, professionals have raised their voices due to concerns that many who are genuinely on the ASD spectrum may be excluded from receiving a diagnosis due to the more rigorous criteria. The *DSM-5* divides seven symptoms of ASD into two main groups, which include a shortfall in both social communication and social interaction, and limited repetitive behaviors and pursuits. In line with current research, the *DSM-5* has included diagnostic criteria of heightened or blunted sensitivity to touch, taste, smell, sound, or visual stimuli due to the recognition of this being a core feature within ASD.

Assessing a child for possible ASD is normally performed by a combination of professionals within a multidisciplinary team, which includes a pediatrician or a child and adolescent psychiatrist, a speech and language therapist (SALT), and a clinical or educational psychologist. As a part of the assessment, information in relation to pregnancy, birth, and a developmental history is taken along with the age at which the parents or carers first became concerned. Included in the overall assessment would be gathering information around sleep and eating habits, along with hypersensitivity or hyposensitivity to light, touch, noise, food texture, and clothing, and a family history, especially in relation to any neurodevelopmental disorders. A commonly used tool in the UK is an ADOS, which is an Autism Diagnostic Observation Schedule (Katherine Gotham, 2012).

The ADOS comprises a series of tasks that affords the examiner an opportunity to pinpoint the core symptoms of ASD. The results of the ADOS are then used in conjunction with parental, carer, nursery, and school reports. The ADOS includes a construction task, imaginative play, a demonstration task, conversation, a description of a picture, relating a familiar story, free and specific play, verbal and nonverbal interaction, anticipation of a routine, and sensory test observations

Full parental involvement for an assessment of autism is fundamental to the correct diagnosis. The child's or young person's parents or carers are of paramount importance in allowing the ASD assessors into the child's behaviors when at home, at school, within the family unit, and within all other settings. They can chart us through the behavioral developmental stages, and tell us what they started to notice and when. They allow us into those moments where initially a problem is perceived, and how they respond and manage this as individuals and as a family.

A 2012 review of autism data worldwide reported an average of 62 cases per 10,000 people (Elsabbagh et al., 2012). More recently, in March 2016, the Centers for Disease Control and Prevention (CDC) estimated that 1 in 68 children have autism in the United States. Recent studies suggest a ratio of four times as many males to females being diagnosed with ASD (Lai et al., 2011; Werling & Geschwind, 2013). "Recent meta-analysis suggests that the widely reported 4:1 ratio of boys to girls is quite consistent across studies, geographical regions, ethnicities and time" (Elsabbagh et al., 2012).

Early Screening and Treatment for ASD Recommended

The American Academy of Pediatrics recommends screening for autism at 18 and 24 months of age. In the UK, this is also the case and the screening tool used here is the M-CHAT™ (Modified Checklist for Autism in Toddlers) as the diagnostic tool. To understand and support individuals on the spectrum, Europe recently initiated a new program: ASDEU (ASDs in the European Union, 2015–2018) and piloted it across many European countries. The findings highlighted a lack of resources to help detect ASD along with difficulties around obtaining an ASD diagnosis. García-Primo et al. (2014) study highlighted that early detection of ASD, along with a corresponding therapeutic intervention, leads to a far better prognosis for the child, and may prevent secondary developmental disturbances and reduce family stress.

Autism and Theory of Mind Research

Professor Simon Baron-Cohen provided the first researched evidence that the Theory of Mind was defective or delayed in children with autism. The Theory of Mind is that ability to attribute to both oneself and others: beliefs, desires, intentions, perspectives, emotions, and unique motives that are different from our own. When that Theory of Mind is impaired, this then affects the individual's ability to understand that others have plans, purposes which are different from their own. This absence of Theory of Mind commonly identified in those with autism leads to a lack of understanding as to why others do certain things. This can precipitate anger outbursts within the person with autism who genuinely does not understand the perspective of the other. It ordinarily then has a negative impact upon relationships (Baron-Cohen, Tager-Flusberg, & Cohen, 2000). Theory of Mind defect in our character Christopher helps to explain his fixations and lack of understanding of how others might be considering events.

Cultural Competence and Diagnostic Failings in ASD Assessment in a BME Population

The National Institutes of Health (NIH) describes culture as:

> the combination of the body of knowledge, a body of belief and a body of behaviour. It involves a number of elements, including personal identification, language, thoughts, communications, actions, customs, beliefs, values, and institutions that are often specific to ethnic, racial, religious, geographic, or social groups.

The NIH describes natural difference and invites all health practitioners to acknowledge and value all in a spirit of respectfulness and appropriate response to each person's "health beliefs, practices and cultural and linguistic needs of diverse patients."

> Cultural competence is a set of congruent behaviours, attitudes, and policies that come together in a system, agency or among professionals and enable that system, agency or those professions to work effectively in cross-cultural situations. (Cross, 1988, 1989)

William Taylor's Reflective Competence Model as applied to a Cultural Awareness Cycle by William Howell explores how as health professionals we can begin the cycle:

- By being "unconsciously culturally incompetent" within an ASD assessment and ignorant of the vital differences, which may include attitude, behavior, eye contact, and possibly medicalizing the assessment on first meeting. For the healthcare professional to be unaware of another's culture can cause cultural errors in the assessment and unwittingly alienate us from the child and the family. We are also more likely to misinterpret behaviors as relevant to the assessment when they may in fact be a part of the cultural aspect of the individual and the wider family and cause us to potentially misdiagnose.
- The next step of the cycle explores how in reaching cultural competency, that the assessor may learn a little of how the cultures impact upon one another in an assessment. This may result in the healthcare professional being "consciously culturally incompetent" and recognize that there is a significant cultural difference. This may leave the practitioner feeling very much at a loss in terms of cross-cultural knowledge, thus causing them to struggle through an assessment and perhaps be unsure of the outcome.
- The third step within this cycle is with the assessor being far more aware of the culture of the person being assessed and actively taking this into account during the assessment. This is referred to as being "unconsciously culturally competent," where the healthcare professional trusts their instincts regarding the cultural differences and yet may be struggling to balance the interface between an earlier lack of cultural awareness and newly acquiring a cross-cultural sensitivity and trying to remain objective.
- The fourth part of the cycle is where the healthcare professional is: "consciously culturally competent" in an ASD assessment where the assessor is fully able to recognize what is and is not culturally appropriate, and is also able to recognize the sensitivities and subtle nuances within that culture and how best to respond to this appropriately and how it may impact upon the final outcome. The model looks to address each of these four stances and bring about a positive shift through reflection, thus moving the practitioner toward conscious cultural competence.

The Purnell Model for Cultural Confidence defines 12 key areas with which health-care professionals are challenged to familiarize themselves and to be conversant in conducting an ethical ASD assessment. These are a full knowledge of all aspects of heritage, communication, family role and organization, workforce, biocultural ecology, high-risk behaviors, nutrition, pregnancy and child-rearing practices, death rituals and bereavement, spirituality, health-care practices, and health-care practitioners.

Culture may be defined as:

> the extent to which a group of individuals engage in overt and verbal behavior reflecting shared behavioral learning histories, serving to differentiate the group from other groups, and predicting how individuals within the group act in specific setting conditions. (Sugai et al., 2012, p. 200)

We are each unique and born into our specific culture where we develop a shared understanding of how this operates and affects us. For another to step into our cultural world requires an understanding of how it developed and the appropriate rules of engagement within that culture. "Cultural awareness may be important because behavioral patterns that are viewed as problematic in our own culture may be the norm in other cultures" (Goldiamond, 2002; Vandenberghe, 2008). An article for the Association for Behavior Analysis International offers an example of a young person diagnosed with severe autism whose family attended a church service lasting three hours each week (Hughes Fong, Catagnus, Brodhead, Quigley, & Field, 2016). The family asked the behavioral therapist to teach the child the necessary skills to sit in church over a three-hour period as this was high on their list of behavioral challenges for the child. The behavioral therapist did not consider this to be a high priority as he was not a churchgoer.

> A culturally aware behavior analyst may have been more aware that "the selection of target behaviors is an expression of values" (Kauffman et al. 2008, p. 254) and that parental expectations of children are likely controlled by cultural contingencies. (Akcinar & Baydar, 2014).

The American Psychological Association's (APA) (2003) multicultural guidelines encourage clinicians to:

> recognize that, as cultural beings, they may hold attitudes and beliefs that can detrimentally influence their perceptions of and interactions with individuals who are ethnically and racially different from themselves. (Hughes Fong et al., 2016, p. 382)

Promoting self-awareness in health-care practitioners may act as a preventative measure in relation to limiting how we serve those from other cultural backgrounds.

In light of the above, it may be that there exists cultural complacency within ASD assessment screening. Many children appear to be falling through the net and failing to receive the help that they so desperately require. Prior to screening for those on the autistic spectrum, should there be a requirement for each member of the assessing team to consider cultural implications to ensure cultural competency? It may be that this is adopted as a more formal compulsory measure within health-care settings to ensure equality and as a means of preventing any form of discrimination.

There are clear guidelines in relation to both criteria and assessment of ASD. However, there appears to be an absence of strict cultural competency guidelines in the assessment of ASD. For example, in certain cultures, a firm handshake is seen to be aggressive and direct gaze to be rude. There can be a stigma in certain cultures where a mental health diagnosis such as ASD is held to be a negative thing. The family and patient being assessed may collude to prevent the clinician from seeing the whole picture. In a 2016 article in *Scientific American* entitled "How cultural differences affect autism diagnoses," Bauer, Winegar, & Waxman (2016) tell the reader of how the delineations around autism are very much attributed to culture. The *DSM-5* criteria mainly reflect a European–American perception of what is accepted normality. An example of "abnormalities in eye contact" and meeting the gaze of an adult could be regarded as a mark of disrespect in cultures such as those in Egypt, Kenya, North Korea, and certain Eastern European countries. In certain rural areas of North Korea, some families will go to great lengths to avoid a diagnosis of developmental delay due to the possible stigma and how it may affect their child's future. The parents are more likely to accept a diagnosis of parental neglect rather than the stigma of ASD.

> Most experts agree that methodological and cultural factors explain the bulk of differences in autism prevalence around the world. For example, U.S. prevalence studies show that autism rates in Hispanic communities are lower than in non-Hispanic communities, even when adjusted for socioeconomic factors. One provocative, though unstudied, explanation is that in Hispanic cultures, where gregariousness is highly valued, having features of autism could affect one's reproductive opportunities more than in Asian cultures, which value solitude and seriousness, especially in men. (Hughes, 2011)

Chris Papadopoulos, principal lecturer in public health at the University of Bedfordshire, wrote an article in October 2016 entitled "Autism stigma and the role of ethnicity and culture." He stated:

> We know ethnicity is a key determinant of health inequalities in England, where Black, Asian and Minority Ethnic communities face poorer access to healthcare (The King's Fund, 2015) including autism services (Slade, 2014). If minority groups access services but experience poor cultural awareness from service providers, they may reject these services. Health care and autism service providers may also be unable to identify and diagnose autism due to language and cultural differences. With progress hampered, services lose the opportunity to engage with the community, raise awareness and understanding of autism and mitigate against the production and effects of stigma. (Papadopoulos, 2016)

An article published in *Pacific Standard* in May 2016 on "autism's race problem" highlights the plight of many disadvantaged black children who require an ASD assessment and the subsequent support but appear to be denied this opportunity. This article reported:

> The autism world prides itself on honoring neurodiversity, but it has been less successful at recognizing racial and ethnic diversity. The statistics are stark: Studies by the Centers for Disease Control and Prevention (CDC) show that rates of autism are essentially identical across racial and ethnic groups. But when you look at children and adults actually diagnosed with autism, white children are 30 percent more likely to receive an autism diagnosis than blacks, and 50 percent more likely than Hispanics, according to 2014 data from the CDC. Minority children are also diagnosed significantly later than white children. (Arnold, 2016)

> Also, Mandell et al., in their study in 2009, identified that a disparity in diagnosis existed among a BME population, showing that black children are diagnosed with ASD at a later age than are white children. (Mandell et al., 2009)

Venessa Bob writes in "Girls and Autism" that "in her community along with other Black, Asian and Minority Ethnic (BAME) communities, there is a problem of under-diagnosis of ASD." She recounts how it took 10 years for her daughter to receive her ASD diagnosis. Venessa Bob lamented on how "every minute that her diagnosis was delayed, her daughter's mental well-being deteriorated" (Carpenter, Happé, & Egerton, 2019).

A study published in August 2019 in *The Journal of Autism and Developmental Disorders* found that the prevalence of autism in blacks and Hispanics is now surpassing those in whites. It concluded that autism prevalence in Hispanics aged three to five years rose 73% in comparison to rates among blacks that increased 44% with 25% increase among whites (Nevison, 2019). Nevison's conclusion reports that both black and Hispanic groups within the Individuals with Disabilities Education Act 3–5-year-old data set have now caught up and surpassed white prevalence in the majority of states within the United States.

Diane Abbott MP wrote a foreword for The National Autistic Society's Report on "Diverse Perspectives, The challenges for families affected by autism from Black, Asian, and Minority Ethnic communities" by Guy Slade. In it, she said that:

> Policy-makers and commissioners must properly assess the needs of BAME communities when producing autism policy and commissioning autism services. The evidence is that communities typically need more accessible information, culturally sensitive support and innovative forms of engagement, whether to improve diagnosis or ensure families can access services.

This report reinforced previous research that families affected by autism struggled around seeking an ASD diagnosis for their child and support for themselves.

This report highlights how society is failing these children and their families and possibly preventing these children from integrating more within society.

Tackling Inequalities

A partial way forward in addressing cultural competency in ASD assessment was highlighted in a recent study using a pictorial assessment effectively (Perera, Jeewandara, Seneviratne, & Guruge, 2017). This research tested an ASD screening tool called a Pictorial Autism Assessment Schedule (PAAS), which was modeled from previously documented ASD screening checklists. Its aim was to help overcome a cultural bias in the assessment of ASD. The results appear to be effective in discriminating between ASD and non-ASD developmental disorder to 88.8% accuracy, and 88% in ASD and typical development. The researchers indicated that the PAAS takes 20 minutes to complete and makes use of photos, each of which illustrates the meaning of the assessment question within the photo.

Neuroscience-led ASD Assessment for the Future

In 2017, a research study by Dr Joseph Piven of the University of North Carolina at Chapel Hill showed the images of the baby's brain at 6, 12, and 24 months using magnetic resonance imaging technique, also showed that infants with older siblings with autism would then go on to be diagnosed with autism at 24 months (Piven, 2017). The study demonstrated that the researchers correctly predicted 80% of the infants who would be diagnosed with autism at 24 months. It has been very difficult in the past to identify those children who will go on to develop autism before the age of 24 months when all the ASD characteristics are clearly observable. This research means that theoretically infants who will later be diagnosed with autism can be identified prior to ASD symptoms emerging.

ASD: Treatment and Therapeutic Interventions

Once a diagnosis of ASD has been confirmed, research clearly shows that therapies are beneficial in enabling the child to better manage the condition. Recent research is showing that with earlier treatment, even better outcomes can be sustained. Reaven, Blakeley-Smith, Culhane-Shelburne, & Hepburn (2012) demonstrated the effectiveness of cognitive behavioral therapy (CBT).

Anxiety is a commonly occurring comorbid feature in children and young people with ASD and can also be an intrinsic element of ASD. Reaven et al. (2012) ran a research trial utilizing a modified CBT treatment program entitled "Face Your Fear". They ran a trial alongside this randomized control trial named "Treatment As Usual." The results clearly evidenced the benefits of the modified CBT approach and showed 71% recovery in the "Face Your Fear" group as opposed to 27% recovery with the "Treatment As Usual" group. The rationale behind the study was that existing CBT treatment for those with a dual diagnosis of ASD and anxiety disorder was too verbal and abstract. The researchers wished to hold to the main elements of CBT in the "Face Your Fear" group and adapted CBT to suit the client group. Their aim was to deliver a treatment package which was more autism friendly. "Face Your Fear" focused on defining anxiety, and identifying fearful situations, breathing strategies, emotional regulation, and helpful thoughts. There was a combination of one-to-one sessions with the children and young people or with one or both parents or carers. The study focused on the standard treatment model adapted for ASD over the first seven weeks, and then over the next seven weeks created a stimulus hierarchy of fears, before then taking graded steps to face these within a group setting. The fears to be faced gradually included fear of the dark, fear of elevators, fear of talking to others, and fear of dying.

A study published in *The Lancet* shows the clinical value of the Pre-school Autism Communication Trial (PACT) as an effective early intervention tool (Pickles et al., 2016). The PACT intervention is a one-year developmentally focused social communication intervention program for young children that consists of 12 therapy sessions (each session being 2 hours long) over 6 months, followed by monthly support and extension sessions for a further 6 months. Additionally, the parents agreed to do planned practice activities for 20–30 minutes each day with their child. Professor Johnathan Green of the University of Manchester said in relation to the results of this study: "The advantage of this approach over a direct therapist–child intervention is that it has potential to affect the everyday life of the child." He went on to say:

> This is not a cure, in the sense that the children who demonstrated improvements will still show remaining symptoms to a variable extent, but it does suggest that working with parents to interact with their children in this way can lead to improvements in symptoms over the long term.

Research tells us that those who are on the autistic spectrum are both visual and literal thinkers, they have difficulty in shifting their focus and are commonly resistant to change. They tend toward a black-and-white thinking style, with a strong moral stance on what is right and wrong (Paxton & Estay, 2007). However, other research indicates that very early intervention when the brain is more plastic and susceptible to change produces good long-term results and recovery in some cases (Dawson, 2008).

The Early Start Denver Model (ESDM) is a socially focused developmental model for toddlers and preschoolers on the autistic spectrum. It emphasizes educating parents over 12 sessions with trained therapists on behavioral strategies involving imitation, communication, and social development. To measure the effectiveness of the ESDM, a randomized control trial was conducted. It identified that a child on the ESDM after two years demonstrated greater improvement in language and cognitive skills, with greater adaptive behaviors and fewer autistic symptoms, than a child with ASD routinely referred for treatment.

From Mandell et al. (2010) study, we know that parents voice concerns about possible autism in their child at a mean age of around 18–19 months, and the actual ASD diagnosis is made at 34–61 months. Rogers et al. piloted a study in 2014 called "Infant Start," offering treatment to seven infants as young as six months with

ASD symptoms. The parents were taught positive reinforcement strategies already accepted as reducing symptoms in older children. In all, 6 out of the 7 infants showed accelerated development by the age of 18 months. By the time, these children were aged three, their development was in the normal range. Lonnie Zwaigenbaum, director of autism research at the University of Alberta in Canada, calls it "a significant study because it demonstrates the ability both to detect symptomatic infants and provide a meaningful intervention prior to 12 months of age" (Roehr, 2014).

Those with ASD have a very individual style of behavioral and cognitive structuring which may fluctuate depending upon the severity of symptoms. The comorbidities most commonly experienced by those with ASD are anxiety, social anxiety, obsessive compulsive disorder, depression, violent aggression, and sleep problems. CBT is a style of therapy which utilizes a strong, fully researched evidence base to produce results. For each of these comorbidities, there is a prescribed treatment plan which a CBT therapist would commonly follow and adapt accordingly. In all cases, trust, respect, and a warm therapeutic relationship are vital prior to embarking on any treatment protocol. Identifying goals can also take the ASD client on a journey of discovery into what was considered impossible but can now be manageable. As control is a key feature in working with those with ASD, it may be helpful to offer a quiver full of coping strategies to help manage and better control their world.

An initial focus when engaging with an individual on the autistic spectrum may be to work with enabling greater emotional literacy. A reduced level of Socratic questioning with a greater focus on rules and self-statements would be a helpful adaptation. Engaging with the parents or carers alongside the child or young person can facilitate improvement. The therapist may model social skills to a child or young person on the autistic spectrum to help build this naturally and fluidly. As social anxiety is another common difficulty in ASD, it is helpful to explain "the rules of the game" and test out this new way of engaging with others to create improved social engagement.

It may be necessary to incorporate a sense of the ASD client "not fitting in" or being that "little bit different" into a case conceptualization to enable a shared understanding of perceived difficulties to help reach a successful outcome. When working with ASD clients, there is an added requirement to assess the style to which the individual is best suited, and to adapt the treatment plan to best accommodate this feature. As is often the case with ASD, there can be a level of rigid and concrete thinking, which may mean that the therapist will opt to use a more behavioral approach. The upside of this may be in cases of obsessive-compulsive disorder, where the individual catches the solution and actively cuts down on their compulsions without necessarily having to fully understand the key obsessions and cognitions that go alongside. Challenging behavior within an ASD population can be treated using a cognitive behavioral model. The therapist, working alongside the client, parents, and carers, can agree tested coping strategies which can lead to positive outcomes.

Another really helpful strategy for treating those with autism is Applied Behavior Analysis (ABA) first applied to autism by Dr Ivor Lovaas at UCLA in 1987. ABA is taught by using a system of rewards and consequences. ABA is designed to "extinguish" undesirable behaviors and encourage desirable behaviors. The use of a rewards chart is very helpful in motivating improved behaviors.

ent advances with an app
lp foster social inclusion
Another fresh approach
hington University, with
ate social skills. Interface
he ASD brain to engage

atekeeper for treatment.
ut for their parents, fam-
cultural issues are being
incumbent upon society
that these children from
more culturally focused
h from Sweden informs
of 54 years, whereas for
he age is 70 years (Gris-
etails a far higher rate of
for more stringent ASD
opulation generally and
dentified early enough in
undiagnosed ASD look
ard nor understood with
th difficulties.
n the ASD Spectrum:

to recognize that it's

es for reassurance
others

thinking
tness

utine is suddenly altered

- Goes to safe area like a tent at ho
- Has a few people that are "safe pe
- Can jerk head, face, and body whe
- Won't eat certain foods/or texture s
- Rigid about eating habits with so
- Regularly displays uncontrollable
- Comorbidities include anxiety, se
- Tends to be rigid around spontan
  to prepare
- Hyperactivity or hyperactivity
- Your child may struggle to feel ho

Helpful hints for parents with childr

- Seek help as soon as you recognize
- Learn about autism
- Become an expert on your child a
- Enjoy your child's difference and
- Be their advocate through difficult
- Create consistency within your cl
  safety
- Create a tent space at home for you
- Reward positive behavior with th
  child's behavior

  https://www.freeprintablebehavior

- Seek an Early Intervention approa
  Pre-School Autism Communicatio
- Speak with nursery or classroom s
  your child
- Request a referral for an Educati
  your child's educational needs and
  your child's education
- Make an appointment with your
  Pediatrician or alternatively seek
  consider an ASD diagnosis
- If you notice problems with your
  Physician refers your child to a SA
- Speak with your GP or Physician a
  to check that your child is hearing w
- Request that your local GP or Phy
  cent Mental Health Services (CA
  child to be assessed by a Psychiatri
- An ASD diagnosis shall then facili
  Tier 3 Specialist CAMHS

The Future

In a world of such diverse technology, there have been recent advances with an app called "Sit With Us" invented by Natalie Hampton to help foster social inclusion within school settings for those lacking in social skills. Another fresh approach to help those with autism is being piloted at George Washington University, with 24 children with autism using interactive robots to facilitate social skills. Interface with the robots is less threatening and can help prepare the ASD brain to engage in evidence-based therapy (Pelphrey, 2017).

Conclusion

Within the therapeutic world, an ASD diagnosis is the gatekeeper for treatment. The young child with undiagnosed ASD has no voice but for their parents, family, and carers. Within our work, we strongly suspect that cultural issues are being mixed into the actual ASD diagnostic framework. It is incumbent upon society in the light of the research outlined above to make sure that these children from mainly BME backgrounds are treated fairly and given a more culturally focused ASD assessment with corresponding treatment. Research from Sweden informs us that those with ASD are likely to die around the age of 54 years, whereas for those within the matched control group without ASD, the age is 70 years (Griswold, 2015; Hirvikoski et al., 2016). The research also details a far higher rate of suicide among those with ASD. It is therefore imperative for more stringent ASD early assessment/diagnosis to help support the ASD population generally and also those within a BME population that are not being identified early enough in terms of early diagnosis. In the main, these children with undiagnosed ASD look forward to a bleak future where their voice is neither heard nor understood with very possibly increasing and misunderstood mental health difficulties.

Key indicators to help recognize if your child may be on the ASD Spectrum:

- Struggles to make friends with peers
- Won't look at you or others directly in the face
- Struggles to read social cues
- Can say embarrassing things without being able to recognize that it's inappropriate
- Can take everything literally
- Can ask adults the same thing repeatedly multiple times for reassurance
- Tends to lack being able to understand the feelings of others
- Avoids going out and meeting new people
- Struggles around understanding what others might be thinking
- Lines things up and put things in rows with great neatness
- Can have a real fixation for certain toys or facts
- Socially naïve and can trust strangers easily
- Can run out on the road without thinking of dangers
- Perfectionistic over certain things
- Obsessional compulsive disorder traits
- Demonstrates severe anger and/or anxiety when the routine is suddenly altered

- Goes to safe area like a tent at home when feelings become too much
- Has a few people that are "safe people" and clings to them
- Can jerk head, face, and body when anxious or about to have an anger outburst
- Won't eat certain foods/or textures of food
- Rigid about eating habits with some foods never being eaten
- Regularly displays uncontrollable anger outbursts
- Comorbidities include anxiety, separation anxiety, and social anxiety
- Tends to be rigid around spontaneous events and requires planning and time to prepare
- Hyperactivity or hypoactivity
- Your child may struggle to feel how you feel and identify with those emotions.

Helpful hints for parents with children on or suspected to be on the ASD spectrum:

- Seek help as soon as you recognize that your child may be on the ASD spectrum
- Learn about autism
- Become an expert on your child and what triggers challenging behaviors
- Enjoy your child's difference and celebrate their positive characteristics
- Be their advocate through difficult times
- Create consistency within your child's schedule to enable predictability and safety
- Create a tent space at home for your child to help them feel safe and calm down
- Reward positive behavior with the use of charts and help to manage your child's behavior

   https://www.freeprintablebehaviorcharts.com/discipline_and_autism.htm

- Seek an Early Intervention approach in terms of accessing something akin to a Pre-School Autism Communication Trial (PACT) (Green et al., 2010)
- Speak with nursery or classroom staff to put in place supportive strategies for your child
- Request a referral for an Educational Psychologist through school to assess your child's educational needs and to offer recommendations to help support your child's education
- Make an appointment with your GP and request that your child be seen by a Pediatrician or alternatively seek a private consultation with a Psychiatrist to consider an ASD diagnosis
- If you notice problems with your child's speech, then request that your GP or Physician refers your child to a SALT
- Speak with your GP or Physician and request that a hearing test be carried out to check that your child is hearing well if a SALT Referral was thought necessary
- Request that your local GP or Physician refers your child into Child & Adolescent Mental Health Services (CAMHS) and request that you would like your child to be assessed by a Psychiatrist for a possible ASD diagnosis
- An ASD diagnosis shall then facilitate possible treatment for your child within Tier 3 Specialist CAMHS

- Within CAMHS, parents are likely to be referred to an Autism Awareness Group to support you and your child after a diagnosis is given
- Your child may be offered the most appropriate treatment within CAMHS, dependent upon symptoms. These include individual therapy for anxiety, social anxiety, separation anxiety, improved social communication skills, or anger management. Your child may be offered a group program initially and if necessary, will possibly receive individual therapy
- Once an ASD diagnosis is given, then speak with your child's teachers to help put in place strategies to help your child better cope and learn in school
- Contact your local council Special Education Needs Team who will let you know of what they can offer you and your child, both financially and educationally. They will help you speak to school to put in place additional support. This support is crucial to enable your child to meet their potential
- Apply for an Educational Health and Care Plan for your child from the local Council. If accepted this funding will help support your child throughout their educational journey
- Get support for the whole family through the National Autistic Society, www.autism.org.uk
- Team Around the Child involving all professionals participating in the care of the child along with the parents and close family members
- Where difficulties arise within any of these processes, then a meeting of professionals with the parents is advised to address delays
- Join an online support group for autism.

Screening Measures for Autism:

- Autism Diagnostic Observation Schedule
- Autism Diagnostic Interview
- Screening Tool for Autism in Toddlers & Young Children
- The Childhood Autism Rating Scale
- The Gilliam Autism Rating Scale-Second Edition
- The modified checklist for Autism Screening for Toddlers-Revised
- Autism Spectrum Quotient
- The Social Communication Questionnaire
- Autism Spectrum Screening Questionnaire.

Helpful Websites:

- National Autistic Society
- Autism Speaks
- Autism Now
- Autism on the Seas
- Autism Resources for Families
- Child Autism UK
- Autism Research Centre
- Ambitious About Autism

- Research Autism
- Gemiini
- Oxford ADHD & Autism Centre
- National Professional Resources, Inc.

References

American Psychiatric Association (APA). (2013). What is autistic spectrum disorder? Retrieved from https://www.psychiatry.org/patients-families/autism/what-is-autism-spectrum-disorder

American Psychological Association (APA). (2003). Guidelines on multicultural education, training, research, practice, and organizational change for psychologists. *The American Psychologist, 58*(5), 377–402. https://www.ncbi.nlm.nih.gov/pubmed/12971086

Anekwe, L. (2020). Harnessing the outrage: It's time to tackle racial bias. British Medical Journal, *368*, 230–231.

Arnold, C. (2016). Autism's race problem. Pacific Standard. May 25. Retrieved from https://psmag.com/news/autisms-race-problem"https://psmag.com/news/autisms-race-problem

Baron-Cohen, S., Scott, F. J., Allison, C., & Williams, J. (2009). Prevalence of autism-spectrum conditions: UK school-based population study. *The British Journal of Psychiatry, 194*(6), 500–509.

Baron-Cohen, S., Tager-Flusberg, H., & Cohen, D. J. (Eds.). (2000). *Understanding other minds: Perspectives from developmental cognitive neuroscience* (2nd ed.). Oxford University Press.

Bauer, S. C., Winegar, J., & Waxman, S. (2016). How cultural differences affect autism diagnoses. Scientific American. Retrieved from https://blogs.scientificamerican.com/guest-blog/how-cultural-differences-affect-autism-diagnoses

Carpenter, B., Happé, F., & Egerton, J. (Eds.). (2019). Girls and *autism*: Educational, *family and personal perspectives* (pp. 36–47).London: Routledge.

Cross, T. L. (1988). *Services to minority populations: Cultural competence continuum*. Portland, OR: Focal Point, Portland State University.

Cross, T. L. (1989). Towards a culturally competent system of care. A monograph on effective services for minority children who are severely emotionally disturbed. Retrieved from https://archive.org/stream/towardscultural100un#page/n1/mode/2up

Dawson, G. (2008). Early behavioral intervention, brain plasticity, and the prevention of autism spectrum disorder. *Development and Psychopathology, 20*(3), 775–803.

Elsabbagh, M., Divan, G., Koh, Y.-J., Kim, Y. S., Kauchali, S., Marcín, C., ... Fombonne, E. (2012). Global prevalence of autism and other pervasive developmental disorders. *Autism Research, 5*(3), 160–179.

García-Primo, P., Hellendoorn, A., Charman, T., Roeyers, H., Dereu, M., Roge, B., ...Canal-Bedia, R. (2014). Screening for autism spectrum disorders: State of the art in Europe. *European Child & Adolescent Psychiatry, 23*(11), 1005–1021.

Goldiamond, I. (2002). Toward a constructional approach to social problems: Ethical and constitutional issues raised by applied behavior analysis. *Behavior and Social Issues, 11*(2), 108–197.

Green, J., Charman, T., McConachie, H., Aldred, C., Slonims, V., Howlin, P., ... PACT Consortium. (2010). Parent-mediated communication-focused treatment in children with autism (PACT): A randomised controlled trial. *The Lancet, 375*(9732), 2152–2160.

Griswold, A. (2015). Large Swedish study ties autism to early death. Retrieved from https://spectrumnews.org/news/large-swedish-study-ties-autism-to-early-death/

Hirvikoski, T., Mittendorfer-Rutz, E., Boman, M., Larsson, H., Lichtenstein, P., & Bölte, S. (2016). Premature mortality in autism spectrum disorder. *The British Journal of Psychiatry, 208*(3), 232–238.

Hughes, V. (2011). Researchers track down autism rates across the globe. Spectrum. Retrieved from https://spectrumnews.org/news/researchers-track-down-autism-rates-across-the-globe/

Hughes Fong, E., Catagnus, R. M., Brodhead, M. T., Quigley, S., & Field, S. (2016). Developing the cultural awareness skills of behavior analysts. *Behavior Analysis in Practice, 9*(1), 84–94.

Katherine Gotham, A. P. (2012, November, Pediatrics). Trajectories of autism severity in children using standardized ADOS scores. *Official Journal of the American Academy of Pediatrics, 130*(5), e1278–e1284.

Lai, M.-C., Lombardo, M. V., Pasco, G., Ruigrok, A. N. V., Wheelwright, S. J., Sadek, S. A., … Baron-Cohen, S. (2011). A behavioral comparison of male and female adults with high functioning autism spectrum conditions. Retrieved from http://journals.plos.org/plosone/article?id=10.1371/journal.pone.0020835

Mandell, D. S., Morales, K. H., Ming Xie, M. S., Lawer, L. J., Stahmer, A. C., & Marcus, S. C. (2010). Age of diagnosis among Medicaid-enrolled children with autism, 2001–2004. *Psychiatric Services, 61*(8), 822–829.

Mandell, D. S., Wiggins, L. D., Arnstein Carpenter, L., Daniels, J., DiGuiseppi, C., Durkin, M. S., Giarelli, E., …, Kirby, R. S. (2009). Racial/ethnic disparities in the identification of children with autism spectrum disorders. *American Journal of Public Health, 99*(3).

Nevison, C. (2019). Race/ethnicity-resolved time trends in United States ASD prevalence estimates from IDEA and ADDM. *Journal of Autism and Developmental Disorders, 49*, 4721–4730.

Papadopoulos, C. (2016). Self-stigma among carers of autistic people. *Network Autism*. Retrieved from https://www.beds.ac.uk/research-ref/ihr/staff/chris-papadopoulos

Paxton, K., & Estay, I. A. (2007). *Counselling people on the autism spectrum: A practical manual*. London: Jessica Kingsley Publishers.

Pelphrey, K. (2017). Robots, apps and brain scans: New tools to help the autistic child. *Scientific American*, January 17. Retrieved from https://www.scientificamerican.com/article/robots-apps-and-brain-scans-new-tools-to-help-the-autistic-child

Perera, H., Jeewandara, K. C., Seneviratne, S., & Guruge, C. (2017). Culturally adapted pictorial screening tool for autism spectrum disorder: A new approach. *World Journal of Clinical Pediatrics, 6*(1), 45–51.

Pickles, A., Le Couteur, A., Leadbitter, K., Salomone, E., Cole-Fletcher, R., Tobin, H., … Green, J. (2016). Parent-mediated social communication therapy for young children with autism (PACT): Long-term follow-up of a randomised controlled trial. *The Lancet, 388*(10059), 2501–2509.

Piven, J. (2017). *First-of-its-kind study accurately predicts autism in infants*. Chapel Hill, NC: The University of North Carolina at Chapel Hill. Retrieved from http://www.unc.edu/spotlight/first-kind-study-accurately-predicts-autism-infants

Reaven, J., Blakeley-Smith, A., Culhane-Shelburne, K., & Hepburn, S. (2012). Group cognitive behavior therapy for children with high-functioning autism spectrum disorders and anxiety: A randomized trial. *The Journal of Child Psychology and Psychiatry, 53*(4), 410–419.

Roehr, B. (2014). Early autism intervention speeds infant development. New Scientist. Retrieved from https://www.newscientist.com/article/dn26181-early-autism-intervention-speeds-infant-development

Rogers, S. J., Vismara, L., Wagner, A. L., McCormick, C., Young, G., & Ozonoff, S. (2014). Autism treatment in the first year of life: A pilot study of Infant Start, a parent-implemented intervention for symptomatic infants. *Journal of Autism and Developmental Disorders, 44*(12), 2981–2995.

Salomone, E., Beranová, Š., Bonnet-Brilhault, F., Briciet Lauritsen, M. B., Budisteanu, M., Buitelaar, J., ..., Charman, T. (2016). Use of early intervention for young children with autism spectrum disorder across Europe. *Autism*, *20*(2), 233–249.

Vandenberghe, L. (2008). Culture-sensitive functional analytic psychotherapy. *The Behavior Analyst*, *31*(1), 67.

Werling, D. M., & Geschwind, D. H. (2013). Sex differences in autism spectrum disorders. Retrieved from https://www.ncbi.nlm.nih.gov/pmc/articles/PMC4164392/

Chapter 12

Moving Young Black Men Beyond Survival Mode: Protective Factors for Their Mental Health

Ivan Juzang

Introduction

This chapter will focus on preventing and reducing mental health issues among young black men; specifically, the upstream, primary prevention of mental health diagnoses of black male youth who experience trauma. Using a "protective factors framework" with black males as an inoculation against the stressors they will face early on in life will arm them with the skills needed to thrive even in the face of repeated exposure to extreme poverty and adverse childhood experiences. Promoting protective factors to cope with stress and trauma is not a new recommendation. The axiom, "risk factors are not predictive factors due to protective factors," is derived from *Youth Violence: A Report of the Surgeon General* (U.S. Department of Health and Human Services, Public Health Service, Office of the Surgeon General, 2001) and is often referenced by experts in mental health. Clearly, a protective factors framework is not a novel idea; yet, it has not been implemented in scale and evaluated with low-income young black males.

Background

MEE Productions was founded in 1990 and has researched, developed, and implemented a number of primary prevention campaigns around the toughest public health issues in America's hardest-hit communities. In 2005, Dr Deborah Prothrow-Stith, a violence prevention expert from Harvard University's School of Public Health, recommended MEE to get involved in *The Blueprint for a Safer Philadelphia*, a major citywide campaign to reduce youth violence, for which MEE developed a community education campaign and behavioral health interventions. Over the course of three years, nearly 175 low-income black youth were hired to conduct community and peer-to-peer outreach throughout the city. It was in the third year of the campaign that behavioral health issues began to emerge: angry, quick tempered, and unfocused youth, and parents collecting their children's paychecks to use for their own purposes. Subsequently, several behavioral and mental health experts were consulted, including Dr. Joseph White, Dr. Carl Bell, and Dr Mark Rosenberg.

The Experts

Dr Joseph White is considered one of the founding fathers of black psychology. The former dean of education at San Francisco State University is also a professor emeritus at University of California, Irvine. He has researched and written about the psychological strengths that black males need to be successful in a racist America, including *Black Man Emerging: Facing the Past and Seizing a Future in America.*

Dr Carl C. Bell is a renowned psychiatrist and leading expert on the mental health of black people. He served as the director of the Institute for Juvenile Research at the University of Illinois and is a clinical psychiatrist emeritus in the Department of Psychiatry, School of Medicine, University of Illinois at Chicago. He is the former CEO of the Community Health Council, Inc. and provided first-hand mental health treatment and recovery services to large populations of low-income blacks on the south side of Chicago.

Dr Mark Rosenberg served as the first director of the National Center for Injury Prevention and Control at the Centers for Disease Control and Prevention (CDC). He is also former executive director of the Task Force for Child Survival and Development. He espouses that one of the biggest lessons a parent teaches the child is how to cope with stress.

Drs White, Bell, and Rosenberg assessed that what was being observed in MEE's violence prevention work was manifestations of stress and trauma due to the negative effects of poverty, violence, and a tumultuous home life. All three encouraged MEE to gain a better understanding of the mental health needs in the low-income black community. In 2007, MEE embarked on collecting primary data to understand stress, trauma, and the perceptions of mental health in poor, inner-city black communities. This two-year institutional research board approved community-participatory research project aimed to increase knowledge about the need for culturally relevant strategies to promote mental wellness aimed at educating the black community, local service providers, and national policymakers. This project led to the 2010 release of *Moving Beyond Survival Mode: Promoting Mental Wellness and Resiliency as a Way to Cope with Urban Trauma* (MEE Productions, 2010).

Stressors and Coping

The research showed that growing up in poverty surrounded by violence, death, police harassment, and unemployment is the major stressor for poor black urban youth. As one male focus group participant explained:

> If you don't have the money to maintain, you might go out and do whatever you need to do in order to survive, which could cause you to end up in prison or dead. (MEE Productions, 2010, p. 11)

The research also revealed how low-income black males were coping with the constant, reoccurring stressors, and unrelenting trauma they experienced in their communities. Many of the focus group participants had lost friends and/or family to violence and were used to dealing with death – it was something they had learned to live with.

Some of the young people coped negatively by using drugs and alcohol to deal with or to escape their reality. Others reacted with violence or responded to violence with violence. Several others internalized or denied the stress altogether, unaware that the buildup of stress creates serious physical or chronic diseases. But there were also young people who coped positively through rapping, journaling, using their creativity, listening to music, or doing other positive things to take their mind off of the stressors. There was also a group who accepted the stress (i.e., "it is what it is"), letting it slide off their backs.

The identification of negative and positive coping was on par with what the research team expected to find. Surprisingly, MEE observed about 10–15% of the young black males were not only surviving their environment but actually thriving – exhibiting better mental and emotional wellbeing than their peers. These youth had a sense of self and a strong mind-set, being more resourceful in generating alternatives to negative coping. In fact, the research identified very specific thriving coping skills with a number of the low-income black males who had managed to excel. They were connected to non-parental adults in their community, hung around with positive people, and believed in a higher purpose/power. Many also focused on goals instead of barriers, and had a plan for what they wanted to do with their lives beyond the environment in which they lived. MEE's efforts to understand stress and mental health problems in the black community uncovered a solution to the problems – thriving through protective factors.

After the *Moving Beyond Survival Mode* (2010) research, MEE promoted protective factors as a way to counter structural and health conditions that keep young black men in survival mode in low-income urban communities in several other major projects. In 2011, MEE used the approach to train and deploy more than 2,000 young people to conduct community outreach around mental health topics for the *Neighborhood Recovery Initiative* in Chicago. The same year, MEE used the protective factors approach in the development and implementation of a youth suicide prevention campaign for the Washington, DC, Department of Mental Health, called *I Am the Difference*. In 2015, the approach was applied to the opioid epidemic in Baltimore, Maryland – the heroin capital of the United States (Alamiri, 2016). MEE's most recent application of the approach was used in *Heard, Not Judged: Insights into the Talents, Realities and Needs of Young Men of Color* (2016), a national research project with 18–24-year-old men of African and Hispanic descent. The project sought to hear directly from the audience what they needed, and how they needed it, to make better, healthier daily decisions (MEE Productions, 2016). These research and intervention opportunities provided enough evidence and antidotes to support the hypothesis that the risk factors that continue to keep young black males at a disproportionate disadvantage for survival should be addressed through the application of a protective factors framework.

Failure Is Built In

An understanding of the conditions young black males are up against is necessary to understand why a protective factors framework must be researched. The social determinants, generally defined as the environmental realities of where people live, work, and play that affect a broad range of quality-of-life outcomes and risk (U.S. Department of Health and Human Services, Office of Disease Prevention and Health Promotion, 2010), have set young black males living in poor urban communities up for failure in terms of diagnoses for all major health disparities, including mental health issues. Being born into poor neighborhoods exposes them to America's unique brand of "urban trauma," characterized by high levels of sustained poverty, ineffective public education, even worse housing conditions, negative media images, institutional racism, criminalization, and regular traumatic episodes such as violence in the home and the community. Inevitably, these environmental conditions shape the worldview of young black males. MEE developed the eight variables model to understand the environments where black males spend most of their time and how the social determinants influence their worldview and learned behaviors.

The MEE Eight Variables Model

The eight variables represent black males' worldview – the social determinants as they see and live them day to day. The MEE eight variables model was initially developed to understand how young people viewed the world through the context of a national CDC-commissioned intervention campaign developed around dating violence, *In Search of Love: Dating Violence Among Urban Youth* (MEE Productions, 1996). The framework helped uncover reasons low-income youth were opting out of public service announcements, public health brochures, and other public health strategies dealing with violence, teen pregnancy, and substance abuse. The MEE eight variables model focuses attention on unhealthy influences that create health, educational, and economic disparities for low-income black urban youth (see Fig. 1). The eight factors the model examines to understand the daily reality for black urban youth are the streets, education/public schools, economics, healthcare and public health, government, mass media, family/community, and mainstream society.

The streets. Violence plays a major role in the lives of young black males, in their homes and on their street corners, and in the images they see on television, movie screens, video games, and social media. With the availability of guns in America's cities, the streets remain a dangerous place for urban teens, and the stakes are rising continuously. In 2015, of all homicides of black males between the ages of 15 and 24, 94% were caused by firearms (Centers for Disease Control

Failure Is Built In:
THE CHALLENGES FACING LOW-INCOME BLACK YOUTH

For effective communication, it is vital to understand the target audience's worldview. In the context of low-income Black youth in urban environments, this includes understanding:

The Streets:
A Matter of Survival
Personal survival and safety is the number one issue for many low-income urban youth.

Education/Public Schools:
The Miseducation of Urban Youth
Educator motives – good and bad – are apparent to low-income urban youth.

Economics:
The Poverty Problem
When youth live in poverty, poverty makes them angry.

Healthcare and Public Health:
The "Injured" Body, Mind, and Soul
Healthcare is not on the radar of many youth. Treatment is often unacceptable and it is unrealistic for practitioners to expect clients who have negative experiences to return for care.

Government:
The System
The Lenses Are Only Pointed at Us – Perceptions of the government meant to "serve and protect" are often symbolized by police injustice or brutality, and juvenile and/or family court.

Mass Media:
The Messages to Impressionable Youth Consumers
Low-income urban youth consume huge amounts of largely negative, exploitive entertainment media.

Family/Community:
The Disappearing Village
A loss of extended family and community necessitates the creation of support systems among youth peer groups, which often leads low-income urban youth to negative/risky behaviors.

Mainstream Society:
The Dominant Culture
Mainstream, dominant society does not appear to include them, so youth seek pleasure from instant consumption and immediate gratification.

MEE
MOTIVATIONAL EDUCATIONAL ENTERTAINMENT
www.meeproductions.com

Fig. 1. The MEE Eight Variables Model. Developed by MEE Productions Inc.

and Prevention, 2015). Relative to the overall number of blacks in America, the numbers of black males affected by gun violence are staggering.

Another major driver for violence in the lives of young black males is a fear of being perceived as weak or vulnerable. Violence as a negative coping behavior has become a normal part of urban teens' lives, and even though most young black males do not subscribe to using violence or joining gangs, if it helps them avoid becoming a target and being re-traumatized, they will do what they feel they need to do to protect themselves.

Education/public schools. The educational system has failed black youth. America's underfunded public education has not provided a way out of poverty for black teens. Historically, urban school systems have been at the bottom of the totem pole when it comes to funding, even though the students they serve have some of the most pressing needs. The government perpetuates the cycle of poverty by distributing school funding based on race (White, 2015), among others. MEE's research has also found that many young low-income black males hold a negative view of attending public schools, reporting that they encounter three types of teachers: teachers who genuinely care for them, teachers who are there just for a paycheck, and teachers who fear their students.

Furthermore, schools are not culturally sensitive and many do not account for different learning styles. For example, without understanding the root of aggressive reactions to typical classroom directives, teachers may end up afraid to engage with young black males. You cannot effectively teach a child you're afraid of. Jens Ludwig, professor and director of the Crime Lab at the University of Chicago, suggests that disadvantaged urban boys are challenged to navigate the different sets of rules in their neighborhoods and ones imposed in the classroom,

> Telling a poor kid "never fight" is the wrong thing to do. There really are situations, unfortunately, in these neighborhoods where sometimes you need to do that. That's an example of a skill that a rich kid doesn't need to have. (Badger, 2015)

Economics. MEE's work in low-income urban communities around the country reveals poverty as the number one stressor for black people. Poverty has become more concentrated over the years as blacks who successfully took advantage of societal changes resulting from the 1960s civil rights movement continued to "move on up" and out of inner-city communities, leaving those who could not afford to escape surrounded by others in the same dire circumstances. Research shows that nearly 30% of urban black males are living in poverty (U.S. Census Bureau, 2015). Employment data paint a bleak picture for their chances to escape. Among 20–24 year olds in the United States, Illinois and Chicago black males had the lowest rates of employment in both 2005 and 2014, at 39% (Cordova & Wilson, 2016). Limited access to employment opportunities keeps many of these young men stuck in the cycle of poverty. Growing up in poverty, facing unemployment and unfair low wages, and not being able to make ends meet were all considered very stressful and sources of shame by young black men MEE interviewed. "I don't want to [ask] this person for money," said one participant, "because it's going to make me feel like less of a man" (MEE Productions, 2010, p. 12). Not having any money, trying to get money, and finding ways to earn money also cause a significant stress for this audience, including several black males who discussed having children they want to take care of but cannot afford to.

Healthcare and public health. Healthcare and public health should be considered assets for black males but they are not. Primary healthcare services are not provided on a consistent basis in the black community. Over time, this manifests itself as a large gap between black and white mortality rates. In 2015, the mortality rate among black infants was more than twice (11.7 vs 4.8 per 1,000 births) that of white infants (Riddell, Harper, & Kaufman, 2017). Additionally, cuts in funding limit the availability of services, particularly in communities with the highest health disparities. The dysfunctional and confusing healthcare system leaves black youth with a slim chance of receiving specialized services to deal with issues such as family violence, child abuse, and intimate partner violence.

The idea of access as a major barrier for black youth seeking health services remains the focal point for many government and social service agencies. MEE's two plus decades of research working with low-income urban youth has found that access to healthcare is not the issue. The main issue is how they are treated when they access the healthcare. Extensive audience research and unannounced youth audits of local health clinics have uncovered three types of experiences black males have as they navigate the healthcare system:

- *Lack of respect:* One focus group participant stated, "If they don't treat you with the respect you deserve ... you walk back out ... you don't go back. Because they're not going to take care of you the way they should" (MEE Productions, 2016). Negative experiences like these with healthcare institutions create negative word of mouth in the community.
- *Lack of trust:* The low levels of trust and confidence in healthcare institutions that black people have is based on their experiences. One Washington, DC, mental health provider said her white colleagues don't know about basic historical events such as the Tuskegee Experiment or Jim Crow. She also stated, "They need to understand that our black kids' anger and low self-esteem is not just a myth .... We're still dealing with racism. They don't get the history, the historical context of why we don't trust" (MEE Productions, 2010, p. 32).
- *Institutional trauma:* In some cases, black males actually experience "institutional trauma" at the hands of medical and healthcare providers and will avoid using them unless it is an emergency. Additionally, as the largest group of youth in foster care, black males aged 13–17 believe that judgmental and uncaring adults, including foster parents and social workers, are "in it for the money" and leave many of these young men feeling as though they have nowhere to turn for help and no one they can trust.

Government. Black urban youth feel that the government ("the system") continues to oppress rather than serve – that the lenses of criminal justice are *only* pointed at them. The government is symbolized by police harassment or brutality, juvenile and/or family court, then incarceration. Black boys are profiled and harassed every day. They are targeted and incarcerated, and then the system monetizes their sentences. For example, in New Orleans in 2014, 81% of all juvenile arrests were for non-violent offenses; 97% of juvenile arrests involved black youth (Townes, 2015). Even after serving time and being released from jail, they are still excluded from mainstream society. In the majority of states, black males with felony convictions cannot vote even after serving their time (Chung, 2016).

Among urban youth there is a deeply held suspicion of the justice system charged with serving and protecting all of its citizens. When black youth commit crimes, they go directly to jail; when white youth commit crimes, they are often sent to treatment programs or receive community service or probation. It says a lot about a government willing to spend money to incarcerate a young black man but not to commit funds to enroll him in a trade school, general education diploma program, or summer job opportunity. California was poised to spend more than $62,000 on each prison inmate in 2014–2015 – almost seven times the $9,200 it would spend for each K-12 student (Hanson & Stipek, 2014). With these levels of negative encounters with government and criminal justice systems, how can young black males be expected to think they will be treated fairly?

Mass media. Urban black youth are the largest consumers of media entertainment (Cohen, 2015). They have little control over the media and messages targeted at them, as negative, stereotypical and exploitive images are continuously reinforced. As Dr Asa Hilliard, a prominent educational psychologist and expert on black child development, put it, "you can't objectify or thing-ify a girl or dog-ify a boy for decades and think it's not going to show up in the culture" (MEE Productions, 2004).

MEE primary audience research indicates that young people spend more time consuming entertainment and social media than they spend in school, reading, in church, and with their parents, combined. The direct impact of this violent, sexist, and negative imagery is influencing their attitudes and behaviors. But the real concern about black males consuming such a huge amount of entertainment and social media is that they are buying into someone else's value system of material consumption and instant gratification.

The indirect impact media has on black males via educators and other service providers is even more damaging than the direct impact. Media affects black male youth indirectly through its impact upon the perceptions of society at large. These distorted views penetrate settings where white adults deal with black youth – schools, courts, and employment locales. These stereotypes make it possible for adults to believe that the negative messages they see and hear are accurate. When adults buy into the myths and stereotypes about urban youth, they lower their expectations, increase their fear and alienation of black youth, or in more severe cases become afraid to communicate with youth, even those within their own communities.

Family/community. Politicians often draw attention to the high percentage of children born to single-parent households as the foundation of many negative social issues. From a historical perspective, single black women have been raising and supporting families for more than 400 years. So, the problem is not single black women raising children, it's the residual effects of the disappearing village – disintegrating social fabric. As middle-class black family members leave the inner city, they take with them essential financial and emotional support, as well as vital images of positive, successful black males. The black church, once a cornerstone of survival, is no longer the beacon of hope. While a core group of committed black women remains, churches have been unwilling to or unsuccessful in addressing the needs of young adult males. Many of the young people MEE has interviewed feel that the church serves to condemn and criticize, not to support and uphold.

The African proverb, "It takes an entire village to raise a child," is as relevant today as it ever was in describing the need for adult involvement in the low-income black community. As middle- and upper-income families pay for social fabric (village) in terms of daycare, after-school programs, tutors, camps, and other youth development experiences, in the absence of the supportive village, low-income black families struggle to manage without the social fabric needed to survive. Without the supportive village, active parenting is compromised. By the time black latchkey kids get to their teens, their peer group is their primary family. To be accepted by one's peers provides a sense of belonging and boosts self-esteem. Noted from the *Heard, Not Judged* report, "A good, close friend holds a familial, loving place in the hearts of BMOC [black males of color]". These bonds are so powerful that the peer group becomes the steering force in the urban teen's life. "They are at once trusted allies in times of need, while also being the source of potentially debilitating distractions" (MEE Productions, 2016, p. 7).

Mainstream society. There is no seat at America's table for black youth. Racism is institutionalized and poor black males are especially targeted for exploitation and monetization. Cities and counties are actually incentivized to hold young black men in custody (Liberman & Fontaine, 2015). Drug runners, low men on the totem pole, are often targeted by police, emphasizing the focus on supply versus demand, which disproportionately affects young men of color in poor neighborhoods (Liberman & Fontaine, 2015).

Racism indirectly underlies much of the political discourse in the United States. For example, the government spends billions of dollars each year on corporate welfare – subsidizing for-profit company activities. This dwarfs any amount of money provided to individuals who need financial assistance to survive. Black single mothers living in the ghetto are only part of the picture, yet in today's conservative political climate, these are the predominant images in the picture pundits paint. Images of low-income whites rarely appear.

When you live in poverty, poverty makes you angry. For young black males to learn to thrive in spite of their environmental conditions, they must have effective behavioral interventions that take their worldview and influences from their unhealthy environment into account.

The Mental Health Treatment System Is Broken

The mental health system could be included in the healthcare and public health variable, but it is such a huge issue for the black community that it warrants its own discussion. The existing mental health delivery model, which favors a treatment-oriented versus prevention-oriented approach, is a barrier to a protective factors approach to mental health. When asked why black males do not access mental health treatment services, Dr Bell suggested,

It's stigma, it's racism, it's that Black people go in and they get insulted, [it's] the American medical model that's focused on what's broken, instead of how to strengthen and prevent it from ever breaking (MEE Productions, 2010, p. 2).

The "fixes" are rooted in understanding why black people aren't using the existing mental health systems in urban cities, why the black community isn't actively talking about the beneficial outcomes of mental health treatment, and what are black inner-city residents' perceptions of and experiences with existing mental health services near or in their communities.

Stigmas within the Black Community

The black community needs an honest and open dialogue about mental illness and mental wellness in order to counter stigmas, myths, and misinformation about utilizing mental health treatment services. Black people are not raised to value or see the benefits of mental health treatment services. Instead, many take offense at being asked whether they need to "talk to someone," fearing that they are being labeled as weak or crazy. One Chicago mental health provider described it this way, "They're afraid of being overmedicated … they're afraid of being strapped down and put in a padded room and all these things you see on television" (MEE Productions, 2010, p. 27).

Knowledge and Attitudes about Mental Health Programs and Services

MEE's research has found that low-income black male youth have a low level of awareness about existing mental health treatment resources. Those who are aware have primarily heard about the services through interactions with the justice system or child welfare – if they have been detained or have been in foster care – or the educational system – if they have been assessed for alleged behavior problems. Of the mental health organizations our research participants were aware of, many had negative reputations in the community. "When my son went to an in-patient facility, he said it was horrible. They treated him like a prisoner, with the doors locked," reported one black mother (MEE Productions, 2010, p. 23). Competent, compassionate, and culturally sensitive services are hard to find. The current tenor of mental health services for young black males is punitive and institution based rather than preventive and community based, increasing resistance to getting help for emotional issues, stress, and trauma.

Mistrust of Mental Health Treatment Services

Black youth are opting out of or avoiding mental health services mainly due to mistrust and mistreatment. There is a general mistrust of mainstream America's medical institutions as a result of institutional racism and the historical mistreatment of black people within the medical research space. Black parents fear losing their children to child protection agencies for issues identified in the home, believing that medication is the preferred method of treatment for providers who treat black children with emotional or behavioral issues. They internalize horror stories about the treatment process and what's been heard in the neighborhood about how bad treatment it is, what kinds of things therapists do, and the drugs they prescribe. For those who have actually accessed the services, the mistreatment they received keeps them from returning.

How Mental Health Providers View Protective Factors

Mental health providers site a lack of scientific evidence about protective factors methods among both low-income black parents and other mental health providers. They report that black people cannot effectively advocate for alternative treatment models because they don't know enough about them and are therefore overwhelmingly prescribe drugs for their children's emotional or behavioral issues. MEE research has shown that black parents feel drugs were often administered before a complete assessment was even completed, and that psychotherapy or counseling were relegated to second-tier options. Ignorance on the part of providers about protective factors leaves parents without enough information to make informed decisions about alternate treatments for their children's mental health.

Resiliency – Moving Beyond Survival Mode

As mentioned, promoting protective factors is not a new concept. The original seven resiliencies were developed decades ago as a strength-based approach to working with people struggling to deal with hardships. They were insight, independence, relationships, initiative, creativity, humor, and morality. Dr Bell and Dr White developed their own versions of the seven resiliencies to specifically address the black experience in America, including slavery. Dr Bell uses "protective factors" terminology as a way to describe resiliency in the face of traumatic events. He identified seven major protective factors that can positively impact young black males dealing with stress and trauma: social fabric/village, minimization of trauma, adult protective shield, connectedness to a larger group or goal, access to modern and ancient technology, social and emotional skills, and sense of self (esteem)/sense of models. Similarly, Dr White uses "psychological strengths" as a way to "successfully master the journey." His seven psychological strengths are resilience, spirituality, connectedness to others, emotional vitality, improvisation, sense of humor, and healthy suspicion of white folks (i.e., the government).

Findings from MEE's large-scale population health interventions with low-income communities of color helped reframe and rebrand the concept of resiliency, including the use of new digital channels to deliver mental wellness education to low-income black males. The contemporary and repositioned version of the seven resiliencies, "thriving coping skills," serve as protective factors for young people in low-income communities exposed to urban trauma and are illustrated in Fig. 2.

The Seven Resiliencies	The Seven Protective Factors (Dr. Carl Bell)	Seven Psychological Strengths (Dr. Joseph White)	MEE's Thriving Coping Strategies for Millennials
Insight	Strong Village / Social Fabric	Resilience	Take Care of Self / Take Care of Others
Independence	Calming (Minimization of the Effects of Trauma)	Spirituality	Sense of Self (Self-Esteem)
Relationships	Adult Protective Shield	Connectedness to Others	Improvisation
Initiative	Connectedness to a Larger Group or Goal	Emotional Vitality	Connectedness to Positive People, Places and Things to Do
Creativity	Access to Ancient & Modern Technology	Improvisation	Having a Plan & a Plan B
Humor	Social and Emotional Skills	Sense of Humor	Higher Purpose
Morality	Self-Esteem	Healthy Suspicion of White Folks	Navigating Systems

Fig. 2. The Evolution of Resiliency Factors. Developed by MEE Productions Inc.

Take Care of Self / Take Care of Others

Low-income black boys are using positive coping strategies to take care of themselves, which is automatically protective. Encouraging young black males to volunteer to take care of others helps youth recognize that they aren't they only ones experiencing challenges. Being present through someone else's problems shifts the focus from their own stressors and helps them see that they may not have it as bad (relatively) as they think; that they are not victims.

Sense of Self (Self-esteem)

A keen sense of self-efficacy helps young black males get through most traumatic events, even if they seem insurmountable. Believing they can get through trauma or anything they put their mind to, makes this one of the most powerful thriving protective factors. Several young men reported that by "using their heads" they manage their emotions and negative feelings pretty well. "I think about my shit. I've seen too many people react just off of emotion, so I think about what I'm going to do," said a Philadelphia male (MEE Productions, 2010, p. 21). "I sit back, think about it [a problem] and revise my strategy," said an Oakland male (MEE Productions, 2010, p. 21). Thinking through the issue, conflict, or stressor versus just reacting serves as an alternative to feeling and behaving like a victim.

Moving Young Black Men beyond Survival Mode 269

Improvisation

Black people consistently demonstrate the ability to improvise whether they are thriving or not. Living in poverty forces low-income black male youth to work with what they have and make the best of dire situations. The act of spontaneously creating something from nothing is a skill transferred to young black males from parents, grandparents, and community members. Within their communities they witness single parents and grandparents raising grandchildren and finding ways to "make it work" for their children – working multiple jobs, cohabitating to share expenses; and they encounter peers who style themselves in the latest trends and hairstyles as a method of status and control over a sliver of their uncontrolled environments.

Connectedness to Positive People, Places, and Things to Do

Having a caring, non-judgmental, non-parental adult involved in their lives is a prime reason why black male youth exposed to urban trauma are able to move beyond survival mode. They report that these "old heads" who live in their community and have also experienced through tough times help them cope by just being there. These older black males serve as informal mentors and help them see beyond the immediate, telling and/or showing them that "you can do it." Creating an environment of caring adults – a new village – provides young black males with positive people to be around, places to go, and things to do. This new village includes service providers, formal mentors, and spiritual leaders trained to develop and maintain solid relationships with black males to help them cope with traumatic experiences.

Having a Plan and a Plan B

Having a plan to cope with stress or trauma and establishing goals allows young black males to see beyond their immediate situation. It helps them focus and figure things out to stay on track, even when trauma hits. Most girls have plans; they write them down and track their to-dos. Many boys, however, are rudderless – they have no plans. "You have to set goals. If you don't have goals that you set for yourself, you are lost," said one young Chicago black male (MEE Productions, 2010, p. 21). Young black males who thrive take the time to develop measurable goals as a way of creating the life they want, instead of reacting to the life they don't want.

Higher Purpose

Higher purpose or higher power wards off the feeling of helplessness during traumatic events for young black males because they realize that their actions have consequences in the universe. For those who may not be spiritual, their form of a higher purpose centers on having people who count on and depend on them, such as their children. That responsibility motivates them to keep going after a traumatic event or to bounce back from hard times.

Navigating Systems

Young people who understand their environment and how things work in America exhibit high levels of mental wellness. They have a level of consciousness about the ills surrounding them and how to navigate them. An awareness of how to take control of the social determinants that lead to health disparities within their communities is a social justice issue, and navigating these systems empowers young black males to expect quality treatment from services and demand respect and cultural sensitivity as tax-paying citizens.

Current State of Resiliency

Several of these protective factors are already evident in significant ways among low-income black communities; yet, they will still need to be reinforced. There are factors that are innate or have been learned via life experiences – they don't necessarily require anyone else's input or assistance. Others, the community has lost, as the safety net associated with the traditional "village" concept has unraveled; these elements must be rebuilt. These factors are usually passed down through intergenerational sharing. Finally, there are protective factors that must be introduced in our communities in a culturally relevant manner. These include navigating systems, which involves dealing with the stigma of having conversations about mental illness and mental wellness. Using these protective factors as a framework will allow a shift from mental health treatment as a focus of funding and programs to one that "inoculates" young people against traumas they will face – a prevention focus.

Evaluate This

Conducting protective factors interventions provides the research and evidence necessary to support the theory that promoting and reinforcing protective factors will help black youth survive and thrive within communities set up to fail them. The Surgeon's General youth violence report was published in 2001. Since that time, the CDC, the Substance Abuse and Mental Health Services Administration, nor the National Institutes of Health has developed or implemented proven, evidence-based interventions based on the report's recommendations. Culturally relevant population health interventions that can provide better outcomes for larger numbers of people for less cost are not being studied in academia or funded by large foundations. And with public health funding having decreased over the past 15 years, these large organizations need to innovate and improvise. MEE Productions recently developed a state-wide social marketing campaign promoting positive and thriving coping strategies for the state of Ohio. This protective factors population health intervention will be evaluated by the University of Colorado at Denver's School of Public Health in 2021.

Population health is traditionally defined as "the health outcomes of a group of individuals, including the distribution of such outcomes within the group" (Kindig & Stoddart, 2003). It is a way for stakeholders to improve health outcomes of a defined community at the lowest cost to that community. Hawe and Potvin (2006) define population-level health interventions as "policies or programs that shift the distribution of health risk by addressing the underlying social, economic and environmental conditions" (p. I8).

Low-income black communities want mental health agencies to go beyond using them for publishing findings. They already know that stressors, trauma, and other mental health issues are negatively impacting their communities, so they want to focus on solutions. They want strategies, tactics, and tools that will work on the "front lines" of their communities – an alternative to the existing mental health treatment system. These communities need evidence-based population health interventions "that will equip young Black males with the psychological tools they need" – without labeling them as having "mental problems" (MEE Productions, 2009, p. 4). Primary prevention, faster recovery, addressing other health disparities, and trends in funding are presented as reasons why protective factors interventions need to be evaluated.

Primary Prevention

Primary prevention strategies that promote thriving coping skills are necessary to prevent or minimize the impact of trauma on young black males. Those strategies work to balance the protective factors against the risk factors. Dr White calls for a "resilience training" strategy for black youth:

> We need to teach these kids problem solving, opportunity finding skills, resilience, how to bounce back from setbacks, incorporating the seven psychological strengths – before negative coping behaviors or mental illness problems. (MEE Productions, 2009, p. 4)

Service providers, family members, educators, and mentors are perfectly positioned to serve as the first line of defense and must understand the psychological strengths required to insulate black youth from the onslaught of traumatic events in their communities.

Faster Recovery

Promoting protective factors that have resilient qualities helps individuals heal faster when trauma does occur. The most powerful of these protective factors, according to Dr Bell, is a keen sense of self-efficacy that helps black people "get through" most traumatic events, even if they seem insurmountable.

> [There's a sense of] "I can figure this out, I can do something about this, I can fix this," whether you actually can or not. Even if you just feel you can is protective. (MEE Productions, 2009, p. 2)

Focusing on wellness from the prevention side as opposed to the treatment side is an opportunity for black male youth to learn and incorporate skills to become stronger in the broken places by providing a positive means to cope, heal, and thrive.

Addressing Other Health Disparities

Beyond mental illness prevention, a protective factors intervention is a solution to physical health disparities in the black community. A comprehensive approach to prevention and treatment that encompasses a protective factors strategy teaches alternatives to negative coping such as violence, youth suicide, and drug abuse; and it also addresses disparities associated with a number of chronic diseases, including obesity and hypertension. Dr White states:

> and as they move into their 20s, if the brother isn't super careful he's going to start to experience high blood pressure. And then high blood pressure throws the whole system off, because the longer you have high blood pressure, which is a Black male disease, the more you are in danger of an early stroke, heart failure, exacerbate diabetes, and so on. So not only are you not dealing with mental health issues, eventually, if you don't deal with them they start to be physical health issues. (MEE Productions, 2009, p. 4)

Trends in Funding

Public funds for treatment services are dwindling and institutions have to be smart about how they spend their dollars. City and state mental health agencies can no longer afford to "treat their way" to a solution to urban trauma. Consider the current opioid epidemic. Public dollars are being poured into increasing access to treatment for heroin addicts and the wider availability of Naloxone to combat overdose deaths; yet, the national crisis continues to grow in nearly every state. Just as public health experts like Dr Prothrow-Stith have said "you can't arrest your way to reducing violence," you also will not be able to Naloxone your way to reversing the opioid epidemic. The only viable, cost-effective solution to the heroin epidemic, and all social determinants of health in poor urban and rural communities is a population health protective factors intervention that puts skills directly into the community by providing capacity building to the organizations with their boots on the ground – community-based organizations, non-profits, and faith-based institutions.

Conclusion

Preventing and reducing mental health issues among young black males who experience trauma is the only way to move them out of survival mode into thriving. The current mental health system, rooted in exploitation through the monetization of poverty, doesn't work for them. As difficult as it may be for mainstream America to do, it is imperative that a health and wellness model that refrains from labeling and demonizing black youth is actualized. If 10–15% of these young men are thriving without formal intervention, what would the percentage be if we developed, implemented, and evaluated a protective factors population health intervention? What would be the tipping point to shift low-income black boys from survival mode to thriving mode and ultimately self-sufficiency? Therefore, population health interventions should be studied and evaluated because of their potential to provide better outcomes in a cost-effective, culturally relevant way.

References

Alamiri, Y. (2016, August 12). The crisis in Baltimore: How heroin and opioids have turned "charm city" into the heroin capital of America. Retrieved from http://rare.us/rare-news/across-the-u-s-a/the-crisis-in-baltimore-how-heroin-and-opioids-have-turned-charm-city-into-the-heroin-capital-of-america/

Badger, E. (2015, June 3). Young black men face daunting odds in life. These programs can help. Retrieved from https://www.washingtonpost.com/news/wonk/wp/2015/06/03/young-black-men-face-daunting-odds-in-life-these-programs-can-help/

Centers for Disease Control and Prevention. (2016). 10 leading causes of death, United States, 2016, Black, Males. Retrieved from CDC. https://www.cdc.gov/healthequity/lcod/men/2016/nonhispanic-black/index.htm

Chung, J. (2016). *Felony disenfranchisement: A primer*. Washington, DC: Sentencing Project.

Cohen, D. (2015, February 23). STUDY: African Americans watch more TV, multiscreen more. Retrieved from http://www.adweek.com/digital/study-ipsos-media-ct-facebook-iq-african-americans/

Cordova, T., & Wilson, M. D. (2016). *Lost: The crisis of jobless and out of school teens and young adults in Chicago, Illinois and the U.S*. Chicago, IL: Great Cities Institute.

Hanson, K., & Stipek, D. (2014). Schools v. prisons: Education's the way to cut prison population. *Mercury News*. Retrieved from http://www.mercurynews.com/2014/05/15/schools-v-prisons-educations-the-way-to-cut-prison-population/

Hawe, P., & Potvin, L. (2006). What is population health intervention research? *Canadian Journal of Public Health, 100*(1), I8–I14.

Kindig, D., & Stoddart, G. (2003). What is population health? *American Journal of Public Health, 93*(3), 380–383.

Liberman, A. M., & Fontaine, J. (2015). *Reducing harms to boys and young men of color*. Washington, DC: Urban Institute.

MEE Productions Inc. (1996). *In search of love: Dating violence among urban youth*. Philadelphia, PA: MEE Productions Inc.

MEE Productions Inc. (2004). *The price of sex: An inside look at black youth sexuality and the role of media*. Philadelphia, PA: MEE Productions Inc.

MEE Productions Inc. (2009). What the experts say: Violence and the impact on mental health. *Urban Trends, 16*(2), 2–4.

MEE Productions Inc. (2010). *Moving beyond survival mode: Promoting mental wellness and resiliency as a way to cope with urban trauma*. Philadelphia, PA: MEE Productions Inc.

MEE Productions Inc. (2016). *Heard, not judged: Insights into the talents, realities, and needs of young men of color*. Philadelphia, PA: MEE Productions Inc.

Riddell, C. A., Harper, S., & Kaufman, J. S. (2017, July 3). Trends in differences in US mortality rates between black and white infants. *JAMA Pediatrics, 171*(9), 911–913. doi:10.1001/jamapediatrics.2017.1365

Townes, C. (2015, August 27). New Orleans is locking up hundreds of traumatized kids. Retrieved from https://thinkprogress.org/new-orleans-is-locking-up-hundreds-of-traumatized-kids-83e2c70c7873/

U.S. Census Bureau. (2015). Poverty status, 2011–2015 American community survey 5-year estimates. Retrieved from https://factfinder.census.gov/faces/tableservices/jsf/pages/productview.xhtml?pid=ACS_15_SPT_B17001&prodType=table

U.S. Department of Health and Human Services, Office of Disease Prevention and Health Promotion. (2010). Social determinants of health. Retrieved from https://www.healthypeople.gov/2020/topics-objectives/topic/social-determinants-of-health

U.S. Department of Health and Human Services, Public Health Service, Office of the Surgeon General. (2001). *Youth violence: A report of the Surgeon General*. Rockville, MD: Department of Health and Human Services, U.S. Public Health Service.

White, G. B. (2015, September 20). The data are damning: How race influences school funding. Retrieved from https://www.theatlantic.com/business/archive/2015/09/public-school-funding-and-the-role-of-race/408085/

Chapter 13

African Americans and the Vocational Rehabilitation Service System in the United States: The Impact on Mental Health

Julie Vryhof and Fabricio E. Balcazar

African Americans and Mental Health

In the United States, individuals of color are more likely to have disabilities than those who are White (Mwachofi, Broyles, & Khaliq, 2009). Additionally, African Americans experience increased severity in their disability. Across all age category groups, African Americans are also more likely to have a higher proportion of individuals with severe disabilities when compared to their White counterparts (Capella, 2002). Although many researchers attribute socio-economic status to the prevalence of mental health diagnoses in people of color, it is apparent that race needs to be considered when discussing mental health prevalence and services (Smith, 2015). While substantial work has been done to increase cultural competency in services provided for assessing and treating mental illness, the professions that provide those services (e.g., social work, psychology, and psychiatry) were deeply influenced and created by and for Western European male individuals (Smith, 2015). Additionally, African Americans experience multiple barriers when accessing mental health services for both diagnosis and treatment, including financial barriers, barriers for seeking help, and barriers in receiving high quality culturally competent services (Holden & Xanthos, 2009).

The seminal report to the Surgeon General of the United States on Mental Health (U.S. Department of Health and Human Services, 2001) pointed out that historical adversity, which included slavery, sharecropping, and race-based exclusion from health, educational, social, and economic resources, translates into the socio-economic disparities experienced by many African Americans in the United States. Socio-economic status, in turn, is linked to mental health – poor mental health is more common among those who are impoverished than among those who are more affluent. Also related to socio-economic status is the increased likelihood of African Americans becoming members of high-need populations, such as people who are homeless, incarcerated, or have substance abuse problems, and have children who come to the attention of child welfare authorities and are placed in foster care. Racism is another aspect of the historical legacy of African Americans. Negative stereotypes and rejecting attitudes continue to occur with measurable, adverse consequences for the mental health of African Americans (Lukyanova, Balcazar, Oberoi, & Suarez-Balcazar, 2014). Therefore, a number of historical and contemporary negative circumstances have led many African Americans to mistrust the system of care and to face many contextual and personal barriers to mental health treatment and rehabilitation. We will discuss some of these factors in the next section.

African Americans and Employment

Meaningful employment is a desired goal for working-age adults. However, for individuals with disabilities this goal is often unattainable. Individuals with disabilities often face discrimination (Wilson, Alston, Harley, & Mitchell, 2002), have insufficient training and job experiences (Beveridge, Fabian, & Ethridge, 2009), encounter inadequate employment supports (Kaye, Jans, & Jones, 2011), or have limited experience in job-seeking skills (Rhodes, Hergenrather, Barlow, & Turner, 2008).

Historically, individuals with disabilities have experienced lower rates of employment than individuals without disabilities, a disparity which is seen across all socio-demographic groups (Steinmetz, 2006; U.S. Department of Labor, Bureau of Labor Statistics, 2012). The July 2015 young adult unemployment rate was 12.2%, more than double the national average of 5.3% (U.S. Department of Labor, Bureau of Labor Statistics, 2015, August). Unemployment is even more acute for young people of color, particularly for African American young adults, who have an unemployment rate of 20.7%. A report by the Great Cities Institute at the University of Illinois at Chicago (Cordova, Wilson, & Morsey, 2016, January) concluded that in 2014, 47% of the 20–24 years old Black men in Chicago were out of school and out of work in 2014 compared 20% of Hispanic men and 10% of White men in the same age group.

While people with disabilities as a whole experience higher rates of unemployment, examining race and mental illness diagnosis seems to intensify these disproportionate rates. Individuals of color with disabilities are more likely to be unemployed than their White peers and individuals with severe mental illnesses can have unemployment rates as high as 95% (Burns et al., 2007; Stuart, 2006). Several studies suggest that among individuals with mental health diagnoses, individuals of color experienced less favorable outcomes in their participation in the competitive labor force as compared to their White peers (Burke-Miller et al., 2006).

Findings in research surrounding race, mental illness, and employment are often nuanced. Wewiorski and Fabian's (2004) meta-analysis of research found that individuals who were White had greater success at gaining employment, but people of color were more likely to be employed six months after their initial job placement. Burke-Miller et al. (2006) examination of the Employment Intervention Demonstration Program dataset did conclude that individuals of color work more hours in a month. However, this could be attributed to working in lower paying jobs. This finding is supported by research that has concluded that White individuals are more likely to get higher paying jobs (Mwachofi et al., 2009).

Several individual and contextual factors contribute to this pervasive high rate of unemployment of people with disabilities. Individuals with disabilities are a heterogeneous group and employment-related outcomes appear to be associated with individual-level factors. Poor employment outcomes tend to increase with severity of the disability (Balcazar, Taylor-Ritzler, et al., 2012; Crisp, 2005; Meade, Lewis, Jackson, & Hess, 2004; Ozawa & Yeo, 2006; Phillips & Stuifbergen, 2006; Walker, Marwitz, Kreutzer, Hart, & Novack, 2006), being a member of a minority race or ethnic group (Arango-Lasprilla et al., 2009; Balcazar & Taylor-Ritzler, 2009; Gary et al., 2009), being less educated (Crisp, 2005; Krause & Terza, 2006; Ozawa & Yeo, 2006; Randolph & Andresen, 2004), and having low earnings or limited previous work experience (Mwachofi et al., 2009).

Environmental factors can also drastically limit community/employment participation for individuals with disabilities. These factors include the physical, social, and the attitudinal environment in which people live (Schopp et al., 2007). Products and technology for personal use in daily living, attitudes of community members, and the availability of health and social support services are examples of such environmental factors (World Health Organization, 2013). Additionally, even without considering disability, racial disparities exist in the US labor market (Mwachofi et al., 2009). Overall, individuals of color make less and have higher unemployment rates than Whites (Mwachofi et al., 2009). Thus, individuals of color with disabilities are susceptible to those same discriminatory practices when seeking employment as individuals of color without disabilities (Burke-Miller et al., 2006).

Individuals with mental illness face unique attitudinal and structural barriers when seeking and sustaining employment (Stuart, 2006). They often experience both direct and indirect discrimination in the workplace, including prejudicial attitudes, low expectations, and neglect (Stuart, 2006). Scheid (1999) found that half of US employers were hesitant to hire someone with a history of a mental illness and more than half were reluctant to hire someone currently taking antipsychotic medication. Even if employed, individuals with mental illness are often employed in jobs which are part-time or temporary and they experience significant barriers in career advancement (Stuart, 2006). Additionally, research has suggested that employers are more likely to hire someone with a physical disability and, compared to individuals with physical disabilities, twice as many people with mental illness anticipate experiencing stigma in the workplace (Stuart, 2006). Individuals with mental illness who are also unemployed often experience combined social stigmatization for both their status as mentally ill and their status as unemployed. In an attempt to avoid this stigmatization, individuals with mental illness often chose not to disclose their disability. This lack of disclosure can prevent many of them from receiving the supports and/or accommodations they may be entitled to and/or that they need in order to perform their job effectively (Stuart, 2006).

While the data support the disproportionate unemployment rates of individuals with mental health diagnoses, research has also suggested that individuals with mental illness have a desire to and can work in the competitive job market with appropriate supports (Burke-Miller et al., 2006; Catty et al., 2008; Cook et al., 2005). Active employment has also been correlated with several positive outcomes, including increases in quality of life, promoting self-esteem, and facilitating the gaining of skills for individuals with mental illness (Cook et al., 2005). Dunn, Wewiorski, and Rogers (2008)'s qualitative analyses found that individuals with mental illness reported that employment had both personal meaning and promoted recovery. In fact, while individuals with mental illness often experience unemployment or underemployment, these conditions can increase the risk for mental illness (Stuart, 2006).

In the United States, several national programs and policies have been implemented to address the unemployment rates of individuals with disabilities, including the Rehabilitation Act of 1973; followed by the Americans with Disabilities Act of 1990; amendments to the Rehabilitation Act of 1992 and 1998; and the Ticket to Work and Work Incentives Improvement Act of 1999. Although some of these federal policies have mandated non-discriminatory hiring practices and reasonable accommodations in the workplace (Cook et al., 2005), most working-age adults with disabilities continue to be at a significant disadvantage in the current labor market as reflected in their low labor force participation rate, generating severe economic, social, and psychological consequences. We now examine the characteristics of one of the programs created to promote employment among people with all types of disabilities.

The Vocational Rehabilitation Program

In accordance with the Rehabilitation Act of 1973, the Rehabilitation Services Administration (RSA) administers state formula grants to provide vocational rehabilitation (VR) services designed to prepare people with disabilities for gainful employment (U.S. Department of Education, 2012). Individuals who are eligible for VR services are individuals who have physical and/or mental impairments that impede their ability to obtain and maintain employment (Mwachofi et al., 2009). Eligible individuals are offered an array of services (22), including vocational guidance, assessment, information and referral, job search assistance, job readiness, treatment, occupational training and education, and on-the-job training and supports (U.S. Department of Education, 2012). In the United States, there are a total of 80 VR agencies: 24 states have separate programs for the blind and individuals with other types of disabilities; and 26 states, the District of Colombia, and five territories have combined blind/general disability agencies. The program also administers the funds that support the national network of Independent Living Centers, which provides advocacy training, personal care attendant services and housing assistance to people with disabilities so they can enjoy independent and productive lives in their communities.

The VR program can have a significant impact on the lives of people with disabilities hoping to become employed. However, the US Government

Accountability Office (U.S. GAO, 2005) prepared a report to Congress reviewing the VR program which found that of the more than 650,000 individuals exiting the state programs in fiscal year 2003, only one-third (217,557) obtained a new job or maintained their existing job for at least 90 days after receiving services (successful closure or status 26). The RSA's data from FY 2003 (U.S. GAO, 2005) showed that two-thirds of VR consumers exited the VR program without employment (unsuccessful closure or status 28) most often because the individual refused services or failed to cooperate with the VR counselor (46% of the time) or could not be located or contacted (24%) for follow up. The report pointed out that the VR program purchased more than $1.3 billion in services for all individuals who exited the program in fiscal year 2003, two-thirds of which were used to provide services to individuals exiting without employment. In addition to this financial cost, there is the human cost of failure and hopelessness for all those individuals who were not able to attain their rehabilitation goals. The report also found that employment, salary earnings, and the amount of purchased services received while in the VR program varied significantly by individuals' disability type and race/ethnicity, among other characteristics. Additionally, state VR agencies varied substantially in the employment rates they achieved, the characteristics of the individuals they served, their frequency of providing certain services, and their service expenditures (U.S. GAO, 2005, p. 2). These findings indicate the need for continued efforts to improve VR services and outcomes for individuals with disabilities.

In a more recent report (U.S. GAO, 2018), the agency found that state VR agencies reported expanding services for employers in order to promote hiring individuals with disabilities in mainstream employment (where they are integrated with employees without disabilities and earn competitive wages); however, the US Department of Education has not fully addressed related challenges. Most VR agencies in the last GAO's survey reported providing specific employer services under the Workforce Innovation and Opportunity Act; but many agencies reported challenges meeting employers' needs and promoting mainstream employment. For example, some did not fully understand when they are allowed to help employed individuals with career advancement. Additionally, employers with whom the GAO spoke cited challenges navigating workforce programs, yet few agencies reported documenting roles and responsibilities of the agencies they partner with to work with employers.

VR Services for African American with Mental Health Diagnoses

Individuals from racial and ethnic minority backgrounds experience many challenges when receiving services from VR (Alston, Wilson, & Harley, 2001; Capella, 2002; Mwachofi et al., 2009; Taylor-Ritzler, Balcazar, Suarez-Balcazar, & Garcia-Iriarte, 2008; Wilson, Edwards, Alston, Harley, & Doughty, 2001; Yamada & Brekke, 2008). The U.S. GAO (2005) report also highlighted that only 13% of African Americans receiving VR services achieved competitive employment while 11.6% achieved non-competitive employment compared with 85.2% and

87.3% of Whites, respectively. Kaya (2018) noted similar disparities in competitive employment based on their analysis of youth with intellectual disabilities. Research suggests that African Americans experience disparities throughout their involvement with the VR program. They are significantly less likely to be accepted for services, to be successfully rehabilitated (i.e., obtain gainful employment) and, if employed, they receive lower salaries (Capella, 2002; Olney & Kennedy, 2002; Wilson, 2000; Wilson et al., 2001; 2002; Yamada & Brekke, 2008). Additionally, Mwachofi et al. (2009) concluded that VR spending per person was greater for Whites than for individuals of color.

Ethnic minority individuals with disabilities are underserved by rehabilitation service agencies, including both the independent living and VR programs, and as a result, they are more likely to experience more social, economic, educational, and vocational disadvantages than their White counterparts (Alston, 2003; Fujiura, 2000; Granados, Puvvula, Berman, & Dowling, 2001; Olney & Kennedy, 2002; Rosenthal, 2004; Suarez-Balcazar & Balcazar, 2007). These disparities have persisted despite the fact that the US Congress passed amendments to the Rehabilitation Act in 1992 and 1998 to ensure equal treatment to all persons with disabilities regardless of their race and other characteristics (Capella, 2002; Mwachofi et al., 2009). Furthermore, positive independent living outcomes are less favorable for African Americans, Latinos and other minorities with disabilities than for Whites (Garcia-Iriarte, Balcaza, Taylor-Ritzler, & Suarez-Balcazar, 2008; Granados et al., 2001; Lillie-Blanton & Hudman, 2001; Suarez-Balcazar, Friesema, & Lukyanova, 2013).

African Americans can also face barriers in accessing VR counselors that are culturally competent in their service delivery (Capella, 2002). While research has supported the importance of culturally informed practices, considerations of the socio-cultural needs of minority groups are often not well integrated into the assessment and delivery of rehabilitation services for individuals with mental illnesses and there is often a disconnect between the cultural understanding of the provider and minority consumers (Burke-Miller et al., 2006; Kaya, 2018). This disconnect can lead to service delivery that is less consumer-driven, creating less satisfaction with the services among the recipients (Yamada & Brekke, 2008). Research has suggested that a lack of cultural competence when delivering services can be correlated with a decrease in the quality of care and negative outcomes from that care (Yamada & Brekke, 2008). Due to the increasing number of minorities in the United States and the increased prevalence of disability among African Americans, the need for culturally competent VR counselors will likely continue to outnumber the available supply.

Our research team has conducted several studies that examine service delivery for African Americans with mental health diagnoses in VR. These studies illustrated that individual and contextual-level factors are predictors of employment-related outcomes. For example, Lukyanova et al. (2014) examined the VR records from a Midwestern state that included 2,122 African American and 4,284 Caucasian consumers who reported mental illness as their primary disability. We found that African Americans had significantly more closures at referral (before their cases could be opened) and overall were closed as non-rehabilitated more often than Caucasians. Logistic regressions indicated that African American VR consumers were less likely to be employed compared to Caucasians. The regression also found differences by gender (females were more likely to find jobs than males). This particular finding was surprising, since previous literature consistently attributes better employment outcomes to males than females (e.g., Arango-Lasprilla et al., 2009; Coutinho, Oswald, & Best, 2006). We also found differences by age, as middle-age consumers (between 36 and 50 years old) were more likely to find jobs than younger consumers (18–35 years old).

In a similar study, Balcazar, Oberoi, Suarez-Balcazar, and Alvarado (2012) examined a VR database that included 37,404 African Americans who were referred or self-referred over a period of five years. Logistic regression analyses indicated that age and disability type were significant predictors of successful VR. Consumers older than 20 years had a higher likelihood of successful rehabilitation outcomes. The likelihood of rehabilitation increased by about 10% for every 10 years in age and the odds increased by 80% for consumers between 51 and 60 years old. In terms of type of disability, African American consumers with physical disabilities had 15% less likelihood of a successful closure but those with a sensory disability had a 72% higher likelihood of successful rehabilitation. The chances of VR of African American consumers with chronic health problems or mental illness were not significantly different from those with a learning disability and/or behavioral disorder.

In another study, Balcazar, Oberoi, and Keel (2013) examined a VR database from a Midwestern state that included 26,292 transition cases. Transition outcomes were identified for 4,010 youth (15.3%) and analyzed based on factors of gender, race, and disability type. Logistic regression analyses for predictors of employment and college enrollment indicated that females had a higher chance of going to college. However, despite their lower rates of college attendance, males had a greater proportion of competitive employment outcomes compared to females. Regarding race, White and Asian youth had a significantly higher percentage of identifiable transition outcomes than African Americans. Finally, disability type was also found to be predictive of transition outcomes; individuals with sensory and physical disabilities were attending college in a larger proportion compared to individuals with other disabilities. Balcazar, Oberoi, et al. (2012) also found that providing appropriate support services (intensive case management) to youth in transition can have a positive impact in the attainment of their transition goals.

Studies of VR consumers conducted by our research team have also identified contextual factors that impact rehabilitation outcomes, and often explain a large proportion of the variance. For example, Lukyanova et al. (2014) found that VR case expenditures between $1,000 and $4,999 were significantly lower for African Americans than for Whites, which explains, in part, the differences in employment outcomes between the two groups of consumers. Balcazar, Oberoi, et al. (2012) found that when analyzed alone, none of the 22 types of VR services available was a significant predictor of rehabilitation for African Americans with disabilities. However, the number of services a consumer received was a significant predictor, such that, each additional service received by a consumer increased his/her chances of rehabilitation by 47%. Furthermore, the logistic regression suggested that as the amount of money spent on a case increased, the chances of successful rehabilitation increased such that each additional thousand dollars spent on a case doubled the consumers' likelihood of successful rehabilitation. Most importantly, according to the analysis, spending between $5,000 and $8,000 per consumer is associated with the maximum rate of rehabilitation (a 1,360% higher likelihood of getting rehabilitated). Balcazar et al. (2013) also found that the chances of a youth in transition gaining competitive employment increased as the amount of money spent by the VR counselor on the case increased. Furthermore, youth who received vocational guidance and on-the job supports had higher chances of obtaining competitive employment than of going to college.

While past research has substantiated racial disparities in various aspects of the VR system, recent research has demonstrated progress in racial equity for individuals with other disability categories. In a study by Giesen and Lang (2018), African American males with visual impairments were more likely to have closure earnings exceeding substantial gainful activity for Social Security Disability Insurance. Kang, Nord, and Nye-Lengerman (2019) found that African American VR consumers with intellectual disabilities were earning a higher weekly wage than White consumers. However, under close examination, the authors found that they were working more hours than White consumers, but at a lower hourly wage.

Recommendations

The disparities in the VR system along racial lines require an examination and possible modification of current policies and practices in order to create and maintain a system that ensures equitable access to services and better employment outcomes for individuals of color with disabilities (Mwachofi et al., 2009). As Wilson et al. (2001) asserted, individual and societal factors surrounding race make it extremely challenging for minorities with disabilities to find employment through VR services. They emphasized the need to explore multiple strategies and models to achieve employment for minorities with disabilities. Such strategies include supported employment and self-employment.

Supported Employment

Supported employment is one strategy that can help individuals with mental illnesses access and sustain competitive employment (Burke-Miller et al., 2006; Burns et al., 2007; Catty et al., 2008; Cook et al., 2005; Drake & Bond, 2008). Additionally, supported employment has been correlated with increased numbers of hours working and higher pay (Cook et al., 2005). Supported employment, sometimes referred to as "place and train," involves assisting an individual with finding employment in an integrated settings and then providing training and support to both the individual with a disability and the employer/co-workers as appropriate (Burns et al., 2007; Cook et al., 2005). This employment strategy emphasizes the preferences and autonomy of the individual with the disability;

research has suggested that supported employment has long-term benefits for people with disabilities (Burns et al., 2007).

In a longitudinal follow-up study of 38 individuals with severe mental illness that participated in supported employment, 82% of participants reported working in competitive employment and the majority of participants reported working more than half of the years since their participation in the supported employment program (Becker, Drake, Whitley, & Bailey, 2007). Participants also reported increased self-esteem, relationships, and management of their mental health symptoms as other benefits of their employment experience (Becker et al., 2007).

Despite its benefits, supported employment does have some limitations. Primarily, supported employment operates on the idea that all individuals with disabilities want to work. Some individuals with mental illness may autonomously decide that they do not want to work, while others do not want to work for fear of losing their federal and/or state benefits (Drake & Bond, 2008). The Social Security Administration, the US federal agency in charge of these programs is aware of the potential disincentive impact of the Social Security Disability Insurance program and is trying to modify the policies so consumers can only start losing benefits after reaching a certain monthly income threshold. Similar policies are being implemented to prevent consumers with disabilities from losing their federal health insurance benefits, since most of the jobs available to them do not include private insurance benefits and there is no national insurance health program in the United States.

Additionally, people with mental illnesses still experience barriers to success, such as psychiatric symptoms and inadequate mental health services that can challenge the effective implementation of the supported employment program (Drake & Bond, 2008). Furthermore, recent research suggests that access to educational opportunities is also necessary for success in supported employment. Waynor, Gill, Reinhardt-Wood, Nanni, and Gao (2018) analyzed employment outcomes for individuals with severe mental illnesses in supported employment and found that educational level was a significant predictor of continued engagement in work at six-month follow-up.

Self-employment

One aspect of the VR program that has not been studied very much is self-employment. VR counselors can use self-employment to help address the employment disparities for individuals with disabilities (Ashley & Graf, 2018). Revell, Smith, and Inge (2009) presented a summary of the RSA-911 database regarding state-by-state closures for self-employment compared to closures for regular employment (status 26) for FY 2003, FY2005 and FY2007. The total results indicated a slightly decreasing tendency from 4,067 cases of self-employment in 2003, to 3,388 cases in 2005 and 3,246 cases in 2007. These cases represent only 1.93%, 1.69%, and 1.63% of the total closed cases in the United States during those fiscal years. As the numbers indicate, self-employment is not widely used in the VR system, with great disparities from state to state. For instance, the state of

Mississippi reported the highest number of cases in 2007 (572) while the District of Colombia reported no cases in 2003.

Arnold, Seekins, and Spas (2001) reported the results of a survey from 330 self-employed individuals with disabilities. A total of 66% of the respondents were male, 88% White, 2% were African Americans, and 2% were Hispanics. A total of 80% were between 30 and 59 years old, and 79% had more than high school education. Among the top reasons identified for self-employment, respondents indicated: Wanted to work for myself (56%); identified need for product/service (48%); wanted to make more money (46%); wanted to own a business (46%); needed to create own job (44%); and to accommodate a disability (i.e., flexible hours and/or working conditions) (43%). More than half of respondents made initial investments of less than $10,000. Initial investments came from one or more sources, such as personal savings (59%), credit card purchases/cash advances (30%), loans from family members (25%), lending institution loans (18%), and/or state VR agency funding (16%). A total of 30% of respondents' businesses supplied over half of their total household income; 39% reported that their business incomes were adequate to maintain their desired standard of living. Finally, 34% of respondents earned $5,000 or less annually. A total of 10% earned between $5,001 and $10,000; 10% earned between $10, 001 and $20,000; 8% earned between $20,001 and $30,000; 10% earned between $30,001 and $100,000; 14% earned between $100,001 and $500,000; and 6% earned $500,000 or more. Clearly, some of these businesses were very profitable.

A limitation of the study was that the respondents to the survey were members of the Disabled Business Persons Association (DBA) and/or individuals who had sought assistance from state VR agencies. Their responses may not be representative of all people with disabilities who are self-employed/business owners. It is very difficult to conduct such a "population-based" study. Other self-employed people with disabilities who have not received VR services or who are not DBA members may or may not be similar to these respondents.

Entrepreneurship can be a viable career option for many people with disabilities and is increasingly being promoted as an effective employment strategy for person with disabilities (Arnold & Ipsen, 2005; Arnold & Seekins, 2002; Griffin & Hammis, 2014; Ipsen, Arnold, & Colling, 2005; Office of Disability Employment Policy, 2005). Kaufmann and Stuart (2007) added that entrepreneurship is a strategy that can lead to economic self-sufficiency and is particularly important for people with severe disabilities that have frequently been denied equal access to traditional labor markets. However, many people with disabilities can lose their aspirations to become entrepreneurs through lack of customized entrepreneurship assessment services that could help them make personally meaningful choices about what it takes to become a business owner. They often lack access to entrepreneurship training or the financial resources needed to start a business and many individuals do not understand or get sustained assistance in business planning (Parker-Harris, Renko, & Caldwell, 2014). These factors, as well as a variety of systemic disincentives, have limited the number of people with disabilities who become successful business owners (Shaheen & Killeen, 2009). Research evidence also indicates that minority consumers are likely to encounter more difficulties and barriers to self-employment when compared with Whites. These include challenges obtaining support, start-up capital, and developing marketable ideas (Stodden, Conway, & Chang, 2003).

Unfortunately, little research has been conducted in the area of self-employment and individuals with disabilities, particularly in the context of VR. In a recent study, Ashley and Graf (2018) interviewed 18 individuals with disabilities who participated in self-employment. Seven participants noted that their VR counselors discouraged them from self-employment. Six of the participants described how their VR counselors helped support them pursue self-employment, but three of the six later described how the support was insufficient. Because the research is so limited in this area, additional quantitative and qualitative studies need to be conducted to garner a better understanding of the role of VR counselors in support self-employment for their consumers.

Beginning in 2006 and continuing through 2009, the US Department of Labor/Office of Disability Employment Policy (ODEP) sponsored three national demonstration projects to research effective policies and practices that improve self-employment outcomes for people with disabilities. These "Start-UP USA"[1] projects represented a diversity of locations, economic environments, and stakeholder groups and resulted in local policy and program improvements that could provide more individuals with disabilities a way to achieve their entrepreneurship career goals. The programs, however, targeted individuals with disabilities in the general population and have not generated sufficient information about factors that predict successful self-employment among individuals receiving VR services. Unfortunately, self-employment remains a marginal practice in VR agencies from across the United States and the implementation and the promotion of entrepreneurship skills among VR customers is very limited. Previous research indicates that individuals with disabilities who had frequent contacts with VR counselors with experience in entrepreneurship and who targeted the consumer's individual employment plan to self-employment (Arnold & Seekins, 1998; Hayward & Schmidt-Davis, 2003; Lustig, Strauser, & Weems, 2004), and completed trainings and followed up, were more likely to be successful in achieving self-employment outcomes (Keim & Strauser, 2000; Patrick, Smy, Tombs, & Shelton, 2012). Other components associated with self-employment success include the presence of family and community support (Parker-Harris et al., 2014); mentoring and support from savvy local business owners who can assist in completing the business plans (Wallen et al., 2010); and individuals who are highly motivated and have clear business ideas (Katz, 2006).

One approach for entrepreneurship development is through *business incubators*. This is a business support process that accelerates the successful development of start-ups by providing entrepreneurs with an array of targeted resources and services (National Business Incubation Association, 2013). A business incubator's main goal is to produce successful businesses that will leave the program

---

[1] More information about Start-UP USA can be found on its website: http://www.start-up-usa.biz/about/index.cfm.

financially viable and freestanding. Incubator graduates have the potential to create jobs, revitalize neighborhoods, commercialize new technologies, and strengthen local economies. Incubators vary in the way they deliver their services, in their organizational structure and in the types of clients they serve. Incubators can be highly adaptable. Some incubator sponsors have targeted programs to support micro-enterprise creation, the needs of women and minorities, and environmental endeavors. Unfortunately, this model has rarely being used to support people with disabilities.

One example was implemented by the "Chicago Add Us In (AUI) Initiative" sponsored by the US Department of Labor, ODEP (Balcazar, Kuchack, Dimpfl, Sariepella, & Alvarado, 2014). The initiative created an entrepreneurship program for people with disabilities in order to counteract the barriers they faced to secure employment, while seeking to promote empowerment and facilitate their economic self-sufficiency. The model includes a course on how to write a business plan, one-on-one business mentoring, technical assistance, and start-up business grants from the VR agency (for an average of $10,000 but could be more funding depending on the business plan). In addition to the core program components, there was an emphasis on facilitating systemic change in the Illinois Vocational Rehabilitation Agency to ensure program sustainability, which led to the development of a business incubator for people with disabilities in the Chicago area. The incubator, which required an investment of over a million dollars, provides multiple trainings, equipment, office space, phones, and computers for the business start-ups. The incubator also has equipment to train interested consumers in areas like computerized embroidery, heat pressing, and graphic design. Our experiences with this project suggest that trusting relationships, insightful analysis of program data, and desire to improve and find effective solutions were essential to foster systemic changes in the state VR agency. Finally, the Chicago AUI Initiative also explored the creation of cooperatives as a way to include groups of individuals with disabilities who could participate as co-owners of the business in a cooperative business arrangement (Balcazar et al., 2014).

The strategy of supporting groups of individuals with disabilities in the process of starting their own businesses through *cooperatives* is another way to promote self-employment. A worker cooperative has members who are both workers and owners of their enterprises. As worker-owners, members have a large degree of flexibility not only in defining the economic and social benefits of their enterprise, but also in establishing conditions of work that cater to their specific needs (International Labour Organization [ILO], 2012). Disabled workers' cooperatives are found around the world. In Eastern Europe numerous factories are managed and operated by them. Similarly, workers with disabilities in developing countries have formed several industrial workers', artisan, and handicraft cooperatives to maximize their individual talents and to engage in joint production, purchasing, marketing, and sales at local and international markets.[2] Cooperatives can engage

---

[2] See http://www.abilis.fi/ for a comprehensive list of projects sponsored by the Abilis Foundation.

in a diverse array of products and services. As these cooperatives grow, they often expand their services to the provision of skills training, health care, financial services, transportation, and other activities.

As the ILO (2012) argues, job creation for people with disabilities is often at the heart of these types of cooperatives. Members can include people with disabilities, their families, volunteers, disability associations, local government agencies, and others that have a stake in the care and/or support of the members with disabilities. Referred to as multi-stakeholder cooperatives, these businesses can engage in a wide range of productive activities and services. They can contribute to increase the wellbeing of persons with disabilities not only economically and socially, but also can play a role in advocacy, reducing discrimination and promoting social integration (ILO, 2012).

Cooperatives put people at the heart of their business because they are owned and democratically controlled by their members. The decisions taken by cooperatives balance profitability with the needs of their members and the wider interests of the community. Found in many different forms, serving many different needs, resilient to crisis and thriving within diverse societies, the cooperative way of doing business provides a wide range of opportunities to address the economic, social, and cultural needs of persons with disabilities (ILO, 2012). Cooperatives of disabled persons exist in many countries around the world; however, in the United States, these cooperatives are rarely implemented. The ILO (2012) concludes that the development of cooperative enterprises continues to be hampered by a lack of knowledge and understanding of the cooperative business model, as well as insufficient awareness about how cooperatives can respond to the needs of specific groups of people, like individuals with disabilities. One limitation in the United States is that the VR program that could fund cooperative start-ups for individuals with disabilities only considers individual plans for employment and the policies do not include any type of group ownership. Additionally, the ILO (2012) report also cautions that even when the cooperative form of business is introduced to potential members, promoters often underestimate the need for capacity building, business management skills, and specific training in cooperative governance. These are particularly important factors for cooperatives that cater to the needs of disabled people where expectations are often higher.

Conclusions

African Americans experience more barriers and challenges when applying for VR services and in their efforts to attain vocational and occupational outcomes compared to Whites. While some researchers refuse to discuss race openly, it is necessary to determine and understand the racial disparities in the VR system in order to work toward a more equitable system with more equitable outcomes for all its users (Alston, Harley, & Middleton, 2005). It is important to ensure equitable access to research opportunities to all recipients of VR services in order to promote best practices that benefit individuals of all racial identities. The wider dissemination of programs like supported employment that has been empirically validated as an effective strategy to support community-based employment among individuals with severe mental illness is necessary. Self-employment is another venue that is not often considered by VR counselors, in part because it requires a lot of work in the absence of community partners who can provide training, mentoring, and technical assistance in the development of the business plan. The creation of business incubators at the local level could address these limitations and expand the opportunities and supports for individuals with disabilities interested in entrepreneurship. Finally, cooperative arrangements could allow groups of individuals with disabilities and their supporters to own and operate their own businesses. These are some of the possibilities available to people with mental illness who are eager to work, and attain independence and self-sufficiency like anyone else.

References

Alston, R. J. (2003). Racial identity and cultural mistrust among African-American recipients of rehabilitation services: An exploratory study. *International Journal of Rehabilitation Research, 26*(4), 289–295.

Alston, R., Harley, D., & Middleton, R. (2005). The role of rehabilitation in achieving social justice for minorities with disabilities. *Journal of Vocational Rehabilitation, 24*(3), 129–136.

Alston, R. J., Wilson, K. B., & Harley, D. A. (2001). Race as a correlate of vocational rehabilitation acceptance: Revisited. *Journal of Rehabilitation, 67*(3), 35–41.

Arango-Lasprilla, J. C., Ketchum, J. M., Flores-Stevens, L., Balcazar, F. E., Wehman, P., Foster, L., & Hsu, N. (2009). Ethnicity/racial differences in employment outcomes following spinal cord injury. *NeuroRehabilitation, 24*, 37–46.

Arnold, N. L., & Ipsen, C. (2005). Self-employment policies: Changes through the decade. *Journal of Disability Policy Studies, 16*(2), 115–122.

Arnold, N. L., & Seekins, T. (1998). Rural and urban vocational rehabilitation: Counselors perceived strengths and problems. *Journal of Rehabilitation, 64*(1), 5–13.

Arnold, N. L., & Seekins, T. (2002). Self-employment: A process for use by vocational rehabilitation agencies. *Journal of Vocational Rehabilitation, 17*(2), 107–113.

Arnold, N., Seekins, T., & Spas, D. (2001). *First national study of people with disabilities who are self-employed*. Missoula, MT: University of Montana Rural Institute.

Ashley, D., & Graf, N. M. (2018). The process and experiences of self-employment among people with disabilities: A qualitative study. *Rehabilitation Counseling Bulletin, 61*(2), 90–100.

Balcazar, F. E., Kuchak, J., Dimpfl, S., Sariepella, V., & Alvarado, F. (2014). An empowerment model of entrepreneurship for people with disabilities in the United States. *Psychosocial Intervention, 23*(2), 145–150.

Balcazar, F. E., Oberoi, A., & Keel, J. (2013). Predictors of employment and college attendance outcomes for youth in transition: Implications for policy and practice. *Journal of Applied Rehabilitation Counseling, 44*(1), 38–45.

Balcazar, F. E., Oberoi, A., Suarez-Balcazar, Y., & Alvarado, F. (2012). Predictors of outcomes for African Americans in a rehabilitation state agency: Implications for national policy and practice. *Rehabilitation Research, Policy and Education, 26*(1), 43–54.

Balcazar, F. E., & Taylor-Ritzler, T. (2009). Perspectives of vocational rehabilitation counselors on the factors related to employment outcomes of racial and ethnic minorities with disabilities. *Journal of Social Work in Disability and Rehabilitation*, *8*(3–4), 1–16.

Balcazar, F. E., Taylor-Ritzler, T., Dimpfl, S., Portillo-Peña, N., Guzman, A., Schiff, R., & Murvay, M. (2012). Improving the transition outcomes of low-income minority youth with disabilities. *Exceptionality*, *20*(2), 114–132.

Becker, D., Drake, R. E., Whitley, R., & Bailey, E. L. (2007). Long-term employment trajectories among participants with severe mental illness in supported employment. *Psychiatric Services*, *58*(7), 922–928.

Beveridge, S., Fabian, E. S., & Ethridge, G. (2009). Differences in perceptions of career barriers and supports for people with disabilities by demographic, background and case status factors. *Journal of Rehabilitation*, *75*(1), 41–49.

Burke-Miller, J. K., Cook, J. A., Grey, D. D., Razzano, L. A., Blyler, C. R., Leff, H. S., ... Carey, M. A. (2006). Demographic characteristics and employment among people with severe mental illness in a multisite study. *Community Mental Health Journal*, *42*(2), 143–159.

Burns, T., Catty, J., Becker, T., Drake, R. E., Fioritti, A., Knapp, M., ... EQOLISE Group. (2007). The effectiveness of supported employment for people with severe mental illness: A randomised controlled trial. *The Lancet*, *370*(9593), 1146–1152.

Capella, M. E. (2002). Inequities in the VR system: Do they still exist? *Rehabilitation Counseling Bulletin*, *45*(3), 143–153.

Catty, J., Lissouba, P., White, S., Becker, T., Drake, R. E., Fioritti, A., ... Burns, T. (2008). Predictors of employment for people with severe mental illness: Results of an international six-centre randomised controlled trial. *The British Journal of Psychiatry*, *192*(3), 224–231.

Cook, J. A., Leff, H. S., Blyler, C. R., Gold, P. B., Goldberg, R. W., Mueser, K. T., ... Burke-Miller, J. (2005). Results of a multisite randomized trial of supported employment interventions for individuals with severe mental illness. *Archives of General Psychiatry*, *62*(5), 505–512.

Cordova, T. L., Wilson, M. D., & Morsey, J. C. (2016, January). *Lost: The crisis of jobless and out of school teens and young adults in Chicago, Illinois and the U.S.* Chicago, IL: Great Cities Institute, the University of Illinois at Chicago.

Coutinho, M. J., Oswald, D. P., & Best, A. M. (2006). Differences in outcomes for female and male students in special education. *Career Development for Exceptional Individuals*, *29*(1), 48–59.

Crisp, R. (2005). Key factors related to vocational outcome: Trends for six disability groups. *Journal of Rehabilitation*, *71*(4), 30–37.

Drake, R. E., & Bond, G. R. (2008). The future of supported employment for people with severe mental illness. *Psychiatric Rehabilitation Journal*, *31*(4), 367–376.

Dunn, E. C., Wewiorski, N. J., & Rogers, E. S. (2008). The meaning and importance of employment to people in recovery from serious mental illness: Results of a qualitative study. *Psychiatric Rehabilitation Journal*, *32*(1), 59–62.

Fujiura, G. T. (2000). The implications of emerging demographics: A commentary on the meaning of race and income inequity to disability policy. *Journal of Disability Policy Studies*, *11*(2), 66–75.

Garcia-Iriarte, E., Balcaza, F. E., Taylor-Ritzler, T., & Suarez-Balcazar, Y. (2008). Conducting disability research with people from diverse ethnic groups: Challenges and opportunities. *The Journal of Rehabilitation*, *74*(1), 4.

Gary, K. W., Arango-Lasprilla, J. C., Ketchum, J. M., Kreutzer, J. S., Copolillo, A., Novack, T. A., & Jha, A. (2009). Racial differences in employment outcome after traumatic brain injury at 1, 2, and 5 years postinjury. *Archives of Physical Medicine and Rehabilitation*, *90*, 1699–1707.

Giesen, J. M., & Lang, A. H. (2018). Predictors of earnings enabling likely roll departure for SSDI beneficiaries with visual impairments in vocational rehabilitation. *Journal of Disability Policy Studies*, 29(3), 166–177.

Granados, G., Puvvula, J., Berman, N., & Dowling, P. T. (2001). Health care for Latino children: Impact of child and parental birthplace on insurance status and access to health services. *American Journal of Public Health*, 91(11), 1806–1807.

Griffin, C., & Hammis, D. (2014). *Making self-employment work for people with disabilities* (2nd ed.). Baltimore, MD: Paul H. Brookes Publishing Co.

Hayward, B. J., & Schmidt-Davis, H. (2003). *Longitudinal study of the vocational rehabilitation services program. Final report 2: VR services and outcomes*. Durham, NC: Research Triangle Park.

Holden, K. B., & Xanthos, C. (2009). Disadvantages in mental health care among African Americans. *Journal of Health Care for the Poor and Underserved*, 20(2A), 17–23.

International Labour Organization. (2012). *A cooperative future for people with disabilities*. Geneva: Issue Brief, Cooperative Branch, ILO.

Ipsen, C., Arnold, N. L., & Colling, K. (2005). Self-employment for people with disabilities: Enhancing services through interagency linkages. *Journal of Disability Policy Studies*, 15(4), 231–239.

Kang, Y., Nord, D., & Nye-Lengerman, K. (2019). Weekly wage exploration of vocational rehabilitation service recipients: A quantile regression approach. *Journal of Rehabilitation*, 85(1), 4–14.

Katz, J. A. (2006). And another thing. 2006 Coleman paper on Entrepreneurship Education presented at the Annual Meeting of the US Association.

Kaufmann, B., & Stuart, C. (2007). *Road to self-sufficiency: A guide to entrepreneurship for youth with disabilities*. Washington, DC: National Collaborative on Workforce and Disability for Youth, Institute for Educational Leadership.

Kaya, C. (2018). Demographic variables, vocational rehabilitation services, and employment outcomes for transition-age youth with intellectual disabilities. *Journal of Policy and Practice in Intellectual Disabilities*, 15(3), 226–236.

Kaye, H. S., Jans, L. H., & Jones, E. C. (2011). Why don't employers hire and retain workers with disabilities? *Journal of Occupational Rehabilitation*, 21(4), 526.

Keim, J., & Strauser, D. R. (2000). Job readiness, self-efficacy and work personality: A comparison of trainee and instructor perceptions. *Journal of Vocational Rehabilitation*, 14(1), 13–21.

Krause, J. S., & Terza, J. V. (2006). Injury and demographic factors predictive of disparities in earnings after spinal cord injury. *Archives of Physical Medicine and Rehabilitation*, 87(10), 1318–1326.

Lillie-Blanton, M., & Hudman, J. (2001). Untangling the web: Race/ethnicity, immigration, and the nation's health. *American Journal of Public Health*, 91(11), 1736–1738.

Lukyanova, V. V., Balcazar, F. E., Oberoi, A. K., & Suarez-Balcazar, Y. (2014). Employment outcomes among African Americans and whites with mental illness. *Work (Reading, Mass.)*, 48(3), 319.

Lustig, D. C., Strauser, D. R., & Weems, G. H. (2004). Rehabilitation service patterns: A rural/urban comparison of success factors. *The Journal of Rehabilitation*, 70(3), 13.

Meade, M. A., Lewis, A., Jackson, M. N., & Hess, D. W. (2004). Race, employment, and spinal cord injury. *Archives of Physical Medicine and Rehabilitation*, 85(11), 1782–1792.

Mwachofi, A. K., Broyles, R., & Khaliq, A. (2009). Factors affecting vocational rehabilitation intervention outcomes: The case for minorities with disabilities. *Journal of Disability Policy Studies*, 20(3), 170–177.

National Business Incubation Association. (2013). Retrieved from http://www.innovation-america.us/associations-61466/innovation-organizations/35-affiliates/68-national-business-incubation-association-nbia

Office of Disability Employment Policy. (2005). *Self employment training and employment guidance letter*. Employment and Training Administration Advisory System, U.S. Department of Labor, Washington, D. C. Retrieved from: https://oui.doleta.gov/dmstree/tegl/tegl2k4/tegl_16-04.htm.

Olney, M. F., & Kennedy, J. (2002). Racial disparities in VR use and job placement rates for adults with disabilites. *Rehabilitation Counseling Bulletin, 45*(3), 177.

Ozawa, M. N., & Yeo, Y. H. (2006). Work status and work performance of people with disabilities: An empirical study. *Journal of Disability Policy Studies, 17*(3), 180–190.

Parker Harris, S., Renko, M., & Caldwell, K. (2014). Social entrepreneurship as an employment pathway for people with disabilities: Exploring political-economic and sociocultural factors. *Disability & Society, 29*(8), 1275–1290.

Patrick, J., Smy, V., Tombs, M., & Shelton, K. (2012). Being in one's chosen job determines pre-training attitudes and training outcomes. *Journal of Occupational and Organizational Psychology, 85*(2), 245–257.

Phillips, L. J., & Stuifbergen, A. K. (2006). Predicting continued employment in persons with multiple sclerosis. *Journal of Rehabilitation, 72*, 35–43.

Randolph, D. S., & Andresen, E. M. (2004). Disability, gender, and unemployment relationships in the United States from the behavioral risk factor surveillance system. *Disability & Society, 19*(4), 403–414.

Revell, G., Smith, F., & Inge, K. (2009). An analysis of self-employment outcomes with the federal/state vocational rehabilitation system. *Journal of Vocational Rehabilitation, 31*, 11–18.

Rhodes, S. D., Hergenrather, K. C., Barlow, J., & Turner, A. P. (2008). Persons with disabilities and employment: Application of the self-efficacy of job-seeking skills scale. *The Journal of Rehabilitation, 74*(3), 34.

Rosenthal, D. A. (2004). Effects of client race on clinical judgment of practicing European American vocational rehabilitation counselors. *Rehabilitation Counseling Bulletin, 47*(3), 131–141.

Scheid, T. L. (1999). Employment of individuals with mental disabilities: Business response to the ADA's challenge. *Behavioral Sciences & the Law, 17*(1), 73–91.

Schopp, L. H., Clark, M. J., Hagglund, K. J., Sherman, A. K., Stout, B. J., Gray, D. B., & Boninger, M. L. (2007). Life activities among individuals with spinal cord injury living in the community: Perceived choice and perceived barriers. *Rehabilitation Psychology, 52*(1), 82–88.

Shaheen, G., & Killeen, M. (2009). *A primer on the StartUP NY four phase model*. New York makes work pay comprehensive services Medicaid Infrastructure grant. Retrieved from http://nymakesworkpay.org/

Smith, J. R. (2015). Mental health care services for African Americans: Parity or disparity? *The Journal of Pan African Studies (Online), 7*(9), 55–63.

Steinmetz. (2006). *Americans with disabilities: 2002 (Current population reports)* (pp. 70–107). Retrieved from www.sipp.census.gov/sipp/p70s/p70-107.pdf

Stodden, R. A., Conway, M. A., & Chang, K. B. T. (2003). Professional employment for individuals with disabilities. Unpublished manuscript, Honolulu, HI.

Stuart, H. (2006). Mental illness and employment discrimination. *Current Opinion in Psychiatry, 19*(5), 522–526. https://doi.org/10.1097/01.yco.0000238482.27270.5d

Suarez-Balcazar, Y., & Balcazar, F. E. (2007). Empowerment approaches to identifying and addressing health issues in minorities with disabilities. In C. Dumont & G. Kielhofner (Eds.), *Positive approaches to health* (pp. 153–168). New York, NY: Nova Science Publishers.

Suarez-Balcazar, Y., Friesema, J., & Lukyanova, V. (2013). Culturally competent interventions to address obesity among African American and Latino children and youth. *Occupational Therapy in Health Care, 27*(2), 113–128.

Taylor-Ritzler, T., Balcazar, F. E., Suarez-Balcazar, Y., & Garcia-Iriarte, E. (2008). Conducting disability research with people from diverse ethnic groups: Challenges and opportunities. *Journal of Rehabilitation, 74*(1), 4–11.

U.S. Government Accountability Office (GAO). (2005). *Vocational rehabilitation: Better measures and monitoring could improve the performance of the VR program*. GA0-05-865. U.S. GAO, Washington, DC.

U.S. Government Accountability Office (GAO). (2018, September). *Vocational rehabilitation: Additional federal information could help states serve employers and find jobs for people with disabilities*. GAO-18-577. U.S. GAO, Washington DC.

U.S. Department of Education. (2012). *Guide to US Department of Education Programs*. Office of Communications and Outreach Washington, D.C. Retrieved from: https://www2.ed.gov/programs/gtep/gtep.pdf

U.S. Department of Health and Human Services. (2001). *Mental health: Culture, race, and ethnicity – A supplement to mental health: A report of the surgeon general*. Rockville, MD: Substance Abuse and Mental Health Services Administration, Center for Mental Health Services.

U.S. Department of Labor, Bureau of Labor Statistics. (2012, December). Current Labor Statistics, (December Tables). Retrieved from https://www.bls.gov/opub/mlr/2012/12/cls1212-tables.pdf.

U.S. Department of Labor, Bureau of Labor Statistics. (2015, August). The National Longitudinal Surveys of Youth: research highlights. Monthly Labor Review, Retrieved from https://www.bls.gov/opub/mlr/2015/article/the-national-longitudinal-surveys-of-youth-research-highlights.htm.

Walker, W. C., Marwitz, J. H., Kreutzer, J. S., Hart, T., & Novack, T. (2006). Occupational categories and return to work after traumatic brain injury: A multicenter study. *Archives of Physical Medicine and Rehabilitation, 87*(12), 1576–1582.

Wallen, G. R., Mitchell, S. A., Melnyk, B., Fineout-Overholt, E., Miller-Davis, C., Yates, J., & Hastings, C. (2010). Implementing evidence-based practice: Effectiveness of a structured multifaceted mentorship programme. *Journal of Advanced Nursing, 66*(12), 2761–2771.

Waynor, W. R., Gill, K. J., Reinhardt-Wood, D., Nanni, G. S., & Gao, N. (2018). The role of educational attainment in supported employment. *Rehabilitation Counseling Bulletin, 61*(2), 121–127.

Wewiorski, N. J., & Fabian, E. S. (2004). Association between demographic and diagnostic factors and employment outcomes for people with psychiatric disabilities: A synthesis of recent research. *Mental Health Services Research, 6*(1), 9.

Wilson, K. B. (2000). Predicting Vocational Rehabilitation acceptance based on race, education, work status, and source of support at application. *Rehabilitation Counseling Bulletin, 43*(2), 97–105.

Wilson, K. B., Edwards, D. W., Alston, R. J., Harley, D. A., & Doughty, J. D. (2001). Vocational rehabilitation and the dilemma of race in rural communities: Sociopolitical realities and myths from the past. *Journal of Rural Community Psychology, 4*(1), 55–81.

Wilson, K., Alston, R., Harley, D., & Mitchell, N. (2002). Primary source of support at referral among African-Americans and European-Americans in vocational rehabilitation: Why pays the bills? *Journal of Rehabilitation Administration, 26*, 35–41.

World Health Organization. (2013, October). *How to use the ICF: A practical manual for using the International Classification of Functioning, Disability and Health (ICF). Exposure draft for comment*. Geneva: WHO.

Yamada, A.-M., & Brekke, J. S. (2008). Addressing mental health disparities through clinical competence not just cultural competence: The need for assessment of sociocultural issues in the delivery of evidence-based psychosocial rehabilitation services. *Clinical Psychology Review, 28*(8), 1386–1399.

Chapter 14

Targeted Intervention in Education and the Empowerment and Emotional Well-being of Black Boys

Cheron Byfield and Tony Talburt

The Challenges Affecting Black Boys in Schools in the UK

The stark realities of underachievement and disengagement from schools, that have affected many Black boys in education over the last few decades, have been the subject of a number of studies and public discussions (Byfield, 2008; Demie & Mclean, 2015; NEA, 2011). This is often brought into sharp focus in communities in the UK where there are significantly large proportions of Africans and African Caribbean minority ethnic groups. The overused adage that Black men are under-represented in the top universities, but over-represented in prisons and mental health institutions in the UK, sadly, continues to be more than just words, but a reality. For example, in the London borough of Lambeth, where the proportion of African Caribbean people is the highest in the UK, according to a report in *The Guardian* newspaper, nearly 70% of the borough's residents in secure psychiatric institutions are of African or Caribbean heritage (Davie, 2014). Furthermore, according to the Social Mobility and Child Poverty Commission (reported in *The Guardian*, 14 August 2014) there is a definite educational elitism operating in Britain that disadvantages and disempowers children and young people from poor backgrounds and from minority ethnic groups. Given the fact that many Black people in these communities are from lower socioeconomic backgrounds, being Black, as well as coming from poorer socioeconomic backgrounds may help to contribute to the behaviour traits and low achievements in schools among some Black boys. The study by the Lambeth Local Authority, led by Feyisa Demie and Christobel Mclean (2015), on the Under-achievements of Black Caribbean Heritage Pupils in Schools, highlighted a number of bleak statistical data. Their study, citing data from the Department for Education (DFe) in 2014, showed that Black Caribbean pupils were three times more likely to be excluded from secondary schools than their White counterparts. Furthermore, only 16% of Black

Caribbean boys went to university, and the rates of admissions and detentions in mental health institutions were higher for Black Caribbean and African groups than the rest of the population, with about 70% of the inpatients being from these groups (Demie & Mclean, 2015).

Very often, and as will become clear in the discussions below, many Black boys found themselves excluded from primary and secondary schools, due in large part, to their manifested variety of disruptive behaviour. In 2006 in the UK, the Department for Children, Schools and Families, which later became the DFe, carried out a study into the reasons for the large number of exclusions of Black boys from schools. The report found that Black pupils were punished more harshly, praised less and told off more often in schools than other pupils. The report went on to point out that 'staff in many schools are unwittingly racist' (Ranger, 2008, p. 2).

In short, this means, that for a number of Black boys, the UK school system is a very negative experience which plays a significant part in contributing to, or causing their low levels of educational achievement and social and emotional well-being. Therefore, part of the rationale for this study centres upon the need to help prevent young Black boys from developing attitudes and behavioural symptoms which results in them being excluded from secondary schools. More specifically, the study seeks to examine specific intervention strategies employed in schools which serve the dual purpose of raising social and academic aspirations and also contributing towards the emotional well-being of Black boys in the UK education system.

It was in recognition of these challenges that Excell3, the umbrella organisation that operates the nationwide Black Boys Can project, was established in 1999 Birmingham, UK. This was, from its inception, a community-led positive action educational initiative, which constituted a response by the Black community to address the educational needs of Black boys. These projects seek to supplement the educational provision of mainstream schools by acting as a bridge to help empower Black boys to raise their educational achievement and aspirations, and also to help them develop their emotional and social well-being so that they can participate more fully initially in the school environment, and then more broadly and subsequently in the wider society. The organisation works on the principle that children and young peoples' educational attainment is adversely affected if their social and emotional well-being are seriously impaired. So, although not equipped with mental health experts, or seeking to address mental health issues in children and young people specifically, the approach taken by Excell3 has been to focus on their holistic health and social and emotional well-being to improve their educational achievement.

Because some aspects of the negative behaviour traits displayed by some Black boys have often been linked to their emotional imbalance, it is important to briefly discuss the relationship between mental health and education, more broadly. There is a worrying trend of increasing mental health conditions in England's schools of which the majority are presented as behavioural and emotional conditions. Some typical symptoms of mental health behaviour in children include, depression, anxiety and conduct disorder. This situation has risen very sharply in recent years. Mental health disorders are very strongly related to family history and background and also by major adverse life events such as the death of a friend or serious illness or injury (Johnston, Propper, Pudney, & Shields, 2011). Other significant causes for emotional disturbances among children are associated with biological and environmental factors (Kutash, Duchnowski, & Lynn, 2006).

That there is a link between mental health and well-being on the one hand, and educational achievement in schools, on the other, has been established by a number of independent studies. According to Thorley (2016) mental health was selected as the fifth most important topic in the 2014 Make Your Mark Youth Referendum, in which 876,000 young people across the UK were balloted, as part of the Youth Parliament. He also pointed out that in a 2015 survey of 1,180 headteachers, two-thirds of them identified the mental health of pupils as their top concern. Furthermore, a survey of 2,000 parents found that 40% worried about their children's mental health more than they did about any other health concern (Thorley, 2016).

Catherine Ross and Chia Ling Wu found that people from well-educated backgrounds had a greater sense of control over their lives and their health, and, very importantly for our study, also had higher levels of social support. They concluded that high educational attainment directly helps to improve health and also indirectly helps to improve health through work and economic conditions, social psychological resources and health lifestyle (Ross & Wu, 1995). The study by Johnston et al. (2011) found that by using unique UK survey data together with expert diagnoses, mental health conditions are more closely associated with the young people from lower socioeconomic backgrounds (Johnston et al., 2011). Rather than relying upon data pertaining to children's mental health from parents and teachers and the children themselves, they used diagnostic-style assessments from a panel of psychiatric assessors to carry out their research into the prevalence of psychiatric problems among people aged between 5 and 16. They focussed on the three main categories of mental health, namely: conduct, disorder and emotional disorders and hyperkinetic disorders (Johnston et al., 2011). In addition, Kutash et al. (2006), based on their studies of the situation in America, not only stressed the importance of the US government attempting to improve the levels of school-based mental health services to raise the emotional well-being of all children as well as their academic achievement, but also noted that the outcomes for students with mental health conditions from the most disadvantaged backgrounds, generally received the lowest levels of support. There seems to be general agreement, however, that specific targeted intervention is needed to improve the overall social and emotional well-being and educational achievement of deserving students.

Specialist education groups such as the Mulberry Bush Outreach organisation in the UK, clearly recognise that where there is evidence of emotional and mental health issues in children and young people in schools, there is an equal demand and need to engage in meaningful intervention strategies. Their purpose and aim is to work collaboratively with education, social care and health providers to develop outstanding outcomes for vulnerable children across the country. This is achieved through the promotion of professional staff and organisational development underpinned by research (Mulberry Bush Outreach, 2019). This recognition and educational emphasis on a more holistic targeted approach, involving the schools, parents and the wider community, all working for the common interest of the child or young person, have long been part of the aim of Excell3 and was the reason for the establishment of the organisation in Birmingham, UK in 1999, with its signature Black Boys Can project.

Excell3's Black Boys Can Intervention Programmes

Excell3, a leading community-led national educational charity, has, since its establishment in 1999, demonstrated unfailing commitment to the empowerment and emotional well-being of Black boys. The network of Black Boys Can projects has a distinctive mission of raising the academic aspirations and attainment, as well as the well-being, of Black boys throughout the UK, by providing targeted or bespoke additional support to mainstream education through such provisions as: additional lessons, personal skills, aspirational sessions on career and university applications, as well as mentoring. In response to high levels of demand for the services of Excell3's Black Boys Can project, the organisation replicated its best practice throughout the country by supporting local communities to set up and manage their own Black Boys Can projects, through its offer of a community franchise package of training and support.

Excell3 grew out of the Black churches and some of its local Black Boys Can projects are church-based while others are non-faith-based community initiatives. In recent years, increasing attention has been given to the relationships between religiosity and mental health, with many studies demonstrating positive associations between the two (Koenig, King, & Carson, 2012). On balance, those who are more religious have better indices of mental health, more hope and optimism and life satisfaction (Koenig, 2009), less depression, lower rates of suicide (Van Praag, 2009), and reduced delinquency (Johnson, Li, Larson, & McCullough, 2000). The important role that Black churches and faith make to the empowerment and mental well-being of Black boys is often overlooked. However, many of the Black male students in Byfield's study (2008) attributed their faith and the support from Black churches, as being a contributory factor to their educational achievement. Access to 'Divine Capital' (a person's connectedness to God), a concept coined by Byfield (2008), was found to: enhance some Black boys' self-confidence, provide them with a sense of direction, enabled them to remain focussed in the face of peer pressure and other adversities, helped to develop their character, endowed them with moral values, shielded them from adverse situations and associations, and through prayer, they were able to draw strength and solicit support from God (Byfield, 2008). Hence religion gave these students solace, confidence and strength when they needed it and provided them with a sense of acceptance and belonging. In addition, 'progressive' churches were known to empower Black boys through, for example, publicly celebrating their success in church, profiling them on the church noticeboards, providing them with a strong personal, social and community identity, offered social and psychological support, and gave them a sense of belonging, reassurance and self-validation. In this sense, therefore, many of the

Black boys interviewed in Byfield's study were able to relate their educational achievement and emotional well-being to the support and intervention, not only from the Black Boys Can Programmes which were often church-based community groups, but from the church and their Christian faith.

In recognition of the fact that Black boys are not a homogeneous group, Excell3 has developed a range of programmes to meet their diverse needs. Their Black Boys Empowerment Programme is a generic one which is accessible and beneficial to all Black boys who undertake to engage on the programmes. There is the School Exclusion Risk Reduction Programme, which specifically targets boys who are at high risk of being permanently excluded from school, while the university programmes specifically target Black boys who are academically gifted and talented, irrespective of whether they are recognised as such. One of the key features of the Black Boys Can projects is its interconnected four-pillar strategy of: empowering Black boys; upskilling and supporting parents to be effective co-educators of their sons; challenging and supporting schools and other educational institutions in educating Black boys; and engaging Black professionals from the community to engage in mentoring and training programmes that help in the empowerment of Black boys.

There are a number of different intervention programmes employed by Black Boys Can. One of these is focussed around the provision of positive Black role models for the boys. Several of the students in Byfield's study (2008) made reference to the significance of having access to positive role models both within their church congregation, as well as from Black male professionals more generally. More often than not, these role models were professional Black men and women who had been successful either in their field of employment or in business. These students aspired to be like the people who inspired them, and, therefore, valued the opportunity they had to interact with these professionals.

These role models (teachers, mentors and coaches) supported Black boys to overcome the challenges which adversely impacts on their mental health and educational outcome. Typically, these professionals are ethnically empathetic, able to reassure the boys that they understand the challenges they face in society and also at school, and its power or ability to reinforce inequality and affect educational outcomes. Furthermore, these mentors were also aware of the structural and institutional discrimination that Black boys face because of their ethnicity, and were able to offer advice, some of which were based on their own experiences. Black Boys Can provides Black boys with the emotional support and cultural understanding which they often craved for. The identity, culture and experiences of these role models enabled Black boys to connect culturally with them, and, when necessary, to speak frankly about racist incidents. Sam and Albert (not their real names) Black boys in Byfield's study (2008) recalled:

> In my school, I was the only Black person. There were some teachers who didn't know how to relate to you. Whenever race issues came up they felt uncomfortable. I always felt in the middle of it all, so I tended to withdraw from the discussion (Sam).

> It was good having them (Black mentors) 'cause they can relate to you, so if I had a problem, even a personal problem or discrimination problem I felt I could go to them because they've probably been through it before (Albert).

Excell3's Amos Bursary Scheme, developed by Baroness Amos of Brondesbury (former UK Cabinet Minister) was established in 2012 to provide fair access to professional careers for ambitious Black boys with the potential of becoming the leaders of tomorrow. The Black boys selected to join the programme receive professional mentoring to get into top universities, ensuring that they get a great spring-board to embark on their career as well as bursaries and support through their university degree programmes. Many of these Black boys successfully secure internships in top organisations including: Google, Goldman Sachs, Linklater's, EY and Deutsche Bank. In addition, these boys gained access to a range of opportunities including support to attend the Democracy and Youth European Conference in Seville Spain in 2012 (which inspires a sense of citizenship, solidarity and tolerance among young Europeans, as well as to involve them in shaping the Union's future). They also get access to sponsorship to gain work experience abroad, and also opportunities to host and share experiences with international students, such as one event where they hosted 40 Martin Luther King Scholars from the United States in 2014.

Additionally, they get plenty of networking opportunities. For example, one student was able, through networking, to secure one week's work experience at the Institute of Directors Business Ethnicity Summit. These students also receive encouragement and support to profile themselves, resulting in a student being selected as the runner up from the Anne Frank Trust for peacemaker of the year, and another student being listed in the Powerful Media Future Leaders publication in September 2014. Typical comments about the experiences of being on the programme is captured by a student who described how it was such a rare experience to be in a room with so many young Black men whose drive and potential is completely unshackled. It not only helped to make them feel more optimistic and excited about the possibility of working with fellow students in the future, but also helped to create or enhance their emotional self-esteem and emotional well-being.

Excell3 has developed a programme specifically to address the needs of Black boys who have been excluded from school, or who are at high risk of being excluded. The programme, known as the School Exclusion Risk Reduction Programme, is based on the premise that many of the problems associated with Black boys and criminality is located within an educational context. These include such issues as; as racism, poor attainment, and low teacher expectations which pushes some Black boys to the margins of the school community, providing an exit strategy from school and an entry point into criminality. The programme seeks to address some of the key issues affecting Black boys such as Black male self-concept and anger. W. E. B. Du Bois (1994), the renowned pan Africanist, educationalist and criminologist, referred to the problem of Black male self-concept as 'double consciousness', where he stated that the problem of

Black males self-actualising is as a consequence of having: two souls, two thoughts and two unreconciled strivings two warring ideals in one body (Du Bois, 1994). Another key concept which the programme addresses is anger. The cumulative impact of social problems and identity concerns often results in Black boys being angry with parents, siblings, peer group, schoolteachers and society at large. This unbridled anger, coupled with a failure in schools to provide effective anger management intervention, often results in eventual exclusion from school as a result of some form of inappropriate violent behaviour.

Central to the success of the Black Boys Can project is the pedagogy and philosophy of the organisation which includes positive student self-esteem, academic values and skills and also life and career planning. Julius, who progressed to university after completing the programme at Black Boys Can, recalls:

> My mum and my Sunday school teacher encouraged me and my brother to go to Black Boys Can. It was a nice environment. It influenced my thinking about my ability to achieve and opened up new possibilities for me. We covered many areas ranging from Black culture to goal setting, and we learnt to cook as well!. What I found most amazing was the lessons' we had on the Black presence in the Bible. That was the first time I ever learnt about Black people in the Bible so I found it fascinating. I also enjoyed lessons on Black inventors – some I had learnt about though TV and Black history month, but a lot of it was new to me. I think we should cover these types of subjects in school. Our parents don't teach us these things because they didn't know either; they learned British history at school, not Black history.

The programme helped to compensate for the racialised or colonialised nature of the school environment and curriculum which failed to reflect the racial identities and cultural tastes of Black boys. This often contributed to a physical and emotional disconnect from the mainstream school system by some Black students. Bill, who succeeded in getting into Oxford University observed:

> I've gone through the education system though to Oxford but I never studied Black history, I never studied a Black author, I've never studied any Black philosophers, I never did any form of Black music; they don't value you.

The proactive pedagogy of the Black Boys Can Programmes, however, helped to make Black boys feel valued. It helped to counteract negative media stereotypes of Black men and provides a much-needed supplement to the characteristically monocultural state schools' curriculum. The programmes also encouraged Black boys to embrace the achievement ideology associated with the dominant cultural environment while valuing and embracing Black culture, and teaching them the skills of being able to 'culture switch' when it was in their interest to at any point in time. Racial connectedness, a taken for granted phenomena among

White teachers and White children in schools does aid interpersonal relationships between Black boys and the Black workers. The very presence of Black male role models helped to affirm the sense of pride and a positive sense of identity of the boys.

The Black Boys Can programmes motivated the boys, made lessons fun, interactive and challenging, kept them focussed, instilled hope in them, built their confidence in their ability to achieve, provided them with opportunities to excel, and gave them respect and in return commanded their respect. By focussing on the boys' talent and maximising their potential, they are able to channel their energies positively thus acting as a buffer against 'self-elimination', from the education system. These targeted programmes, therefore, helped to provide the boys with a higher level of self-esteem and also boost their emotional well-being.

One of the interviewees in Byfield's study made reference to the environment of Black Boys Can being a 'nice environment'. This creation of a positive environment is a typical feature often noted in other studies about community interventionist programmes. Chevannes and Reeves (1987), for example, describes the environment of such programmes as having a strong group solidarity based on common experiences of being Black in a White society. They therefore help in providing an environment for 'insulating, protecting and supporting the individual against the unpredictability of White behaviour and constant difficulty of interpreting outcomes in a context of widespread White prejudice and discrimination. Typically, displays and walls are covered with images of Black success and this serves to inspire, challenge and empower Black boys. The boys are able to experience a positive sense of community where they feel a sense of belonging and inclusion and valued for who they are, thus promoting positive mental health and well-being, connectedness, inclusivity and positive relationships.

Black boys are among the most disadvantaged in society who do not have a voice. The needs of those who are silent tend to be overlooked or misunderstood and they tend to have restricted access to goods and services that supposedly represent their interests. All too often Black boys are written off as individuals who show no interest or little motivation to engage in processes designed to assist them in some way. The Black Boys Can Programmes challenge those notions and replaces them with understanding free from bias, labelling and judgement. In recognition of the fact that those who are in positions of power are hard to access and reach, Excell3 actively seeks to give Black boys a voice by opening doors for them to reach the powerful. Hence, in addition to Excell3's proactive early intervention work with Black boys at grass roots level, they also operate at national strategic level lobbying to effect change for Black boys. The organisation has seized opportunities to engage with government minsters at round table events, as well as contribute to various government reports, including the *Reach Report* (2007) the UK Conservative Party's *Breakthrough Britain Report* (2007) and also through hosting high profile national conferences. Through these events Excell3 has opened doors for Black boys to have a voice in the public arena which would otherwise not have been possible. Some of these Black boys have, in turn, seized the opportunities Exell3 has given them, to co-chair national Gala Award events, national parents' conferences, a national conference for Head teachers (sponsored by the National Union of Teachers), and a cross-party event held at the House of Commons.

The boys on the Black Boys Can programmes received training to develop their skills and confidence to be able to address people at every level of society. Sean, for example, a 16-year old boy, was selected to address over 100 Members of Parliament at the cross-party event at the House of Commons in 2005 where he articulately spoke on behalf of the Black boys in the UK. Sean's presentation is so powerful that the excerpt below is quoted here in full:

> I am appealing on behalf of all Black boys in this country who haven't been heard. For the boys in prison, who haven't been heard. For the boys on the streets, who haven't been heard. For the Black boys who've been excluded from school, who haven't been heard. For the Black boys who, against all odds, achieved and are successful who haven't been heard. For too long we've been written off by the education system. Society's expectations of us are low. However, no Black boys want to be an underachiever, so please give us a chance. So, if you're serious about our education, our achievements, our opportunities, now here's your chance to make a difference. Isn't it time for us as Black boys to put back into society? We don't want to be a drain on our society! So, what we require from you is equal access to education, to be heard and to be given a chance to show our capabilities. Teachers today only see us as rappers, 100m runners and graffiti artists, but if you look through our eyes you'd see that we want to be doctors, lawyers, teachers etc. However, in order to achieve our ambitions, we need to successfully get through the education system. I am just an ordinary Black boy who joined the Black Boys Can project in 1999. This year I took my GCSE's and I got, not 1, not 2 not 5, but 11 GCSE's grades A*-C. I want all other Black boys to at least be given the opportunity to get access to the type of support I received from Black Boys Can.

As a result of Excell3's expertise in working with boys who have been, or are at risk of being excluded from school, when the Department for Education's High-Level Group on Race Equality identified exclusions of Black pupils as a priority area for action, senior government officials approached the organisation to be involved in the Priority Review. Excell3 invited several of the Boys from their programmes, who had been excluded from school to have face-to-face conversations with government officials. The boys spoke openly, confidently and honestly about their experiences and articulated very clearly what they considered to be key changes required in the education system. Before the report was published, the chair of the Review wrote to Excell3 in 2006 thanking them for their input into the review and commented on and meeting they had had with the organisation. They commented on how invaluable the conversation was on the issue of exclusions as well as a broader understanding of what the policy implications for Black boys might be, across a much wider range of areas.

The finding of the Priority Review culminated in the *Getting It, Getting It Right Report* (DFes, 2006) which reflected the concerns raised through the review process that: the exclusions gap is part of a larger set of issues affecting Black pupils within the system, the system does not give this issue the same weight as Black communities do; those working in the system need support to improve their knowledge and understanding of the issue to deliver; and the compliance levers are so far failing to address this. The report was presented to Ministers and shared with Excell3 alongside those organisations that contributed to the study. From this, the DFes developed a forward-looking strategy to address the underlying causes of disproportionate exclusions among Black children, especially Caribbean boys. This was only possible because of the successful interventionist work of Excell3.

Schools have been criticised for the under-representation of Black pupils in gifted and talented programmes. Furthermore, while intellectual abilities are undoubtedly an asset in the pursuit of high academic attainment, many gifted and talented pupils still underachieve. In Byfield's study (2008), a grammar school Black boy failed to achieve the national standards of 5 GCSEs grade A*-C at the end of compulsory school leaving age, attributing his underachievement to the institutional racism that pervaded his school. Furthermore, Gillborn (1990) argued, ability and dedication are not in themselves enough for Black boys to achieve highly at school. Excell3's university programmes, therefore, actively seek to identify and provide appropriate training and support to gifted and talented Black boys.

Excel 3's university programme incorporates an Open College Network accredited course that empowers boys to aspire to university and equip them with the tools to overcome barriers along the way. The course also includes a complementally workbook for parents to enable them to work alongside their sons and provide effective support for them along their journey. Excell3 formed partnerships with Russell Group universities, including the Universities of Oxford, Cambridge, Imperial College London, Warwick and Birmingham, to run the programme for Black boys, raise their aspirations, their confidence and resilience to successfully apply to, and graduate from, top universities. These programmes also deliver academic master classes to help drive-up their attainment levels thereby improving their chances of securing a place at a top university, provide information, advice and guidance on practical aspects of the application process (e.g. the admissions process) and empower their parents to enable them to provide effective support to their sons. At least 50% of the boys who join Excell3's University programme, gain a place at a Russell Group University, including Oxford and Cambridge.

The Impact of Targeted Intervention for Disadvantaged Pupils

These types of holistic approach to disadvantaged groups of students, carried out by Excell3, have not only helped raise educational achievement and enhance emotional well-being for Black boys in the UK, but are also observed in other countries. For example, some schools across America now find themselves very concerned with ensuring that their role of preventing emotional and behavioural challenges and identifying risk factors considered potential barriers to academic success, is given a very high priority (Kutash et al., 2006). The authors also make reference to a model of intervention based on a four-stage framework comprising the significance of youth, family, community and culture (Kutash et al., 2006). These important stages also relate to the Excell3 model of school, family, community, all of which play an important role in the development of the child and young person as well as in their educational and emotional well-being.

Furthermore, the authors make reference to the importance of interconnected systems or a 'continuum of services' which includes such areas of specialisation as mental health promotion, prevention programmes, early detection and treatment, and intensive intervention as well as maintenance and recovery programmes (Kutash et al., 2006, p. 23). They also stressed the importance of positive behaviour support, which they suggest should be whole school centred rather than simply applied to individual cases (Kutash et al., 2006).

Additionally, and very important in terms of the Excell3 approach and philosophy, specific selective interventions also can be offered in small group settings for students exhibiting similar behaviours. Examples include membership in a social skills club in which specific replacement behaviours are taught, modelled and used by the students (Kutash et al., 2006). This is also similar to the intervention strategy used by Excell3 for students at risk of being excluded from school, due to inappropriate behaviour.

An article by the National Education Association (NEA, 2011) argued that the real problem affecting Black boys in education is that most schools are addressing the issue as an academic problem. The New Jersey's Newark Tech High School, which is regarded by U.S. News & World Report Magazine, as one of the best high schools in the United States, has been leading the way in helping to carry out intervention strategies to help raise the aspirations, achievements and overall wellbeing of their students. Of the 700 mostly Black and Hispanic students attending Newark Tech in 2010, 88% of the student body tested proficient in math, 100% tested proficient in reading and 100% graduated (NEA, 2011).

As they quite rightly point put, a much more holistic approach is needed as, according to the report, 'we can't address a crisis of self-image, self-esteem, self-discipline and self-respect, as an academic problem' (NEA, 2011, p. 2). One of their strategies employed in schools, in its attempt to address the issue affecting such disadvantaged groups of students, was to blast a positive daily message on the public address system to help counteract the effects of some of the negative message students receive outside of the school. They also have weekly classes on manhood with specially arranged small group sessions with men from the community. They also use culturally appropriate material in some of their teaching.

The study by Sharples, Slavin, and Chambers (2011) was particularly important in that its central purpose was to examine the best available international evidence on what works in terms of improving services and outcomes for children living in poverty, including White working-class boys. Although a substantial part of their research methods and findings involved practices in the United States, some of their overall findings were nonetheless very significant and applicable within a British context. Their study highlighted the fact that examples of effective intervention strategies used for pupils from one ethnic group or socioeconomic group, can generally be applied in a wider context for other groups.

They also argue that a fundamental cause for lower levels of attainment in schools, based on GCSE results, is the extent of poverty levels (Sharples et al., 2011). One of the major issues they highlighted was that there was very little understanding of what actually works to improve educational attainment of children from disadvantaged groups. A number of key effective strategies were highlighted which included: rigorous monitoring and use of data, raising pupil aspirations using engagement/aspiration programmes, engaging parents, and developing social and emotional competences (Sharples et al., 2011). In addition, they suggested targeted intervention and support in primary schools, especially in numeracy and literacy, changing teaching practices through extensive continuing professional development, as well as cooperative teaching methods, especially in mathematics were found to be very effective.

According to Craig Thorley (2016) there is a serious crisis with regard to mental health provision in secondary schools in England due to such issues as inadequate funding, the inconsistency of mental health support as well as 'insufficient external checks on the appropriateness and quality of the particular "professional mix" that individual schools bring together to meet their pupils' mental health needs' (Thorley, 2016). One of the key recommendations offered by his research was for all secondary schools to be guaranteed access to at least one day per week of onsite support from a Child and Adolescent Mental Health Services professional who is able to provide targeted mental health interventions to pupils, rising to two days per week by 2022/2023 (Thorley, 2016). However, and more specifically, with regard to this study, additional support to vulnerable students, especially from poor backgrounds is important. Targeted intervention strategies, as used by Excell3, are important tools in the quest to improve the academic performance of Black boys and also help to enhance their overall emotional well-being.

Conclusions

What this study has done, is to provide an examination of the different kinds of intervention strategies that have been used by Excell3 in its attempts to raise the level of academic performance in Black boys as well as their emotional well-being. The main claim being made is that targeted intervention is crucial, especially for disadvantaged groups of children and young people, especially Black boys, if they are to achieve successful academic results in schools and also positive emotional well-being. The chapter has shown that where the emotional well-being is impaired, these could lead to lower levels of educational achievement, and eventual disengagement from the education system. Although some studies suggest the issue of poverty is the main factor responsible for low attainment in schools, for many Black boys, added to the issue of their low socioeconomic background, is the issue of their ethnicity. If you are poor and Black, your chances of success could be far worse. These holistic programmes use self-development and empowerment strategies to enable boys to develop coping strategies, enhance their mental well-being and personally transform them and raise their social and academic aspirations and achievements.

References

Byfield, C. (2008). *Black boys can make it, how they overcome the obstacles to university in the UK and USA*. London: Trentham Books Ltd.

Chevannes, M., & Reeves, F. (1987). The black voluntary school movement: Definition, context and prospects. In B. Troyna (Ed.), *Racial inequality in education*. New York, NY: Routledge.

Davie, E. (2014). It's time to tackle mental health inequality among black people. Retrieved from https://www.theguardian.com/healthcare-network/2014/oct/28/tackle-mental-health-inequality-black-people. Accessed on July 17, 2017.

Demie, F., & Mclean, C. (2015). The underachievement of Black Caribbean Heritage Pupils in schools. Retrieved from https://www.lambeth.gov.uk/rsu/sites/www.lambeth.gov.uk.rsu/files/The_Underachievement_of_Black_Caribbean_Heritage_Pupils_in_Schools-_Research_Brief.pdf. Accessed on July 13, 2017.

DFes. (2006). *Getting it, getting right: Exclusion of Black Pupils: Priority review*. London: Department for Education and Skills.

Du Bois, W. E. B. (1994). *The souls of black folk*. New York, NY: Dover Publications.

Gillborn, D. (1990). *Race, ethnicity, and education: Teaching and learning in multi-ethnic schools – Key issues in education*. London: Unwin Hyman.

Johnson, B., Li, S., Larson, D., & McCullough, M. (2000). A systematic review of the religiosity and delinquency literature: A research note. *Journal of Contemporary Criminal Justice, 16*, 32–52.

Johnston, D., Propper, C., Pudney, S., & Shields, M. (2011). *Child mental health and educational attainment: Multiple observers and the measurement error problem*. Institute for Social and Economic Research: No. 2011 – 20 August.

Koenig, H., King, D., & Carson, V. (2012). *Handbook of religion and health* (2nd ed.). New York, NY: Oxford University Press.

Koenig, H. G. (2007). Religion and remission of depression in medical inpatients with heart failure/pulmonary disease. *Journal of Nervous Mental Disease, 195*, 389–395.

Koenig, H. G. (2009). Research on religion, spirituality, and mental health: A review. *Canadian Journal of Psychiatry, 54*, 283–291.

Kutash, K., Duchnowski, A., & Lynn, N. (2006). *School-based mental health: An empirical guide for decision-makers*. Tampa, FL: Research and Training Center for Children's Mental Health Dept. of Child & Family Studies, Louis de la Parte Florida Mental Health Institute, University of South Florida.

Mulberry Bush Outreach. (2019). Retrieved from https://mulberrybush.org.uk/learning-research-centre/outreach/. Accessed on June 21, 2017.

National Education Association (NEA). (2011, February). Focus on Blacks: Race against time, educating black boys. Retrieved from http://www.nea.org/assets/docs/educatingblackboys11rev.pdf. Accessed on July 24, 2017.

Ranger, J. (2008). *Challenging exclusions: Handbook for parents. Principle and Partnership for Achievement* (2nd ed.). Birmingham.

Reach Report. (2007). *REACH: An independent report to government on raising the aspirations and attainment of Black Boys and Young Black Men*. London: Government Response Communities and Neighbourhoods.

Ross, C. E., & Wu, C. L. (1995, October). The links between education and health. *American Sociological Review, 60*(5), 719–745.

Sharples, J., Slavin, R., & Chambers, B. (2011). *Effective classroom strategies for closing the gap in educational achievement for children and young people living in poverty, including white working-class boys*. London: Centre for Excellence and Outcomes in Children and Young People's Services (C4EO).

The Conservative Party. (2007). *Breakthrough Britain … Ending the Costs of Social Breakdown Volume 6: Policy Recommendations to the Conservative Party*.

Thorley, C. (2016). *Education, education, mental health: Supporting secondary schools to play a central role in early intervention Mental Health Services*. London: Institute for Public Policy Research.

Van Praag, H. M. (2009). The role of religion in suicide prevention. In D. Wasserman & C. Wasserman (Eds.), *Oxford textbook of suicidology and suicide prevention*. Oxford: Oxford University Press.

Part IV

Theory and Practice

Chapter 15

Toward Positions of Spiritual Reflexivity as a Resource: Emerging Themes and Conversations for Systemic Practice, Leadership, and Supervision within Black Mental Health

Maureen Greaves

Introduction: The Significance of Spirituality for Black Mental Health Professionals and Service Users

There is no one universally agreed upon definition of spirituality. However, there has been increasing reference to it within mental health services for a number of years, taking many forms in assisting practitioners to consider how individual beliefs might shape behaviors, relationships, and communication patterns (Cook et al., 2010). This increase and acceptance in attending to the spiritual and religious needs of service users has come after a continuous onslaught of radical attention to race relations and anti-discriminatory practice from the 1970s and has been associated mostly with the religious practice and cultural experiences of black families and communities. Religion and the multiplicity of faith (described in Appendix 1), are also terms that are sometimes used interchangeably alongside spirituality; however, religion is largely assumed to be congruent with a community of organized rituals and practice that influences individual and relational culture concerning the associated doctrine.

There have been numerous historic examples of how religion and spirituality have been segregated from the cultural practice of western counseling and psychotherapy, largely due to skepticism expressed by scholars such as Freud, who have rendered them as examples of delusional hysteria or neurosis (O'Hagan, 2001). This has left a great deal of reluctance and skepticism within the psychotherapy and counseling profession as one of the main arenas for treating mental illness. In addition, there have been several facets contributing to the reluctance for engaging service users in conversation regarding religious and spiritual practice that include an overreliance on scientific knowledge; the role of religion in perpetuating racist colonial practices among indigenous and enslaved peoples; the perception of religion as overly controlling, sexist, and abusive; and the growth of religious fundamentalists and cults in western society (O'Hagan, 2001).Nevertheless, the appetite for considering how spirituality and religion might be a helpful resource for black families appears to be gaining momentum as part of an overall framework for developing culturally competent practice within health and social care services (Cook et al., 2010).

Spirituality does not necessarily require association with a religious denomination, although, there is historic evidence that closely links Christianity with the cultural expression and identity of black African and Caribbean people through a long and tumultuous relationship of slavery and colonialism. There has also been evidence of a growing number of black people that have rebelled against this association, seeing Christianity as a *white man's religion* and adopting religious beliefs of Islamic charismatic leaders such as Louis Farrakhan in the late 1980s and the 1990s (Brown, 2001). This historical legacy places Christianity and Islam at the center of spiritual and religious underpinnings that have developed within the political, social, relational, economic, and health cultures of black families (Boyd-Franklin, 1989).

Critical race theory offers a theoretical framework for the examination and analysis of culture and society, and the marginalization of black people through discourse, policy, practice, and subordination. Developed in the late 1980s within the United States of America's response to critical legal studies in which themes of white supremacy, racial power, and practice dominated in society, its founders – Patricia Williams, Richard Delgardo, Derrick Bell, and Kimberie Williams-Crenshaw sought to address the growing instances of racism, oppression, and mistreatment of black people within American society in response to a *color-blind* approach often adopted within and after the civil rights movement. The theory analyzes the law and legal traditions which often support such practices, attempting to transform the legal landscape of overrepresentation within mental health institutions and prisons, similar with the UK context. Similarities and comparisons between the UK and the US contexts do not end there, and in addition to the close economic and political relationships between the prime minister of the UK and the American president (regardless of who sits in office), there are lived experiences which resonate for black people in relation to their cultural context and instances of racism ingrained in the fabric of society (Gordon, 1999).

Critical race theory therefore has some significance in relation to exploring how concepts of racial division and minimization further shape discourse around the marginalization of some communities in various practice contexts, in addition to how experiences of spirituality, Christianity, and religion have been marginalized as something being practiced once a week in a distinct community or location. The reality is, many Christians acknowledge their faith is in existence wherever they are and can be integrated into their practice while acknowledging God's influence (1 John 3:20, Holy Bible – King James Version, 1998). Themes of mental, emotional, and economic emancipation therefore, continue to be at the forefront of transformation for black community members and the words of Bob Marley's "Redemption Song" (Marley, 1980) have resonance here.

Addressing spirituality has the potential to be relevant when considering assessment models, safeguarding well-being, developing cultural competence, and managing diversity in positive ways, particularly in relation to an increase in emerging issues of religious intolerance, religious delusion in psychosis, and the prevalence of hate crime, which are under scrutiny in negative ways (Drew, 2016). The prevalence of a history of using strength-based spiritual approaches and support systems inherent within the dimension of cultural identity (Boyd-Franklin, 1989) and affiliations to Christianity and Islam should therefore not be overlooked.

The language of spirituality as a phenomenon, juxtaposed to the use of religion, is used recursively in the text to include and address aspects of hope, possibility, and connection to a greater source of power (internal, external, and relational power) to facilitate change in individuals and families. While this term is privileged, this is not to agree with the many and varied sources of literature that have sought to disable the connection of religion from the state and mental health practice in derogatory ways, i.e., referencing oppression, abuse, and lack of tolerance (Drew, 2016), but as a more creative and adaptable resource that can manage diversity of belief and corresponding behavior to transform the lives of others, irrespective of religion. The inclusion of spirituality as a transformative practice is therefore resonant in reflexive and responsive ways, requiring further research and didactic training methods to implement it within clinical work, including the supervision of psychotherapists and counselors (Jafari, 2016.)

In systemic practice and training, the Social GRRACCESS (gender, race, religion, ability, culture, class, ethnicity, spirituality, and sexuality – Burnham in Divac & Heaphy, 2005), is a common model used to orientate practitioners around the complexities of the various belief systems, values, and corresponding behaviors impacting the communication and assessment process as a form of cultural competence. Within this model, spirituality and religion are referenced as separate entities or aspects of the relational practice and have the propensity to be more than a checklist of questions to note demographic or statistical information on case notes. These paradigms are often used as discussion points for avoiding discrimination and for helping practitioners pay attention to the aspects of the client context which they privilege and highlight as important in conversation, thus producing a more positive outcome for the dilemmas about which they are seeking consultation. With the introduction of a recursive and relational aspect, addressing spirituality, within practice, communication, and learning can be enhanced and therefore produce (sometimes unexpected or anticipated) change.

The inclusion and joining together of spirituality with reflexivity within the various practice territories, as discussed later, brings an opportunity to create an environment for recursively shaping perception and behaviors incumbent within the organizational structures that provide mental health services, with the added *lived experience* of service users producing a more integrated and effective environment to respond to mental health concerns for black families. A narrative approach that privileges the voice of black experiences within psychiatry can accommodate this flexibility (Cook, Powell, & Sims, 2016).

Discussions around representations of spirituality associated with religion are central to the discussion of clinical practice in mental health; however, it remains beyond the scope of this chapter to fully deconstruct such nuances. In recognition of this, religious beliefs and associated doctrine are both critically discussed yet respectfully de-centered to facilitate a more coherent and practical application of spirituality as a resource toward culturally competent practice.

What Is Spiritual Reflexivity?

The term spiritual reflexivity (Taylor, 2016) is a developing concept through my own systemic research practice (reframed from reflexive spirituality, a term coined by Wade Clarke-Roof in Besecke, 2014) used to privilege and prioritize spirituality over religion. It also seeks to privilege the relationship with God (identified as a spirit that exists internally, externally, and relationally) as the main lens through which reflexive practice is situated. It does not purport to be readily applicable to all aspects of spiritual representation or affiliation; neither does it seek to exclude any. The term is used as a means of locating the discussion from within the lived experience of the author as a black female Christian CEO, business consultant, systemic psychotherapist, and researcher; attempting to remain coherent, authentic, transparent, and resourceful.

There are many emerging and developing aspects to how spiritual reflexivity is being used in practice, namely: an attempt to deconstruct discourse that is often associated with traditional religious practices and organizations (Van Dijk, 1985); a distinction between how a concept of God (as seen through the many lenses of Christianity through shared community and identity) resonates within practice paradigms in helpful ways (Elliott-Griffith, 1995); considering spirituality as acknowledging God's voice in relationships through internal and external communication; and as collaboration (between concepts, people, and communities) when responding to the stimulus of practice situations in ethical, reflexive, and culturally competent ways. Like reflexive spirituality, it is not imagined as new doctrine to replace old concepts that have dominated traditional religious language and practice but has the creative ability to be applicable to practitioners in a variety of contexts (Besecke, 2014).

There is further resonance in relation to one of the tenets of Christian faith and identity concerning working together (collaboration). Jakes (2007), Francis (2016), and Meyer (1995) all see this collaboration as essential for Christians to practice, and as adding authenticity to the self of the Christian practitioner or person. The metaphor of *the body of Christ* is often used to describe how individuals, doctrine practices, and communities have both individual and collective purpose (or assignments) to be realized in preparation for His (God's) return to the earth. Spiritual reflexivity, working with God and others as a collaborative process, is therefore relevant for evaluating how communities with shared identities or cultures collaborate. This concept also fits in relation to seeing the inherent means through which bodies remain healthy (all components, internal and external, working together) and the challenges of managing complexity within living organisms and territory such as mental health and social care services (Cook et al., 2016).

Spiritual reflexivity is bespoke, personal, and adaptable, as we are as individuals. Our communication patterns, relationships, cognition, and behavior are all interconnected to our dimensions of self and socially constructed and shaped lived experience. The means through which we pay attention to the nuances of dispositional knowledge and experiences in mental health practice and not just line with cognitive and descriptive stories about self but in experiential, analytic, artistic, and creatively embodied stories of the multidimensional self (Rober, 1991).

Spiritual reflexivity can be used as a structure to move toward a greater representation of how reflexive processes might aid practitioners to creatively and boldly embed critical discussions and shape the social construction of diversity in positive ways. Spiritual reflexivity utilizes *stories of spirituality* and *spiritual creativity* as a means of introducing how it might be socially constructed and not just attuned to religion, but how it might also be a useful resource in leadership practice. The language of social construction uses stories of make-believe (created by social scientists); the language of spirituality (represented in Christianity) uses language of *reality* in being and knowing, going beyond what is socially constructed. These positions are not necessarily at odds with each other and finding a way for these languages to coexist will be an interesting tension to hold throughout the practice paradigm (Gergen in Alvesson & Skoldberg, 2009).

In practice, these positions might also be represented through the coexistence of the medical scientific model with the social scientific model of systemic practice within child and adolescent mental health services, alongside the spiritual characteristics of the therapist applying the theory and the cultural or religious context in which the practice is embedded. These parallel processes require further research to explore how best organizations, black communities, and groups work collaboratively with a shared vision, ethic, belief, or spiritual understanding within the mental health arena and the propensity to provide a rich environment to shape the journey toward wellness for black families and communities.

Power, Discourse, and Mental Health

Power within discourse as a phenomenon, may facilitate the empowerment (internal representation of power expressed as confidence or courage) of individuals in a strength-based way. Spiritual reflexivity as a concept seeks to provide access to this relational use of power and as such might become a vehicle through which dilemmas and inspiration presented in the practice and leadership paradigm are accessed. The resonance of inspiration and challenge are two important themes practitioners hold the tension between in clinical and supervisory practice, particularly when there is an impasse. For example, the Bible, seen and described as the inspired word of God (Holy Bible), is a source of potential inspiration for many Christians, and the centrality of the text is regularly emphasized throughout the Christian community. The spirit of the word, the life and relationality of it, is sometimes evoked when *reading* it with expectation that energy, wisdom, and power held in it, as a part of a Christian theory of change, will be transferred to the reader. Recalling the content in times of distress can therefore increase accessibility of solutions for both service users and practitioners. The Bible therefore helps to illuminate aspects of God's character, instructions, language, and desired relationship with humanity, and as a key resource for spiritual beliefs associated with Christianity is central to the reflexive process, through the practice of hermeneutics (Osbourne, 1991).

The Bible is written in many languages and comes in many versions, each with different emphasis and interpretation, filtered through the lenses of the author and the reader alike. It is with a spiritually reflexive lens that we hope to be inspired and challenged, bringing news of difference, (Bateson, 1972) as a means of bringing to life creativity within professional practice and life experience. In addition to this, the internalized voice of God (the Holy Spirit), being congruent with what is written in the Bible, may bring news of difference to what might appear to be a contradiction to His word, but helps to illuminate how seemingly opposing discourse and positions can coexist – death and life; fear and faith; strength and weakness; knowing and curiosity; and movement and stillness.

Inherent in these tensions is where our practice faces the most challenging moments and yet offers a rich opportunity for change and intervention. Critical discussion within the language of Christianity, science, politics, and academia is one in which we aspire to engage to deconstruct dominant ideology about practice tensions, such as blame, responsibility, risk associated with mental health, and safeguarding practice. These are not seen as linear, binary, or hierarchical positioning but as relationally recursive (Liddle & Saba, 1983).

Toward a Representation of Spiritual Reflexivity: Using a Metaphor of the GPS

One of the emerging themes used to foreground how a spiritual reflexive process resonates for myself (and potentially others) is that of the God Positioning System (GPS). This is a metaphoric representation (Garrett, 2007) I developed to consider how Christians might develop their unique relationship with their perception of God and how this shapes individual and cultural identity, honors His presence within our lives, and encourages ethical practice within a variety of paradigms. Having originally thought about the concept, language, and resource in relation to leadership practice for presentation at the International Conference of Qualitative Inquiry, (Taylor, 2016), I created the GPS metaphor, as something I perceive as being God given and *inspired* through a moment of critical decision-making.

In conversation with others, the use of the GPS began to gain momentum and resonance for me in much the same way that I imagine innovation within mental health practice to be recursively shaped. Questions were posed to me such as: how do I know the difference between the voice of God and my own voice? Are there senses in the spirit and if so, are these the same as or different from those in the physical realm? How do I pay attention to the voice of others and their perceptions of God within practice? What is my (and God's) imagined success? Such questions have facilitated a greater exploration of spiritual reflexivity as a practice consideration in helpful ways, similar with the way in which questions form the main means through which meanings are derived within therapeutic and supervisory encounters.

The metaphor of the GPS, as described, is a potential extension and adaptation of the concept of systemic reflexivity (in combination with positioning theory, (Harre, 2012) and conversational discourse (Sawyer & Norris, 2016) to represent spiritual reflexivity in action. The images imagined are representative of the car's electronic version and considers orientation and movement around the territory we find ourselves in, such as: practice, life, and relationships, simultaneously and recursively providing and receiving feedback loops (shaping and being shaped) within the communication process.

One interpretation of the GPS (as one such interpretation of many) externalizes the inner conversations in relationship with God, His ideas, ways of operating, and people or places He is concerned with. An expression of this communication is stimulated through: spiritual senses as opposed to cognitive or physical ones (externalizing the voice, touch, will, and presence of God within the environment and territory we find ourselves in), navigation of the practice territory (guiding interactions and existence within it as part of performing a life journey, relationship, or role), and critical decision-making (having the embedded text of Christianity, i.e., the Bible, at the forefront of the process to recall, implant, or transfer ideas into cognition or behavior). Evocative and transparent accounts of personal experience within practice through auto-ethnography are gaining momentum for practitioners and researchers, providing opportunity for less stigma and division between service users and providers (Bochner & Ellis, 2016).

Externalization of thought process as a systemic concept is useful in relation to analyzing material and information in ways similar with those in which the video-recorded Goal Decision System (GDS) is used to analyze a disputed goal in a football match. Questions that are posed to aide analysis might be: what is going on here? What are people's positions? What are the rules about positioning and the game (or practice) that aide in this decision-making or explorative process? This system is not used to replace systems or undermine authority (such as that of the referee or workplace managers) but to support what is already being considered.

Use of the GPS as a metaphor also fits the global considerations apparent in higher-ordered thinking within Christianity while acknowledging the free will of the believer to choose a destination and feel in control of the process or journey. There is an inherent invitation from us (believers) to be open to aspects of navigation while knowing we can re-orientate ourselves, get on or off course, or be re-orientated at various points. The significance of movement and navigation is embedded not only in the mental health and supervisory journey but also within the practice and performance paradigm, in addition to life itself. The metaphor does not account, however, for the individual, intimate, and bespoke relationship we develop over time with a living deity (imagined as God in this instance); nevertheless, it provides a useful and symbolic representation of faith and Christian identity for use within mental health and supervisory practice (Williams, 2006). As a concept, the GPS metaphor is still in development and further resonance will be highlighted within ongoing research.

Reflexivity in Clinical and Leadership Practice

Reflexivity is described by Mead (1934) as a "bending back" of self and ideas in action. Self-reflexivity, predominantly introduced within systemic psychotherapy training, can invite curiosity into the conversation, internally, externally, and through cognitive and emotive application. Within systemic psychotherapy training and supervision, resonances in reflexivity and associated processes often begin to take shape, which include: aspects of relational risk-taking (Mason, 2005) in conversations; invitations to externalize inherent conversations and attempts to shift therapeutic impasse (Rober, 1991); and creating useful and productive interventions with clients and supervisees.

Neden (2012) reports that reflexivity is produced within the theory application and the various ways theorists have historically constructed reflexive processes. These differences of emphasis illuminate and impact various aspects of reflexive application within practice. Cognition and social construction are both seen as the main means through which reflexivity is recognized, evaluated, and used; however, it fails to address dimensions of reflexivity in relation to aspects of spiritual identity when considering the self of the therapist and the influence on belief, behavior, and relationship (Becvar, 1997). Neden's positioning in relation to spirituality, helpfully, locates it in relation to a creative and useful resource for shaping and enhancing practice that may have resonance for practitioners and supervisors.

Hedges, (2010) talks about the importance of reflexivity in relation to therapeutic practice and paying attention to the strengths clients bring. Stories and conversations are used to embed conversations which influence, change, and bring new meaning to people requiring support; including the discussion about how the therapist may position themselves in the process. However, other aspects central to the mental health arena remain unexplored through research, such as: the polyphonic aspect of including strengths of practitioner, clients, society, and organizations, and the inclusion of spirituality that moves beyond the naming of demographic labels such as gender, religion, or ethnicity, etc.

Leadership and supervisory styles vary a great deal within religious and spiritually orientated environments. There may be evidence of servant and authentic leadership traits blended within hierarchical styles of leadership, and organizational frameworks alongside collaborative models which have seen the phenomena of the *mega church* being created in both the USA and the UK alike. This shift in the landscape of church growth, predominantly in the black evangelical church community, has led to greater visibility and viability of appropriate service provision for black families (although the term *black* is not seen as a homogenous group), in addition to an economic basis for sustainability that has been lacking from mainstream service provision. Service to others has been recognized as the established framework for church, community, and other religious organizations, for growth and development, and as a vital lifeline of support given the economic downturn and withdrawal of services due to the criteria for access and thresholds of intervention increasing. These spiritually orientated environments foster competence in managing change, tolerating difference, reducing isolation, and accepting the coexistence of faith and fear; hope and despair; and joy and pain, among other resources (Becvar, 1997).

Concepts of faith, religion, and spirituality are often entwined in language discourse and faith for many Christians and are both important aspects of religious positioning and characteristic of a relationship with God, while also being an expression of self and ontological framework (Jakes, 2007). Including spirituality within the conversational space for black families can therefore enhance the practice paradigm; however, there may also be a reluctance or tension about discussing such topics for some practitioners for fear of the potential difficulties in navigating such conversations.

> There is a greater appreciation of how a person's spirituality can be a real source of strength, hope and acceptance. It defines who they are, and helps them derive comfort and find meaning in even the bleakest of situations ... are we deterred from raising the topic of religion for fear of wading into waters too deep, tricky and potentially volatile to navigate? (Bee, 2016, p. 15)

A Supervision Case Example: Staying Connected and Repositioning Practice with the GPS

The nature of spiritual communication and understanding may play a significant role in orientating, shaping, and gaining a sense of control within our practice environment and supervisory relationships. As a potential conduit for ethical practice, spiritual reflexivity has the propensity to offer practitioners a framework for evaluating their connections to faith, beliefs, and ideas that shape change. It challenges practitioners not to only privilege cognition as the main source of academic excellence and ways of knowing and includes dispositional learning; seeking to build a bridge between cognition, spirituality, and embodied/physical practice as one tripartite definition to human experience (spirit, mind, and body). Spiritual reflexivity further gives a voice (as an expression of spirit) to a dimension of self that is often reduced to a religious affiliation or demographic description, juxtaposed to bringing to life the recursive influencing between aspects and dimensions of identity (Williams, 2006).

As spiritual reflexivity draws on the relationship with God (imagined as the one that knows everything about our desires, hopes, and dreams) and His hopes and desires for our lives, it opens internal and external conversations about how useful our current experience and tensions are in shaping our career journey, contribution, and destination. Paying attention to our own spiritual voice, expressed personally as God, and represented through the Holy Spirit, is therefore not seen as self-indulgent but as essential to our inner confidence and external success. Reverential power (defined as a respect for and admiration of God) is also used as a backdrop for identifying and practicing in ethical and authentic ways (Jakes, 2007).

Spiritual reflexivity, is a means by which individuals can hope to remain attuned to nuances of practice, paying attention to the intuitive and embodied experiences that compel us to either keep going or step back from a process if it does not feel, seem, or appear right. Such an intuitive and spiritual experience has already shaped the direction of my own practice and has facilitated me to reposition myself within supervision. (A written account of this practice example and exploration can be found in Appendix 2.)

Purposeful conversation through biblical meditation and prayer can also give a sense of confidence, liberation, and empowerment. To maintain these positions, i.e., directly speaking and listening to God, to invite Him into every situation, remains critical to the journey, like keeping the radio turned down a little while we listen to the instructions at a critical point when using the electronic GPS in the car. Access is never prohibited or unavailable, no matter how deep or into a dead end we get (unlike with the electronic version) (Kebbe, 2012). Spiritual reflexivity (God as a resource) is the passion that may give hope to those feeling despondent, suicidal, or depressed, enabling them to continue the journey.

Creating an Environment for Transformative Practice: Potentiality and Possibility

The dominant discourse in mental health provision has left an over-representation of black people within the mental health system (proportionate to the number of people resident in the UK and the USA); an overdiagnosis of schizophrenia for black African-Caribbean men (Cohen, 1995; Helwick, 2012; Schwartz & Blankenship, 2014); an overuse of pharmacology treatment (Cohen, 1995), and associated stigma and isolation for mental health service users (Mind & Rethink, 2010). Transformation of this reality therefore remains one of the greatest challenges for black mental healthcare providers. An overemphasis and reliance on medical models and the context in which mental health provision is practiced does little to change this experience for children and adults alike. With increasing segregation and individualistic service delivery models that separate family members and divide services based on symptoms, age, and behavior presentation, there has been little scope for maintaining a coherent and integrated approach toward mental health support within mainstream provision (Mind & Rethink, 2010). There is therefore scope to find new and innovative ways of supporting mental and emotional well-being for black children and families in environments more culturally and community orientated.

For families that have a church, community, and extended or surrogate family-based existence, there may be a wealth of support and counsel being offered by members of that community, which may not be readily visible to therapists and social workers assessing and seeking to safeguard their well-being. In addition, the impact and influence of these community members are often marginalized or referenced only as a place for spiritual attunement, seen as being outside the scope of inclusion within clinical practice. This positioning within practice may further serve to isolate individuals from finding integrated and coherent narratives that help to explain their circumstances, resulting in lack of trust or disengagement with the therapist if not explored or prioritized (Boyd-Franklin, 1989).

The context and environment in which clinical work is predominantly practiced are crucial in establishing a conversational space for addressing spiritual and family goals, and for exploring differences between family members. These differences and points of conflict may be resonant in generational perspectives relating to religion, spirituality, identity, or other shared family or community lifestyles in which differences in opinion are common between parents and children. There are many examples of how young people have respected their parent's beliefs and traditions yet manage to challenge and create new environments for expressing their spiritual beliefs and faith within church that include: the introduction of peer mentoring, youth groups, street evangelism, writing and performing music and plays, social media marketing, and developing therapeutic communities of faith. Church organizations such as: Bill Winston Ministries, The Potters House, TD Jakes ministries, Ruach City Church, and Kingsway International Christian Centre have all developed innovative programs on an international stage. These environments are critical in maintaining and establishing positive regard and respect for others and have the potential to be further utilized within the therapeutic, supervisory, and leadership coaching process.

The reinforcement of concepts and ideas through group engagement and decision-making often has greater and longer-lasting emphasis on change. Such potential within systemic practice is referenced as third-order positioning (Hirvonen, 2016) and is in increasing use within mental health provision, often fueled by economic restraints. Communities of faith may have access to additional support services provided by the church and ways of embedding helpful coping strategies, such as prayer, meditation, the use of creative and expressive arts, scripture-based study, narrative (didactic storytelling through sermons), reliance on a *divine other* in times of stress and exhaustion, and a myriad of isomorphic processes which facilitate the positive regard of self and others in action. Such intersections of spirituality within everyday existence are often overlooked as being relevant only within the context of religion juxtaposed with mental health practice. A move toward a more inclusive, coherent, and authentic representation of self is therefore essential to include in clinical applications of spirituality (Caplin, 2002).

The community church environment (particularly in black-led evangelical congregations) has also been a place where individuals can physically express their frustrations, hindrances, and successes in any aspect of life, in loud, vibrant, and physically expressive ways. This might include: shouting, falling on the floor, dancing, running, singing, or clapping. Such behavior might be considered grounds for applying external restraint (including mental health sectioning) in most other places, but in the Pentecostal church it is an acceptable form of worship and expression that is commonplace, irrespective of age, profession, economic, or mental health status. Such behavior may also act as a counteractive component to stigma and isolation that black families often talk about. It helps demonstrate a sense of liberation and feeling of connection and acceptance among peers who take care of their needs and minister to them during the service.

Discrepancies between spiritual ideologies may play out within supervision or consultation sessions as taken-for-granted assumptions about the relevance of spirituality, faith, or religion for clinical practice. This may be positive and relevant if raised by mental health service users; less so when brought to the centrality of discussion for practitioners or managers. These conversations can also be excluded from the conversational space altogether, when seen as something separate to the individual. Deconstructing this in relation to the practice territory and significance of spirituality and reflexivity therefore remains a challenge within clinical and supervisory practice and encourages supervisors to maintain positions of humility and equity within practice (Todd & Storm, 2014).

Embodied Spirituality Within a Mental Health Journey

Teske (2000) describes the human spirit as being socially constructed and acknowledges the limitations of neuropsychology, theology, anthropology, and science to account for the human spirit and identity alone. While there is much resonance to this position, social construction also has limitations to the way in which the nature, experience, and relationship of human spirituality are experienced and expressed by many Christians. Transcendence and embodiment are essential components of spiritual attunement; however, many scholars are unable to account for a level of scientifically unexplained expression linked to identity and culture within spirituality. Connection to God is often described as both internal and external to the human spirit and therefore is not dependent on other human connection but is shaped by it.

Ferrer (2008) discusses the meaning of spiritual embodiment, which he suggests has tenets, such as: integration, realization, awakening, pleasure, an urge to create, an integration of matter and consciousness, etc. While these views expressed in the article are not in full alignment with all Christian perspectives, Ferrer does acknowledge the idea that traditional religious practices have marginalized and disembodied individuals from a more coherent spiritual integration through associated language that sees the body as a hindrance to spiritual growth or in opposition to God's will and purpose. God's will may be interpreted in different ways according to the individual or communities that are using it to define or describe a set of certain events. Philosophically, God's will is referred to in relation to mysterious or unexplained occurrences, things outside of cognitive understanding, particularly in relation to death, destruction, or natural disasters.

Embodied spirituality is seen as redressing the power imbalance between dimensions of self and placing all aspects of human existence on equal footing rather than in competition with each other. Ambiguity and mystery as linguistic concepts are helpful discussion points and are to be embraced in much the same way as McNamee (2015) talks about the management of diversity and complexity to aid being in ethical relationships with others. These second-ordered positions are described by Watzlawick, Weakland, and Fisch (1974), and ways of being a therapeutic practitioner, manager, or researcher offer additional coherence as themes for generating and creating new ways of ethical relational practice.

> *Grounded spiritual visions*: As we have seen, most major spiritual traditions posit the existence of an isomorphism among the human

being, the cosmos, and the Mystery. From this correspondence it follows that the more dimensions of the person that are actively engaged in the study of the Mystery – or of phenomena associated with it – the more complete his or her knowledge will be. This "completion" should not be understood quantitatively but rather in a qualitative sense. In other words, the more human dimensions creatively participate in spiritual knowing, the greater will be the dynamic congruence between inquiry approach and studied phenomena and the more grounded in, coherent with, or attuned to the ongoing unfolding of the Mystery will be our knowledge. (Ferrer, 2008, p. 7)

Embodiment as connected to both spirituality and reflexivity is a critical emerging theme to explore further in research to observe questions and considerations such as, the relevance and place for intuitive or spiritual interventions in therapy and supervision; spirituality and reflexivity as a conduit for embodied practice; and how we create environments that facilitate the expression of embodied spirituality and reflexivity in a world of increasing agile working practices (Caplin, 2002; Todd, 1989). Through paying attention to the embodied nature of spirituality and its expression, supervisors can explore how these concepts connect and assist other practitioners as a valuable resource.

In further development, is the connection with Carberry's (2017) ideas in relation to *"isomorphic mattering"* (juxtaposed to how Bateson, 1972, uses the concept of isomorphism) and how we experience *embodied* moments underpinning *mattering*, which are symbolic of the presence of the Holy Spirit (i.e., the embodied identity of God within us) in our lives. This is what moves us, convicts us, what calls us into "action" and what helps us to gain a sense of authenticity and acknowledgment of individual and collective significance: I, we, matter. Consideration of how or why we might deviate from listening to, or following, God's voice; how we get back on track or on course with our perceived assignment; how diversions might lead to more useful (perhaps quicker) routes of practice (possibly avoiding common misperceptions or aspects of practice that are associated with repeated poor outcomes) – also require attention.

Summary

There remains a critical opportunity to develop culturally competent and sensitive practice that illuminates how spirituality can be addressed within practice for the leader and practitioner alike; reflexive practice offers one such framework for starting to address this phenomenon. Reflexivity, as a core component of systemic practice, facilitates the practitioner to stay connected (in the moment) to the nuances of their own and other people's communication styles, values, and context when intervening in and evaluating situations. It is retrospective, introspective, and future orientated, giving the practitioner an instant opportunity to consider appropriate and useful connection to the mental health or relational dilemma.

The complex interplay between belief, behavior, faith, context, and relationality has been given some attention within both systemic professional practice (Boyd-Franklin in Walsh, 2010) and Christian arenas (Jakes, 2007; Meyer, 1995; Munroe, 1992). Perception of religion as a useful phenomenon is often reduced to a set of traditions and rituals located around church (mosque or temple) and goals synonymous to encouraging others to join the community of practice. Additionally, competing values between religion and reason and a declining role of religion in society over the past four decades have further resulted in some Christian practitioners feeling marginalized in the workplace (Besecke, 2014; Williams, 2006). Adopting spiritually reflexive positions within practice may therefore assist practitioners and supervisors to be less constrained within practice territories and to tap into a wealth of unexplored resources to facilitate transformational change.

The attention to spirituality is not intended to have a narrow applicability to practice relevant to church (often described as a building, location, or religious group) but for *church* reframed as a practitioner, i.e., the embodied church in practice. The question of what counts as ethical and culturally competent practice is therefore intrinsic to this concept, providing an opportunity to develop a more inclusive and coherent narrative around spirituality (Cook et al., 2010).

There is some recognition that mental health services for children and adults require a major reorganization and transformation given they are struggling to meet the increasing need and complexity presented by black service users. Quality, design, and creativity, which involve service users, are increasingly being seen as opportunities to develop services in collaborative ways, creating less distinction, and a more participative framework of delivery. This poses a challenge for managers and leaders of mental health services seeking to uphold ethical and suggested evidence-based practices recommended by National Institute for Health and Care Excellence (NICE) in the UK. Nevertheless, there are ambitious plans to invest in mental health services, reduce waiting times for service users, and address the cultural needs of black communities as part of the "*Five Year Forward*" report produced by the Independent Mental Health Task Force (2015). When conversations relating to spirituality are included and explored within the conversational space of therapists, supervisors, trainers, and researchers, it can open up a wealth of possibilities and connections linked to the self of the practitioner, support systems, empowerment, cultural competence, and management of diversity. When used respectfully (as with any other epistemological or ontological framework) within the mental health arena, it can provide a rich context and environment for internal, external, and relational transformation to occur.

Including the matrix of spirituality and reflexivity, provides practitioners with the opportunity to continually develop their practice in ways that are adaptable, responsive, inclusive, and coherent with their own sense of authenticity, recognizing that these are not fixed phenomena and are emerging as significant tenets of psychotherapeutic practice. For black professionals, service users, and families, there are added benefits of integration and recognition that lives are connected, identities evolving and shaping existence, and lived experience is more than a mental health status.

Mental and emotional emancipation, the freedom to be our authentic self, is deeply embedded within black culture, history, relationships, and existence. Spiritual reflexivity seeks to embrace this concept to shed the restrictive, divisive, and reductionist language often ascribed when referencing black and minority ethnic populations (a term I seek to avoid where possible as it brings with it a perception of reduced numerical relevance and significance). Changing professional thinking (theoretical modalities), practice (theoretical application), and associated research (questioning and exploring), is required if we are to realize goals synonymous with transforming for the better the lived experience of black mental health service users and the overall community. These treatment goals are in line with use of systemic and counseling models as evidence-based practice in the UK and invite an alternative perspective for the inclusion of spirituality in a variety of practice and community settings.

It is further hoped that spiritual reflexivity might be equally applicable to those outside of any religious framework and remains relevant for those who may privilege the voice of the universe or other spiritual phenomena associated within black mental health. The conversational style of spiritual reflexivity is also represented in systemic practice as ethical discourse in action as part of the supervisory and leadership paradigm (Todd & Storm, 2014).

Spirituality, addressed as a form of cultural competence, can therefore provide a useful framework, not only for collaboration within the black community but as a historical component of black community cohesion and access to support. Consideration of how these concepts might assist professionals within leadership and organizational development as part of addressing black mental health service provision (in addition to how they might shape the associated discourse) is therefore a much-needed paradigm to consider within further research.

References

Alvesson, M., & Skoldberg, K. (2009). Reflexive methodology. In *New vistas for qualitative research* (2nd ed., p. 30). London: Sage Publications.

Anderson, H. (1997). *Conversations, language and possibilities*. New York, NY: Basic Books.

Bateson, G. (1972). *Steps to an ecology of mind: Collected essays in anthropology, psychiatry, evolution and epistemology*. Chicago, IL: University of Chicago Press.

Becvar, D. (1997). *A spiritual orientation in counselling and therapy*. New York, NY: Basic Books.

Bee, M. (2016). *Professional social work* (pp. 14–15). London: BASW.

Besecke, K. (2014). *You can't put God in a box: Thoughtful spirituality in a rational age*. London: Oxford University Press.

Bochner, A., & Ellis, C. (2016). *Evocative autoethnography. Writing lives and telling stories*. Oxon: Routledge.

Boyd-Franklin, N. (1989). *Black families in therapy*. New York, NY: Guilford Press.

Brown, D. (2001). Quotes from Louis Farrakhan. *The Guardian*, July 31. Retrieved from https://www.theguardian.com/uk/2001/jul/race.world1.

Caplin, H. (Ed.). (2002). *The philosophy of mental representation*. London: Clarendon University Press.

Carberry, K. (2017). Presentation: Workshop certificate in parenting: Haitian families of the Caribbean and isomorphic mattering. The University of Bedfordshire Postgraduate winter conference 2017. Unpublished paper.

Cohen, S. (1995). Over diagnosis of schizophrenia: Role of alcohol and drug misuse. *The Lancet, 346*(8989), 1541–1543.

Cook, C., Powell, A., & Sims, A. (Eds.). (2010). *Spirituality and psychiatry*. London: The Royal College of Psychiatrists.

Cook, C., Powell, A., & Sims, A. (Eds.). (2016). *Spirituality and narrative in psychiatry practice*. London: The Royal College of Psychiatrists.

Divac, J., & Heaphy, G. (2005). Space for GRRAACCES. *Journal of Family Therapy, 27*, 280–284.

Drew, P. (2016). Opportunities and challenges: The intersection of faith and human rights of LGBTI persons. *Wilton Park Newsletter*. UK: Arcus Foundation.

Elliott-Griffith, M. (1995). Opening therapy to conversations with a personal God. In F. Walsh (Ed.), *Spiritual resources in family therapy* (p. 2003). New York, NY: The Guilford press.

Ferrer, J. N. (2008). What does it mean to live a fully embodied spiritual life? *International Journal of Transpersonal Studies 27*(1), 1–11. San Francisco, CA: California Institute of Integral Studies.

Francis, J. (2016). *Walking in your assignment: Finding your purpose and destiny*. Aberdeen: Cross House Books.

Garrett, J. (2007). Aristotle on metaphor: Excerpts from poetics and rhetoric. NP 28 Web 29 September 2014. Retrieved from http://people.wku.edu/jan.garrett/401s07/arismeta.htm

Gordon, R. (1999). A short history of the "critical" in critical race theory. *American Philosophy Association Newsletter, 98*(2). Retrieved from http://readingfanon.blogspot.com/2011/06/short-history-of-critical.html

Harre R. (2012). Positioning theory: Moral dimensions pf social cultural psychology. In J. Valsiner (Ed.), *The Oxford handbook of culture and psychology* (pp. 191–206). New York, NY: Oxford University Press.

Hedges, F. (2010). *Reflexivity in therapeutic practice*. London: Palgrave.

Helwick, C. (2012). *Schizophrenia may be over diagnosed in black patients*. New York, NY: National Mental Association, Annual Convention and Scientific Assembly.

Hirvonen, P. (2016). *Positioning theory and small-group interaction: Social and task positioning in the context of joint decision-making*. Thousand Oaks, CA: Sage.

Holy Bible – King James Version. (1998). Ann Arbor, MI: Michigan World Publishing.

Jafari, S. (2016). Spirituality and social change. Religion and spirituality within a counselling/clinical psychology training programme: A systematic review. *British Journal of Guidance and Counselling, 44*(3), 257–267.

Jakes, T. D. (2007). *Reposition yourself. Living life without limits*. New York, NY: Atria Books.

Kebbe, L. (2012). Keep the conversation going. A study of conversational spaces during family business succession. Ph.D. thesis, University of Bedfordshire. Retrieved from http://uobrep.openrepository.com/uobrep/handle/10547/234472

Liddle, H. A., & Saba, G. W. (1983). On context replication: The isomorphic relationship of training and therapy. *Journal of Strategic and Systemic Therapies, 2*, 3–11.

Marley, R. (1980). *Redemption song. Legend album*. Kingston: Island Records.

Mason, B. (2005). Relational risk-taking and the training of supervisors. *Journal of Family Therapy, 27*, 298–301.

McNamee, S. (2015). Ethics as discursive potential. *Journal of Family Therapy, 36*, 419–433.

Mead, G. H. (1934). *Mind, self and society* (1st ed.). London: University of Chicago Press.

Meyer, J. (1995). *Battlefield of the mind. Winning the battle in your mind.* London: Hodder & Stoughton.
Mind and Rethink. (2010). *A report into attitudes towards mental health problems in the South Asian community in Harrow, North West London.* London: King's College.
Munroe, M. (1992). *Unleash your purpose.* Nassau: Destiny Image Publishers.
Neden, J. (2012). *Reflexivity dialogues: An inquiry into how reflexivity is constructed in IT education.* Newcastle: Northumbria University.
NHS England. (2015). *The five year forward view mental health task force.* London.
O'Hagan, K. (2001). *Cultural competence.* London: Jessica Kingsley Publishers Ltd.
Osbourne, G. (1991). *The hermeneutic spiral. A comprehensive introduction to Biblical interpretation.* Chicago, IL: Intervarsity Press.
Rober, P. (1991). The therapist's inner conversation in family therapy practice: Some ideas about the self of the therapist, therapeutic impasse and the process of reflection. *Family Process, 38*, 209–228.
Sawyer, R. D., & Norris, J. (2016). *Forms of practitioner reflexivity. Critical, conversational & arts-based approaches.* London: Palgrave Macmillan.
Schwartz, R., & Blankenship, D. M. (2014). Racial disparities in psychotic disorder diagnosis: A review of empirical literature. *World Journal of Psychiatry, 4*(4), 133–140.
Taylor, M. (2016). Toward an explanation of spiritual reflexivity: The GPS for Christian practitioners. Presentation at the 12th annual International Congress for Qualitative Inquiry, Chicago, and subsequent unpublished paper/s.
Teske, J. (2000). The social construction of the human spirit. In N. Gregerson, W. Drees, & U. Gorman (Eds.), *The human person in science and theology.* (pp. 189–213). Edinburgh: T&T Clarke Ltd.
Todd, T. (1989). *Becoming isomorphic: A model for family therapy. Retrospective theses and dissertation.* Paper No. 11168. Iowa State University, Ames, IA.
Todd, T., & Storm, C. (Eds.). (2014). *The complete systemic supervisor. Context, philosophy and pragmatics* (2nd ed.). Chichester: John Wiley & Sons Ltd.
Tomm, K., Hoyt, M., & Madigan, S. (1998). Honouring our internalized others and the ethics of caring: A conversation with Karl Tomm. In M. Hoyt (Ed.), *The handbook of constructive therapies* (pp. 198–218). San Francisco, CA: Jossey-Bass Publishers.
Van Dijk, T. A. (Ed.). (1985). *Handbook of discourse analysis.* London: Academic Press.
Walsh, F., (2010). Spiritual resources in family therapy. In N. Boyd-Franklin (Ed.), *Incorporating spirituality and religion into the treatment of African American clients* (2nd ed.). New York, NY: Guilford Press.
Watzlawick, P., Weakland, J., & Fisch, R., (1974). *Change: Principles of problem formation and resolution.* New York, NY: W W Norton & Co.
Williams, R. (2006). What we mean by Christian identity: World Council of Churches address. Retrieved from http://rowanwilliams.archbishopofcanterbury.org/articles.php/1781/what-we-mean-by-christian-identity-world-council-of-churches-address

Appendix 1: Poem

Faith

Faith is a seed, plant it
Faith is a servant, put it to work
Faith is a hope, have it
Faith is a currency, spend it
Faith is blameless, free it
Faith is truth, believe it
Faith dictates time, set it
Faith is a shield, wear it
Faith is your partner, honor it
Faith is gift, receive it
Faith is understanding, get it
Faith is courageous, stand on it
Faith is God, embrace Him!

I allow God to excite my imagination and embrace the challenge.
I bring forth good things by speaking them out, from God!

My future is in my heart and in no one else's hands. No one can stop me or keep me from my destiny.

My heart is my spirit.
This is the diversity of my faith

Maureen Greaves (formerly Taylor) 2015

Appendix 2: A Narrative From My Research Supervision Journal

Within mental health practice we may get into moments of maintaining the momentum of activity, even when it doesn't feel right. How do we end up veering off track? Are we listening to voices that we had previously learned to drown out? Or is it our own voice, wanting to explore new and possibly different paths that look interesting? Whatever the myriad of answers, I have found myself "off track" and ignoring the embodied experience of a voice saying do you really want to go this way?!

One such experience during the research process happened as I began to prepare a work assignment. I remember thinking I had to decide between research focusing on two binary choices of therapeutic practice or leadership, I opted for leadership, as this was the direction of travel I find myself more immersed, in relation to everyday practice as a supervisor and CEO. I had somehow forgotten to incorporate the *both-and* rather than *either-or* dichotomy in trying to meet what I considered to be the assessment requirements. Furthermore, I found myself becoming stuck in a narrative about leadership being the central focus while writing about something else. Not only was it the not yet said (Anderson, 1997) but the not yet named and the not quite relevant! It was like driving around a roundabout several times before noticing the sign that says, "this is the direction you want to take" ... or passing the picturesque village along the way and making an impromptu stop to look around and have lunch. Recognising the focus is just a part of the whole journey and my purpose is greater than the sum of parts, or stops that I make (Bateson, 1972) I came to a critical point in which I needed to hear clearly the voice of God on the journey and to differentiate this from all the other voices I had heard along the way, including my own.

Within supervision several questions were posed in relation to: Where is it I desired to get to? What is it that I want? What is it that's congruent with the voice of God, the spiritual GPS. I too was listening intently and ready to trust the answer (since listening to the voice of the supervisor alone did not appear to be bringing forth the desired congruency). I remember thinking that, for me, congruency without desire and authenticity, that is, staying true to my original desires and goals is not going to bring the desired outcome. Staying connected to what inspires me (the spirit in motion) became central to the desired goal.

I was guided in using the internalized other intervention (Tomm, Hoyt, & Madigan, 1998) by one of my supervisors who respectfully suggested this as a means of connecting with the voice of God. During this moment the story of the original desired destination emerged and I felt an overwhelming senses of relief, power, and revelation at the same time. It was my voice, yet God's words, repositioning me and reminding me of my (and His) original desire on starting the practice journey. It emerged that everything I needed was already given (i.e., the navigation) however, my default position was to seek what was "expected" from others; respectfully adhering to expectations of others that appear to know what is best for me. Whatever the reason/s the important thing for me is: the GPS (or the supervisors) did not interfere with my free will at any point but allowed me to go through the experience and used the learning and journey to not only reposition myself but to bring me back to the place I needed to be. It was like standing at the beginning and being exactly where I needed to be at the same time. Time was not an issue. I already had all the material, I just needed to slightly adjust the language to fit the topic inherent in the conversations I had already had with God.

I will take the lesson of this experience forward as keeping me connected to the practice that drives me. It is not defined as therapy or supervision alone (although these are two of the distinct things I do and enjoy), but a range of practice that is synonymous with collaborating with others to contribute to a range of health and social care practice problems, community growth, and development of new and more integrated services. Practice for me is both autonomous and community-based simultaneously and as such brings the influence and passion of God into daily living by helping others to realize their purpose and passion, respectively. These are not competing goals or goals just relevant to people that identify with a Christian identity but for many communities.

Chapter 16

'Marginal Leaders': Making Visible the Leadership Experiences of Black Women in a Therapeutic Service for Disenfranchised Young People

Romana Farooq and Tânia Rodrigues

> [...] living as we did – on the edge – we developed a particular way of seeing reality. We looked both from the outside and in from the inside out ... we understood both.
>
> (hooks, 1984, p. viii)

Introduction

Delivering effective mental health services for children, young people and families is a key priority in the UK (DoH, 2015a). In line with this there has been significant focus on providing therapeutic services for vulnerable children, young people and their families, in particular those subject to child sexual abuse and child sexual exploitation (CSE) (DoH, 2015b). Following this and the growing public concern around CSE, the government launched a programme to invest significant funding to develop more effective ways of supporting vulnerable, children, young people and their families (DfE, 2014a, 2014b, 2014c). This resulted in funding being allocated to develop a sub-regional delivery model to provide innovative therapeutic support to children and young people at risk of or subject to sexual exploitation in a high risk geographical area.

The proposal included the recruitment, development and support of specific foster carers to provide safe placements for young people across the South Yorkshire sub-region. Intensive wrap-around support and therapeutic services were to be made available to help sustain such placements. A similar offer was made for young people who could safely remain at home with their families. As evidence suggests that a strong supportive parent is one of the best indicators of recovery from abuse and violence (Hill, Stafford, Seaman, Ross, & Daniel, 2007), skilling up professionals to support parents and carers through a range of different interventions was seen as a means to minimise family and placement breakdown. One of the geographical areas for which funding was awarded was Rotherham.

Professor Alexis Jay's inquiry into CSE in Rotherham (2014) recommended that a strategic approach to protecting children who were sexually exploited should be adopted and that cross-boundary solutions should be found. As such, it was felt that by adopting a sub-regional approach to tackling these issues, learning and best practice could be applied across all four authorities and solutions could be adopted to ensure positive outcomes for children and young people affected by these issues.

These proposals had the support of senior leaders and lead cabinet members across all local authorities/trust. The regional police also endorsed the proposal alongside key partners. Governance arrangements had been confirmed through each of the local safeguarding children's boards in addition to the CSE regional forum. A newly established CSE management board was strategically responsible for overseeing the implementation of the proposal with an operational board reporting to them who would manage the day-to-day delivery of the project.

Strategically there was a sound and coherent plan; however, operationally, the lack of understanding or perhaps the lack of awareness to cultural and contextual realities within each of the local authorities/trust leads to significant challenges. It became apparent that despite there being a drive and willingness to improve the lives of vulnerable children, young people and their families and being committed to working in a collaborative and inclusive manner, the understanding of what this process entailed and the systems supporting staff teams achieving such tasks were often contradictory and imbued within a patriarchal, top down and cost-saving approach. This experience was in line with what Bell (2002) highlighted in her research study looking at promoting children's rights through a relationship-based model. The paper highlighted that the 'dominant value-base for social services departments today is business efficiency rather than the human rights of the child' (Bell, 2002, p. 2), emphasising the systemic pressures on professionals when trying to address or work with vulnerable children and young people. In addition to deeply entrenched rigid systems directly affecting professionals practice within each local authority/trust there was also the issue of the moral dimension of sexual abuse/exploitation which has remained implicit rather than explicit. Meaning that common sense morality has often been applied without analysis.

CSE: A UK Context

CSE is a form of child sexual abuse. It occurs where an individual or group takes advantage of an imbalance of power to coerce, manipulate or deceive a child or young person under the age of 18 into sexual activity in exchange for something the victim needs or wants, and/or for the financial advantage or increased status of the perpetrator or facilitator. The child or young person may have been sexually exploited even if the sexual activity appears consensual (DfE, 2017). It can also involve violence, coercion, degradation and intimidation, with threats of actual or perceived physical harm or humiliation. CSE can happen in both online and offline contexts, such as through the use of technology. In law, there's no specific crime of sexual exploitation. Perpetrators are often convicted for associated offences such as sexual activity with a child. Therefore, it has not been possible to obtain accurate figures of the scale of the problem from police statistics (Berelowitz, Firmin, Edwards, & Gulyurtlu, 2012). The lack of clarity in legislation alongside the deeply entrenched patriarchal morality leads both boys and girls to continue minimising their own experiences of abuse. We live in a patriarchal world. We also live in a world where the sexual abuse of children is endemic. These two issues are deeply connected and unfortunately, as a society we will not significantly reduce the incidence of sexual abuse of children – boys and girls – until we challenge the rules and narratives of patriarchy itself.

Although the eradication of sexual abuse of children and young people has been a national priority within the UK for a number of years, it wasn't until 2014 and following a number of Public Inquiries (Casey, 2015; Jay, 2014) in to the systematic sexual exploitation of children and young people, that CSE was placed on the agenda as a national public concern. The Jay Report (2014) found that due to significant failings within the local council, police, and children's services, an estimated 1,400 children were likely to have been victims of CSE. In South Yorkshire, the publication of the report drew a long period of national, political and media attention to the town and local authority of Rotherham.

However, although the independent inquiries highlighted the systematic failures of child protection agencies to protect and safeguard vulnerable young people, they were criticised for marginalising diverse communities and neglecting the experience of minority girls and women subject to sexual violence (Gohir, 2013). The dominant narrative in the UK amongst the public and the media has been around Black and Asian men systematically grooming and exploiting White girls through organised street-based gangs. These dominant narratives have led to moral panic in relation to groups of 'South Asian men', Black and Asian communities and a general hostility towards diverse communities (Harrison & Gill, 2015).

The Diverse Leadership Deficit

A recent article in *The Guardian* (2017) highlighted that there is a lack of diversity at senior levels within social care, in particular that

> it's not that Black, Asian and Minority Ethnic (BAME) people are under-represented in the workforce – they constitute an estimated 17%, rising to 59% in London – but they are few and far between at senior levels.

Leadership, or rather the lack of it, is a recurrent theme in our lives as Black women. We often ask ourselves how are leaders created? How do we overcome the systemic and structural biases that have resulted in our current crisis of leadership? How do we nurture and develop diverse leaders who transmit our values of inclusion and social justice? In a post-Brexit reality of hostility to multiculturalism, to equality and within a climate of economic uncertainty it is important to understand and consider the intersectionality of race, gender and politics when seeking answers and implementing solutions to these fundamental leadership concerns. In addition, it is crucial to accept that the dissonance between ideals and reality is indeed harsh and requires ongoing debate.

Leadership has been defined in various ways often reflecting the professional and personal orientations of their authors. Most definitions share a focus on a process of interpersonal influence that uses power and authority to encourage others to act to achieve goals (Yukl, 2009). Although men and leadership have been studied extensively, women, especially Black women, have only become a topic of research within the last two decades and even then, the influence of race and ethnicity were largely undermined (Chemers, 1997). Although it is beyond the scope of this chapter to discuss or examine the barriers leading to the advancement of (Black) women leaders, it is important to highlight that the racial and gender discrimination that Black women face involves a trajectory of diverse challenges and setbacks rather than following a straight line to the top. Women can achieve leadership positions but only through careful negotiation and compromise as they confront issues associated with pregnancy and child care needs, racism, sexism and discrimination on the basis of religious and sexual identity.

Who Are We?

We are two Black women, feminists, qualified clinical psychologists of differing level of experience, trained in different countries but both practicing in the UK and both passionate about social justice and social empowerment. Despite our age difference and professional trajectory, our personal and professional journey has been one shaped by social injustice and discrimination which has undoubtedly influenced our practice and our narrative.

Romana Farooq – I am a Black woman, Kashmiri, Muslim who works clinically with survivors of human rights-based violations, gender-based violence and sexual violence within the National Health Service. I have worked with children, young people and their families who have been subject to sexual violence both in the statutory and voluntary sectors. I have worked with grassroots communities and community leaders to co-develop services and to support them in influencing existing service provision. I am currently working with children and young people who present with high risk, high harm and high vulnerability in the community as well as those who have been deprived of their liberty within the Children's Secure Estate.

Tânia Rodrigues – I am an African-Euro-Asian Black woman with 15 years' experience working with both men and women experiencing mental health difficulties both working in the community and within mental health forensic settings. I am currently working clinically with women offenders within HMP Services and working clinically with young people in foster care survivors of domestic violence and sexual violence. I also offer training to social care staff on how to develop a trauma informed service and support young people with mental health needs.

How Did Our Paths Cross?

In 2015, a charity organisation was commissioned to develop a therapeutic model to work with 'hard to reach youth' and their families tackling CSE. The advert to recruit a clinical lead for the project was advertised twice during a period of six months as it was difficult to find a match between the role and skill set of those interested in the role. The second role involved a clinical psychologist to support the clinical lead in the development and delivery of the model and service.

At the time the roles were advertised, Tânia was working as the female service clinical lead for a private mental health organisation offering psychological services for females with a dual diagnosis of personality disorder and/or mental illness/forensic history. Year after year women admitted to the services presented with a long-standing history of trauma and abuse, clinicians often highlighted how there had been several missed opportunities during their younger years for interventions to have been delivered with a potentially better long-term impact. In comparison, Romana was in her final year of completing her doctorate in clinical psychology, she was working clinically with refugees and asylum seeking women and children escaping trafficking, human rights-based violations and gender-based violence and had come to the realisation that traditional services were not accessible to the most vulnerable and had a passion to do psychology differently.

The roles and the opportunity to develop an innovative model of working with vulnerable young people and their families as well as having the opportunity of supporting staff teams understand these young people's experiences and needs felt like a chance to practice psychology differently and to develop an inclusive yet curious culture. This was also a huge responsibility. In order to take on just a challenge having a cohesive core team is crucial. Unfortunately, due to timeframes, the recruitment process was done independently and team members joined at different times.

We already met in post. We started talking about our previous work experiences and despite the differences in age and level of experience we were surprised by some of the similarities in both of our professional and personal experiences. We were both fascinated with how our personal journeys had shaped our professional stance and our commitment to social justice. There and then we knew that any therapeutic model had to embrace our previous experiences and be rooted within principles of community psychology and Afrocentric practice.

How we describe ourselves will hopefully reveal aspects of our identities and experiences which we feel have significantly shaped us as professionals but above all as human beings. In sharing parts of our histories and narratives we have undoubtedly consciously or unconsciously processed and ascribed meaning to such experiences and that meaning has created a narrative by which we experience ourselves and others in the world. It is no surprise, that the areas in which we work are inherently linked to our own personal and professional journeys. This chapter presents our own personal reflections on our experiences and we felt it would be helpful to share the process of writing this chapter as we felt it was central to its content. We felt it was important that we didn't present our experiences in a sanitised, clinical or palatable manner, however, we were also mindful that as Black women we often don't talk about our experiences because of our sensitivity to other people's anxieties and feelings of guilt or anger. Therefore, the aim of this chapter was to make visible our leadership experiences as Black women and to facilitate an understanding of how race, racism, gender and class intersect and impact on that experience.

> When I dare to be powerful — to use my strength in the service of my vision, then it becomes less and less important whether I am afraid.
>
> (Audre Lorde, 1984)

Reflections on Becoming *'Leaders'*

Romana Farooq

I am a Muslim, Kashmiri, British-born, working class feminist. I have always identified as a Black working class Muslim woman and recognise that gender and cultural identity are social constructs (Campbell, 2010; Stoltenberg, 2000). I grew up in one of the most deprived and poverty stricken urban areas in the UK, namely Bradford. It is one of the largest and most densely populated areas in the UK outside of London, it has a relatively high population of Black, Asian and minority ethnic (BAME groups, low levels of economic activity and educational qualifications and high levels of social deprivation in the inner city area (Darlow et al., 2005). During the first 15 years of my life, I witnessed significant political unrest, racial tensions and marginalisation. I distinctly remember feeling fearful, anxious and powerless as a child during the Pennine Disturbances in 2001. This involved a series of riots across Northern cities in the UK, one of which included Bradford. The Bradford riots were an intense period of rioting and political and personal unsettlement which occurred between the large and growing British Asian community and the City's White majority. The conflict was initiated and escalated by far rights groups such as the British National Party and the National Front.

Despite this I was raised in a family and community where politics, feminism and being Black were important and embraced. However, in contrast in school and college I experienced profound silencing around issues of gender, ethnicity and race despite the growing tensions in the City. I felt and experienced this as a contradiction, a double bind, a sense that something horrific was happening to my community but that others in positions of relative power (teachers, leaders, etc.) did not 'see' it or want to create a space to talk about it. During my studies, I searched every reading list for a name that resonated with my own, that was 'different' like me and I found none. It wasn't until I started university and experienced some freedom in respect of reading what interested me that I came across authors like Toni Morrison, Paulo Freire, Frantz Fanon and Heidi Safia Mirza. How could I have gone through so many years of schooling and not realised that someone like me could write a book or be a leader?

During my training for the doctorate in clinical psychology, I attended a predominantly White institution, my tutors highlighted how influencing others and systems was one of the core competencies of a clinical psychologist, but I never felt that any of the literature, representations of an influential leader or the teaching ever resonated with me. I didn't see myself as the 'typical leader' that was being presented to us. I'm not White, middle class, loud, powerful, expert or demanding. I believe in restoring hope, resiliency and meaningfulness, I love honesty, diversity and justice, not just for their effect on personal circumstances, but for their effect on the world, the whole human experience. Does that mean that I could never be a leader?

During my life and my studies I regularly had to endure other people's overt and covert prejudices around 'Asian', 'Muslim' and 'Pakistani' people, but in particular their prejudices around 'Asian and Pakistani women'. In school, college and then in professional contexts, I felt unprepared when I realised that most of the White people I studied or worked with saw me as inferior to them and as not worthy of being at college, university or as I discovered later on in my life not good enough to be a clinical psychologist. My peers hid their dismay when I achieved better results in both my GCSE's and A levels and then my university tutor told me not to 'hold my breath' when I expressed interest in becoming a clinical psychologist. Although my family and my immediate community encouraged me to work hard and always held hope that I would do well, that didn't stop me from being plagued with self-doubt. I struggled with my voice, both finding it and using it with confidence. I felt confused about why I was positioned as inferior and why I had to experience so many barriers in comparison to my White peers.

In 1940, almost 60% of employed African-American women were in roles termed 'domestics'. The 1970 census was the first time this category of work did not contain the largest segment of the Black female labour force (Rollins, 1985). So of course for our White colleagues seeing me in a profession that wasn't the stereotypical Black work would appear 'unusual'.

Although I have personal experiences of marginalisation and racism, the primary wounds that I carry of discrimination and racism are as a witness. As a child, I witnessed teachers and other professionals ignore and undermine my mother, for whom English was not her first language. I remember a White teacher who taught my younger brother in primary school who went out of her way to publicly humiliate my mother every time we turned up to collect him from class. I remember asking my mother why she frequently did this to which my mum gently held my hand, softly smiled and said 'don't worry, she's doing her job, teachers do something wonderful, they give us education, they help us learn'. I remember in that moment feeling very cross with my mother for dismissing what I believed as a child to be rude and unacceptable behaviour. However, it wasn't until I grew into adulthood and really understood my parents' simple acts of kindness did I fully understand what they were doing. They were surviving.

So when I first qualified as a clinical psychologist and found myself in a role in which I would be 'leading' or 'shaping' a therapeutic service for disenfranchised young people, I sat with both excitement and dread. I was excited that I would have the opportunity to 'do differently' for disadvantaged and marginalised young people but I also carried with me the overt and covert prejudices I had both experienced and witnessed in my life, could I actually be a leader? Could I influence? Could I make a difference? Are women like me heard? Will my voice matter and do I have power?

Patricia Hill Collins (1986) speaks about the importance of Black women's self-definition and self-valuation and the benefits of placing greater trust in the creative potential of our personal and cultural biographies. I had to draw on my own personal and cultural biography and construct for myself what type of leader I wanted to become. That is not to say that my own experiences of trying to assert myself with my White colleagues didn't influence my understanding of what was 'acceptable' for me to do. I distinctly remember an interaction with a White male middle class supervisor in which I tried to assert myself, we were having a conversation around my job and job planning in which I asked him to be more specific about what he meant by 'developmental and developmental milestones' and what that would look like in my job. He responded by describing my request for clarity as having a 'sense of entitlement' and when I tried to share my confusion around how seeking clarity had anything to do with having a sense of entitlement, he spoke over me and privileged his experience of the interaction. This reminded me of the words of bell hooks (1990):

> No need to hear your voice when I can talk about you better than you can speak about yourself ... I want to know your story. And then I will tell it back to you...in such a way that ... I am still author, authority. I am still the colonizer, the speak subject, and you are now at the centre of my talk. (p. 151)

I can recall multiple examples of interactions in which as a Black woman I have been silenced, undermined and dismissed. It was these experiences that influenced my ability and sense of leadership. However, I have always recognised that my ability to feel safe and reflect on some of the challenges that I experienced in shaping this service as well as my leadership style was only made possible by the fact that I was supervised and mentored by a Black woman. There is significant evidence that Black women supporting other Black women as mentors or supervisors can have a positive impact on career progression as well as aid in developing their full leadership potential (Counts, 2012). For me it was pivotal that I was supported by someone who understood my experience of oppression, microaggressions and marginalisation as well as recognised the importance of giving me permission to develop my own unique leadership style.

During the implementation of this community-based therapeutic service I was mindful that phrases like 'the police are here to protect and serve', 'child and adolescent mental health services are for all children' and 'children's services support and safeguard vulnerable families' are indeed contradictory to the experience of a great proportion of disadvantaged and disenfranchised communities in the UK. Children from BAME communities are more likely to live in neighbourhoods that are afflicted with social problems such as poverty, political unrest, crime and deprivation. These children and young people often don't experience services as accessible and don't feel they can trust professionals that operate within them. I inhabited both a space within these communities and neighbourhoods as well as a space within professional services, making me an 'outsider within'. This gave me access to a special 'insight' into oppressed groups (Hartsock, 1983) due to my own personal and cultural history.

To understand some of the challenges faced when setting up and implementing this innovative therapeutic model as well as having our voice heard and taken seriously, we felt it was important to consider how race, gender and class intersect. King (1988) speaks of the multiple jeopardies and disadvantages that Black women experience due to their multiple disadvantaged and subordinate identities in society. The limitation that our subordinate roles/identities placed on us was evident every time we attended senior management meetings to discuss our service model. Sometimes I wondered if we would have had such difficulty convincing other organisations to work alongside us if we had been White middle class men pitching the importance of the service for vulnerable children and young people. Van Dijk (1993) states:

> Elites have the means to manufacture consent ... this does not mean that all opinions of elites are always adopted by the public at large, but only that their opinions are well known, that they have the most effective means of public persuasion and the best resources for suppressing or marginalising alternative opinions (p. 45)

Tânia Rodrigues

I am an African-Euro-Asian feminist Black woman and I am also a mother, a wife, a clinician, a supervisor, a daughter and a friend. My heritage informs and shapes my every role and reminds me of my greatest responsibilities. My partner is White British and our son was born in Britain. As a Black woman of mixed heritage within a multi-racial relationship I embarked on a journey of self-discovery as well as the ever so daunting responsibility of educating and imparting values, a moral code and a philosophy of life. As a mother of a child growing up in a predominantly White community it is important to me that my son is aware of his heritage and the struggles that many face every day to understand and acknowledge our White privilege. How can a Black woman refer to 'White privilege' one might ask? I am a Black woman with a mixed heritage and brown skin and I am aware that this mixed heritage afforded me the opportunity to experience life from a unique perspective, but this has also heightened my responsibility to use my White privilege to give voice to those that do not have it. Identifying myself as a Black feminist is an act of resistance towards the patriarchal systems and institutions we find ourselves navigating through in the course of our lives.

I feel sick when I see power abused. I feel sick and I feel angry. I 'feel' sick and angry because this abuse triggers old and repressed memories of a reality I haven't been part of for many years now ... or have I? I fled one reality in search of a more liberal, more inclusive, more enlightened reality and what did I find?

A first world country with immense opportunities, scientific advances and economic and social stability. I was born in Southern Africa, Angola. It took me years to understand my identity and that too came with many challenges and struggles. My heritage is diverse. I was born in Africa but I wasn't dark enough to fit in with the other kids in the neighbourhood and my parents, though working class, had far more available resources than most in the neighbourhood so, that too made me 'different'. I spent part of my childhood in Europe and lived with my grandparents. My grandfather was White, but in Europe I wasn't light-skinned enough. Back at home my skin tone was a reminder of colonisation. That sense of being somewhat different became apparent very early on and with that an awareness of injustice, difference, shame and anger. I grew up between Africa and Europe and remained a keen observer of how my appearance and my manner impacted on others. I was always very opinionated. At school I was known by all my teachers because I was as much of a good student as I was a 'rebel' – I spoke out. I lived within a communist regime. I experienced war. And yet, I was privileged, others did not have the same access to safety, health and food. As life unfolded I became more and more aware of the interplay between power, gender, race, class, religion and how these different facets are used to assess and label different groups of people. I found myself navigating through different 'labels' depending on context. A part of me took pride in having this chameleon-like attribute but another part of me felt like a voyeur complacent in the separatism and discrimination of others. Every time I was 'taken in' by a certain group of people I was privy to their perception/discrimination of another group. At times, I found myself powerless and angry but then, I too abused power – I have hurt others, ignored their needs or have controlled and manipulated others to give into my needs, my wants. I noticed how when feeling desperate or afraid I too used my power to control others and this made me feel ashamed and guilty. Maybe, I was no different from those I was angry with. Or, maybe having this knowledge, being reflective about my own use/abuse of power meant there was a chance for me to do things differently. I realised that one person cannot change the world but if I could change/improve one person's experience in the world then I had made a difference. I wanted to make a difference. I still do.

When I finished high school I wanted to be a clinical psychologist but fate would have it that my 'emotional baggage' was holding me back. Academically, I was a strong candidate but emotionally, my repressed anger, shame and guilt seemed to seep through and I was told that I wasn't yet ready to embark on such a demanding and strenuous training. That was a harsh reality to deal with but it opened other doors and I decided to pursue a master's degree in gender studies. This course was an empowering and cathartic experience as it allowed me to make sense of my own experiences but above all it introduced me to a woman that would shape my view of Black women leaders – Professor Amina Mama. Being taught by this confident Nigerian-British feminist, intellectual, researcher and author not only opened my horizons to Afrocentrism and the notion of 'feminisms', but also, it allowed me to take on a more inquisitive approach to learning and more importantly to reflect on the political struggles informing such learning. My previous 'rebellious' identity had finally been given a meaning.

After completing my gender studies at the University of Cape Town, a predominantly White university I was accepted for my clinical training in psychology at the University of the Western Cape, a Black university with a strong history of creative struggle against oppression, discrimination and disadvantage. It was during this time that I was exposed to community psychology and I became increasingly aware of the bias in psychiatry and how clinical psychology as a profession had a responsibility to influence and shape practice, policy and legislation.

Having started my career in South Africa, I was exposed to the works of Frantz Omar Fanon (1967), an Afro-Caribbean psychiatrist, philosopher, revolutionary and writer who was in particular, interested in the psychopathology of colonisation and the human, social consequences of decolonisation. His work interested me on a personal level as it highlighted my personal, inner battles, my own shame and guilt. Equally, Professor Amina Mama's (1995) work offered an insight beyond the concept of Black identity as a 'White mask', placing race and gender at the centre of our understanding of identity.

The answer to my struggles, my atonement as such, came with my new identity as a clinical psychologist. Not just any other psychologist but one that had trained in South Africa and had been exposed to a new social consciousness 'the rainbow nation'. And, through Hussein Abdilahi Bulhan's (1985) work, I reflected on how mainstream psychology as a discipline had too been contaminated by the power imbalance that permeates society and had been used as a means to control, manipulate and oppress people. An example being, Hendrik Frensch Verwoerd, the so-called 'Architect of Apartheid', a South African psychologist who would go on to become Minister of Native Affairs, Leader of the Nationalist Party and later Prime Minister of the Apartheid Regime was a reflection of typical mainstream psychology.

As a foreign, Black woman working in the UK my practice reflects my training and my earlier experiences in a traumatised social context. Placed within an evidence-based driven mental health setting in the UK, I have found myself trying to understand individuals in their context, within their histories and within the narratives that describes them. I have assessed and engaged with clients with the knowledge that our realities are different and therefore our experiences and expectations will be different. An understanding that highlights 'difference' as a given, not as something 'better', 'worse', 'normal' or 'abnormal' but something that will certainly impact our perception of ourselves and others and will inform or guide our behaviour and its consequences. In our differences, we also find similarities in accepting and sharing our positions we co-develop a narrative that allows respect and trust to be built. It was this 'acceptance and respect of otherness' that I felt was an integral part of leading a clinical team working with disenfranchised young people and their families. Although working predominately within a female team our personal experiences and our understanding of social struggle was varied. Introducing the concept of self-reflection in our practice and challenging our bias was met with much resistance. Drawing on Afrocentric practices, the leadership style adopted was one that attempted to promote 'humane-ness' and participatory decision-making in the search of a contextualised management approach. Working with young people subject to sexual exploitation and their families is an emotionally draining job and professionals can feel isolated in their experiences as well as holding on to fear of failure and/or disciplinary action. This approach aimed to open up a space for 'hidden messages', resentments and aspirations to become openly articulated. As a leader, it was important to model to others in the team that it is acceptable to be vulnerable, experience doubts, not understand others experience and challenge and question practices and procedures. It was important to create a culture in which our differences as well as our similarities would enhance and improve our practice. However, it was also important to maintain a working environment where professional ethic and accountability was maintained.

The Clash of the Titans: Pseudo-leadership

There was a clear acceptance and commitment from government and relevant stakeholders that mainstream approaches to working with vulnerable young people and their families were ineffective and more focus should be placed on inclusive and holistic approaches. In principle, the ethos for the project working with disenfranchised young people and their families was culturally sensitive and embraced diversity. The model developed was accepted and its implementation supported at all levels. However, managing people's resistance to engage in reflective practice often meant that the 'hidden messages', the 'elephants in the room' were not being addressed and this perpetuated a narrative of secrecy and lack of trust. As Black leaders attempting to introduce an approach that often left people having to be confronted with their moral and social bias within an organisational system that was experienced as punitive rather than supportive it was a challenging task. Containing individuals fears whilst nurturing their curiosity so they could remain aware of their bias in their practice was often undermined by organisational systems that focussed more on performance management and systematic budget cuts than personal development. The schism between the narrative at grassroots level and at corporate level meant that this was an experience of pseudo-leadership as opposed to true leadership. The leadership role was contained within a system and structure that was often experienced as oppressive and punitive and as such the potential for retaliation from different agencies was a reality. True leadership requires power to drive change and this was not something that existed within our role.

So What Does This Mean?

The benefits of employing and supporting 'outsider within' leaders when transforming children, young people and families mental health services can bring many opportunities for innovation and transformation. Despite the many challenges faced within this project and the barriers for true leadership there have been substantial gains. In introducing a management approach that supported professionals (who subsequently supported clients) to be open about their biases and their blind spots, it created the opportunity for self-knowledge and self-knowledge is power because the more we understand ourselves the more we can understand others. It brings a different kind of power – personal power, the power to name. The more we can be honest and open the better we can communicate. It allowed people to be in touch with their feelings, their emotions and this is vital in maintaining relationships with others. It has been our experience that the changes we achieved through our leadership approach were based on our ability to tolerate discomfort and to name the 'hidden messages' and allow for open dialogue about them without threat of punitive action. This in turn has allowed for a culture of 'curious enquiry about otherness' without fear of being labelled a racist, sexist, homophobe or others.

> We need leaders not in love with money but in love with justice.
> Not in love with publicity but in love with humanity
> – Dr Martin Luther King

References

Bell, M. (2002). Promoting children's rights through the use of relationship. *Child & Family Social Work*, 7, 1–11.

Berelowitz, S., Firmin, C., Edwards, G., & Gulyurtlu, S. (2012). *I thought I was the only one. The only one in the world. The Office of the Children's Commissioner's inquiry in to child sexual exploitation in gangs and groups: Interim report.* London: Office of the Children's Commissioner.

Bulhan, H. A. (1985). *Frantz Fanon & the psychology of oppression.* Boston, MA: Boston University.

Campbell, A. (2010). Cultural identity as a social construct. *Intercultural Education*, 11(1), 31–39.

Casey, L. (2015). *Reflections on child sexual exploitation.* London: Department for Communities & Local Government.

Chemers, M. (1997). *An integrative theory of leadership.* Mahwah, NJ: Erlbaum.

Collins, P. H. (1986). Learning from the outsider within: The sociological significance of black feminist thought. *Social Problems*, 33(6), 14–32.

Counts, S. (2012). *Invisible woman: Narratives of black women leaders in southeastern two year colleges.* Unpublished Doctoral dissertation. Clemson University, USA.

Darlow, A., Bickerstaffe, T., Burden, T., Green, J., Jassi, S., Jackson, S., ... Walton, F. (2005). *Researching Bradford: A review of social research on Bradford District.* London: Joseph Rowntree Foundation.

DfE. (2014a). *Children's social care innovation programme: Overview.* London: Department for Education.

DfE. (2014b). *Rethinking support for adolescents.* London: Department for Education.

DfE. (2014c). *Rethinking children's social work.* London: Department for Education.

DfE. (2017). *Child sexual exploitation: Definition and a guide for practitioners, local leaders and decision makers working to protect children from child sexual exploitation.* London: Department for Education.

DoH. (2015a). *Future in mind: Promoting, protecting and improving our children and young people's mental health and wellbeing.* London: Department of Health and NHS England.

DoH. (2015b). *Vulnerable groups and inequalities task and finish group report.* London: Department of Health.

Fanon, F. (1967). *Black skin, white masks.* London: Pluto Press.

Gohir, S. (2013). *Unheard voices: The sexual exploitation of Asian girls and young women*. Birmingham: Muslim Women's Network – UK.

Harrison, K., & Gill, A. (2015). Child grooming and sexual exploitation: Are South Asian men the UK media's new folk devils? *International Journal for Crime, Justice and Social Democracy*, *4*, 34–49.

Hartsock, N. C. M. (1983). The feminist standpoint: Developing the ground for a specifically feminist historical materialism. In S. Harding & M. Hintikka (Eds.), *Discovering reality* (pp. 283–310). Boston: D Riedel.

Hill, M., Stafford, A., Seaman, P., Ross, N., & Daniel, B. (2007). *Parenting and resilience*. York: Joseph Rowntree Foundation.

hooks, b. (1984). *From margin to center*. Boston, MA: South End Press.

hooks, b. (1990). *Yearning: Race, gender and cultural politics*. Boston, MA: South End Press.

Jay, A. (2014). *Independent inquiry into child sexual exploitation in Rotherham*. Rotherham: Rotherham Metropolitan Borough Council.

King, D. K. (1988). Multiple jeopardy, multiple consciousness: The context of a black feminist ideology. *Signs*, *14*(1), 42–72.

Lorde, A. (1984). The Master's Tools Will Never Dismantle the Master's House. In A. Lorde (Ed.), *Sister Outsider: Essays and Speeches* (pp. 110–114). Berkeley, CA: Crossing Press.

Mama, A. (1995). *Beyond the masks: Race, gender & subjectivity*. London: Routledge.

Rollins, J. (1985). *Between women, domestics and their employers*. Philadelphia, PA: Temple University Press.

Stoltenberg, J. (2000). *Refusing to be a man*. London: Routledge.

The Guardian. (2017). 'We've not broken the barrier': How can social care tackle its diversity deficit? Retrieved from https://www.theguardian.com/social-care-network/skills-for-care-partner-zone/2017/aug/09/bme-bame-people-still-under-represented-at-senior-levels-in-social-care

Van Dijk, T. A. (1993). *Elite discourse & racism*. California, CA: Sage Publications Inc.

Yukl, G. (2009). *Leadership in organizations* (6th ed.). Upper Saddle River, NJ: Prentice Hall.

Chapter 17

Forty Years in the Wilderness: A Review of Systemic Barriers to Reducing the Over-Representation of Black Men in the UK Psychiatric System

Gail Coleman-Oluwabusola

I am a Black British woman who was born in Manchester in the North West of England in the 1970s. My parents are both Jamaican and came to this country in the late 1960s. I grew up in inner-city Manchester in a largely African-Caribbean and South Asian community. Within my experiences of this community, white people were considered as 'racist' and it was 'common knowledge' that as a Black child I would have to work twice as hard to achieve educational or economic 'success' and to avoid being arrested or blamed for something. Not because of any inherent biological deficit we possessed, but simply because of 'racism'. Within the community we were encouraged not to trust 'white people'. I have friends from these communities who have been arrested, beaten up by police, faced discrimination at work or who have been sectioned onto psychiatric wards, mostly black men. In terms of gender roles, I have grown up seeing black women being 'strong' out of necessity (often the breadwinner of the family) and black men who seem to be defeated. As a child in school, I and my female black friend, 'knew' that we would have a better chance at 'success' than our male counterparts. This was particularly relevant in the classroom, where we often witnessed black boys getting into trouble and being placed in lower educational streams. Little was expected of them.

The above statement is taken from the personal reflection I included in qualitative research almost 16 years ago. This was written in the spirit of an Afrocentric researcher presenting sufficient information about myself to enable readers to assess how and to what extent my presence influenced the choice, conduct and outcome of the research. From that research emerged a framework for conceptualising the development of a persecutory framework for black men living in the UK, in the context of social inequality, loss, institutional racism and additional powerlessness, international over-representation and death in the psychiatric system. This is partly represented in Fig. 1.

This chapter briefly summaries research over the past four decades (and prior) associated with black men and mental health in the UK. The chapter also examines some responses to the research. This is because we unfortunately remain in a situation where black men in Britain are 17 times more likely than white counterparts to be diagnosed with a psychotic illness. This is an appalling situation but the sense of shame that this should invoke in the UK seems to dissipate decade after decade.

Research into the mental health needs of black men has been conducted repeatedly in the UK, with each new generation hopeful for change. By briefly exploring some policies that have emerged to address this inequality, this chapter highlights the barriers to change. The argument being that we have conducted the research and we undoubtedly have the answers, but yet progress is at best slow, if at all evident. We need to be honest about why this is.

What We Know

Research into the mental health needs of black men in the UK highlights issues that are well known, such as the use of coercive pathways to care, the overuse of medication, under-representation in access to psychological therapy, the mistrust of psychiatric services amongst black communities in the UK and the subsequent impact on engagement with services.

Recurrent and Repeated Themes

My doctoral research submitted in 2002 (Coleman, 2002) used semi-structured interviews to explore the content and form of delusions experienced by African and African-Caribbean men with psychiatric histories. Additionally, staff members who worked with these groups were interviewed. I reviewed the research available at the time and concluded that it was unfortunately well established that rates of psychotic illness amongst the African-Caribbean population in Britain were elevated compared to the indigenous white British population. I specified that this was first noted by Hemsi (1967) and pointed to a number of subsequent studies indicating the same over-representation (see Bagley, 1971; Bhugra et al., 1997, cited in Gilvarry et al., 1999; Harrison et al., 1989; Leff, Fischer, & Bertelsen, 1976; McGovern & Cope, 1987; Os Van, Castle, Takei, Der, & Murray, 1996; Wesseley, Castle, Der, & Murray, 1991).

I also referred to Professor Robin Murray and researchers at the Institute of Psychiatry in London, who concluded that black people were not genetically more prone to schizophrenia. Furthermore, it was found that although 75% of white patients with schizophrenia had some biological reason for their illness in the black population this was only 25% (BBC News Online, 2000). Prior to this, it was noted that African-Caribbean patients were less likely to be offered psychotherapy and more likely to receive electroconvulsive therapy and higher doses of medication (Littlewood & Cross, 1980). Littlewood and Lipsedge (1988) also reported high admission rates under the Mental Health Act and over-representation of black patients in secure units and special hospitals (Littlewood & Lipsedge, 1981; McGovern & Cope, 1987).

In a classic summary, Littlewood and Lipsedge (1988, p. 950) cite explanations for the excess rate of schizophrenia which included: the experience of migration and 'status striving in a climate of limited opportunity' (Bagley, 1971; Giggs, 1986) and a culturally determined response to adversity (Bebbington, Hurry, & Tennant, 1981); patterns of service utilisation (Cochrane, 1977), that is, depressed African-Caribbean populations were found to be less likely to seek psychiatric treatment, seldom offered admission and if they were admitted they were more likely to be diagnosed as schizophrenic.

At the time, I observed that it had been repeatedly stated in the literature that in the Caribbean, rates for psychotic illness are not similarly elevated. For example, Hickling and Rogers-Johnson (1995) found a restrictive CATEGO[1] schizophrenia diagnosis first contact incidence rates for the black population in Jamaica of 1.16 per 10, 000. This is slightly lower than the rate of 1.4 per 10,000 for the general white population in Nottingham, UK (see Harrison, Owens, Holton, Neilson, & Boot, 1988) and falls within the indicated range of the WHO International Schizophrenia Study (Sartorious et al., 1986). Additionally, it did not compare with Harrison's findings of 13.5 and 36.4 per 10,000 of schizophrenia for first and second-generation African-Caribbeans in Nottingham (predominantly Jamaican origin) respectively. See also Hickling (1991) and Bhugra et al. (1996).

These findings were taken as evidence that the risk is greatest in African-Caribbeans born in Britain (second generation) and indicated that there are adverse environmental factors in operation (see Gilvarry et al., 1999) Wesseley et al. (1991) cite frequent exposure to social adversity. Cochrane and Bal (1989) suggested that this may affect African-Caribbeans born in the UK as much as, or more than their parents.

At the beginning of the twenty-first century, McKenzie, Samele, Van Horn, Tattan, and Van Os (2001) carried out a secondary analysis of 708 patients with research diagnostic criteria-defined psychosis from a two-year randomised control trial of case management. They found that people of Caribbean origin living in the UK were more likely to be diagnosed as suffering from schizophrenia than British whites (AC, 50%; BW 31%). They were also less likely to have A-levels or a degree (AC, 8%; BW, 24%).

These studies were the substance of my review at time. With regards to results of the interviews I conducted, three themes emerged. These are summarised in the next section.

---

[1]This is a computer programme used to classify patients into diagnostic categories.

Being or Becoming Ill

In terms of this particular sample, analysis of data suggested that when a person becomes ill, they often experience a sense of distress, due to certain life events or due to the specific symptoms they are experiencing. Their 'self-trust' may be affected and they may begin to question their own sense of judgement. Alternatively, they may hold firmly to the reality of the experience. However, whether they believe the expereince or not, it may be experienced as overwhelming. Hence, the person becoming ill may then seek others to help.

'Others', such as family members, may themselves feel distressed by what other person becoming ill is going through. They may then feel a need to call additional 'others' such as the police or the psychiatric system who can 'help'. Generally, 'others' may feel torn between wanting to accept what the person becoming ill is experiencing, feeling the need to control the person in some way and fears about potential collusion. However, the first response according to the interviews conducted is more likely to lead to the person [becoming ill] engaging with others. Alternatively, if the person becoming ill is faced with attempts to control them, they may understandably attempt to hide their symptoms or 'play the good patient' once in the mental health system. Other ways of coping, included attempting to regain control outside of psychiatry. This may or may not include taking part in religious activity.

The Persecutory System

The second emergent concept concerned 'persecutory systems'. The dominant persecutory system is described as nameless and appears to be a vehicle of control, oppression, racism, discrimination and social inequality. This system has a number of facets within it. An exception to this system was a spiritual persecutory system based on a Christian framework.

A merge between real persecutory experiences and 'delusional' persecutory experiences at the hands of the social persecutory system was indicated. There were also frequent references to what appeared to be real experiences of persecution, with the police being mentioned frequently in addition to racist name calling from peers or 'mates'. The reason for persecution appeared to be related to the recipient's racial identity.

In terms of racial identity, the impact of rejection in the context of a racist society is perhaps evident in this quote from a staff member, Andrew,[2] a white British staff nurse in the NHS:

> We had this one guy who erm, who thought ... that he'd been poisoned by his *white foster carers*. In order to turn him from a black child, into a white child. He was quite pale. Pale skin. I think his

---

[2]Pseudonym.

mother was white, his father was African I think, erm and he believed that his complexion, his skin colour had lightened as he'd grown up, that he was changing into a white person, but it, a very kind of sad delusional explanation for his kind of experiences as a child really, you know, living in foster care, he was kind of rejected by his mother. Kind of issues, that's one example, but I'm sure there are others.

There appeared to be a strong sense of helplessness and frustration in the face of persecution. However, arguably adaptive responses to persecution included ignoring the persecutors and not fighting back. Occasionally people would fight back, but this tended to be aimed at perceived individual persecutors, rather than persecutory systems.

The persecutory system also included the psychiatric system, housing authorities which were viewed as discriminatory and places of employment. These systems were often linked with institutional racism. With regards to housing, the Grenfell Tower tragedy London is perhaps testament to the impact of inadequate funding decisions and arguably to discrimination (see Hanley, 2017).

Steven an in-patient of African-Caribbean origin stated:

> [...] it's like when you go for a job and if they don't, don't like you, just like, I really want them to say 'oh we don't like you, so leave the premises' I'd like them to say that ... if you go to the workplace and you tell them, 'oh yeah', I'm an advanced student er I'm applying for this job' it's like because of your appearance or something, they won't give you the job.

With regards to housing and a sense of discrimination, Steven also stated:

> [...] even housing and all that, they don't want to give you a place. I went to a housing place one day and said er 'can I have a flat or somewhere?'... I asked for a two storey flat or, so they offered me some flat, a high rise, you know what I mean, and I didn't want it, I didn't want it. But it was the only place they wanted to offer me ... I took the place, I just, I couldn't live in them conditions.

Concerning the police, Steven added:

> [...] he's got nothing to say, a policeman comes up to you ... he just wants to lock you up, so he wants to lock you up 'cause your Black ... in their statement, it said, erm, 'he believed to be a half-caste dood'. Know what I mean so, my dad, my dad's got vex now... said erm, erm, 'How could they say that, how could they say that, when you're black?

Sam, an out-patient of African-Caribbean origin, suggested that one reason for the persecution was a fear of different cultures. He stated, 'Yeah, I had a lot of experiences like that at school, when you get called names and I told my pa and he said, 'don't worry son, it's the same thing happen to us when we just come over into this country'. Used to say we had tails and we were monkeys that we stunk, 'cause we had tails hidden under our coats. It's happening now with the Asians and the rioting and Oldham and being another colour, not only in Britain, but all over the world .... Not only I experienced it, my foreparents experienced it and ... upto this day, we're experiencing it ...'.

Sam also refered to persecution being part of a conspiracy to *wipe out* black people. This was something he dwelt upon particularly when he first began to experience severe mental health difficulties. His distress was compounded by the fact that such practices might be quite overt, but still accepted at the time. He stated:

> Slavery, wondering about slavery, and the conspiracy to erm, to erm, when the holocaust, the holocaust against the Jews and as a young person, you used to think about them things a lot, what if they do wipe out the black race, like they wiped out the Jews, all them things happening, as a youth, it's on the news and it's not hidden, it's there in front of you. I used to think on it a lot, and done me head in. I couldn't study or work or anything. I was less motivated to do anything, than white people are.

Sam later continued:

> I think that's part of what made me ill and all that, 'cause I used to think hard on it, I woulnd't go out and ... fight against people, but it was spinning in my mind, after I'd been called names, what, how should I take, I didn't know how to take it (lowers voice) you know being black ... I used to sit down and write, 'cause I'm black, I can't get this opportunity', 'cause I'm black I can't get that opportunity'.

Mental health staff made the following statements when referring to the African-Caribbean men they have worked with:

> [...] persecutory ideas of abuse by a racist system, a system designed to keep them erm down and locked and incarcerated ... it's a nameless system, but geared with racism, a system designed from a thousand years to keep Black people in their place, you know erm I know it sounds funny, it's a system, but it's nameless and an unidentifiable system of facets which are keeping some people with them ideas down ....Yeah, a system designed which can belittle you and erm reinforced by media, family...schoolteachers, nurseries, doctors, psychiatrists. System designed to erm

reinforce your, your (low position) in life. (Brian[3]; a Black British social worker of African Caribbean origin)

[...] most African-Caribbean men that I've worked with that suffer paranoia delusions, tend to look at it from, a persecution point of view from the 'system' er system including health authority, the doctors and the nurses er social services and particularly the police ... usually it tends to be like the powers that be within the system here in Britain. (Carl[4]; a Black African support worker)

The sense of being silenced and the powerlessness and sense of hopelessness associated with this situation is perhaps highlighted in the quote below, from Sam[5]:

When I was in mental hospital and when I was in prison. I actually got beaten up...some of the screws[6]... I was naked and a pile of them come in the cell and beat me up and put me in a strip cell, chained and cuffed, on a cold floor. I've experienced some bad things but **who listens anyway** so ... I don't want to talk about it anyway so ... I don't want to start no trouble with no authority or anything, you know erm but they've been cases where a lot of Black men have died in custody and all that and I thought I could have been one of them ... I don't know if I've died and come back.

Loss Experiences

The interviews indicated that bereavements and loss of role/status/job at times in the context of migration contributed to the development of mental health problems.

With regards to the loss of a job, Carl (African support worker) stated:

I had a gentleman who I think it started off with a sense of persecution in terms of racism, 'cause he had a very good erm role in (says name of a suburb) which is a very a white area, very middle-class area, and erm because of all this feeling of er racism towards him, he, it eventually led to the loss of job. And I think after a couple of months, he'd (sit down at home) and writing letters to the Queen and to the Prime Minister. He stayed up late nights, er days and nights I think and eventually he developed an illness.

---

[3]Pseudonym.
[4]Pseudonym.
[5]Pseudonym.
[6]A slang term used by prisoners to describe prison officers.

In terms of the impact of migration, Carl also stated:

> They tend to have migrated as well, from one part of the world, where some like never ever had experienced racism, because there is no, there is no other person of a different colour to come and oppress them...I know some of the African cultures ... not racism, but maybe tribalism ... I think, a lot of people that have a break down here, tend to have er grown up within a middle-class environment in their culture and have come here and have found it more or less impossible to fit into a similar kind of erm social class.

The interviews also highlighted the impact of the loss of cultural frameworks in addition to loss of parental figures. For example, John, an in-patient of mixed African and white British descent stated:

> cause I, my first family was Irish family. That was my first family. I was fostered to, adopted ... and I was with them for I think about ten years, then my foster mother died. I got moved on to a Jamaican family, so I've been in (coughs) two different cultures, so it's been a bit of a mixed time for me to get used to one culture, to a next culture.

Previously held beliefs were also lost, for example, Sam stated:

> I come in the winter, snow, first time I seen snow and aeroplanes and big cars and all them lights and it was nice though, it was a nice experience ... coming to see my parents, 'cause I lived with my grandparents in Jamaica. They grew me up, then I come here, met my mother and father, and then found out that they was my mother and father, and that person who brought me up in Jamaica was me grand-parents.

An exception to the loss of a parental figure was the sad experience of Terence, an out-patient of African-Caribbean descent. He stated:

> I had a baby that died ... I can remember I can hear these like, hear him saying to me, 'we, we've never hurt anyone and look what they are doing to us' I feel as if the baby's saying that, the baby said that to me when he died. He died at the age of three.

According to the interviews, losses unsurprisingly had an impact upon their self-esteem, affective state and subsequent behaviour.

Development of the Persecutory Framework

Based on the interviews and emerging themes, a framework was proposed for the development of a persecutory framework. This is partly represented below.

On review and based on experiences of working across adult and child mental health services, I have added experiences of powerlessness in the education system. Hence, this represents an adapted model (see Fig. 1).

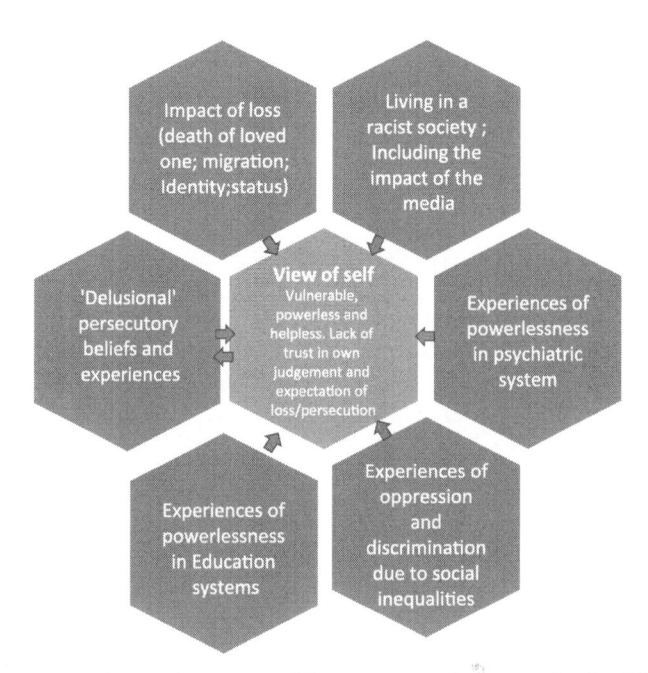

Fig. 1. Proposed Development of Persecutory Frameworks for Black Men Experiencing Persecutory Delusions in the UK.

Still in the Wilderness

Hence, despite the title of this chapter making reference to 40 years in the wilderness, which concerns the plight of oppressed Israelites in the book of Exodus in the Bible, the documentation of over-representation of African-Caribbean men in the UK psychiatric system is at least 50 years old. Unfortunately, there has not been a significant change in these figures despite evidence-based statements such as 'Being black in Britain is bad for your mental health' (McKenzie, 2007).

Kirkbride et al. (2012) conducted a systematic review of incidence rates in England over a 60-year period (1950–2009) to determine the extent to which rates of schizophrenia and other psychoses varied along accepted (age and sex) and less-accepted epidemiological gradients (ethnicity, migration and place of birth and upbringing and time). The researchers found that rates of most disorders were elevated in several ethnic minority groups compared with the white (British) population. For example, for schizophrenia: black Caribbean (pooled RR: 5.6; 95%CI: 3.4–9.2; $N = 5$), black African (pooled RR: 4.7; 95%CI:

3.3–6.8; $N = 5$) and South Asian groups in England (pooled RR: 2.4; 95%CI: 1.3–4.5; $N = 3$). They found no evidence to support an overall change in the incidence of psychotic disorder over time, though diagnostic shifts (away from schizophrenia) were reported.

With regards to the incidence of psychotic disorders and ethnicity, they identified *26 citations* (Baudiš, Matesová, Škoda, Kabešová, & Skodová, 1977; Bhugra et al., 1997; Carpenter & Brockington, 1980; Castle, Wessely, Der, & Murray, 1991; Castle, Wessely, Van Os, & Murray, 1998; Coid et al., 2008; Dean, Downing, & Shelley, 1981; Dean, Walsh, Downing, & Shelley, 1981; Fearon et al., 2006; Giggs, 1973; Goater et al., 1999; Harrison et al., 1997, 1988; Hemsi, 1967; Hitch & Rack, 1980; Kirkbride et al., 2007, 2008; King, Coker, Leavey, Hoare, & Johnson-Sabine, 1994; Leff et al., 1976; Littlewood & Lipsedge, 1978; Lloyd et al., 2005; McGovern & Cope, 1987; Morgan et al., 2006; Rwegellera, 1977; Van Os, Castle, Takei, Der, & Murray, 1996; Van Os, Takei, et al., 1996), which provided incidence data in relation to ethnicity or country of birth. Schizophrenia was included in 18 of these, with 10 primary citations providing 37 overall incidence estimates in minority ethnic groups. Some citations also provided rates in different ethnic groups stratified by age and generation status.

Kirkbride et al. (2012) note that rates of psychotic disorder were most particularly and consistently raised for people of 'black ethnicities' compared with the baseline population in each study (typically those of white or white British ethnicity). The authors performed a random effects meta-analysis on data from five studies which presented overall incidence rates of schizophrenia in different ethnic minority groups. This suggested rates of schizophrenia were elevated in black Caribbean (RR: 5.6; 95%CI: 3.4, 9.2; $I^2 = 0.77$) and black African (RR: 4.7; 95% CI: 3.3, 6.8; $I^2 = 0.47$) migrants and their descendants, compared with the baseline population. This pattern was also evident for the affective psychoses, including bipolar disorder and psychotic depression independently. For substance-induced psychoses, one study reported higher first admission rates of cannabis-induced psychoses in black Caribbean men. However, the authors highlight unpublished data from the ÆSOP study (see later) which indicated that 92.6% of people with a substance-induced psychosis were white British, with the rest of mixed ethnicities.

Notably, they identified five citations (Bhugra et al., 1997; Fearon et al., 2006; Harrison et al., 1997, 1988; McGovern & Cope, 1987) which presented rates of psychotic disorder in different ethnic groups by age. Three of these (Bhugra et al., 1997; Harrison et al., 1988; McGovern & Cope, 1987) distinguished between first- and second-generation black Caribbean migrants and found support for raised rates of psychotic disorder for both generations. Two citations (Fearon et al., 2006; Harrison et al., 1997) presented rates of psychotic disorder by ethnicity across several age groups; rates were elevated at all ages for black Caribbean and black African groups.

Furthermore, Morgan et al. (2017) found that there was evidence that black Caribbean patients experienced worse clinical, social, and service use outcomes, and black African patients experienced worse social and service use outcomes, compared with white British patients. Baseline social disadvantage contributed to these discrepancies. This was part of the ÆSOP-10 Study, a follow-up at 10 years of a cohort of 458 (initially 532) patients with first episode psychotic disorder initially identified in south-east London and Nottingham.

In this study, in order to capture exposure to multiple disadvantage and isolation, the researchers constructed an index by counting the presence of the following: unemployment, living alone, living in rented housing and being single. Service use involved information on contacts with mental health services. This included adherence with treatment (clustered into regular, irregular and none, based on appointment attendance and how frequently medication was taken). Clinical outcomes defined remission as absence of psychotic symptoms for six months. These were categorised into three types: episodic (no episode lasting more than six months) and neither episodic not continuous (at least one episode of more than six months and at least one remission of more than six months). Symptom recovery was defined as sustained remission for two or more years.

It was concluded that:

> [...] one of our most striking findings is the high levels of social disadvantage and isolation, at baseline and throughout the follow-up, among Black Caribbean and Black African patients. This suggests that addressing the social needs of those from these groups should be a priority for mental health services. (Morgan et al., 2017, p. 6)

Whilst we hold this research in high esteem, the findings are arguably not surprising and reflect what people have been saying for decades. The authors also conclude:

> More broadly, our findings mirror wider inequities in health in many marginalised and disadvantaged groups. This perspective draws attention to the social structures and processes, including institutional racism .... (Morgan et al., 2017, p. 6)

This conclusion is again arguably consistent with previous findings. Hence, we have policies such as The Five Year Forward View for Mental Health published by the Independent Mental Health Taskforce (2016) which states:

> Some groups are disproportionately represented in detentions to acute and secure in-patient services, and are affected by long stays. For example, men of African Caribbean ethnic origin are twice as likely to be detained in low secure services than men of white British origin and stay for twice as long in those services on average. This suggests a failure to ensure equal access to earlier intervention and crisis care services (Mental Health Taskforce, 2016, p. 31).
>
> People with acute mental health needs will be able to access appropriate care, as in-patients or through community teams. Their housing, social care and other needs will be assessed on admission and the right support made available on discharge. Use of the Mental Health Act will be monitored, with a focus on black and minority ethnic groups (Mental Health Taskforce, 2016, p. 32).

> Finally, we have placed a particular focus on tackling inequalities. Mental health problems disproportionately affect people living in poverty, those who are unemployed and who already face discrimination. For too many, especially black, Asian and minority ethnic people, their first experience of mental health care comes when they are detained under the Mental Health Act, often with police involvement, followed by a long stay in hospital. To truly address this, we have to tackle inequalities at local and national level (Mental Health Taskforce, 2016, p. 82).

There have been a number of policies and inquiries to address such inequalities over the decades, such as: Inside Outside – Improving Mental Health Service for black and Minority Ethnic Communities in England 2003; The Independent Inquiry into the Death of Rocky Bennett published by the Norfolk, Suffolk and Cambridgeshire Strategic Health Authority & Department of Health (2003). New Horizons: a shared vision for mental health (HM Government, 2009); the fact that we live in an inherently racist society arguably buffers against change. The simplest analogy I can draw is when a parent who has a complex and dramatic life, at times impacted by experiences of abuse, brings their child to Child and Adolescent Mental Health Services and asks clinicians to 'fix' the child. The thinking being that the child will be fixed despite returning to live in an emotionally unstable home environment.

It is important to clarify that in the above analogy, the child is not the individual black male patient, the 'child' is the over-representation of black men in the British psychiatric system. Hence, the unstable home is the racist society commissioned with implementing policies. As such, policies that do not take into account the fact that they are being implemented in a racist society and which are not comprehensively resourced, with long-term investment as a basic requirement, rather than short-term funding will not suffice because in essence they represent an attempt to 'fix'. This is not a 'quick fix' situation, as the decades of research with repeated themes testify. Additionally, good policies that change or are replaced based on the political climate arguably, have no place in addressing this situation.

As the following quote states:

> We have an excellent plan for improving mental health services for black and minority ethnic groups, but we need to go further. If we knew that one group in society were 10 times more likely to develop lung cancer, we would focus on them - perhaps with a targeted anti-smoking strategy. We would not just make lung cancer treatment services more equitable .... Prevention of mental illness in black communities is the sort of complex problem that should attract a high-level government inquiry that leads to action. I am used to hearing politicians say that doing nothing is not an option. This is an area where the phrase has real meaning. The high rates of mental illness in people of Caribbean and African origin are not going to go away. If anything, their legacy will blight a generation and the impact will be felt by us all. (McKenzie, 2007)

Analysis and Conclusions

When we think of the term institutional racism, we often think of organisations, rather than a racist society. However, I often make reference to raising children in a racist society and the need for a conscious awareness of this when I teach trainee Clinical Psychologists, always hopeful that they will inspire change in the profession. I am in essence guilty of the same naivety of a quick 'fix'. If real change is to occur it has to be independent of the political party in power and it has to take into account the fact that we live in a racist society. If not the design and implementation of such policies will be deficient.

In the UK, there have been and remain respected advocates over the decades, Professor Suman Fernando (who famously rejected his OBE) and Dr Kwame McKenzie come to mind in particular. They have championed the cause. Both men, both psychiatrists and both visible minorities. However, according to Walker (2017) we live in a society where *a third of designated Sure Start children's centres have been lost since 2010 in England, with 1,240 fewer than when the coalition took office.* Walker further states:

> The north-east and London witnessed the biggest falls, with more than 40% of centres lost. Two local authorities, Swindon and Solihull, revealed in a freedom of information request that they had no designated centres left. More than 230 centres have been lost in the past year alone.

In response the Walker notes:

> A DfE spokesman said: 'These figures are misleading as they fail to account for children's centres which are still offering vital services, but have been merged with other centres in the area to increase efficiency'.

Having focussed this chapter on the mental health of black men in the UK, the reader may be confused by a sudden focus on the needs of children. The reasoning is this, in a society that wants to rationalise inadequate care and support of children and their families, how can there be an expectation that the needs of marginalised groups will take priority? Additionally, the work to address the over-representation of black men in psychiatric systems has to include work with black children in the UK for generational change. Unfortunately, such focussed work is often viewed as a threat to 'mainstream' society. That is because mainstream society also faces discrimination, often based on *class and social* status. Ideally the needs of both white families living in poverty and marginalised groups based on race will be met. Thus shattering the legacy of divide and conquer, that leads to varying levels of inequality in the UK. On a personal note, how could I know as a child that when there is an economic crisis, 'we' as black communities will be blamed and will be at the bottom of the pile. It is unfortunately because it is a reality I witnessed each day growing up in the UK.

Furthermore, more recently in the current era of austerity measures, I see this played out in politics and the media in the UK as part of a narrative the blames migration for the economic crisis.

In terms of the actual initiative to address the over-representation of black men in the psychiatric system, this has to be community psychology and psychiatry in practice. That is, comprehensive psychological formulations and initiatives that not only consider the impact of social reality, such as housing, employment and educational discrimination but also advocates work with agencies that represent social needs. This again is not a new concept. However, those agencies cannot be under-funded or under-resourced or short-term 'pilots'. The work cannot be an 'add-on' but it has to be mainstreamed and provide an avenue for culturally appropriate psychological *and* social intervention. As stated, this work has to cut across child and adult services too, in order to affect change across the generations.

The initiatives need to be truly joined up, mainstreamed and positioned in such a way that they are not viewed as a threat. In 2012, in his 80th year, Suman Fernando stated, 'You can't mention equalities [within the Department of Health]. There is a sense that race is off the agenda' (O'Hara, 2012). When I think back to the 1990s race was on the agenda, unfortunately in the form of short-term funding, but it was on the agenda. At that time, I was co-chair of the North-West 'Race' and Culture Special Interest Group of the British Psychological Society (BPS). It is perhaps significant that both the national and regional 'Race' and Culture SIGs no longer exists in the BPS. I also conducted research on making clinical psychology services more accessible to black communities in Manchester, North-West England (see, Coleman, Brown, Acton, Harris, & Saltmore, 1998). I was hopeful of change.

As stated, in the current climate of austerity in the UK, it certainly feels that race is no longer prioritised on the mental health care agenda. O'Hara (2012) notes: *Despite being on several mental health advisory boards over the years, including Mental Health Act Commission, Fernando's career is marked by his refusal to accept that a few political initiatives are evidence of real change.* I am unfortunately inclined to agree.

References

Bagley, C. (1971). The social aetiology of schizophrenia in immigrant groups. *International Journal of Social Psychiatry, 17*(4), 292–304.

Baudiš, P., Matesová, A., Škoda, C., Kabešová, L., & Skodová, M. (1977). A comparison of first admissions of mania in Prague, Aarhus and London: A transcultural study linked up with the international pilot study of schizophrenia of WHO. *Social Psychiatry, 12*(1), 185–193.

BBC News Online. (2000, July 14). UK life blamed for ethnic schizophrenia. *BBC News* Retrieved from http://news.bbc.co.uk/1/hi/health/807945.stm

Bebbington, P. E., Hurry, J., & Tennant, C. (1981). Psychiatric disorders in selected immigrant groups in Camberwell. *Social Psychiatry, 16*(1), 43–51.

Bhugra, D., Leff, J., Mallett, R., Der, G., Corridan, B., & Rudge, S. (1997). Incidence and outcome of schizophrenia in Whites, African Caribbeans and Asians in London. *Psychological Medicine, 27*(4), 791–798.

Bhugra, D., Hilwig, M., Hossein, B., Marceau, H., Neehall, J., Leff, J., ... Der, G. (1996). First-contact incidence rates of schizophrenia in Trinidad and one year follow-up. *British Journal of Psychiatry, 169*(5), 587–592.

Carpenter, L., & Brockington, I. F. (1980). A study of mental illness in Asians, West Indians and Africans living in Manchester. *British Journal of Psychiatry, 137*, 201–205.

Castle, D., Wessely, S., Der, G., & Murray, R. M. (1991). The incidence of operationally defined schizophrenia in Camberwell, 1965–84. *British Journal of Psychiatry, 159*, 790–794.

Castle, D. J., Wessely, S., Van Os, J., & Murray, R. M. (1998). *Psychosis in the inner city: The Camberwell first episode study.* Hove: Psychology Press/Erlbaum (UK) Taylor & Francis.

Cochrane, R. (1977). Mental illness in immigrants to England and Wales: An analysis of mental hospital admissions. *Social psychiatry, 12*(1), 25–35.

Cochrane, R., & Bal, S. (1989). Migration and schizophrenia: An examination of five hypotheses. *Social Psychiatry, 24*(4), 2–11.

Coid, J. W., Kirkbride, J. B., Barker, D., Cowden, F., Stamps, R., Yang, M., & Jones, P. B. (2008). Raised incidence rates of all psychoses among migrant groups: Findings from the East London first episode psychosis study. *Archives of General Psychiatry, 65*, 1250–1258.

Coleman, P. G. (2002). An exploratory investigation into persecutory delusions experienced by a sample of African and African-Caribbean men: Implications for cognitive models and for elevated rates of persecutory delusions amongst African and African-Caribbean populations in Britain. Unpublished thesis submitted as partial fulfilment of the degree of Doctorate of Clinical Psychology, Department of Medicine, Liverpool University, UK.

Coleman, P. G., Brown, R., Acton, C., Harris, A., & Saltmore, S. (1998). Building links with a black community: Experiences in central Manchester. *Clinical Psychology Forum, 188*, 43–38.

Dean, G., Downing, H., & Shelley, E. (1981). First admissions to psychiatric hospitals in south-east England in 1976 among immigrants from Ireland. *British Medical Journal Clinical Research Education, 282*, 1831–1833.

Dean, G., Walsh, D., Downing, H., & Shelley, E. (1981) First admissions of native-born and immigrants to psychiatric hospitals in South-East England 1976. *British Journal of Psychiatry, 139*, 506–512.

Fearon, P., Kirkbride, J. B., Morgan, C., Dazzan, P., Morgan, K., Lloyd, T., ... Mallett, R. (2006). Incidence of schizophrenia and other psychoses in ethnic minority groups: Results from the MRC AESOP study. *Psychological Medicine, 36*, 1541–1550.

Giggs, J. (1973). High rates of schizophrenia among immigrants in Nottingham. *Nursing Times, 69*(38), 1210–1212.

Giggs, J. (1986). Ethnic status and mental illness in urban areas. In J. Rathwell & D. Philips (Eds.), *Health, race and ethnicity* (pp. 137–174). London: Croom Helm.

Gilvarry, C. M., Walsh, E., Samele, C., Hutchinson, G., Mullet, R., Rabe-Hesketh, S., ... Murray, R. M. (1999). Life events, ethnicity and perceptions of discrimination in patients with severe mental illness. *Social Psychiatry and Psychiatric Epidemiology, 34*(11), 600–608.

Goater, N., King, M., Cole, E., Leavey, G., Johnson-Sabine, E., Blizard, R., & Hoar, A. (1999). Ethnicity and outcome of psychosis. *The British Journal of Psychiatry, 175*(1), 34–42.

Hanley, L. (2017, June 16). Look at Grenfell Tower and see the terrible price of Britain's inequality. *The Guardian*. Retrieved from https://www.theguardian.com/commentisfree/2017/jun/16/grenfell-tower-price-britain-inequality-high-rise

Harrison, G., Glazebrook, C., Brewin, J., Cantwell, R., Dalkin, T., Fox, R., ... Medley, I. (1997). Increased incidence of psychotic disorders in migrants from the Caribbean to the United Kingdom. *Psychological Medicine*, *27*(4), 799–806.

Harrison, G., Holton, A., Neilson, D., Owens, D., Boot, D., & Cooper, J. (1989). Severe mental disorder in Afro-Caribbean patients. *Psychological Medicine*, *19*(3), 683–696.

Harrison, G., Owens, D., Holton, A., Neilson, D., & Boot, D. (1988). A prospective study of severe mental disorder in Afro-Caribbean patients. *Psychological Medicine*, *18*(3), 643–657.

Hemsi, L. K. (1967). Psychiatric morbidity of West Indian immigrants. *Social Psychiatry*, *2*(3), 95–100.

Hickling, F. W. (1991). Psychiatric hospital admission in Jamaica 1971 and 1988. *British Journal of Psychiatry*, *159*(6), 817–821.

Hickling, F. W., & Rogers-Johnson, P. (1995). The incidence of first contact schizophrenia in Jamaica. *British Journal of Psychiatry*, *159*(2), 817–821.

Hitch, P. J., & Rack, P. H. (1980). Mental illness among Polish and Russian refugees in Bradford. *British Journal of Psychiatry*, *137*(3), 206–211.

HM Government. (2009). New horizons: A shared vision for mental health. Retrieved from http://webarchive.nationalarchives.gov.uk/20130104235147/http://www.dh.gov.uk/en/Publicationsandstatistics/Publications/PublicationsPolicyAndGuidance/DH_109705

Independent Mental Health Taskforce. (2016). The five year forward view for mental health. Retrieved from https://www.england.nhs.uk/wp-content/uploads/2016/02/Mental-Health-Taskforce-FYFV-final.pdf

King, M., Coker, E., Leavey, G., Hoare, A., & Johnson-Sabine, E. (1994). Incidence of psychotic illness in London: Comparison of ethnic groups. *British Medical Journal*, *309*, 1115–1119.

Kirkbride, J. B., Barker, D., Cowden, F., Stamps, R., Yang, M., Jones, P. B., & Coid, J. W. (2008). Psychoses, ethnicity and socio-economic status. *British Journal of Psychiatry*, *193*, 18–24.

Kirkbride, J. B., Errazuriz, A., Croudace, T. J., Morgan, C., Jackson, D., Boydell, J., ... Jones, P. B. (2012). Incidence of schizophrenia and other psychoses in England, 1950–2009: A systematic review and meta-analyses. *PLoS ONE*, *7*(3), e31660.

Kirkbride, J. B., Morgan, C., Fearon, P., Dazzan, P., Murray, R. M., & Jones, P. B. (2007). Neighbourhood-level effects on psychoses: Re-examining the role of context. *Psychological Medicine*, *37*(10), 1413–1425.

Leff, J. P., Fischer, M., & Bertelsen, A. (1976). A cross-national epidemiological study of mania. *The British Journal of Psychiatry*, *129*(5), 428–442.

Littlewood, R., & Cross, S. (1980). Ethnic minorities and psychiatric services. *Sociology of Health and Illness*, *2*(2), 194–201.

Littlewood, R., & Lipsedge, M. (1978). Migration, ethnicity and diagnosis. *Psychiatria Clinica*, *11*, 15–22.

Littlewood, R., & Lipsedge, M. (1981). Acute psychotic reactions in Caribbean-born patients. *Psychological Medicine, 11*, 303–18.

Littlewood, R., & Lipsedge, M. (1988). Psychiatric illness among British Afro-Caribbeans. *British Medical Journal*, *296*, 950–951.

Lloyd, T., Kennedy, N., Fearon, P., Kirkbride, J. B., Mallett, R. M., Leff, J., ... Jones, P. B. (2005). Incidence of bipolar affective disorder in three UK cities: Results from the ÆSOP study. *British Journal of Psychiatry*, *186*, 126–131.

McGovern, D., & Cope, R. V. (1987). First psychiatric admission rates of first and second generation Afro Caribbeans. *Social Psychiatry*, *22*, 139–149.

McKenzie, K. (2007). Being black in Britain is bad for your mental health. *The Guardian*, April 2. Retrieved from https://www.theguardian.com/commentisfree/2007/apr/02/comment.health

McKenzie, K., Samele, C., Van Horn, E., Tattan, T., & Van Os, J. (2001). Comparison of the outcome and treatment of psychosis in people of Caribbean origin living in the UK and British Whites. *The British Journal of Psychiatry*, *178*(2), 160–165.

Morgan, C., Dazzan, P., Morgan, K., Jones, P., Harrison, G., Leff, J., … AESOP Study Group. (2006). First episode psychosis and ethnicity: Initial findings from the AESOP study. *World Psychiatry*, *5*, 40–46.

Morgan, C., Feron, P., Lappin, J., Heslin, M., Donoghue, K., Lomas, B., & Dazzan, P. (2017). Ethnicity and long-term course and outcome of psychotic disorders in a UK sample: The ÆSOP-10 study. *British Journal of Psychiatry*, *211*(2), 88–94.

Norfolk Suffolk and Cambridgeshire Strategic Health Authority & Department of Health. (2003). Independent inquiry into the death of David Bennett. Retrieved from https://www.blink.org.uk/docs/David_Bennett_report.pdf

O'Hara, M. (2012). Black and minority ethnic mental health patients 'marginalised' under coalition. *The Guardian*. Retrieved from https://www.theguardian.com/society/2012/apr/17/bme-mental-health-patients-marginalised

Os Van, J., Castle, D. J., Takei, N., Der, G., & Murray, R. M. (1996). Psychotic illness in ethnic minorities: Clarification from the 1991 Census. *Psychological Medicine*, *21*, 185–196.

Rwegellera, G. G. (1977). Psychiatric morbidity among West Africans and West Indians living in London. *Psychological Medicine*, *7*, 317–329.

Sartorious, N., Jablensky, A., Korten, A., Ernberg, G., Anker, M., Cooper, J. E., & Day, R. (1986). Early manifestations and first-contact incidence of schizophrenia in different cultures. *Psychological Medicine*, *16*(4), 909–928.

Van Os, J., Castle, D. J., Takei, N., Der, G., & Murray, R. M. (1996). Psychotic illness in ethnic minorities: Clarification from the 1991 census. *Psychological Medicine*, *26*, 203–208.

Van Os, J., Takei, N., Castle, D. J., Wessely, S., Der, G., MacDonald, A. M., & Murray, R. M. (1996). The incidence of mania: Time trends in relation to gender and ethnicity. *Social Psychiatry and Psychiatric Epidemiology*, *31*, 129–136.

Walker, M. (2017). A third of Sure Start children's centres in England lost, says labour. *The Guardian*, April 5. Retrieved from https://www.theguardian.com/society/2017/apr/05/sure-start-childrens-centres-cuts-labour

Wesseley, S., Castle, D., Der, G., & Murray, R. (1991). Schizophrenia and Afro-Caribbeans. A case control study. *British Journal of Psychiatry*, *159*(6), 795–801.

Chapter 18

Oppositional and Defiant Behaviours Among Black Boys in Schools: Techniques to Facilitate Change

Steve Clarke

The main theme of this chapter is raising awareness and improving insights and planning abilities in relation to problems faced by people of colour, as individuals and in institutions. In promoting these skills, there is a need to recognise the role played by personal perceptions and emotions in the way in which we construe problems. Here, the author presents a personal construct psychology (PCP) (Kelly, 1955, Ravenette, 1997) derived approach, which offers a way through the conceptual confusion clouding our thinking about aspects of our lives that concern us, and often leaves us lacking the energy and ability to loosen our thinking and move in the direction of rewarding new attitudes and behaviours.

The question of educational performance and racial propensity has stirred emotions from as early as the 1950s in Great Britain, when West Indian migrants grew concerned about their children's education. For many, Great Britain was supposed to be a promised land and the British education system the best in the world – but that system failed to deliver.

They encountered widespread racism which perfused schools, fuelling the widely held belief that black children were somehow educationally inferior. For teachers in Britain's state schools, black under-achievement was not an anomaly that needed to be addressed; it was to be expected.

None of the initiatives, from the 1985 Swann report Education for All, to Ofsted's 1993 Access and Achievement in Urban Education or the Labour Party's 2007 REACH report which highlighted the need, specifically for black boys, to have middle class professional role models, have achieved the desired effect.

When data from exam results are analysed, the statistics show that black children are trailing behind every other racial group, despite having the same talent and potential. Even though the performance of black children is improving at a faster rate than white British children, collectively they are still under-performing. Clearly, there is something happening that is holding them back.

Over the last few decades, there has been considerable debate and discussion in the areas of 'race', ethnicity and schooling in Britain. Amongst the development of concepts such as 'multicultural' and 'anti-racist' education, one issue – 'underachievement' – has dominated research and policy (Rampton, 1981; Sewell, 2009; Swann, 1985). Indeed, the documentation of inequality of opportunity and the resultant 'under-achievement' by some black groups has been the driving force behind 'multi-cultural' and antiracist education. The impact of such initiatives over the last two decades has been regarded, by some, as piecemeal and largely ineffective (Tomlinson, 1987; Troyna, 1987).

Research evidence over the last three decades has consistently shown some black young people, notably African-Caribbean, Pakistani and Bangladeshi, to under-achieve in schools (Eggleston, Dunn, & Anjali, 1986; Rampton, 1981; Swann, 1985). Strand (2012) reported a white British–black Caribbean achievement gap at age 14 which cannot be accounted for by socio-economic variables or a wide range of contextual factors.

There can be no doubt that school exclusion has an adverse effect on young people's education and on their subsequent life chances. Racial inequality continues to impact the life chances of young black people. Black Caribbean students are almost four to six times more likely to be excluded than their white counterparts and eleven times more likely than white British girls, according to a report by the Children's Commissioner and Department for Education and Employment. Eighty-three per cent of the permanent exclusions in 1995–1996 (Department for Education and Employment, 1999) were boys.

Majors, Gillborn, and Sewell (1998) argue that, in the paucity of national statistics on fixed-term exclusions, it is likely that the official statistics underestimate the true level of exclusions amongst black boys. Moreover, it is feared that black boys may be more susceptible to be victims of 'informal' or 'back-door' exclusions, that is, where parents are asked to withdraw their child before a formal exclusion occurs (Majors et al., 1998). Circumstances under which African-Caribbean boys become excluded appear to be anchored in a 'race' and ethnicity framework. As mentioned above, research evidence over the last two decades has pointed to the under-achievement levels of African-Caribbean boys, and the role of racism as a contributory factor in schools and in society at large (Eggleston et al., 1986; Rampton, 1981; Swann, 1985). Low expectations on the part of teachers and negative stereotyping of black boys have been shown to be an important factor (Eggleston et al., 1986; Wright, 1987). Parsons (1996) found that different peer and teacher influences may increase African-Caribbean boys' resistance to school, leading to serious disciplinary measures such as exclusion. Moreover, once excluded, the majority are unlikely to return to mainstream education, thus being further disadvantaged. Research studies have found that black boys are often excluded from schools for exhibiting 'culture-specific' behaviours (e.g. hair styles, eye behaviour and walking styles) in the classroom (Majors et al., 1998). School can become a battleground in which black boys seek recognition and affirmation of their racial and cultural identity (Majors et al., 1998). Such conflict is clearly not conducive to learning and good educational attainment.

Barn (2001) concluded that it is crucial to have an adequate conceptualisation of the areas of risk and vulnerability for different groups and that such conceptualisation can begin to influence policy and provision to reduce disadvantage and discrimination.

Clearly many black Caribbean students are failing to engage with the schools and the curriculum. What is needed is an approach which can help to discover why this is the case and at the same time help such students to re-engage with the curriculum on their own terms. PCP offers a range of techniques to elicit the individual's perspective and has a model for change which is integral to its theoretical perspective.

Personal Construct Psychology

Given that black males are frequently overrepresented in terms of figures for exclusions and back-door exclusions (Majors et al., 1998), it is imperative that we can develop a methodology for working with those who are struggling to cope with the education system. A poor education leads to poor life chances (Home Office Development and Practice Report, 2004; Rutter, Maughan, Mortimore, & Ouston, 1979). Using theory and techniques derived from PCP can provide such a framework.

It is essential to recognise the role played by personal perceptions and emotions in the way in which we construe problems. Adopting this stance is not easy; we all at some time in our lives drift on and are overwhelmed by a welter of emotions which seem attached to our construction of a particularly challenging problem. Developing an ability to step outside the constraints of the thinking which ensnares us and prevents insightful and creative experimentation is the theme of this chapter.

PCP sometimes referred to as personal construct theory, was conceived by George Kelly (1955, 1969). Writing at a time when there were two predominant psychological theories: psychodynamics and learning theory, he rejected the historic dichotomy between cognition and emotion. Instead, he viewed individuals as being in control of their behaviours, views and attitudes in response to events they encountered (Björklund, 2008), as opposed to being passive victims of such things as their past, their culture, their race or personality. According to Kelly, we do not respond to a stimulus, we respond to our interpretation or perception of a stimulus. For instance, whilst many debate the influence of gangs on the everyday choices gang members make, Kelly would have argued that gang members behave according to their construal of the gang's messages, and do not have to slavishly conform. Kelly acknowledges the existence of a 'reality' outside the individual, but asserts that contact with this reality will never be interpretation-free (Bannister & Fransella, 1971). There is, according to Kelly (1955), always a choice; he calls this construct alternativism:

> No one needs to paint himself into a corner; no one needs to be completely hemmed in by circumstances; no one needs to be a victim of his biography, there is always an alternative.

Kelly (1969) argues that 'all of our present interpretations of the universe are subject to revision or replacement' and that our behaviour is our way of elaborating our construct system (Bannister & Fransella, 1971; Chiari & Nuzzo, 2003) concerning ourselves, other people and the world we live in (Bannister, 2003). We validate our constructs by using the feedback we receive from our behaviour experiments to improve our understanding of our reality and confirm or modify our initial theories.

Kelly explains that we, like scientists, all have theories of our own reality and experiences. We hypothesise what will happen and then we test our predictions or anticipations through the behaviours we adopt, similar to scientists, engaged in experimentations (Boeree, 2006). Through the lens of PCP, our hypotheses are generated from 'constructs' – patterns or templates.

There is no room for despair in a PCP approach, as there may be for those who take a more deterministic approach. The person is an agent, who is capable of reconstructing his world. This is not to underestimate or ignore the often horrendous experiences that have led to the individual construing the world as they do. However, change is possible through the generation and adoption of alternative theories. Kelly (1955), considers that this can't be generated from without, as behavioural interventions would have us believe, but can only come from within. Just as the person can make choices which lead to their placement in a specialist provision, they can equally make choices which will lead to a reversal of that process. The purpose of PCP intervention is to ensure that the person has access to a full range of alternatives and that they make an informed choice in order to facilitate a reconstruction of their world. The person's theories are central in this process. If attempts are made to force the student to change from without and the student has no real desire to change, change, if any, will be superficial. As Dalton and Dunnett (1992, p. 152) warn professionals:

> It is not your function to tell your client how to be, or what constructs to keep or discard like teaching them to play cards. You are not there to provide 'advice', good or otherwise.
>
> Your role is one of assistance, almost that of a catalyst, encouraging reactions in your client without imposing anything of yourself into the reaction.

Any change which occurs because of PCP intervention is generated from the individual and therefore is more likely to succeed, and to be maintained for as long as the individual sees the utility of their new theories.

The author would argue that the processes outlined above are universal, as Kelly was outlining a psychological theory of human nature, and can therefore be applied in a range of multicultural circumstances, from the perceptions of Syrian refugees (Naffi & Davidson, 2016) to the personal constructs of convicted terrorists (Sarangi, Canter, & Youngs, 2013).

We can apply this logic to how the construct systems that individuals use control their interpretation of their educational experiences. As Solas (1992) argued, 'Personal Construct Theory has a role to play in education. The theory offers ways of seeing and doing which are potentially applicable to many teaching and learning issues'.

The way the individual uses language is important in this process, as it may be the case that the meaning of a phrase or word, is ascribed in an idiosyncratic way, and may mean something completely different to what is assumed. Take for example the word 'boring', this could mean that something is not interesting, but equally it could mean it is not exciting. One student the author worked with told him that he found high school 'boring'. After elaborating this concept, it appeared that when not in high school, the student had unlimited access to his Xbox and movies. In contrast, high school was perceived as not being fun, and as having to do things other people wanted him to do. Having a clearer understanding of the nature of the problem allows for appropriate strategies to be considered. There is a need to have a life conversation (Harri-Augstein & Thomas, 1991) to see whether the student has any higher aspirations which would make education more meaningful. The education establishment could look at designing a curriculum more allied to his interests and parents could impose restrictions on his access to entertainment when he is not attending. Ravenette (1997) implores to 'never, never, never, give advice'. Therefore, the solutions need to come from the people who are to implement them, to ensure ownership of the strategies employed. A skilled practitioner, aware of the nature of change, as outlined by Kelly (1995), will lead individuals involved in the problem, to reflect on their own constructs and to experiment with new behaviours, which derive from a re-examination of those constructs. The practitioner acts like a mirror, to aid in this self-reflection. Self-reflection in itself may be enough to stimulate change. Often individuals get stuck in behaviour patterns, the origins of which become forgotten. Reflecting on one's constructs and resultant behaviour can reveal that the behaviour is redundant and no longer serves its original purpose. This can allow for adjustments in behaviour to align it with the way a person construes the situation in 'real time', as opposed to historically.

PCP has a range of techniques in its repertoire to help elicit and elaborate a person's constructs. Kelly (1995) outlined several techniques, including triadic sorting, self-characterisation sketches and fixed role techniques. Hinkle (1965) provide the laddering technique which is particularly efficacious in eliciting higher order and core constructs by asking the 'why question'. Landfield (1971) introduced the pyramid technique which helps to elaborate how constructs are applied by asking the 'how and what' questions. Neimeyer (1992) provided the downward arrow technique which asks the 'so what, question', in order to elaborate what a particular experience or event, means to the individual. These techniques are used to understand and elaborate a construct and how it is related within a person's construct system. Tschudi (1977) suggested that the ABC network could be used to help individuals examine why they were finding it difficult to make choices, and what the implications of change may be for them.

The author has used the theory and techniques of PCP throughout his career as an educational psychologist and in his experience, it has proved to be an effective way of working (Clarke, 1999). The author has trained other psychologists in the theory and techniques of PCP, and as part of the course he ran, would ask the trainees to try out the techniques with their clients, and feedback their experiences to the group. One example will serve to illustrate the simplicity and efficacy of the PCP approach. One of the course participants was working with a pupil of Afro-Caribbean descent, in a school for students excluded from the education system. The pupil in question, who I shall call Cody, was on the verge of being excluded from his new school after a few weeks. The issue was that Cody refused to remove his baseball cap when in school and that was in breach of school rules. Cody would arrive, usually late, and then when told to take his hat off, would refuse. He wasn't allowed into class and either spent his time in isolation or was sent home. Both Cody and the school were locked in a battle of wills and the school was losing patience. The psychologist was asked to speak to Cody to see whether she could help change his behaviour. One of the techniques the author taught was to enter into the invitation mode (Fransella & Dalton, 2000); this means, putting it simply, being puzzled by the client and asking them to help you to make sense of their behaviour. Cody obliged, as people often do, being happy to give his side of the story. Cody explained that his baseball cap was his identity and being told to take off his cap, was in his opinion, disrespectful. From Cody's perspective, being commanded to take of his cap denied; his culture, which he was proud of, denied his right to be different, and his right to be in control of his own behaviour. He was also not going to lose face, as he perceived this to be an insult to his manhood.

The school position was that there were few rules on what the students should wear, but that there should be some rules, which needed to be strictly enforced, otherwise they would have no control over the students. Cody's repeated refusal to comply signalled to them that he was not ready to enter their school. His behaviour was seen as challenging, confrontational and disruptive to the smooth running of the school.

Faced with this apparent impasse, the psychologist asked the simple question, 'what would it take to get you to take off your cap?' Cody replied that he had no problem removing his hat, if he was asked and not told to take it off.

The psychologist reported this, with Cody's permission, to the school and the deputy principal agreed to ask Cody, rather than tell him to remove his cap. Cody returned to school and when asked in a respectful manner to remove his cap, complied. Occasionally, he might be found wearing his cap in school, but if asked, he always complied. Clearly, this was not going to be the end of the story, but a potential serious conflict which could have led to permanent exclusion from the school was resolved.

This example serves to illustrate several points. Firstly, the school had made many assumptions about the meaning of Cody's behaviour which were inaccurate. They saw him as stubborn and confrontational. They did not recognise the significance of the baseball cap to Cody, nor the implications for Cody if he complied. The psychologist had recognised that some of Cody's core constructs (Kelly, 1955) were being challenged and that these were notoriously difficult to change (Hinkle, 1965).

Secondly, Cody did not recognise the school's position and underestimated their capacity to be flexible and change.

By taking the approach that all behaviour has meaning, and that all behaviour is an experiment, the psychologist was able to understand the purpose of Cody's behaviour and to elicit the underlying constructs. By sharing these constructs with the school, they in turn were able to reconstrue Cody's behaviour and adjust their strategies. The solution required both parties to make slight changes in the way they construed the problem and slight changes in their behaviour. However, these subtle changes enabled a solution to the problem to be found.

The psychologist did not attempt to map out Cody's entire construct system, nor did she elaborate individual constructs to any great extent, but she was able to get a glimpse of the constructs pertinent to Cody's behaviour.

By communicating Cody's viewpoint to the school, they were able to examine their own response to Cody. They were encouraged to examine their own purposes and this led to the school changing their approach. The school's response had the purpose of instilling good order and discipline, but they were reminded of a higher, superordinate purpose, that is, the need to engage with pupils to enable positive change, which in turn leads to positive outcomes and the wellbeing of their students.

People working within institutions often become 'stuck' engaging in repetitive behaviour which does not achieve the results they want. In the above example, the school was frustrated that they were not getting Cody to engage and yet repeated their response to his behaviour as they could see no other way forward. They were engaged in what Harri-Augstein and Thomas (1991) call robotic thinking, that is, the automatic repetition of behaviours which do not get the desired results. By getting the school to reflect on their hierarchy of purposes, the psychologist was able to facilitate change.

This would not be something the psychologist would have done prior to being introduced to PCP. The psychologist would have tried to find an incentive to reward Cody for complying, that is, a simplistic behaviourist approach, but that in my opinion, would have been doomed to failure, as it would not have addressed the issue, namely that Cody would not want to lose face, wanted to be treated with respect and was not prepared to compromise. Without an understanding of the significance of wearing a baseball cap to Cody, it is difficult to see how the situation could be resolved.

Ravenette (1997) suggests that educational psychologists can work both with individual students and significant adults in order to foster change. He used personal construct techniques to elicit the individual's perspective. The class teacher's and parents' constructs are also seen to be of significance and he proposes that change can be fostered by working with the student, the teacher, the parent or a combination of all three.

Change talk tends to be associated with successful outcomes. This strategy elicits reasons for changing from the young person, by having them give voice to the need or reasons for changing. Rather than the adult lecturing or telling the young person the importance of and reasons why they should change, change talk consists of responses evoked from the individual. Young people's responses usually contain reasons for change that are personally important for them. Change talk, like several motivational interviewing strategies, can be used to address discrepancies between words and actions (e.g. saying that they want to become engaged, but continuing to opt out) in a manner that is nonconfrontational.

Importantly, change talk tends to be associated with successful outcomes.

This is not to say that the solution lies solely with the student, change should involve everyone concerned with the student. As Ravenette (1997) indicates, it isn't just the student's perspective that is important, but also the perspective of the adults involved with the student.

> The important aspect ... is to remind the client (teacher, child or parent that the responsibility for change is theirs...
> (Ravenette 1997, p. 181)

Self-organised Learning, A Model of Change

The problem of meaning is central to educational change. Fullan (2001) states that the neglect of the phenomenology of change (i.e. how people actually experience change) is key to the failure of new initiatives. There is the need to understand the *what* and the *how* of change. Meaning is accomplished in relation to both these aspects, with those involved in change needing to know what should change and how best to accomplish this. In addition, all changes involve an element of loss, anxiety and struggle to varying degrees. Some of this will arise from reflection and the challenge to dominant constructs, discourse and paradigms.

Approaches to change at whatever level (individual, group or organisation) can fail if the above caveats are not heeded. People are unlikely to respond to requests for change imposed from the outside unless they can agree to the underlying principles and philosophy behind the change (Fullan, 2001). The approach described below has at its heart the assumption that individuals must be consulted, and involved, if change is to take place (Clarke, 1996).

Self-Organised Learning (SOL, Harri-Augstein & Thomas, 1991) is a conversational science dedicated to the elaboration of meaning and to promoting change. It is the author's opinion that the processes underlying SOL dovetail nicely with theory and techniques derived from PCP and the wider social constructionist approach of Foucault (1967, 1977). By reflecting on the paradigms of people engaged in the consultation, underpinning discourse and paradigms can be revealed.

Kelly believed that human beings, by their very nature, are constantly learning. We are in the business of making sense of the world. We conduct experiments to test the validity of our theories and modify our constructs/theories accordingly. Learning is not therefore simply that structured activity which takes place in the classroom. In this model, no distinction is made between learning and behaviour, as this would be a false dichotomy (Kelly, 1969).

Central to the SOL model is the unique concept of a learning conversation, where the learner, in a structured inquiry, is consulted about their own theories on the nature of the problem and what action might be taken. In a joint venture, the person 'leading' the consultation (learning coach) and consultee (client), construct strategies to tackle what is perceived to be in need of change. The strategies are implemented, after having considered outcomes and constructed methods of evaluation. The learning coach must suspend their own constructs in order to subsume the constructs of the learner and therefore help the learner to develop purposes and strategies that work for them. The learning coach is akin to a sports coach, in that he/she has knowledge about how to develop and enable the person's skills and expertise, but the strategies and actions undertaken are ultimately owned by the person.

In an SOL consultation the client, usually teacher, parent and child, individually or together, can expect to be asked about the nature of the problem, their perceptions of it, what would need to change and why they perceive change to be necessary. Eliciting constructs, elaborating the nature of the problem and sharing different perceptions in order to arrive at a conjoint understanding of the problem and what needs to be done, would normally take up a significant part of the consultation. In terms of strategies, the consultee/s would be asked to note when the problem did not occur, as a pointer to further understanding the nature of the problem, and would be asked to look at what is working well at the moment. In addition, the consultee/s would be asked to identify what resources (e.g. financial, personnel, etc.) may be available.

Once strategies have been agreed, expected outcomes can be negotiated and a review date set. The consultation process follows the PSOR model described below. It is a methodology allowing for learning conversations to occur within a structured framework.

The PSOR Model

Purpose, Strategy, Outcome, Review (PSOR)

At the core of SOL is the PSOR cycle (Harri-Augstein & Thomas, 1991; Harri-Augstein & Webb, 1995), which consists of:

1. Identifying the task/behaviour to change.
2. Identifying the purpose.
3. Designing a strategy and identifying resources.
4. Deciding on expected outcomes.

This is explained further in the model and explanatory text below.

Reviewing the Process

Purposes

Purposes are defined as the individual's underlying resources/rationale for attitudes, events and behaviours. These can reflect deeper paradigms where that discourse is challenged.

When purposes are examined, they can challenge our existing constructs and establish new attitudes and personally valid ways of thinking, feeling and behaving. It is often the case that strategies, both individually and collectively, that are currently employed have become so automatic, that they are no longer under conscious control. The theories which underlie these strategies, whether the person is aware of them or not, influence the way they act. It is therefore of supreme importance that people become aware of the underlying theories/discourses which influence their behaviour, if they wish to change behaviours. Reflective skills are needed to challenge these theories, and underlying constructs/discourses, bringing them back into awareness and thus opening them to revision and development.

From the identification of purposes, strategies, objectives and review processes can be established.

Strategies

Strategies are conceived as being subordinate to purposes. Strategies describe actions to be carried out by the consultee. In the planning stage of the PSOR cycle, reflection on strategies used in the past, in relation to a long-standing problem, often reveal automatic thinking and semi-conscious forms of action, with accompanying negative feelings and emotions. Repeating the same behaviour and making the same mistakes, without ever reflecting on the nature of the difficulties, typify this.

Often hard-pressed practitioners would tend to begin at this stage, suggesting pre-formed strategies, which are often imposed, rather than ones reflecting change after consideration of underlying constructs, discourse and paradigms. However, the difficulty with such an approach is that a great many assumptions are being made about; common goals, commitment to change, that no confusion over purposes exists and that the parties involved have achieved consensus about what they are striving to achieve. If there is no agreement concerning common aims, values, beliefs and purposes, then the strategies, suggested or imposed from the outside, are more likely to fail.

Having elicited the purposes, the strategies that follow are related directly to them and the system of reviews at each level ensures that the strategies do reflect purposes. The desired outcomes and achieved outcomes also reflect the original purposes. If a mismatch occurs, a modification of purposes, strategies or expected outcomes can take place. This cycle of reflection and action ensures that the teacher employing a PSOR approach can be flexible, adjusting their approach according to circumstances and a perceived need to change.

If there is a mismatch between purposes and strategies, this can be experienced as being psychologically uncomfortable. This can range from feelings of unease to acute distress, for example, the parent of a reluctant reader who forces their child to spend hours every evening and weekend painfully plodding through text.

The more central/core a purpose is to that individual, the more likely that a perceived mismatch between purposes, strategies and outcomes, will be regarded as a negative experience. If a purpose is backed by the discourses around a person, then this is more likely to be central and core.

Outcomes

By discussing outcomes, we access the part of our value system that governs our expectations and the way we consciously or more usually unconsciously, judge the effectiveness of our behaviour. Each outcome should be related to a purpose and if mismatch occurs: either the purpose has not been clearly elaborated, the expected outcome is unrealistic or the strategies used were inappropriate. People are not always aware of how unrealistic their goals are. They are largely unaware of what causes feelings of dissatisfaction, which result from this mismatch and previous failures.

Review

Defined purposes will affect strategies and are in turn affected by the outcomes that derive from them. Strategy leads to outcomes, and the outcomes, when related to purpose, provide the criteria for measuring effectiveness. Together these components provide the structure for conversing about the learning process. Review extends more widely than simply reviewing purposes; it involves an appraisal of the whole process.

Review involves checking the quality of the outcome and how this relates to the original purpose. The effectiveness of each strategy is evaluated and a decision as to whether new strategies need to be employed is made. The expected outcomes may also need to be reviewed to determine whether the goals that were set are actually related to the original purpose, and whether they are realistic. In one sense, review takes place at each level of the PSOR cycle (Fig. 1).

In addition to a review at each stage of the model, the PSOR cycle also provides a review of the whole process, assessing the effectiveness of the purpose-strategy-outcome conversation. If the outcome did not match expectations or did not seem to relate to intended aims, then the cycle will need to be critically examined, to decide why a mismatch occurred. As a result, the consultee may have to review their purposes and ask several questions: are their purposes still relevant, are they realistic given the current circumstances, can they be more clearly stated, is there any confusion of purposes, such that what appears to be one purpose, actually contains a number of individual purposes, could their purposes be further elaborated? With regard to strategies, the person leading the consultation could ask: whether the strategies related to purposes and outcomes, was the strategy appropriate, might an alternative strategy have achieved the desired outcome, how might the relationships between purpose and strategy be altered so that a mismatch is not repeated, was there a thorough review of the alternative strategies or was a hasty choice made? Any evidence of robotic thinking (i.e. we have always done it this way)? These types of questions lead to the potential to explore deeper, underlying paradigms.

The relationship between outcomes, strategies and purpose could also be reviewed, in order to place the outcomes as a result of purposes. For instance, were outcomes considered before the strategies were employed and did they, for instance, reflect the purposes?

In summary, if anticipated outcome is different from actual outcome, then the discussion and interpretation of these differences can be used as a basis for encouraging the individual or institution, to reconstruct their system of beliefs

Purposes – elicit and elaborate purposes, arrange in order of importance and conduct a resource check.

Strategy – must be related to purpose and expected outcome. Negotiate and adjust strategy where necessary.

Outcome – what is the expected outcome? Is it realistic? Does it relate to the original purpose?

Review – check the quality of the outcome against the purpose. Check the effectiveness of the strategy. Revise the expected outcomes where necessary.

Assess the effectiveness of the Purpose Strategy Outcome cycle

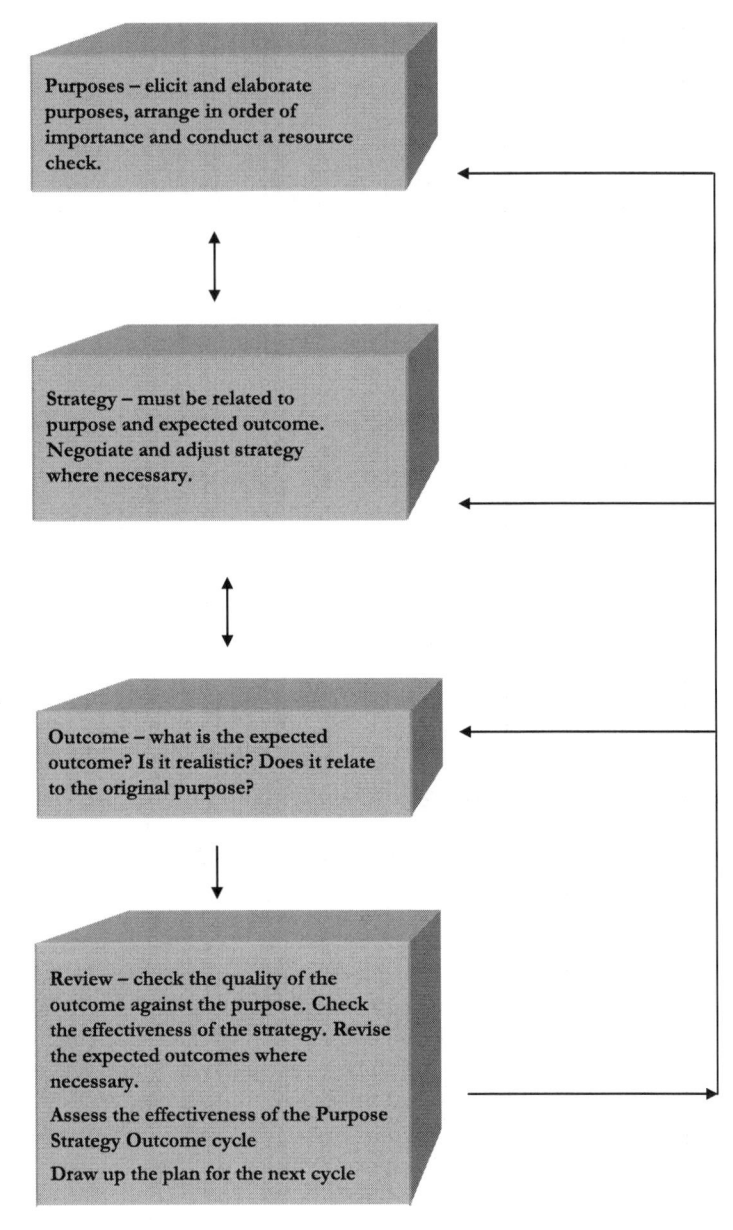

Draw up the plan for the next cycle

Fig. 1. An Algorithm of the PSOR Model. *Source:* Author's creation, based on Learning Conversations theory by Harri-Augstein and Thomas (1991).

or knowledge structure that informed the original plan. Therefore, underlying discourses and paradigms are challenged. Alternatively, they could revise their strategies and expected outcomes, so that they reflect the purposes.

The PSOR cycle is designed to help the learner set achievable goals that are related to the group or individual purposes. The learner is encouraged to establish ways of evaluating progress and to define more realistic ways of measuring success. The outcome provides the criteria for evaluating effectiveness. The self-organised learner is self-critical and uses their own experiences as a test bed for evaluating their effectiveness.

By investigating purposes in an open way, the paradigms, assumptions and constructs that people work within are elicited. The information gathered at this stage directly influences the conduct of the subsequent three stages of the process.

It is a Friday morning in a junior high school provision for students who have behaviour, social, and emotional difficulties, as defined by the education system. If you were to visit on any other day you may witness one or maybe two students struggling to cope with the school day. On other days, the school may be peaceful, all the students settled and working.

However, this Friday morning is the same as any other Friday morning, absolute mayhem! In every class two or even three students are misbehaving, being confrontational and disruptive. The normal routine is shattered and the teachers are struggling to maintain control. Even those students who have behaved perfectly for the majority of the week are causing problems. Some are taking advantage of the mayhem, encouraging others to even greater heights of disruption. Others are apparently undergoing a major behavioural shift.

If you speak to the teachers, they have their own theories about what causes Friday mornings to be so bad. It's the cycle of the moon, high winds, something has happened at the student's home. These theories are delivered half-jokingly but reveal consternation as to what is the real cause of the Friday pandemonium.

Discussion with the principal and deputy principal reveals that the school runs a reward system, which culminates in a Friday afternoon reward session. Students are awarded points during the week for good behaviour. For each lesson, students can earn points for behaviour and application to the tasks set by the teacher; bonus points can also be awarded. If a student reaches their target, they can choose an activity at the end of the week. Activities take place on a Friday afternoon.

The choice of activities is extensive and highly valued by the individual students. It includes trips to the ice skating rink, Laser Quest, a bowling alley, a soccer academy, etc. Some students choose to go to MacDonalds.

The behaviour of those students who don't achieve the desired number of points appears to make sense from their perspective. They know that they will be staying in, being made to work, whilst their peers are out enjoying themselves. They are clearly angry and find it hard to control such a strong emotion. To the principal their behaviour makes sense. He would predict that they would behave in this way. However, he is prepared to manage their behaviour on a Friday afternoon, detailing his most competent staff to contain them. When questioned about his strategy, he reveals that it is his firm belief that there should be consequences for poor behaviour, and encouragement for good behaviour. His purpose is to encourage all students to conform and make the right choices concerning behaviour. He feels his strategy is partially successful, as for four days a week the vast majority conform. Some, if not most of those who do not earn their rewards are gradually enticed into changing their behaviour in order to earn the coveted rewards. He has consulted with the students and designed a reward system which they clearly value.

When asked about how they explain the behaviour of those students who have achieved their reward, the principal and deputy share the same theory. They believe that this group of students are resting on their laurels. Having achieved their target, they know they will be receiving their reward. They know that the school policy is not to remove rewards once they have been achieved. They therefore can revert to more disruptive behaviours, ones well practiced and firmly stored in their behavioural repertoire, without fear of consequence.

When asked what would happen if those who behaved badly did not receive their rewards, the principal and deputy agreed that the whole reward system would collapse and the situation would be worse than it is now. They are perplexed and don't know how to solve this dilemma. The current system works, but not on a Friday. If they punish those who misbehave on a Friday morning, the whole system would be in jeopardy. It goes against their principles to remove hard earned rewards, and disregard the efforts students have made.

Individual students' perspectives confirm that Friday morning is perceived as an opportunity to have some fun. Why should they conform if there is nothing in it for them? Their reward is assured, and anyway, it is good fun to taunt those students who are sulking because they have not earned their reward. Most students agree that the reward scheme is good and that they would try hard to earn their reward during the week. Those that are going to stay in on a Friday are angry; they perceive an injustice, they think it is not 'fair'.

The school is clearly in a dilemma. Something needs to change, but what? In order to move the problem on, we need to look at the parameters of the problem and underlying assumptions. Is there any evidence of automatic thinking which assumes something should be this way because it always has been this way? By inviting the principal and deputy to suspend their assumptions and revisit their theories, eventually a new strategy emerges. They are convinced that a reward system works; they think that awarding points for good behaviour which can be used to earn a reward is a sound strategy. They are also convinced that removing rewards would be a disastrous strategy. The current points system runs from Monday to Thursday with Friday being a rewards day. When asked why 'Monday to Thursday?' the principal and deputy look slightly embarrassed and reply, 'because it seemed the best way to do it'.

However, this system leaves a gap on Friday which is being exploited by the students. The next question 'what if the system was constructed differently?' The principal and deputy suggest that, if Friday becomes the start of a new points week running for five days, that is, Friday until Thursday, the problem of a Friday hiatus is removed. All other aspects of the school's reward system would be in place and the school would not be compromised in their purpose.

The solution appears simple, with hindsight, but when you are immersed in the problem, it is often difficult to distance oneself and check one's assumptions. After all, this difficulty had been going on for some time and the solution had not emerged.

We witness this automatic behaviour every day. The fuel cap on a car is located on the left or the right-hand side. Pumps at gas stations have a long reach and usually can easily accommodate the width of a car. However, you frequently see long queues of people waiting to get to a gas pump which is on the same side as their fuel cap. The author has even seen people reverse when they realise the pump is on the wrong side. Harri-Augstein and Thomas (1991) have coined the term robotic thinking to describe this behaviour. It often can be at the heart of the failure to make change and to becoming stuck in a cycle of under-performance or failure.

Concluding Thoughts

The aim of personal constructs, put at its most pious, is liberation through understanding. (Bannister & Fransella, 1971, p. 201)

The author hopes to have conveyed to the reader a sense of the way in which personal freedom to change and increase one's level of performance or experience a heightened sense of satisfaction with life, in its fullest sense, is related largely to the way in which we are able to construct and reconstruct our experience. In order to become proficient in this skill, Harri-Augstein and Thomas (1991) would suggest that we need to be capable of thinking about our own thinking along a number of different dimensions. Perhaps the most important insights we might gain, stem from the realisation that we might best view ourselves as being motivated by sets of personal values, beliefs and theories. These will have been acquired in our families initially, and later through our experiences of education and the community. These govern such basic features of our behaviour and the way we conduct ourselves. Some might argue that we are robots, in the sense that early learning shapes such behaviour, and this early conditioning is difficult to shake off. A more optimistic stance, the author considers to be worth pursuing, is that such beliefs and values can be constructed and reconstructed in response to experience. By making ourselves aware of these aspects of our thinking, we are better able to pursue goals that are intrinsically meaningful and allow our expectations and anticipations to be influenced by the experience of their pursuit.

References

Bannister, D. (2003). Kelly versus clockwork psychology. In F. Fransella (Ed.), *International handbook of personal construct psychology* (pp. 33–40). New York, NY: John Wiley & Sons Ltd.

Bannister, D., & Fransella, F. (1971). *Inquiring man: The theory of personal constructs.* Harmondsworth: Penguin.

Barn, R. (2001). *Black youth on the margins: A research review.* York: Joseph Rowntree Foundation.
Björklund, L. (2008). The repertory grid technique: Making tacit knowledge explicit: Assessing creative work and problem-solving skills. In H. Middleton (Ed.), *Researching technology education: Methods and techniques* (1st ed., pp. 46–69). Rotterdam: Sense Publishers.
Boeree, G. C (2006). Personality Theories e-text book.
Chiari, G., & Nuzzo, M. L. (2003). Kelly's philosophy of constructive alternativism. In F. Fransella (Ed.), *International handbook of personal construct psychology* (pp. 41–50). New York, NY: John Wiley & Sons Ltd.
Clarke, S. (1996). *Principles and purposes in EBD provision: An alternative model.* Unpublished Ph.D. Thesis, University of Manchester.
Clarke, S. (1999, September). Using personal construct psychology with pupils who have emotional and behavioural difficulties – A case study. *Journal of Child Psychology and Psychiatry Child Psychology and Psychiatry Review, 4*(3), 109–116.
Dalton, P., Dunnett, G. (1992). *A psychology for living: Personal construct theory for professionals and clients.* Chichester: Wiley.
Department for Education and Employment. (1999). *Statistics of education, schools in England.* London: Defer.
Eggleston, S. J., Dunn, D., & Anjali, M. (1986). *Education for some: The education and vocational experiences of minority ethnic groups.* Stoke-on-Trent: Trentham Books.
Foucault, M. (1967). *Madness and civilisation: A history of insanity in the age of reason.* London: Tavistock.
Foucault, M. (1977). *Discipline and punish: The birth of the prison.* London: Allen Lane.
Fransella, F., & Dalton, P. (2000). *Personal construct counselling in action* (2nd ed.) London: Sage Publications, Centre for Personal Construct Psychology.
Fullan, M. G. (2001). *The new meaning of educational change* (3rd ed.). New York, NY: Teachers College Press.
Harri-Augstein, E. S., & Thomas, L. F. (1991). *Learning conversations – The self-organised way to personal and organisational growth.* London: Routledge.
Harri-Augstein, E. S., & Webb, I. A. (1995). *Learning to change.* Maidenhead: McGraw-Hill Book Company.
Hinkle, D. (1965). *The change of personal constructs from the viewpoint of a theory of implications.* Ph.D. dissertation, Ohio State University.
Home Office Development and Practice Report. (2004). *The role of education in enhancing life chances and preventing offending.* London: Home Office.
Kelly, G. A. (1955). *The psychology of personal constructs.* New York, NY: Norton.
Kelly, G. A. (1969). *Clinical psychology and personality: The selected papers of George Kelly.* New York, NY: Wiley.
Landfield, A. (1971). *Personal construct systems in psychotherapy.* Chicago, IL: Rand McNalley.
Majors, R., Gillborn, D., & Sewell, T. (1998). The exclusion of black children: Implications for a racialised perspective. *Multicultural Teaching, 16*(3), 35–37.
Naffi, N., & Davidson, A.-L. (2016). Examining the integration and inclusion of syrian refugees through the lens of personal constructs. *Psychology Personal Construct Theory & Practice, 13,* 200–209.
Neimeyer, G. J. (1992). *Constructivist assessment. A casebook.* Counseling Psychologist Casebook Series, #2. London: Sage Publications.
Parsons, C. (1996). Permanent exclusions from schools in England in the 1990s: Trends, causes and responses. *Children and Society, 10*(3), 177–186.
Rampton, A. (1981). *West Indian children in our schools, Cmnd 8273.* London: HMSO.
Ravenette, A. T. (1997). Tom Ravenette: Selected papers: Personal construct psychology and the practice of an educational psychologist. Farnborough: EPCA Publications.
Rutter, M., Maughan, B., Mortimore, P., & Ouston, J. (1979). *Fifteen thousand hours: Secondary schools and their effects on children.* London: Open Books.

Sarangi, S., Canter, D., & Youngs, D. (2013). Themes of radicalisation revealed through the personal constructs of Jihadi terrorists. *Personal Construct Theory & Practice*, *10*, 2013.

Sewell, T. (2009). *Generating genius: Black boys in love, ritual and schooling*. London: Institute of Educational Press.

Solas, J. (1992). Investigating teacher and student thinking about the process of teaching and learning using autobiography and repertory grid. *Review of Educational Research*, *62*, 205–225.

Strand, S. (2012). The White British–Black Caribbean achievement gap: Tests, tiers and teacher expectations. *British Educational Research Journal*, *38*(1), 75–101.

Swann, L. (1985). *Education for all: Final report of the committee of inquiry into the education of children from ethnic minority groups, Cmnd 9453*. London: HMSO.

Tomlinson, S. (1987). Towards AD 2000: The political context of multicultural education. *New Community*, *14*, 96–104.

Troyna, B. (Ed.). (1987). *Racial inequality in education*. London: Tavistock.

Tschudi, F. (1977). Loaded and honest questions. In D. Bannister (Ed.), *New perspectives in personal construct theory* (pp. 321–350). London: Academic Press.

Wright, C. (1987). The relations between teachers and African Caribbean students: Observing multiracial classrooms. In G. Weiner & M. Arnot, (Eds.), *Gender under scrutiny: New enquiries in education* (pp. 173–186). London: Open University/Unwin Hyman.

Chapter 19

Black Therapists – White Families, Therapists' Perceptions of Cultural Competence in Clinical Practice

Karen Carberry and Belinda Brooks-Gordon

Introduction

Caribbean Migration and Acculturation

Following the Second World War, West Indians helped to rebuild the UK by working in factories, transportation and the National Health Service. They became known as the 'Windrush Generation' named after the first 500 people who sailed on the Empire Windrush ship in 1948. The intention of many was to make money and return 'home' within a few years. Difficulties such as obtaining accommodation, lower job status, and dealing with racism were often withheld from the extended family in their countries of origin (Braithwaite, 1998; Ferron, 1995; Fryer, 1991; Goulbourne & Chamberlain, 2001; Sirett, 2004). Garfield (2002) highlights that in nursing, some White patients refused to allow Black nurses to treat them, whilst other patients provided encouragement in the form of letters, gifts, and invitations, which helped to redress the imbalance of power, and enable nurses to develop new scripts (Byng-Hall, 1995). By sending money home, and withholding details of their acculturation experiences, the nurses became parentrified, and created consensus role images – an unchallenged agreement that each one fulfils the family myth – that life in Britain was good. This avoided discussions around the complex dynamics initiated by migration, influencing how a family coped with the natural stresses present at every family life cycle (Ali, 2003; Byng-Hall, 1995; Carter & McGoldrick, 1999; Sirett, 2004).

Second Generation Socialisation

The second generation differed from the previous one, and Tatum (1987) found that Black families have had to guide their children through conflicting developmental tasks, during which the child must internalise the dominant views of our society, and at the same time learn to recognise and reach his or her potential within these conflicting constraints. In developing new scripts, Black therapists can draw reflexively on the transgenerational experiences of the family system; crossing theoretical borders to make sense of their 'outsider' position in cross-cultural interactions with the dominant 'insider' group (Banks, 1999; Carter & McGoldrick, 1999; Cavener & Spaulding, 1978; Cross, 1971; Fooks, 1973; Harrison, 1975; Helms, 1984, 1990, Helms & Cook, 1999; Lago & Thompson, 2002; Moodley & Dhingra, 2002; Pomales, Clairborn, & LaFromboise, 1986; Taylor-Muhammad, 2001; Tolendo, 1996; Wright, 1975).

There are arguments which state that family therapy does not need to be adapted to be culture specific, yet there is increasing evidence which supports the inclusion of cultural contexts both in training and clinical practice (Abela, Frosh, & Dowling, 2005; Burck, 2005; Erskine, 2002; Falicov, 1995; Killian, 2002; Laszloffy & Hardy, 2000; Lidchi, 2002; Ma, Chow, Lee, & Lai, 2002; Nath & Craig, 1989; Nwoye, 2000; O'Brian, 1990b; Papadopoulos, 2001; Sveaass & Reichett, 2001; Tolendo, 1996). Crossing theoretical borders challenges the observer to enhance their lens of curiosity in order to achieve a meta perspective that will test variables associated with process, patterns, themes, and differences and levels at which these may be enacted. Whilst circular questioning puts the speaker into the position of expressing their perceptions about the similarities and differences between client and therapist (Boyd-Franklin, 1989; Cecchin, 1987; Falicov, 1995; Hoffman, 1990; Imber-Black, Roberts, & Whiting, 1988; Lidchi, 2002 Rober, 1999). In this chapter, second generation Black therapists have been given an opportunity to test their perception of their White clients experience in therapy, using categorical variables associated with cross-cultural efficacy, racial identity statuses, socialisation and acculturation experiences, cross-cultural training, and reports of successful outcomes associated with change.

Early qualitative studies sought to illuminate subjective experiences via individual case studies. Research by Cavener and Spaulding (1978) and Thomas (1992) present examples of analytical cross-cultural therapy from the Black therapist/White patient perspective. Their findings show that unintentional racism, symmetrical relationships, and cultural variables can successfully be worked with, and provides a reflexive framework, which can be understood in part by the therapist's use of self (Boyd-Franklin, 1989; Rober, 1999). Working systemically from the White therapist/Black client dyad, O'Brian (1990) raises the importance of the 'insider' therapist acknowledging the impact of racism on 'outsider' families living in an 'insider' dominant culture that affect the self. In their work with refugees, Papadapolous (2001) and Sveaass and Reichett (2001) agree that powerful and emotional experiences occur when working cross culturally. For example, Indian therapists feel that some of the systemic concepts require modification prior to use in an Indian context, in particular, ideas of 'self' (Daneshpour, 2016) and in both cultures, anxiety is raised about which variables to address first (Nath & Craig, 1989). As an 'outsider' working with the dominant Chinese 'insider' culture, the importance of paying attention to cultural metaphors is highlighted by Ma et al. (2002). Subsequent research illustrates that getting to know the culture helps to demystify possible over-generalised cultural stereotyping that certain cultures are unresponsive to family therapy (Ma, 2005).

Cultural Perception Study Design Choice

Although qualitative studies are rich in terms of linear information, and can lead to hypotheses testable in quantitative terms, there are examples of quantitative analysis preceding a qualitative major design, such as Reicher and Emmler (1986) who conducted qualitative interviews on groups originally identified through a quantitative survey. This clearly offers a promising route for such cultural research. Mixed designs are not uncommon either; in Pearce's (2002) study on twelve White female counselling psychology students, a questionnaire and paper for comments were used to measure the biases of respondents when confronted with identical case histories of clients, with the cue of ethnic group (White, Asian, Jewish, and West Indian). Results showed that participants showed more favourable patterns of attribution for White clients with descriptions of 'warm', 'friendly', 'helpful', and possibly stereotyped the other ethnic groups. A redesign of Pearce's study encompassing a culturally educative variable, or repeated measures design, pre- and post-cross-cultural training, would reframe the possibility of 'stereotyping' as an indication of a need for future cultural competence, cross-cultural training, and examination of trainees beliefs about their insider position, drawn from a multidimensional approach (Falicov, 1995; Guanipa, 2003).

One of the few empirical studies of White counsellors in training Banks (1999) used a questionnaire, semi-structured interviews, and video response rating scale of counsellors; and drew on Helms racial identity interaction model. This model defines the way in which racial identity is formed differently for Black and White clients. It also explains that changes in attitudes occur as a result of social interaction with other racial groups (Carter, 1990; Cross, 1971, 1978; Cross, Parham, & Helms, 1991; Erskine, 2002; Helms, 1990, 1994; Helms & Cook, 1999). Banks (1999) achieved a high response rate (338 out of 360, p. 153) and results suggests that 'emotions were more heightened in the cross-cultural encounter or sensitive to ethnic differences than other emotions and that specific training in the counselling needs of Black clients did appear to enable White therapists to perceive Black clients' needs. The design omits the impact of variables such as the 'outsider' researcher on the dominant 'insider' group, but concedes that 'being a Black interviewer may have affected the response rate of interviewees who may have tended to give a "politically correct" or guarded answers. It could be argued that Helms' (1990) quantitative research on the formation of racial identity statuses could lead therapists to develop a prejudicial lens when working with clients (Cecchin, Lane, & Ray, 1994). However, in focussing on the effect of social interaction between cultures, Helms and Cook (1999) releases information that can act as another cross-cultural lens with which to view the 'insider' and 'outsider' position with sensitivity and understanding of the powerful emotions involved. The literature suggests, therefore, that a questionnaire is the most efficient method of assessing client satisfaction with race/therapy (Helms, 1990).

Black Racial Identity Status

- The first status consists of Conformity (Pre-encounter) stage. At this level, a Black person conforms to the Eurocentric and White orientated world view, with the support of a colour-blind outlook. They will deny racism exists, and is oblivious to the socio-political histories of socioracial groups.
- At the Dissonance (Encounter Stage), the person now experiences a situation that brings them face to face with racism. The experience is so shattering that it forces the individual to re-interpret and redefine their world view, resulting in ambivalence and confusion concerning one's own socioracial group and self-definition.
- During Immersion Stage, idolisation of one's own social group and denigrating of that which is perceived to be White occurs, and the individual uses their own racial group (in-group) to self-define and own group commitment and loyalty.
- Emersion/Immersion encompasses the most sensational aspects of Black Identity development – a euphoric sense of well-being and solidarity that accompanies being surrounded by people of one's own socioracial group.
- Internalisation finds the individual in a place of positive commitment to and acceptance of one's own socioracial group. In addition, a person at this stage relies on internal cues to define their racial attributes, together with the capacity to objectively assess and respond to members of the dominant group.
- During Integrative Awareness, one has the capacity to express a positive racial self, and to recognise and resist the multiplicity of practises that exist in one's environment, to discourage positive racial self-conceptions and group expression. In addition, when this status is accessible, the person is able to accept, redefine, and integrate in self-enhancing ways, those aspects of himself/herself that may be deemed to be characteristic of other socioracial and cultural groups – conceptualisation is complex and needed to ensure healthy intrapsychic and interpersonal functioning (Helms & Cook, 1999).

White Racial Identity Status

- During the Contact status, the individual is satisfied with the racial status quo, and displays obliviousness to racism and one's participation in it. The individual may approach Black people with feelings on interest and curiosity. Helms (1990) suggest in the Contact stage a White person may become aware of negative reactions of Whites towards Black people, and White people in interracial relationships.
- Disintegration status raises the White person's awareness, and forces them to both realise that they are White, and what Whiteness means in terms of privileges in a racist society. Helms suggests that this stage is characterised by guilt and anxiety as the individual is forced to acknowledge their role in White society. Individuals react in different ways, for example, compensating by taking

on the 'Black struggle' or shying away from contact with Black people and reintegrating into (racist) values and belief.
- Reintegration finds that the White individual becomes more positively biased towards their own culture and may develop anti-Black sentiments. Depending on how the individual copes with their feelings (as discussed in the previous stage by becoming personally active or uninterested in challenging of racist values), the individual may be happy to keep the status quo, and protect the dominant group, return to the previous stage or move on.
- Pseudo-Independence stage begins where White people start to possess an intellectual curiosity about Black and White relations. A person at this stage begins to reject the 'bad' racist Whites and identify with the 'good' Whites. In this stage social contact becomes possible and interaction is no longer characterised by the emotional curiosity of the Contact stage or the resentment of Reintegration.
- At the stage of Immersion the White person searches for a new, humanistic, non-threatening definition of Whiteness. In addition, the individual seeks to find accurate information about race and racism in order to recover from the prior racist distortion, and search for either internally defined racial standards, or re-education of oneself.
- The Emersion status is the appreciation of and withdrawal into the community of re-educated White people for the purpose of rejuvenating oneself and solidifying one's goal of seeking new self-knowledge.
- In the final stage of Autonomy the individual develops from having an intellectual curiosity about Black and White relations and racial differences to understanding the differences at both a thinking and feelings level. White people in this stage can seek out and enter interracial contact due to being secure in the own racial identity and appreciative of cultural difference. When a person is operating from the Autonomy status, they no longer have to impose arbitrary racial definitions on others nor must succumb to others' arbitrary racial criteria.

Racial identity theory provides an initial language to cement one's own experience, but also an indication of areas in which one can also be curious. It shows that in many therapeutic relationships, people may find it possible to switch between symmetrical and complementary responses that keep the sequence moving, within safe limits, and without the other person losing out to stereotyping. This is borne out in Ben-David's (1996) research on therapists' perceptions of their assessment and treatment of new immigrant families from two populations: the former Soviet Union and Ethiopia. Their findings indicated that the wider the gap between the cultural background of the therapist and the immigrant families, the more sensitive and contextual the therapist's assessment and intervention choices. Abela et al. (2005) in their investigative study on marital satisfaction among Maltese couples has shown that by exploring how cultural beliefs shape marital relationships, findings included the influence of a child-oriented family in the level of marital satisfaction, and the predominance of a constructive style of conflict resolution, which differed from those we normally found in the

Anglo-American literature. In addition, the importance of taking into account the cultural context when working with couples was highlighted, together with the implications for practice of the various beliefs embedded in the culture. The literature thus raises questions about the impact on the self of the therapist in cross-cultural exchanges, effect of socialisation, training, and curiosity regarding variables associated with beliefs around successful therapy between the 'insider' and 'outsider' therapeutic dyad.

Authors' Therapeutic Experience

During the penultimate session with the parents of a White family, with whom the first author (K.C.) had been working with for six months, conversation centred around change in the relationships between the family members as a result of therapy. The husband likened the positive outcome to a change in attitude, and in attempting to give this change meaning, he stated that in the past, if he had seen three groups of boys comprising from the Black, Asian, and White racial groups, he would have believed 'that the White group of boys were simply hanging about, having a laugh', and he said he would 'have been uncomfortable in the presence of the latter two groups, presuming that they were up to something'. Reflecting on White racial identity attitudes, we postulated that the family may have moved from 'Contact', to the Disintegration/Reintegration stage of Helms and Cook's (1999) Interactional model. Using cues to deconstruct the narrative, via curiosity and circular questioning, the couples were asked to explore in what way working with a Black therapist also contributed to this change in attitude (Cecchin, 1987). They revealed that the experience had highlighted the absence of Black people within their social system, and that working with a Black therapist had contributed to a change in their attitude towards Black people. She was able to cross theoretical borders, drawing on systemic theory, and knowledge of Black and White racial identity statuses, and cultural theory whilst utilising a reflexive stance to help continue to facilitate a reciprocal relationship with the family from a position of safe uncertainty (Birch, 1996; Du Gay, 1997; Hoffman, 1991; Mason, 1993; Rober, 1999). What is clear from the research is that in order to work effectively with White clients, who are likely to move back and forth, fluidly between different racial identity stages, it is crucial for the therapist to continue to their level of cultural awareness (Abela et al., 2005; Banks, 1999; Ben-David, 1996; Boyd-Franklin, 1989; Laszloffy & Hardy, 2000; Taylor-Muhammad, 2001). The hypothesis leads to the prediction that cultural contexts such as acculturation and socialisation experiences of second generation Black therapists are associated with successful outcomes with White clients. This study aimed to answer the following questions:

1. What is perceived to be the most common identity status of White clients at the beginning of therapy with Black therapists?
2. Do the socialisation experiences of Black therapists positively influence the therapy?

3. Do Black therapists experience successful outcomes in therapy with White clients?
4. Does cross-cultural training assist Black therapist in dealing with intentional and unintentional racism in therapy?

Method

In order to conduct effective race-culture research, information on factors that constitute good outcomes is required, and surveys have been frequently used to report outcome issues, and relate to client satisfaction (Banks, 1999; Devillis, 1991; Helms & Cook, 1999; Punch, 1998; Reicher & Emmler, 1986). A quantitative design is clearly a suitable way of initially exploring this field and to prepare the ground for future research. The central hypothesis, therefore, was that the socialisation map of Black therapists enables the employment of cultural reflexivity when working with White clients, which helps towards delivering successful outcomes.

Materials

Materials included a 28-item data form which provided therapists' profiles (Appendix 1) along with a summary of the Black and White racial identity stages developed by Helms (1990) (Appendix 2). Each participant completed a questionnaire that was developed to explore Black therapists' perception of White clients experience in therapy with them (Appendix 3). The scale consists of 10 items to which subjects are asked to respond using a five-point Likert Scale (Likert, 1932) (1=strong disagreement and 5=strong agreement) (Appendix 3). A stamp addressed envelope was supplied for the return of the data. For the purposes of statistical analysis and a measure of association a chi-squared (χ^2) test was used on SPSS for Windows Version 10.1.

Participants

A total of 56 therapists (15 male and 41 female) were approached at family therapy conferences, workshops, peer supervision groups, academic institutions, and therapeutic organisations agreed to participate in the research. Two participants wanted to participate anonymously. Of the 56 packs containing instruments sent out, 29 (51.8%) were returned from 21 females and 8 males. Participants therefore comprised a stratified sample ($n=29$) of second generation Black, Asian, and Mixed Heritage therapists.

Demographic Characteristics

The Counsellor age range was between 30 and 64 years (mean 42 years), this is shown in Fig. 1.

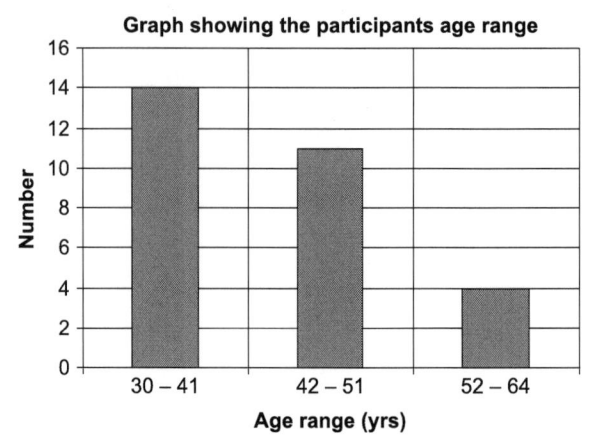

Fig. 1. Therapists' Age Range.

Participants had various lengths of residence in the UK. One participant had lived in the UK for 12 years, one (3.4%) for 20 years, fourteen (48.2%) between 30 and 40 years, nine (30%) between 41 and 44 years, and three (10.3%) between 46 and 57 years.

The majority of therapists' parents migrated from the West Indies (n=18): two were from Africa; four from Asia, one from America, one from the Middle East, and four were either born in the UK or migrated from Europe. Their self-described cultural backgrounds are detailed in Table 1.

All participants except one were second generation British subjects whose parents had migrated to the UK between 1945 and 1991 as detailed in Table 2. It is clear from this table that the majority migrated in the 1950s and 1960s with migration tailing off in later decades.

Eight therapists described their socio-economic status as middle class, and five as working class. Two therapists described themselves as 'spiritual' and

Table 1. The Cultural Background of Therapists.

Country of Origin	No.	Percentage
Black African-Caribbean	18	62
Black African	4	13.7
Asian	4	13.7
Mixed Heritage	2	6.9
Middle East	1	3.5

Table 2. Dates in which First Generation Parents Migrated to the UK.

Year of Migration	1940s	1950s	1960s	1970s	1980s	1990s	Unanswered
No.	1	12	6	3	0	1	6

Table 3. Parents' Occupation on Arrival in the UK.

Parents' Occupation	No.
Professional	14
Skilled/manual	12
Manual	2
Unemployed	2
Unanswered	27

Table 4. Therapist's Occupation.

Therapist's Occupation	No.
Consultant – NLP master practitioner	1
Psychotherapist – Family therapist/ systemic practitioner/psychologist	14
Health visitor/child mental health Therapist/social worker/family worker	10
Counsellor	4

Table 5. Therapist's Therapeutic Qualifications.

Therapeutic Qualification	No.
Doctorate: Masters	17
Degree: Diploma	10
Certificate: A-level	2

'professional' respectively, and 44% declined to respond to this question. The parents' and the therapists' occupations are depicted in Tables 3 and 4.

The majority of participants had been educated to doctoral or post-graduate level, followed by degree or diploma level study, with just two participants educated to British 'A' level standard. This can be seen in Table 5.

Procedure

The questionnaire was developed after previous research suggested that the process with therapy and outcome was relevant to client satisfaction. The questionnaire was piloted with a sample of 10 qualified and trainee Black and Asian family therapists, who offered critical comment on the items and determined the clarity of questions. Black and Asian therapists were approached at venues and therapeutic organisations in which Black and Asian therapists were employed. A total of 56 Black and Asian therapists agreed to participate. The refined questionnaire was sent by post and a summary of the Black and White racial identity stages was developed by Helms (1990).

There were four parts to this study. The first part analyses the characteristics of the Black therapists together with aspects of familial migrational history. The second part analyses the perception of the White client's experiences. The third part draws on the Black therapist's use of socialisation experience and beliefs about dealing with intentional and unintentional racism in therapy. The final part examines the impact of both client and therapist's racial identity statuses, the significance of the therapist's years of experience and training to aid in positive outcomes.

The Chi-square test (χ^2) was used for cross-tabulation comparison of data to investigate whether the relationship between given variables arose by chance or whether there was a statistically significant relationship unrelated to chance. The (χ^2) test allowed a comparison of actual frequencies with those which would be expected to occur on the basis of chance alone. The greater the difference between the observed and expected frequencies, the larger the resulting (χ^2) value, and taking into account the degrees of freedom, the greater the significance value.

Design

A between-subjects design was used and participants were allocated to their groups categorically on the basis of cultural background. The approach taken in this survey-based research is a quantitative analysis which fits the survey questionnaire-type design (Banks, 1999; Devillis, 1991).

Ethical Issues

Ethical approval was granted by the ethics committee at Birkbeck, University of London. During the study it was emphasised that the participant did not have to answer any question with which they felt uncomfortable, and could withdraw from the study at any time during the study. The possibility of participants becoming anxious whilst completing the questionnaire, particularly around items that may have triggered stressful memories regarding racist communication that have been widely documented as an experience of most Black people living in the UK was anticipated. A list of counselling organisations was, therefore, offered to all participants who engaged in the research, should it be required by them at the time or in the future.

Significant Findings

The association of significant independent variables on the dependent variable can be seen in Table 6.

Table 6. Association of Significant Independent Variables on the Dependent Variable.

Question	n	P Value	X^2	Sig.
Age of therapist associated with a level of therapeutic training	29	75.99	(1,n = 29)	0.03
Age of therapist associated with years of therapeutic work with White clients	29	175.96	(1,n = 29)	0.03
Good eye contact associated with all White racial identity statuses	28	14.77	(1,n = 28)	0.04
Age of therapist and belief that it is possible to work with unintentional racism in therapy	26	54.45	(1,n = 26)	0.04
Race of therapist and during the first session you find that White clients make good eye contact	28	37.48	(1,n = 28)	0.04
Black therapists perceive White clients as more likely to be at the contact and reintegration status in the early stages of therapy	21	23.46	(1,n = 21)	0.05
Black therapists tend to perceive their racial identity status to be at least two stages in advance of their White clients	21	84.00	(1,n = 21)	0.05
Therapist perception of client and own racial identity statuses	21	4.08	(1,n = 21)	0.10

1. Analysis revealed that the age was associated with level of therapeutic training X^2 (1,n=29) = 75.99, p=0.03. p<0.05.
2. The age of therapist was associated with years of therapeutic work with White clients X^2 (1,n=29) = 175.96, p=0.03. p<0.05.

3. Good eye contact was associated with all White racial identity statuses X^2 (1,n=28) = 14.77, p=0.04. p<0.05.
4. The race of therapist was associated with good eye contact X^2 (1,n=28) = 37.48, p=0.04. p<0.05.
5. The age of therapist was associated with belief that it is possible to work with unintentional racism in therapy X^2 (1,n=26) = 54.45, p=0.04. p<0.05.
6. White clients tend to be at the Contact and Disintegration statuses at the beginning of therapy with Black therapists X^2 (1,n=21), p=0.05. p<0.05.
7. Black therapists tend to perceive their racial identity status to be at least two stages in advance of their White clients X^2 (1,n=21)= 84.00, p=0.05. p<0.05.
8. The perception of White clients racial identity statuses was associated with the therapist's perception of their own racial identity statuses was not statistically significant, but close enough to be worth exploring further in future with a larger sample size X^2 (1,n=21)=4.08, p=0.10. p>0.05.

A table of further relevant findings is given in Table 7.

1. Analysis revealed that (18) 85.7% perceived to be between Contact and Reintegration.
2. Analysis revealed that (14) 48.3% stated that their parents provided advice on dealing with racism at work.
3. Analysis revealed that 6.9% (2) self-identified as Emersion, 17.2% (5) as Internalisation, and 65.5% (19) Integrative Awareness statuses. 10.35 (3) did not answer.
4. Analysis revealed that 11 therapists had between 2 and 5 years' experience (37.9), 11 had between 6 and 10 years (23.8%), 5 had between 15 and 18 years (17%), and 2 between 23 and 38 years (6.8%).
5. Analysis revealed that 72.4% reported that they did not receive training.
6. Analysis revealed that 12 therapists had between 1 and 5 years' experience (41.4%), 10 had between 6 and 10 years (34.5%), 5 had between 15 and 18 years (17.3%), and 2 between 23 and 30 years (6.8%).
7. Analysis revealed that 13.8% (2) of Black families attend therapy in the Conformity Status, 17.2% (5) in Dissonance, 20.7% (6) in Emersion, 13.8% (4) in Internalisation, and 10.3% (3) in Immersion.
8. Analysis revealed that 42.4% reported that they had received training, compared to 57.6% who responded that they did not.

Discussion

This study aimed to answer four research questions: (1) Contact and Disintegration appear to be the most common identity statuses met by the Black therapist, who (2) draw on their own socialisation experiences when working with White clients in therapy. (3) A large number (n=21) of Black therapists experience successful outcomes in therapy with White clients, who respond to challenge and report change. However, 6 (21%) therapists felt that this was not the case. A total of 74% have not received cross-cultural training for working with White clients. (4) A total of 48% of Black therapists received transgenerational advice from their parents in dealing with racism at work, while 44.8% did not receive any advice from their parents.

Our findings suggest an association between the therapists and therapeutic training, and may indicate an increasing number of Black and Asian trainee therapists. The results also show that the largest group had 2–5 years' experience of working with White clients. The next largest group had between 6 and 10 years' experience and reflect the research literature in that due to the training and background of Black counsellors, they are more likely to be geared to working with White people and not with Black people (Moodley & Dhingra, 2002). Our study also shows that 41% had more experience in working with Black families, having between 1 and 5 years' experience, followed by 34% between 6 and 10 years' experience, and may be a result of more Black therapists entering the training profession.

Table 7. Relevant Findings.

Question	n	Mean	SD
What is your general perception of the racial identity stage of most clients whom you have worked with therapeutically?	21	2.1	5.1
Advice from parents/primary carers on dealing with racism at work?	27	1.48	5.1
What do you perceive to be your racial identity status?	26	4.65	6.3
Number of years you have worked with therapeutically with White families?	29	9.3	7.82
Have you received cross-cultural training for working with White families?	29	9.3	0.44
Number of years you have worked therapeutically with Black families?	29	8.9	6.96
What is your general perception of the racial identity of most Black clients who you have worked with?	22	3.0	1.57
Have you received cross-cultural training for working with Black families?	28	1.57	1.57

Eye Contact

Eye contact is highly regarded in western society, and results suggest that Black therapists found that White clients give good eye contact in the first session. It is not uncommon for clients to display that they are uncomfortable in the first session and it is invariable the first time that they have shared their difficulties with someone outside of the familial and social network and the shifting of the body, and indirect eye contact is one way in which this is communicated to the therapist. The expectation that the therapist is from one's own racial group is information from the outside world filtered by our own constructs, which helps to develop a personal representation of the outside world. Social constructionism adds a further dimension to the theory, arguing that we do not construct these representations in isolation with others, which can leave the client wondering whether therapists who are outsiders to the surrounding dominant culture can relate to them therapeutically (Hayward, 1996; Lidchi, 2002). Our findings suggest that avoidance of eye contact was significant for White clients working with Black therapists, and sensitive strategies, such as circular questioning help the joining process.

The Impact of Curiosity

Dependent upon their racial identity status, some clients may deny any differences between a Black therapist and themselves, in order to preserve politeness (Thomas, 1992, p. 140). In attempting to move on the joining process, Black counsellors have been reported as using a proactive approach by asking 'How do you feel about working with me, a Black therapist?' and received the following responses from White clients: 'I'm not prejudiced', 'You seem all right', 'You speak good English', and 'I didn't realise you were Asian'. Another counsellor who confronted a client found herself at the end of a barrage of negative perceptions about 'race'. This was difficult for the counsellor to receive initially, but with good supervision and being clear about her therapeutic approach provided an opportunity for this counsellor to understand her client (Moodley & Dhingra, 2002). The results suggest that Black therapists draw on their socialisation experiences to explore the impact of race and culture on the client, together with advice from parents, rather than cross-cultural training. The work of Banks (1999) show that White therapists with longer years of experience did influence counsellors in their greater use of family network, in that counsellors with longer experience used this facilitating mechanism more than counsellors with fewer years of experience. Interestingly, the Black therapists within the younger age group appeared to be more optimistic that unintentional racism could be worked with than the older Black therapists, and perhaps the socialisation experiences provide much more support than those of the older therapists.

Reflexivity When Working within the Insider/Outsider Position

Falicov (1995) raises the dilemma of too much focus on cultural difference and cultural specificity, citing that one loses track of human similarities and may create division. Although not enough focus of differences, and acceptance of the view of the 'universal mainstream culture', Falicov suggests that one can also miss important cultural specificity and power differentials that make the difference between mental health treatment success and failure. In responding to the dependent variable, therapists may have employed the concept of 'reflexivity', the involvement of the therapist in the therapeutic process, as they are clear that the White clients' racial identity status affects the way in which they react to Black clients (Hoffman, 1991). Lidchi (2002) states that:

> although the reaction to the therapist's represented identity may vary from caution, distrust, disrespect, insulting behaviour and hostility, the situation has to be managed, framed and understood differently, taking account of prejudices.

This entails stepping back, recognising that consequences of the represented identity in the local environment and gaining a fresh perspective on what might be otherwise a disrupting experience for the outsider therapist. The process of getting to know helps reveal both client and therapist, the boundaries and perspectives that are reimposed on clients' perceptions and on the therapists understanding. With 43% of therapists perceiving White families to be at Contact, and 24% at the Disintegration stage, the Black therapists are usually aware of the representations of their own culture, as well as those that their culture holds about people from outside, and appreciate the insider/outsider dimension but from the inverse perspective. This includes what the therapists represent, their 'embedded' identity, what this signifies for the outsider client and how it structures the interactions. Sensitive to the complexity, confusions surround the issues of 'race', culture, and ethnicity, and thus, with this knowledge, good supervision, peer support, religion, and spiritual beliefs one can begin to sensitively address any power differential that pervades interactions (Lidchi, 2002; Moodley & Dhingra, 2002; Prest, Russel, & D'Souza, 1999; Taylor-Muhammad, 2001).

Status of Clients and Therapists' Own Racial Identity

Our results suggest that Black therapists were able to significantly perceive the statuses of their clients and their own racial identity. A culturally competent counsellor, using positive aspects of themselves offers clients the opportunity to 'risk take', challenge previously held assumptions, and transform themselves in counselling, and that skilful handing of therapy will prevent clients from the shame of some of the emotions associated with the early White racial identity statuses (Hardman, 1996). In addition to the theory maps which Black therapists employ, awareness of the convergence of multiple cultural contexts and collective identities empowers trainees to deal with families from different ecological niches, and raises consciousness about professional and personal biases (Falicov, 2002; Pearce, 2002). Abela et al. (1995) addresses the importance of taking into account the cultural context when working with interracial couples; particularly when one partner is more or less understanding of the other person's reality, and the therapist can use both reflexivity, and socialisation map in processing some of the difficult emotions associated with cross-cultural and interracial therapy.

Importance of Working with a 'Not Knowing' Position

The results show that the importance of working with a not knowing position will help work within a second order stance (Mason, 1993). One can use a blend of theories to hypothesise, and cultural theories provides an inspiration in two complementary approaches to cultural meaning, semiotic and discursive, from a structural and post-structuralist approach. Ideas that describe structural and processes cut across therapeutic schools and paradigms acknowledging the use of crossing borders.

> The insight from examining what a therapist represents to the other and how the other feels and so reacts provide a way to accept and resolve ambiguous or conflicted reactions from insiders. (Lidchi, 2002)

The use of informed knowledge thus helps the client and therapist to co-create different meanings about difference, raise awareness, and consciousness about professional and personal biases, and 'opens the door for cultural bridges and connectedness between family and the therapist' (Falicov, 1995).

Limitations and Future Directions

Banks' (1999) empirical study had limitations with the postal questionnaire which became the cultural awareness inventory, and this study was similarly affected by this method of receiving responses. Participants may have been dissuaded from participating due to confidentiality concerns as there were more therapists educated at the diploma and master's levels, and those who were at doctoral level may have felt exposed. A distinction could have been made between Black clients born in Britain and those who were not, in order to ascertain any association with migrational and residential variables. Falicov (1995) cites such limitations thus:

> Ethnic values and identity are strongly modified by a host of within-group variables: education, social class, stage of acculturation ... many ethnic traits are in flux, stimulated by cultural evolution and by exposure to or imposition of the dominant culture.

A qualitative study might have brought richness to Black therapists' experience, however, due to strain within training organisations and the emotional states of participants, a quantitative study was felt to be a less emotive experience.

The questionnaire was a useful mechanism from which one could extrapolate variables for further research. For example, future research could redesign the study using a mixed methodology to give the respondents the opportunity to make attributions in their own words as this would be more natural and less subject to reactivity of instruments (Bryman, 1992).

The therapists in this study felt that White clients' own racial identity status affects the way in which they respond to Black therapists, and this is an area for further exploration, particularly in relation to the theory of unconscious bias (Lee, 2005).

Black therapists feel that their socialisation experiences have helped them to explore the impact of race and culture on the families' therapeutic experience, and this is an important message that there are processes that may not have been taught, but may have evolved out of acculturation. Although Black therapists mainly agree that unintentional racism can be worked with, research on how process takes place is recommended. With an increasing number of Black therapists in training, information on the lens of unintentional racism in therapy would help in developing strategies to process this, rather than reliving the traumatic effect of racism within the confines of therapy, as well as outside the therapy room.

The outcome of this study has already had policy implications in terms of clinical practice, in particular, risk assessment when working with intentional racism, and unintentional racism in therapy and supervision, as well as strategies to strengthen the use of self. Organisations such as the Black African and Asian Therapeutic Network and the Association of Black Psychologists UK have emerged and provided training and support groups for therapists of colour.

Conclusion

During the study, the first author watched her septuagenarian 'outsider' parents prepare to return 'home' to Jamaica after 60 years in England, she was reminded that their map was to only stay a few years, and return home. Their map reminds us that in the interaction between clients and therapist trust occurs when people are ready, and that the evolution of new ideas takes time and can change shape. Since the study was concluded these parents of the 'Windrush generation' are now in their 80's and decided to remain in England in close proximity to their children and grandchildren, What lessons they have taught us about patience stating the Jamaican proverb 'nothing never happens before its time'.

The time is ripe for Universities and Institutions in the business of training psychotherapists, psychologists and psychiatrists to incorporate cultural competent methods within their curriculums is well overdue. Following the over-represented impact of COVID-19 on the black and brown communities in the developed world, the importance of working with culturally expressed emotional distress, together with adequate service provision, highlights that it is time for a change.

References

Abela, A., Frosh, S., & Dowling, D. (2005). Uncovering beliefs embedded in the culture and its implications for practice: The case of Maltese married couples. *Journal of Family Therapy*, 27(1), 3–23.

Ali, Y. (2003). *Nurses of the Commonwealth*. Unpublished dissertation, Royal College of Nursing, London.

Banks, N. (1999). *White counsellors – Black clients. Theory, research and practice*. Farnham: Ashgate.
Ben-David, A. (1996). Therapists' perception of multicultural assessment and therapy with immigrant families. *Journal of Family Therapy, 18*(1), 23–42.
Birch, J. (1996). Borderlines. *Journal of Family Therapy, 18*(3), 285–290.
Boyd-Franklin, N. (1989). *Black families in therapy: A multi-systems approach* (pp. 97–97). New York, NY: Guilford Publications.
Braithwaite, E. R. (1998). Paid servant. In O. Wambu (Ed.), *Empire Windrush: Fifty years of writing about Black Britain* (pp. 105–112). Guernsey: Guernsey Press.
Burck, C. (2005). Living in several languages: Implications for therapy. *Journal of Family Therapy, 26*, 314–318.
Bryman, A. (1992). Quantitative and qualitative research: Further reflections on their integration. In J. Brennen (Ed.), *Mixing research: Qualitative and quantitative research* (pp. 505–518). Aldershot: Avesbury.
Byng-Hall, J. (1995). *Rewriting family scripts: Improvisation and systems change* (pp. 138–141). New York, NY: The Guilford Press.
Carter, B., & McGoldrick, M. (1999). *The expanded family life cycle: Individual, family, and social perspectives*. Boston, MA: Allyn & Bacon.
Carter, R. T. (1990). Does race or racial identity influence the counselling process in Black and White dyads. In J. E. Helms (Eds.), *Black and White racial identity: Theory, research and practice* (pp. 145–163). Santa Barbara, CA: Praeger.
Cavener, J. O., & Spaulding, J. G. (1978). When the psychotherapist is Black. *American Journal of Psychiatry, 135*(9), 1084–1087.
Cecchin, G. (1987). Hypothesising-circularity-neutrality revisited: An invitation to curiosity. *Family Process, 26*, 405–413.
Cecchin, G., Lane, G., & Ray, W. (1994). Theory of the cybernetics of prejudice. In *The cybernetics of prejudice in the practice of psychotherapy* (pp. 7–26). London: Routledge.
Cross, W. E. Jr. (1971). The Negro-to-Black conversion experience: Toward a psychology of Black liberation. *Black World, 20*(9), 13–57.
Cross, W. E. (1978). Black family and Black identity: A literature review. *Western Journal of Black Studies, 2*(2), 111–124.
Cross, W. E. Jr., Parham, T. A., & Helms, J. E. (1991). The stages of Black identity development: Nigresence models. In R. L. Jones (Ed.), *Black psychology* (pp. 319–338). Berkeley, CA: Cobb & Henry.
Daneshpour, M. (2016). *Family therapy with Muslims*. London: Routledge.
Devillis, R. F. (1991). *Scale development: Theory and application*. London: Sage.
Du Gay, P. (Ed.). (1997). *Production of culture/cultures of production*. London: Sage/The Open University.
Erskine, R. (2002). Exposing racism, exploring race. *Journal of Family Therapy, 24*, 282–297.
Falicov, C. J. (1995). Training to think culturally: A multidimensional comparative framework. *Family Process, 34*, 373–388.
Ferron, E. (1995). *Man, you've mixed: A Jamaican comes to Britain*. London: Whitting & Birch.
Fooks, G. M. (1973). Dilemmas of Black therapists. *Journal of Non-White Concerns, 1*, 181–190. In Carter. R. T. (Eds.), *The influence of racial identity in psychotherapy: Towards a racially inclusive model*. Hoboken, NJ: Wiley.
Fryer, P. (1991). *Staying power: The history of Black people in Britain*. London: Pluto Press.
Garfield, J. (2002). *Black angels from the empire*. Austin, TX: Eastside Community.
Goulbourne, H., & Chamberlain, M. (2001). *Caribbean families in Britain and the trans-Atlantic world*. London: Macmillan Education.
Guanipa, C (2003). Sharing a multicultural course design for a marriage and family therapy programme: One perspective. *Journal of Family Therapy, 25*, 86–106.
Haraway, D. (1991). *Simians, cyborgs and women: The reinvention of nature*. New York, NY: Routledge.

Hardman, V. (1996). Embedded and embodied in the therapeutic relationship: Understanding the therapist's use of self systemically. In C. Flaskas & A. Perlesz (Eds.), *The therapeutic relationship in systemic therapy* (pp. 71–89). London: Karnac.

Harrison, D. K. (1975). Race as a counsellor – Client variable in counselling and psychotherapy a review of the research. *The Counselling Psychologist, 5*, 124–133.

Hayward, M. (1996). Is second order practice possible? *Journal of Family Therapy, 18*, 219–242.

Helms, J. E. (1984). Toward an explanation of the influence of race in the counselling process: A Black – White model. *The Counselling Psychologist, 12*(4), 153–165.

Helms, J. E. (1990). *Black and white racial identity: Theory, research and practice*. Westport, CT: Greenwood Press.

Helms, J. E., & Cook, D. A. (1999). *Using race & culture in counselling & psychotherapy* (pp. 175–283). Boston, MA: Allyn & Bacon.

Hoffman, L. (1990). Constructing realities: An art of lenses. *Family Process, 29*, 1–12.

Hoffman, L. (1991). A reflexive stance family therapy. *Journal of Strategic and Systemic Therapies, 10*, 4–17.

Imber-Black, E., Roberts J., & Whiting, R. (1988). *Rituals in families and family therapy*. London: W. W. Norton & Company.

Killian, K. D. (2002). Dominant and marginalized discourses in interracial couple's narratives: Implications for family therapists. *Family Process, 41*(4), 603–616.

Lago, C., & Thompson, J. (2002). Counselling and race. In S. Palmer (Ed.), *Multicultural Counselling* (pp. 3–20). London: Sage.

Laszloffy, T., & Hardy, V. H. (2000). Uncommon strategies for a common problem: Addressing racism in family therapy. *Family Process, 39*(1), 35–50.

Lee, J. A. (2005). Unconscious bias theory in employment discrimination litigation. *Harvard Civil Rights – Civil Liberties Law Review, 40*, 481–503.

Lidchi, V. G. (2002). Lessons for an outsider: A family therapist's in Bolivia. *Journal of Family Therapy, 24*(2), 150–166.

Likert, R. (1932). A technique for the measurement of attitudes. In *Archives of psychology and group behaviour* (Vol. 22, pp. 140, 55). New York, NY: Wiley.

Ma, J. L. C. (2005). The diagnostic and therapeutic uses of family conflicts in a Chinese context: The case of anorexia nervosa. *Journal of Family Therapy, 27*(1), 24–42.

Ma, J. L. C., Chow, Y. M. M., Lee, S., & Lai, K. (2002). Family meaning of self-starvation: Themes discerned in family treatment in Hong Kong. *Journal of Family Therapy, 24*(1), 57–71.

Mason, B. (1993). Towards positions of safe uncertainty. *Journal of Systemic Consultation & Management, 4*, 189–200.

Moodley, R., & Dhingra, S. (2002). Cross-cultural/racial matching in counselling and therapy: White clients and Black counsellors. In S. Palmer (Ed.), *Multicultural counselling* (pp. 191–200). London: Sage.

O'Brian, C. (1990a). Family therapy with Black families. *Journal of Family Therapy, 12*(1), 3–16.

O'Brien, C. (1990b). Issues arising from intra-cultural family therapy. *Journal of Family Therapy, 18*, 289–302.

Nath, R., & Craig, J. (1989). Practising family therapy in India: How many people are there in a marital subsystem? *Journal of Family Therapy, 21*(4), 390–406.

Nwoye, A. (2000). Building on the indigenous: Theory and method of marriage therapy in contemporary Eastern and Western Africa. *Journal of Family Therapy, 22*, 347–349.

Papadolpoulous, R. K. (2001). Refuse families: Issues of systemic supervision. *Journal of Family Therapy, 23*(4), 405–422.

Pearce, A. (2002). Investigating biases in trainee counsellor's attitudes to clients from different cultures. In S. Palmer (Ed.), *Multicultural counselling* (pp. 203–215). London: Sage.

Pomales, J., Clairborn, C. D., & LaFromboise, T. D. (1986). Effects of black students' racial identity on perceptions of White counselors varying in cultural sensitivity. *Journal of Counselling Psychology, 33*(1), 57–61.

Prest, A. L., Russel, R., & D'Souza, H. (1999). Spirituality and religion in training, practice and personal development. *Journal of Family Therapy, 21*(1), 60–77.

Punch, K. F. (1998). *Introduction to social research: Quantitative and qualitative approaches.* London: Sage.

Reicher, S., & Emmler, N. (1986). Managing reputations in adolescence: The pursuit of delinquent and non-delinquent identities. In H. Beloff (Ed.), *Getting into life* (pp. 3–20). London: Methuen.

Rober, P. (1999). The therapist's inner conversation in family therapy practice: Some ideas about the self of the therapist, therapeutic impasse, and some of the process of reflection. *Family Process, 38*, 209–228.

Sirett, P. (2004). *The big life.* London: Oberon Books.

Sveaass, N., & Reichett, S. (2001). Refugee families in therapy: From referrals to therapeutic conversations. *Journal of Family Therapy, 23*(2), 119–135.

Tatum, B. V. (1987). *Assimilation blues: Black families in White communities: Who succeeds and why?* New York, NY: Basic Books.

Taylor-Muhammad, F. (2001). Follow fashion monkey never drink good soup: Black counsellors and the road to inclusion. *Journal of Counselling and Psychology, 12*(6), 10–13.

Thomas, L. (1992). Racism and psychotherapy: Working with racism in the consulting room – An analytical view. In J. Kareem & R. Littlewood (Eds.), *Intercultural therapy* (pp. 146–160). Oxford: Blackwell Scientific.

Tolendo, A. (1996). Issues arising from intra-cultural family therapy. *Journal of Family Therapy, 18*, 289–302.

Wright, W. (1975). Relationships of trust and racial perception towards therapist-client conditions during counselling. *Journal of Negro Education, 44*, 16–19.

Appendix 1: Personal Data Sheet

Age	Gender	City/county of residence	
Race and ethnicity		No. of years in UK	
Country of origin			
Parents/Primary carer's country of origin.		Year of Migration	
Parent/Primary carer profession on arrival in UK			
Parent/Primary carers current, or profession prior to retirement			
Socialisation: Advice from parent or primary carers on dealing with racism at work			
Your occupation			
Educational level			
Professional level of therapeutic training:			
Have you received specific cross-cultural training for working with			
White clients/families YES/NO Or			**Black clients/families YES/NO**
No of years working therapeutically			
No of years you have worked therapeutically with	White clients/families		Black clients/families
What is your general perception of the racial identity status of most Black and White clients who you worked with therapeutically (Please refer to attached sheet)	White clients/families		Black clients/families
Your socio-economic status/class			
What do you perceive to be your racial identity status (Please refer to attached sheet)			
Pre-encounter	Encounter	Immersion	Emersion	Internalisation
Integrative Awareness			
Date:			
Thank you for completing this form. Your personal details will remain confidential			

Appendix 2: Summary of the Black and White Racial Identity Statuses (Helms & Cook, 1999)

Black Racial Identity Status

Conformity (Pre-encounter) stage

At this level a Black person conforms to the Eurocentric and White orientated world view, with the support of a colour-blind outlook. They will deny racism exists, and is oblivious to the socio-political histories of socioracial groups.

Dissonance (Encounter Stage)

The person new experiences a situation that brings them face to face with racism. The experience is so shattering that it forces the individual to re-interpret and redefine their world view, resulting in ambivalence and confusion concerning one's own socioracial group and self-definition.

Immersion Stage

Idolisation one's own social group and denigrating of that which is perceived to be White. Use of own group to self-define and own group commitment and loyalty.

Emersion

This stage encompasses the most sensational aspects of Black Identity development – a euphoric sense of well-being and solidarity that accompanies being surrounded by people of one's own socioracial group.

Internalisation

Positive commitment to and acceptance of one's own socioracial group. In addition a person at this stage, relies on internal cues to define their racial attributes, together with the capacity to objectively assess and respond to members of the dominant group.

Integrative Awareness

The capacity to express a positive racial self and to recognise and resist the multiplicity of practises that exist in one's environment to discourage positive racial self-conceptions and group expression. In addition, when this status is accessible, the person is able to accept, redefine, and integrate in self-enhancing ways those aspects of himself/herself that may be deemed to be characteristic of other socioracial and cultural groups – conceptualisation is complex and needed to ensure healthy intrapsychic and interpersonal functioning.

White Racial Identity Status

Contact

Satisfaction with racial status quo, obliviousness to racism and one's participation in it. The individual may approach Black people with feelings on interest and curiosity. Helms suggests in the Contact stage a White person may become aware of negative reactions of Whites towards Black people, and White people in interracial relationships.

Disintegration

The White person's awareness forces them to realise both, that they are White and what Whiteness means in terms of privileges in a racist society. Helm suggests that this stage is characterised by guilt and anxiety as the individual is forced to acknowledge their role in White society. Individuals react in different ways, for example, compensating by taking on the 'Black struggle' or shying away from contact with Black people and reintegrating into (racist) values and belief.

Reintegration

Here the White individual becomes more positively biased towards their own culture and may develop anti-Black sentiments. Depending on how the individual copes with their feelings (as discussed in the previous stage by becoming personally active or uninterested in challenging of racist values), the individual may be happy to keep the status quo, and protect the dominant group, return to the previous stage or move on.

Pseudo-Independence

Helms saw this stage as one where White people start to possess an intellectual curiosity about Black and White relations. A person at this stage begins to reject the 'bad' racist Whites and identify with the 'good' Whites. In this stage social contact becomes possible and interaction is no longer characterised by the emotional curiosity of the Contact stage or the resentment Reintegration.

Immersion

At this stage, the White person searches for a new, humanistic, non-threatening definition of Whiteness. In addition, the individual seeks to find accurate information about race and racism in order to recover from the prior racist distortion, in order to search for either internally defined racial standards, or re-education of oneself.

Emersion

The Emersion status is the appreciation of and withdrawal into the community of re-educated White people for the purpose of rejuvenating oneself and solidifying one's goal of seeking new self-knowledge.

Autonomy

In the final stage, the individual develops from having an intellectual curiosity about Black and White relations and racial differences to understanding the differences at both a thinking and feelings level. White people in this stage can seek out and enter interracial contact due to being secure in the own racial identity and appreciative of cultural difference. When a person is operating from the Autonomy status, he or she no longer has to impose arbitrary racial definitions on others nor must succumb to others' arbitrary racial criteria.

Appendix 3: Questionnaire

Thank you for taking the time to complete this form. Please return the completed questionnaire to Karen Carberry in the attached stamped addressed envelope as soon as possible.

This questionnaire is designed to research the resiliency and strengths of second generation African and Caribbean therapists who work, or have previously worked with White clients; together with their perception of the experiences that White clients and families have from the therapeutic service they receive from you. The term clients are used interchangeably to denote the wide range of individuals, couples and families with whom you work with. The term 'Black' is used to collectively describe Black, Bi-racial and Multi-racial and Asian therapists for the purpose of this questionnaire. A breakdown of the cultural and racial backgrounds of all participating therapists will be included in the research.

The attached form simplifies the different identity attitudes for Black and White people for use with this questionnaire. In addition please circle the number that best suits your answer to each statement, using the following scale.

1 – Strong Disagreement. 2 – Disagreement. 3 – Mainly Agree. 4 – Agree 5 – Strong Agreement. For example, if you felt that in all cases White families tend to make good eye contact in the first session, circle number 5. For 'strongly agree' – See example below

| 3. | White clients respond well to challenge and subsequently report a change in attitude to the problem for which therapy has been sought. | 1 | 2 | 3 | 4 | 5 |

If you have any questions regarding this questionnaire, please telephone.

This is a confidential questionnaire, and your personal identity will remain anonymous.

	How Would You Rate the Following Statements?	Strong Disagreement				Strong Agreement
1.	White client's racial identity status affect the way he/she reacts to a Black therapist	1	2	3	4	5
2.	My socialisation experiences have helped me to explore the impact of race and culture on the families therapeutic experience	1	2	3	4	5

	How Would You Rate the Following Statements?	Strong Disagreement				Strong Agreement
3.	White clients respond well to challenge and subsequently report a change in attitude to their problem	1	2	3	4	5
4	It is not possible to work with unintentional racism in therapy	1	2	3	4	5
5.	Exploring the impact of your race on the families therapeutic experience has not been helped by my own socialisation experiences	1	2	3	4	5
6.	White Clients do not make good eye contact in the first session?	1	2	3	4	5
7.	The White client's racial identity status does not affects the way he/she reacts to a Black therapist	1	2	3	4	2
8.	It is possible to work with unintentional racism in therapy	1	2	3	4	5
9.	White clients do not respond well to challenge and subsequently terminate therapy prematurely	1	2	3	4	5
10.	During the first session you find that White clients make good eye contact	1	2	3	4	5

Chapter 20

Transracial Adoption and Mental Health

Nicholas Banks

This chapter considers historical and current perspectives on transracial adoption mainly, but not exclusively, from a British perspective. The term 'transracial adoption' refers to the adoption of children who are from a different ethnicity than that of the adoptive parents (e.g. white parents and black children). In this chapter, the focus is on children of black British origin, including African-Caribbean, black African children and children of mixed 'race' with a black parent. The term black children is used as a generic term unless otherwise specified. Mixed 'race' families, where one parent is black and one parent is white are seen as a 'variant of the black family'.

The difference of skin colour tends to be the focus in transracial adoption, with this placement context seen as having more complexities due to the racialised imbalances in white society with this effected through skin colour as a demarcation of social status and hierarchy. The significance of 'race' and culture in the UK cannot be denied and is evidenced by the difference in health outcomes, education and employment opportunities between various ethnic groups (Community Care, 2011; Gillborn, 2005; Powell, 2017; Rehman & Owen, 2013). Race effects an unequal social and political relationship in negotiating one's belonging, sense of self and social status (Smith & Juarez, 2015). For many white adopters, if not all, it may be argued that race does not matter, with them potentially taking a colour-blind or, at times, a colour-mute position. Most white adopters would be expected to have very different social and personal experiences related to race, as they experience this from a different side of the coin effecting a different perspective to black groups (Feagin, 2010; Smith & Juarez, 2015). White adopters have their own distinctive collective histories and experiences and, importantly, interpretation of those experiences. Few studies find that race and its social status reality do not effect and structure life opportunities (Gillborn, 2005). Importantly, as Smith and Juarez (2015) identify, white adoptive parents do not raise black children in a race neutral social vacuum, with negative notions of race and racism likely to be reflected in historical relationships involving power and domination. White adoptive parents will experience challenges of managing external influences impacting on their internal family dynamic in how to better equip their black adopted children with coping strategies that help the children form adaptive and resilient ethnic identities (Barn & Kirton, 2012; Boivin & Hassan, 2015; Docan-Morgan, 2011).

Ethnic identity is typically seen as having a sense of connection with one's cultural past and one's current heritage (Huh & Reid, 2000). Early research identified ethnic identity development as involved a process in which a person is continually assessing the fit between the self and their position in the varying environmental social systems (Spencer & Markstrom-Adams, 1990). Yoon (2004) makes the important distinction that ethnic identity is conceptually and functionally distinct from the individual's personal identity, even though there is a clear overlap and influence between the two. For black children adopted into a white family, there are likely to be complications in identity development in the context of how they perceive themselves in white society and as a black child within a white family, with this also interacting with how they are perceived by both black and white others. Existing research identifies that black children form their ethnic identity by a connection to their ethnic backgrounds and also imbibing or assimilating aspects of the dominant culture (Docan-Morgan, 2011; Hamilton, Samek, Keyes, McGue, & Iacono, 2015; Hughes, 2003). Again, this dynamic process may show complexities and different influences with black children in their biological families, when compared to black children in an adoptive family with different influences in their experiences and cultural understandings from their family. This is because the parents have a key position in influencing a child's identity formation through sharing their own attitudes and value systems. Unclear and confused approaches to parenting as regards ethnicity and the child's position in a white society, are likely to produce children who themselves are unclear and confused. For example, in an international adoption perspective, earlier research (Westhues & Cohen, 1997), discovered that out of 86 international adoptees from South Korea, South America, Bangladesh, Jamaica, the Philippines, Hong Kong, China and Zambia, ranging from 12 to 25 years of age, 10% believed they were white.

Changes in Law and Political Backtracking

The law on adoption of children in England was altered in 2014 through an amendment which removed the specific earlier legal requirement of 'due consideration' being given to the 'child's religious persuasion, racial origin and ethnic and linguistic background' in adoption placement matters. The UK political view was that by removing this requirement, the number of transracial adoptions would increase, with the goal being to reduce the number of black children in care who were awaiting adoption (Sargent, 2015). This change negated the ethos of the Children Act, 1989 and the Adoption and Children Act, 2002, where it was explicitly stated that due consideration of the child's religious persuasion, racial origin and cultural and linguistic background should be taken into account in placement decision-making. Earlier legal changes occurred in the USA with the Multiethnic Placement Act, 1994 and the Interethnic Adoptions Provisions, 1996, as a colour-blind policy, prohibiting considerations of race and ethnicity in the placement of children. UK politicians also took the view that any consideration of ethnicity in placement criteria was a barrier which prevented children being adopted. Interestingly, one assumption for the change of the UK law, was that it was well-meaning social workers who were attempting to stop black children being adopted, rather than the overrepresentation of black children being the result of potential adopters seeing black children as less attractive to adopt (Barn & Kirton, 2012). This political change was in the context of there being relatively few black or mixed 'race' families available to adopt and an overrepresentation of black and mixed 'race' children in the care system. It would appear that the changes to the UK law were intended to be seen as 'race' neutral and work to provide black children a long-term family placement opportunity. The change in the UK law was based on several assumptions, one of these being that black children would do well and thrive in white families and the second assumption being that white families would want to adopt black children (Barn & Kirton, 2012). A further likely motivation to the legal change was that of an integrationist perspective where, at that time, there were frequent references in the media to multiculturalism having failed due to a lack of integration into white or mainstream British society by various ethnic groups. The view of 'integration' may be better seen as one of an assimilation of any differing values of non-white groups into the white mainstream values and priorities. 'Integration' was arguably a one-way street.

A hidden political agenda of assimilation as a one-way process, rather than integration, appears to remain as shown by more recent developments in the UK media in August 2017, at the time of writing this chapter, in a *Daily Mail* newspaper headline of 29 August 2017; 'MPs anger as Christian girl forced into Muslim foster care; call for enquiry over a 5 year old's plight'. The further detail in this newspaper article describes a 'distressed Christian 5 year old'. The UK government was urged to examine the case, where the child was said to be placed in two Muslim households in the previous six months against the wishes of her family. The *Daily Mail* also noted that the child was white. The reader may have some suspicion that the identification of the child's ethnicity and her Christian religion was the spark for the media outcry. Here, this is an indication that one white Christian child placed transracially, albeit in a short-term foster placement, is sufficient to trigger a public outrage. In contrast, the permanent placement of black children in white families is seen by national government as an altruistic and desirable positive act to be actively legislated for. It is expected that the irony of UK government view is not lost on the reader. The newspaper also identifies the unbearable plight of this 'reverse' transracial placement in further detail:

> Social workers said the child sobbed and begged not to be returned to one foster mother who wore a face veil in public, as the household spoke no English. She also claimed her foster carer had said she should learn Arabic and had taken away her Christian cross necklace.

Another UK newspaper, *The Times* (28 August 2017) reported:

> The child, who is white, was born in Britain and has a UK passport... Her current foster mother wears a burqa in public which completely hides her face.... Last night MPs said the five year old's apparent distress over her foster homes raised disturbing questions over the council's decision to place an English speaking Christian child in Muslim households. Robert Halfon, Chairman of the Commons Education Committee, urged the government to examine the case. He said the child should have the right to be placed with people who reflect her heritage and background... Andrew Bridgen, Tory MP for North West Leicestershire, added: 'This is the wrong decision for the long-term welfare of the child. My constituents will wonder what world they're living in, in Tower Hamlets.... Imagine the outcry from the Muslim community if this had been a Muslim child adopted by a white Christian family.

Former Justice Minister Shailesh Vara, Tory MP for North West Cambridgeshire said the decision was 'completely wrong' adding 'The Local Authority should have ensured that in placing the child in a foster home, her religion and cultural background would be totally respected'.

The media and government outcry suggests that there is a political view of one rule for one group, and another rule for the more dominant group. The media reported that the day after this public outcry, the unnamed girl was returned to her family after a court hearing with the *Daily Mail*, on 30 August 2017, reporting that:

> The girl was taken to her grandmother's house yesterday after a judge urged councils to seek culturally matched placements for vulnerable children.... The judge even went as far as to order the East London Council to conduct an urgent investigation....

and Judge Sapanara told lawyers representing the council that her 'overriding concern (was) the welfare of the little girl'. The judge added 'You would presumably accept that the priority should be an appropriate culturally matched placement?' The lawyers representing the Local Authority agreed, but argued that no white British foster carers were available when the girl had come into care. Incredibly, just two days after the so-called scandal of the placement broke, on 31 August 2017, it transpired that the five-year old 'Christian girl' had Muslim grandparents with the grandmother not speaking English.

This moral outrage appears in stark contrast to the principles fuelling the change of law aimed at black children in 2014. One can clearly see the dynamics of race and power where once the 'tables are turned' on the more powerful white group, the same arguments historically put forward by less powerful black groups in society are used as a rationale against the 'reverse' transracial placement. This sets the current social context, where a public outcry exists for a white child, but not the position of black children in transracial placements. Transracial adoption could be argued to be a matter of white privilege through the political assumption that this would be one-way traffic of black children to white families. It is only when the traffic becomes two-way that the media and politicians are seen to protest and argue that the direction should be reversed, essentially describing the Muslim foster carers as not worthy or fit to parent white Christian children and that white Christian children need to be rescued and protected from non-white carers. This is about ownership and an exercise of white power and white colonialist control.

The Historical Position

In turning the page to set the historical scene of the 1960s and 1970s, it was the National Association of Black Social Workers (1972) in the USA which argued against transracial adoption in the USA by making the policy statement:

> Black children belong physically and psychologically and culturally in black families where they receive the total sense of themselves and develop a sound projection of their future. Only a black family can transmit the emotional and sensitive subtleties of perceptions and reactions essential for a black child's survival in a racist society. Human beings are products of their environment and develop their sense of values, attitudes, and self concept within their own family structures. Black children in white homes are cut off from the healthy development of themselves as black people. (pp. 2–3)

Butler-Sweet (2011) has more recently argued that whether in the USA or UK, the transracial adoption debate has focussed fears that white families, regardless of how well-intentioned, are not psychologically well-placed to help black children thrive in a white racist society and further, that white families will not be able to help black children develop a healthy sense of self and their racial identity (McRoy & Zurcher, 1983; Simon & Alstein, 2002). The positive socialisation practices within black families are said to help insulate from racism and support black children's development of a resilient and positive sense of black self. Although these positive practices have not been well-identified or researched, the adaptive life experience of black parents is said to be transmitted through role modelling to black children to support children's navigation and survival in a racist system. Related to this survival in a racist system are the wider arguments around the negative impact of transracial adoption on black children and the literature on black identity and the significance of being safely embedded in a black family to help achieve a positive understanding of self and resist stereotypes. Importantly, the experience of being raised/socialised in a black family is said to facilitate and enable a positive sense of self and combat self-denigration and hopelessness, typically seen as characteristics of depression. Knowledge and direct experience of black culture is said to further help the child achieve a positive sense of self and resist the negative impact of racism and prejudice (Bobo, Hudley, & Michel, 2004; Hughes, 2003; McAdoo, 2006; Tatum, 1997). The black British experience of racism appears well-documented with one survey showing that more than one quarter of Caribbean (28%) and close to one-third of Africans (31%) had experienced racism in the 12 months prior to the survey (Rehman & Owen, 2013). The Crime Survey for England and Wales in 2013/2014 recorded an increase of 9% in prosecutions for racially and religiously aggravated crimes (Institute of Race Relations).

Looked After Black Children in Social Services Care

The term 'looked after' was introduced by the UK Department of Health in 1989 to describe all children in public care, including those in foster care or residential homes and those still with their own parents, but subject to legal Care Orders. Information about the ethnic origin of children was first collected in 2000. At that time, the numbers of white children looked after were 82%, black or black British 7% and the mixed population was 6%. The figures for black and mixed 'race' children were disproportionate to the numbers in the overall population which were in the region of approximately 1% in the 2001 census (Office for National Statistics (ONS), 2005).

Recent UK government statistics (Department for Education, 2016) identified that 75% of children in care were white and children of mixed ethnicity, that the next largest group at 9% with black or black British children being 7% and Asian or Asian British children being 4% of the population of looked after children. The same statistics identifies that some 34% of these children returned home to their parents or relatives with some 15% being adopted. The total number of children adopted in 2016 decreased for the first time in recent years, with 4,690 looked after children being adopted in 2016 and 5,360 adopted in 2015, showing a downward turn of 12%. More males were adopted than females, with 53% being adopted from care compared to 47% of females, although this figure reflects there being more males looked after than females. In all, 83% were white, with 11% being of mixed ethnicity, with the government report identifying that this is very similar overall trend over the last five years. Looking separately at the Adoption Register statistics for England in the year April 2016 to March 2017, reveals that 72% of the children referred to the Adoption Register were white, with 28% being categorised as black minority ethnic children. Children of black minority ethnicity are also categorised as being harder to place (Kirton, 2000), along with children over three years of age, and those children who are part of a sibling group or who have special needs.

The disproportionate representation of black and mixed 'race' children in the care system has existed since the early 1950s (Bebbington & Miles, 1989; NCH, 1954; Owen & Statham, 2009; Rowe & Lambert, 1973). In the year ending 31 March 2015, some 69,540 children were in care in local authorities in England. Of these, the ethnic breakdown was 77% white, with mixed groups forming some 9% and black or black British groups forming some 7%. Black and mixed 'race' children continue to be overrepresented in the looked after population as only 5%

of the child population of Great Britain were black or mixed in 2015 (Zayed & Harker, 2015). Of these children in care, some 13% were being freed for adoption. The majority of the mixed population in care were white and black Caribbean ($n = 2,270$), with the smallest group of the mixed population in care being white and black African. The largest group in care for the black or black British category, were of African background ($n = 2,490$). Although Owen and Statham (2009) discovered that children of black mixed parentage tended to have the highest rates of adoption relative to any other ethnic group, many are adopted into mainly white families (Selwyn et al., 2010).

The UK placement statistics of 2016 identify that some 11% of children who were adopted were mixed, with these figures being similar to the previous five years. Whether the remaining 6% were black children, is not clearly identified in the 2016 statistics (Department for Education, 2016). If this speculation is so, it would appear that for some reason, children of non-mixed, black background, are less adoptable in practice. This would appear to contradict the government's belief and reason for the amendment to the adoption law in 2014.

The Mental Health of Looked After Children in the UK

Sempik (2007) noted that the mental health of looked after children in the UK was poorer than the general population and that the difficulties with mental health that looked after children faced had not altered despite changing policies and practices in looked after children. Some 45% of children in care in the UK were said to have a diagnosable psychological disorder, with some 70%–80% having recognisable psychological difficulties. These difficulties relate not only to the care and separation from birth parent impact process, but also the reasons for coming into care and the experiences of neglect and abuse prior to care.

Boivin and Hassan (2015), in a review of the psychological adjustment of transracial adoptees, found no clear evidence on the relationship between ethnic identity, racial socialisation by the parents and the psychological adjustment of the children. Boivin and Hassan's (2015) paper identified that the initial response to the previously mentioned 1972 statement of the National Association of Black Social Workers produced a number of studies to test the view (McRoy & Zurcher, 1983; Shireman & Johnson, 1986; Simon & Alstein, 1987). Those studies showed little difference in the general adjustment of transracial adoptees (Bagley, 1993a). This was also the same for a British study, where the focus was on self-esteem (Gill & Jackson, 1983). However, the focus of the Gill and Jackson study appeared to miss the earlier point that the National Association of Black Social Workers were making in the specific comments on the child's racial identity and the child's sense of self as a black child being able to navigate their way in a white racist society. Self-esteem and ethnic identity are conceptually distinct. Importantly, when the issue of ethnic identity was assessed, the results confirmed the perspective of the National Association of Black Social Workers (Friedlander et al., 2000; Hollingsworth, 1997). Those few studies which focussed on transracial placements appeared to confirm ethnic identity developmental status as a separate issue to general psychological wellbeing. The issue here was one of white adopters not apparently being able to provide the black child with sufficient information and positive socialisation experience to support their adopted black child's ethnic identity development. Thus, black children who were transracially adopted had weaker ethnic identities and/or experienced identity confusion more than their same race, non-adopted peers. A potential significant influence here may be that of society's discrimination and its impact on black and white families and the white family's inability to successfully identify and counter this rather than anything necessarily pathological within the white family (Banks, 1992).

In the USA, Hollingsworth (1997) assessed the effect of transracial adoption on the variables of ethnic identity and self-esteem in 238 transracial adoptees, either African-American or Mexican-American with 182 same race placed adoptees and 28 biological offspring as a control group. Hollingsworth found that transracial adoption was likely to predict a weaker ethnic identity for transracial adoptees compared to the same race placement adoptees and non-adopted children. There was no difference in the three groups for self-esteem. From this, Hollingsworth took the view that there was insufficient evidence for a predictive association between ethnic identity and self-esteem and that self-esteem may not be the most appropriate measure of psychological adjustment. This finding appeared to shift the debate from the issue of self-esteem as being a significant single determinant of psychological wellbeing in adopted black children. Similarly, an investigation by Friedlander et al. (2000), also found, with its 8 families with children between the ages of 6 and 15 years, that there was overall good psychological adjustment with clear attachments to the family, although ethnic identity confusion existed. There was a sense of being ethnically different and distinct with the adoptees, with the children typically identifying with white American culture rather than their own black American culture.

In other studies, ethnic socialisation is seen as likely to contribute to positive ethnic identity and an enhanced sense of self-esteem and wellbeing (Baden, 2002; Lee, 2003; Lee, Grotevant, Hellerstedt, Gunnar, & the International Adoption Project Team, 2006). Baden (2002) in a study of 51 transracial adoptees from African-American, Latino national adoptees, South Asian and South American international adoptees, found little difference in psychological adjustment with adoptees who reported higher levels of identification with their birth heritage culture compared to those adoptees reporting higher identification with the culture of their white adoptive parents. Baden (2002) argued that the more influential variable in psychological adjustment of transracial adoptees was the level of their overall identity integration or clarity in their belonging and sense of self, rather than their ethnic or cultural identification. Of interest was that Baden argued that the adoptive parents' awareness and openness of the adopted child's birth origin was likely to have supported the adopted children in developing clarity around their sense of self. This appears to be a specific skill and approach which needs further research enquiry. It is not certain whether these white adoptive parents lived in mixed communities which facilitated this greater sense of clarity, or had social networks which enabled this. However, it appears that the active acknowledgement of the child's birth culture helped enable improved psychological adjustment. Baden (2002) also identified that it was important for children to have clarity in their identity to reduce the child's confusion, as this was a significant influence on a child's psychological wellbeing.

An earlier study by De Berry, Scarr, and Weinberg (1996), involving 88 African-American transracially adopted children with structured interviews at ages 7 and 17, found that the variable of racial socialisation did not predict 'same group' or 'white group' orientations during childhood, but did influence black group orientation during adolescence. The researchers also found that the parents' openness and efforts to promote the racial awareness and identity of their children decreased over time, with some evidence that the parents adopted an increasingly ambivalent and resistant position with the child's increasing age. This ambivalence was found to increasingly negatively impact on the adoptees' psychological wellbeing. As De Berry et al. noted:

> Unresolved racial identity issues could exacerbate the transracial adoptees' difficulties, rendering them more vulnerable.... Potentially compounding unresolved racial identity issues, and increasing the risk, is the multifaceted issue of loss. Perhaps the grieving process for transracial adoptees reflects both a loss of biological parents and a loss of culture and heritage. Although transracial adoptees evidence signs of intellectual and academic competence, suggesting that their esteem needs are met, other needs involving belongingness remain unfulfilled. (p. 2390).

De Berry et al. found the transracial adoptees' psychological adjustment declined over the 10-year period from 7 to 17 years of age. At age 17, some 50%–60% of the transracial adoptees were described as maladjusted. Factors such as the quality of the adoption experience, perceived transracial adoption stress, perceived racial stress, lack of belongingness and racial appearance were found to negatively affect psychological adjustment. With those adoptees who had greater affiliation with their parents' white culture, there was increased difficulty in feeling at ease in both white and black ethnic groups. It also became difficult for the adoptees to develop a sense of their total identity due to their adoptive parents seeing their adopted children's black heritage as a potential threat for family emotional connection. From the studies of De Berry et al. and Baden, the significance of the adoptive parents' influence on the adopted child's psychological wellbeing over time appeared clear. This is particularly so in the context of insecurities in identity development being most marked in adolescence, which is well-documented as an important time for identity development and its integration for psychological wellbeing (Brodzinsky, 2005; McAdoo, 2006).

In considering the impact of discrimination and racism on transracial adoptees, Feigelman (2000), in a longitudinal study with groups of white, East Asian, Latino and black adoptees, found clear evidence, as would be expected, that discrimination and lack of self-acceptance of the adoptees' appearance were connected with psychological adjustment difficulties in their early 20s (mean age of 23). The study found that black adoptees, being highly visible in a white environment, were more vulnerable to being targets of discrimination and racism.

Those adoptees living in a racially mixed environment were much less vulnerable to experiencing a lack of self-acceptance of their physical appearance. From this, one can see that those adoptees who did not perceive themselves to fit in with their neighbourhood peers, were more vulnerable in their psychological adjustment. Importantly, it would seem that the adoptive parents had difficulties in supporting their children's identity needs and also did not provide them with a good understanding of racism and discrimination and how to manage this. It was not only management strategies that were lacking, but also the adoptees' difficulties with coping with their difference, not only within the family, but also the wider neighbourhood, making them feel disconnected and distinct, which impacted on their sense of psychological wellbeing.

Vroegh (1992) in a longitudinal adoption study of 35 transracial and 20 in-racial (black children adopted by adopters of their own race) 17-year old adoptees summarised the research findings as:

> The majority of the adopted adolescents were doing well. The rate and type of identified problems were similar to those found in the general population. The majority of the adoptees, both transracial and in-racial adoptees had good self-esteem; self-esteem was independent of stated race. Eighty-three percent of the in-racial adoptees said they were black; 33% of the transracial adoptees said they were black; 55% of them said they were 'mixed'. Stated race was related to race of birth parents; stated race was independent of variables thought to promote black race identity. The majority of the transracial adoptees had one birth parent identified as black and one identified as white; the majority of the in-racial adoptees had two black birth parents. Seventy-three percent of the transracial adoptees lived in primarily white neighbourhoods; 55% of the in-racial adoptees lived in primarily black neighbourhoods. One half of both groups attended multiracial schools.

When the adolescents were asked how frequently they experienced racial incidents such as name calling, insults, slurs, etc. in their school and in their neighbourhood, 3 of the 35 transracial adoptees reported that they frequently experienced racial incidents in their schools. Twelve said they infrequently experienced such incidents. More than half of the transracial and almost all of the in-racial adoptees said they never experienced such incidents. Regardless of the self-report, parents of transracial adoptee parents believed their children had more experiences than the children actually reported. Only one-third of the teens experiencing racial incidents talked to their parents about them. Parents generally advised ignoring racial incidents rather than confronting the perpetrator. This stance has significant impact as will later be discussed when considering the work of Smith and Juarez (2015).

A review by Boivin and Hassan (2015) concluded that there are too few studies to be conclusive about the impact of transracial adoption on psychological wellbeing, and the results were mixed, this may be because Boivin and Hassan reviewed adopted children from a number of different ethnic groups with studies with differing results. In those studies that included children of black African heritage, the results, regardless of the number of studies, appear clearer, where there was distinct and definite negative impact on psychological wellbeing over time. What may have been missed by Boivin and Hassan is the relative importance of perceived social status, where children of black African origin are likely to have a lower perceived social status and to be more visibly distinct than their Latino and mainly Korean study participants in research. Boivin and Hassan (2015) make this point when identifying that East Asian groups tend to be linked to positive stereotypes of academic achievement, while black adoptees are more likely to experience overt discrimination and negative stereotypes.

Although, in the present writer's knowledge, there has been no UK investigation or study of what white adoptive parents do in providing adequate socialisation experience for black children, in the USA the Evan B. Donaldson Institute (2008) identified that most white adoptive parents did not provide significant cultural socialisation opportunities with their adopted young black children. Those opportunities that were provided were at relatively low levels, through books or cultural events. The result of this was that the black children's experience and opportunities for cultural socialisation decreased with increasing age into adolescence. This appeared to impact on the adopted children's views about their ethnic identity and their practical ability to cope with racial discrimination. Other research has identified that those white adoptive parents who did actively promote their children's racial identity, enabled their children to have much more positive experiences (De Berry et al., 1996). Lee (2003) made the point that:

> Adoptive parents with a belief in enculturation typically provide children with educational, social and cultural opportunities to instil ethnic awareness, knowledge, pride, values and behaviour, as well as to promote a positive ethnic identity (p. 772).

Smith and Juarez (2015) posited an interesting means by which white adoptive parents may be helped to promote their black adoptees' ethnic identity, using what they termed 'white racial framing', initially developed by Feagin (2010) and Picca and Feagin (2007). Smith and Juarez identify what is referred to as 'cognitive frames' or patterned ways of thinking and acting which can be collectively held and passed through generations. Patterned ways of thinking and acting, when considering issues of race and privilege, may need to be challenged and altered through new experiences which continually need reinforcing, updating and extending to ensure the needs of transracially placed children can be met. Smith and Juarez (2015) worked with 10 white adoptive parents who had 13 transracially adopted children but, at the time of the study were adults. All of the adopted children were either black or of mixed black and white heritage. Smith and Juarez found that their participants were actively teaching their children how to interact and communicate with others about racial differences. These were referred to as 'race lessons' which formed the interactions of the white adoptive parents with their children. Race lessons were particular practices used by the adoptive parents to teach their children. This suggests an active attempt by the parents to instil a sense of understanding about difference and diversity and how this should be approached by children. The themes that arose in this study were those of 'celebrating diversity', 'caretaking whites' and 'getting along with whites'. The celebrating diversity theme related to the adoptive parents wanting their children to be able to affirm their 'race' and cultural pride. There appeared a consensus that family members should show pride in their adoptive children's cultural and racial backgrounds. Of interest was that this was something that was seen as an individual position for the adoptee to obtain, and not about their connection in the wider black community reflected through loyalty and emotional connection to a wider black social network. This issue existed as the adoptive families had little social or geographical connection with the wider black community. The opportunities that the adoptees had to meet with other black people typically involved, what was termed as 'cultural camps', where there were mainly other black children who themselves were transracially adopted. This may have limited the more natural learning opportunities and experiences for the transracially adopted children despite good intent. Of interest is that Smith and Juarez noted that, again, despite good intentions, the children were limited in their ability to make systemic connections regarding racism and its systemic influence and mainly had individual rather than collective perspectives. The significance here is that if one sees one's experience as individualised, the pressure of recognising, coping and responding to systemic oppression is likely to be exacerbated and compounded, where the perception will be it being one of the individual who is to blame and responsible rather than systemic factors. This conceptually and experientially limits the black adoptees' understanding of external factors which influence their development and opportunity. As Smith and Juarez noted:

> By using meritocracy to understand race, the adoptive parents did not teach about the structural relations within society that enable the hard work of some to pay off more, than that of (racialised) others.

Of interest is that the writers also identified that despite good intentions, the adoptive parents attempted to provide their children 'with blackness minus the burden of racism' by limited exposure of black experiences through films and passive cultural events. In moving on to the theme of caretaking of whites, this appeared to be related to the adoptive parents instructing the children to more consider the emotional needs of white people when they expose the black person to racist experience or taking care of white people as third parties who witness racist experience. Smith and Juarez (2015) saw this in the examples given of 'hair touching' and the adoptive parents explaining that the white people who touch the children's hair were 'just curious'. Here, Smith and Juarez (2015) point out that the needs of the whites were taken care of, while dismissing the emotional consequences of racial mistreatment for the children. Although the parents described the offending whites as ignorant, this was a cognitive response which did not take into account the emotional needs of the black children. In addition, there was a cognitive load or burden placed on the child, where they were expected to objectively evaluate the severity of each racial event and the intent of the offender, before deciding how to respond. This would result in an emotional overload for the child and shifted them into a position of perpetual educator for the white people who intruded into their personal space through psychologically and physically invasive strategies. This placed the child in the position of an educational object for the offending whites. Smith and Juarez argued that by misframing incidents in terms of 'misunderstandings', the adoptive parents themselves took on the norms of white privilege and white ignorance and placed their children in the position of being exotic and external to white normality expectations and as objects of scientific interest. With the third theme of 'getting along with whites', this was said to place responsibility of the adopted children to maintain peace and harmony. Conflict and anger and other related emotions were said to be bad and to be avoided. Children were instructed to be calm, not emotional and to be accommodating. As Smith and Juarez (2015) argue, the potential consequences for not getting along with white people were likely to be much more serious for the black child than for the white family members. The adoptive parent's guidance did not address the impact of the event on the child. As such, many of the black children in Smith and Juarez's study discussed feeling as if their own emotions were not as important as those of the white offenders. They described having no one to discuss their feelings with and being forced to dismiss their feelings to meet the emotional and psychological welfare needs of the white offenders. This required them essentially to repress their own experiences with Smith and Juarez (2015) explaining that this was likely to impact on the child's mental health.

Similarly, in a small-scale UK study of mixed 'race' children, Tizard (1997) found that the families in her sample lived in mainly white neighbourhoods and that the children had significant difficulties with their mixed identity and had difficulties in making friendships with black children. Tizard (1997) also found what was essentially termed as the adoptive parents, having an unconscious racial bias. Other studies in the UK, involving a longitudinal approach of black Caribbean and mixed 'race' children at ages 7 and 11 (Bagley, 1993b; Bagley & Young, 1979) concluded that the white parents showed 'a lack of black consciousness' but in a contradictory conclusion, the writers believed that the adoptive placements were successfully meeting the psychological and developmental needs of most of the children. A later UK study (Thoburn, Norford, & Rashid, 2000) compared adoptive transracial placements with permanent fostering placements and identified additional issues that the parents faced regarding meeting the needs of the children's ethnic identity, and concluded that transracial placements '… should be unusual and should be clearly linked to specific reasons in individual cases' (p. 208). What arises from the UK studies and the international studies is that race, culture and ethnicity matter and the issues require specific and sophisticated assessments of white carers' motivation for caring for a black child and their particular skills and, importantly, the adopters' support needs.

A further issue in transracial adoption is one of colour-blindness or colour-muteness where white adoptive parents are likely to minimise and lack discussion or exploration of the obviously physical differences that exist between them and their child. Due to clear physical differences, children in transracial placements will be aware of their adoptive status at an early age and thus one could argue that it is particularly important for communication about this difference to take place, before the child raises the issue themselves. Indeed, lack of communication may make the obvious difference one of a 'family taboo', where it is perceived by the child that this should not be spoken about. Brodzinsky (2005) has noted that it is important for communicative openness to exist within an adoptive family to develop the psychological wellbeing of children. Brodzinsky (2005) sees communicative openness as:

> A willingness of individuals to consider the meaning of adoption in their lives, to share that meaning with others, to explore adoption related issues in the context of family life, to acknowledge and support the child's connection to two families and perhaps to facilitate contact between these two family systems in one form or another.

Brodzinsky (2005) has argued that communicative openness, and the implied process of achieving a psychological connection with a child about their difference, is positively associated with psychological adjustment and self-esteem in adopted children (Brodzinsky, 2006; Smith & Juarez, 2015). Hamilton et al. (2015) identify that few studies on children of transracial adoption consider the communication patterns between with their white adopters.

With this in mind, Hamilton et al. (2015) and others (e.g., Docan-Morgan, 2010, 2011) have raised the question about whether transracial adoptees may be experiencing higher levels of racism than they were comfortable in discussing with their white parents, where there was a possibility that issues of race and ethnicity were being actively avoided or minimised in the home. Due to the parents not enabling the child to speak about these experiences as openly as the parents perceived, there was a suggestion that the child was likely to experience heightened discomfort in the discussion of race and racism with the adoptive parents. It would seem that the children who were most visibly different and who were likely to experience the most discrimination as a result of their perceived lower social status in the social hierarchy, were less able to confide in their white parents about their experiences. The difficulty being that although parents believe they are attempting to explore issues with their adopted black children, the severity of difficulties the black children experienced, resulted in them trying to avoid or limit discussion as they did not feel comfortable that their parents could cope with this and/or make meaningful suggestions and provide worthwhile strategies. As Hamilton et al. (2015) agree, their sample size of black and mixed 'race' children was small, with it being difficult to make conclusive statements.

In conclusion, the impact of transracial adoption is not so much related to the process of transracial adoption, but more related to lack of understanding and awareness that white adopters may have in combatting systemic issues and how to meet their black children's support needs. This has implications for government actions when making legislative changes to facilitate transracial adoption.

Funding the necessary training to meet the support needs of black children who are in transracial placements is required. If transracial placements are to succeed for black children, it is necessary for the government to fund resources to support the training of prospective white adopters to provide quality ethnically and culturally related parenting experiences from an informed perspective. As the research of Smith and Juarez (2015) identified, although adoptive white parents often understood the significance of 'race', and the impact of racism on their black adopted children, they were, through no direct fault of their own, unable to understand and make meaning of racism, even when directly experienced and heard. Due to their own cultural encapsulation, white adopters often missed the deeper significance of what needed to be done to meet their children's emotional development and provide meaningful strategies for countering racist experience. In interpreting race and racism through their own limited perspectives, the white adoptive parents were said to re-centre on the white racial frame and thus did not challenge the existing racial hierarchy. As Cone (2004) suggests:

> The quality of white life is hardly ever affected by what blacks think and do. However, everything whites think and do impacts profoundly on the lives of blacks on a daily basis. We can never escape white power and its cruelty. (p. 144)

The well-meaning white adoptive parents lacked an understanding of the politicisation of the whiter racist system and its impact on their lives and those of their children. Smith and Juarez (2015) further point out racial socialisation is not about content of what to do with racial differences, but a process of how one interprets and thinks about and engages with the world in ways that are independent of white liberal traditions.

References

Baden, A. L. (2002). The psychological adjustment of transracial adoptees: An application of the cultural-racial identity model. *Journal of Social Distress and the Homeless*, *11*(2), 167–191.
Bagley, C. (1993a). *International and transracial adoptions: A mental health perspective.* Aldershot: Avebury.
Bagley, C. (1993b). Transracial adoption in Britain: A follow-up study with policy considerations. *Child Welfare*, *72*, 285–299.
Bagley, C., & Young, L. (1979). The identity, adjustment and achievement of transracially adopted children: A review and empirical report. In G. Berma & C. Bagley (Eds.), *Race, education and identity*. London: Macmillan.
Banks, N. (1992). Techniques for direct identity work with black children, adoption and fostering. *BAAF*, *16*(3, Autumn), 19–24.
Barn, R., & Kirton, D. (2012). Transracial adoption in Britain Politics, ideology and reality. *Adoption & Fostering*, *36*(3 & 4), 25–37.
Bebbington, A. C., & Miles, J. (1989). The background of children who enter local authority care. *The British Journal of Social Work*, *19*(5), 349–368.

Bobo, J., Hudley, C., & Michel, C. (2004). *The black studies reader*. New York, NY: Routledge.

Boivin, M., & Hassan, G. (2015). Ethnic identity and psychological adjustment in transracial adoptees: A review of the literature. *Ethnic and Racial Studies, 38*(7), 1084–1103.

Brodzinsky, D. M. (2005). Reconceptualising openness in adoption: Implications for theory, research and practice. In. D. Brodzinsky & J. Palacios (Eds.), *Psychological issues in adoption: research and practice* (pp. 145–166). New York, NY: Greenwood.

Brodzinsky, D. M. (2006). Family structural openness and communication openness as predictors in the adjustment of adopted children. *Adoption Quarterly, 9*(4), 1–18.

Butler-Sweet, C. (2011). 'A healthy black identity'. Transracial adoption, middle class families and racial socialisation. *Journal of Comparative Family Studies, 42*(2), 193–212.

Community Care. (2011, May). Ethnic minorities still over-represented in mental health care. Retrieved from www.communitycare.co.uk/2011/04/05ethnicminoritiesstillover representedinmentalhealthcare

Cone, J. H. (2004). *Martin and Malcolm and American: A dream or a nightmare*. Marknol, NY: Orbis Books.

Curtis, C. M. (1996). The adoption of African American children by Whites: A renewed conflict. *Families in Society: The Journal of Contemporary Human Services, 60*, 156–165.

De Berry, K. M., Scarr, S., & Weinberg, R. (1996). Family racial socialisation and ecological competence: Longitudinal assessments of African American transracial adoptees. *Child Development, 67*, 2375–2399.

Department for Education. (2016, 29 September). *Children looked after in England (including adoption) year ending 31st March 2016*. SFR/2016. National Statistics, UK Government.

Docan-Morgan, S. (2010). Korean adoptees retrospective reports of intrusive interactions: Exploring boundary management in adoptive parents. *Journal of Family Communication, 10*, 137–157.

Docan-Morgan, S. (2011). "They don't know what it's like to be in my shoes": Topic avoidance about race in transracially adoptive families. *Journal of Social and Personal Relationships, 28*(3), 336–355.

Evan B. Donaldson Institute. (2008). *Finding families for African American children: The role of race and law in adoption from foster care*. New York, NY: Evan B Donaldson Adoption Institute.

Feagin, J. (2010). *The white racial frame: Centuries of racial framing and counter framing*. New York, NY: Routledge.

Feigelman, W. (2000). Adjustments of transracial and in-racially adopted young adults. *Child and Adolescent Social Work, 17*, 165–183.

Friedlander, M. L., Larney, L. C., Skau, M., Hotaling, M., Cutting, M. L., & Schwam, M. (2000). Bi-cultural identification: Experiences of internationally adopted children and their parents. *Journal of Counselling Psychology, 47*(2), 187–198.

Gill, O., & Jackson, B. (1983). *Adoption and race: Black, Asian and mixed race children in white families*. London: Batsford.

Gillborn, D. (2005). Education policy as an act of white supremacy: Whiteness, critical race theory and education reform. *Journal of Education Policy, 20*(4), 485–505.

Grow, L. J., & Shapiro, D. (1974). *Black children White parents*. New York, NY: Child Welfare League of America.

Hamilton, E., Samek, D. R., Keyes, M., McGue, M. K., & Iacono, W. G. (2015). Identity development in a transracial environment: Racial/ethnic minority adoptees in Minnesota. *Adoption Quarterly, 18*, 217–233.

Hayes, P. (1993). Transracial adoption: Politics and ideology. *Child Welfare, 72*(3), 301–310.

Hollingsworth, L. D. (1997). Effect of transracial/transethnic adoption on children's racial and ethnic identity and self-esteem: A meta-analytic review. In H. E. Gros & M. B. Sussman (Eds.). *Families and adoption* (Vol. 25, pp. 99–130). New York, NY: Haworth.

Hollingsworth, L. D. (1998). Adoptee dissimilarity from the adoptive family: Clinical practice and research implications. *Child and Adolescent Social Work Journal, 15*(4), 303–319.

Hughes, D. (2003). Correlates of African American and Latino parents' messages to children about ethnicity and race: A comparative study of racial socialisation. *American Journal of Community Psychology, 31*, 15–33.

Huh, S. H., & Reid, W. J. (2000). Inter-country, transracial adoption and ethnic identity: A Korean example. *International Social Work, 43*(1), 75–87.

Institute of Race Relations. (2017). Racial Violence Statistics. Retrieved from www.irr.org.uk/researchstatistics/racial-violence. Accessed on August 2017.

Kirton, D. (2000). *Race, ethnicity and adoption*. Buckingham: Open University Press.

Lee, R. M. (2003). The transracial paradox: History, research and counselling implications of cultural socialisation. *The Journal of Counselling Psychology, 31*(6), 711–744.

Lee, R. M., Grotevant, H. D., Hellerstedt, W. L., Gunnar, M. R. & the International Adoption Project Team. (2006). Cultural socialisation in families with internationally adopted children. *Journal of Family Psychology, 20*(4), 571–580.

McAdoo, H. (2006). *Black families*. Thousand Oaks, CA: Sage Publications.

McRoy, R. G. (1994). Attachment and racial identity issues: Implications for child placement decision-making. *Journal of Multicultural Social Work, 3*(3), 59–74.

McRoy, R., & Zurcher, L. A. (1983). *Transracial and inter-racial adoptees: The adolescent years*. Springfield, IL: Charles C. Thomas Publisher.

National Association of Black Social Workers. (1972, September). *Position statement of transracial adoptions*. Unpublished Position Paper, pp. 2–3.

NCH. (1954). The problem of the coloured child: The experience of the National Children's Home. *Child Care Quarterly, 8*(2).

Office for National Statistics (ONS). (2005). *Census 2001: General report for England and Wales*, Loughborough.

Owen, C., & Statham, J. (2009). *Disproportionality in child welfare: The prevalence of Black and minority ethnic children within the looked after and children in need populations and on child protection registers in England*. London: Department for Children, Schools and Families.

Picca, L. H., & Feagin, J. (2007). *Two-faced racism: Whites in the Back Stage and Front Stage*. New York, NY: Routledge.

Powell, A. (2017, August 16). *Unemployment by ethnic background*. Briefing Paper No. 6385.

Rehman, H., & Owen, D. (2013, October). *Mental health survey of ethnic minorities: Research report*. Ethnos Research and Consultancy in Partnership with University of Warwick.

Rotheram, M., & Phinney, J. (1987). Definitions and perspectives in the study of children's ethnic socialization. In J. Phinney & M. Rotheram (Eds.), *Children's ethnic socialization: Pluralism and development* (pp. 10–28). Newbury Park, CA: Sage Publications.

Rowe, J., & Lambert, L. (1973). *Children who wait*. London: Association of British Adoption Agencies.

Sargent, S. (2015). Transracial adoption in England: A critical race and systems theory analysis. *International Journal of Law in Context, 11*(4), 412–425.

Selwyn, J., Quinton, D., Harris, P., Wijedasa, D., Nawaz, S., & Wood, M. (2010). *Pathways to permanence for Black, Asian and mixed ethnicity children*. London: BAAF.

Sempik, J. (2007). *Mental health of looked after children in the UK: Summary*. Loughborough: Loughborough University.
Shireman, J., & Johnson, P. (1986). A longitudinal study of black adoptions: Single parent, transracial and traditional. *Social Work, 31*, 172–176.
Simon, R., & Alstein, H. (1987). *Transracial adoptees and their families: A study of identity and commitment*. New York, NY: Praeger.
Simon, R., & Alstein, H. (2002). *Adoption, race and identity: From infancy to young adulthood*. New Brunswick, NJ: Transaction Publishers.
Simon, R. J., Altstein, H., & Melli, M. G. (1994). *The case for transracial adoption*. Washington, DC: American University Press.
Smith, D. T., & Juarez, B. G. (2015). Race lessons in black and white: How white adoptive parents socialise black adoptees in predominantly white communities. *Adoption Quarterly, 18*(2), 108–137.
Spencer, M. B., & Markstrom-Adams, C. (1990). Identity processes among racial and ethnic minority children in America. *Child Development, 61*, 290–310.
Tatum, B. (1997). *'Why are the black kids sitting in the cafeteria?': And other conversations about race*. New York, NY: Basic Books.
Thoburn, J., Norford, E., & Rashid, S. (2000). *Permanent family placement for children of minority ethnic origin*. London: Jessica Kingsley Publishers.
Tizard, B. (1997). *Adoption: A second chance*. London: Open Books.
Vroegh, K. (1992, April). *Transracial adoption: How it is 17 years later*. Unpublished report. Chicago Child Care Society, Chicago.
Vrogeh, K. S. (1997). Transracial adoptees: Developmental status after seventeen years. *American Journal of Orthopsychiatry, 67*(4), 568–575.
Westhues, A., & Cohen, J. S. (1997). A comparison of the adjustment of adolescent and young inter-country adoptees and their siblings. *International Journal of Behavioural Development, 20*(1), 47–65.
Yoon, D. P. (2004). Inter-country adoption: The importance of ethnic socialisation and subjective wellbeing for Korean born adopted children. *Journal of Ethnic and Cultural Diversity in Social Work, 13*(2), 77–89.
Zayed, Y., & Harker, R. (2015, October). *Children in care in England: Statistics*. Briefing Paper No. 04470. House of Commons Library.

Chapter 21

Dementia and its Impact on Minority Ethnic and Migrant Communities

David Truswell

Introduction

It is often assumed that dementia is an illness that has its greatest impact on the economically developed regions of the world due to the greater human longevity in those regions. The stereotypic picture of an older person living with Alzheimer's disease, the most common form of dementia, is of a white European or North American man or woman. Dementia is often regarded as a less dominant health concern for the world's economically underdeveloped regions and for minority ethnic and migrant populations within the developed world. This chapter will challenge this stereotype, looking at the impact of dementia in economically underdeveloped countries and on minority ethnic and migrant communities in the developed world.

What is Dementia?

Dementia is a generic term covering several diseases that cause neurological damage and deterioration of the brain. More than 100 different types of dementia have been identified, including Parkinson's disease, dementia due to alcohol abuse (Korsakoff's syndrome), and dementia that can develop at the terminal stages of HIV/AIDS. The most common form of dementia is Alzheimer's disease, which affects about two-thirds of all those suffering from dementia worldwide (www.alzheimers.org.uk). A further 20–25% of the dementia worldwide is due to vascular dementia, which can occur because of a stroke. In mainstream news stories, and in many national or scientific reports, the generic term "dementia" is usually used even when these stories and reports refer exclusively to Alzheimer's disease or are mainly concerned with Alzheimer's disease and vascular dementia. The problems created by this interchangeable use of the terms "dementia" and "Alzheimer's disease" in the field of dementia research are explored in some detail by authors such as Lock (2013). This chapter will adhere to the convention of using "dementia" as a generic term unless citing evidence or research reports that are specific to Alzheimer's disease or vascular dementia alone.

Clinicians regard dementia as a terminal illness. Available treatments may have some limited effect in improving symptoms, but the benefits are contingent on the person living with dementia being diagnosed as early as possible. Not everyone responds to the drugs currently used to reduce the early stage effects of dementia, and the side effects in some cases can significantly impair quality of life. Several studies have found evidence that people from minority ethnic and migrant communities are underdiagnosed, and it is often suggested this is due to cultural factors that cause delay in seeking treatment (Cahill, Pierce, Werner, Darley, & Boberstein, 2015; Moriarty, Sharif, & Robinson, 2011; Nielsen, Vogel, Phung, Gade, & Waldemar, 2011). However, some authors have suggested the factors influencing treatment seeking behavior by people from ethnic minority and migrant communities living with dementia and their carers are more complex (Truswell, 2019; Zubair & Norris, 2015)

Many people diagnosed with dementia have mixed forms of the disease, for example, combining Alzheimer's disease with vascular dementia. As most people with Alzheimer's disease are older (70 years and over), a majority will have other chronic physical health problems that also need ongoing treatment. It has been estimated that most older people living with dementia have other physical health comorbidities (Bunn et al., 2014; Scrutton & Brancati, 2016). Mental health issues, most notably depression, may also develop due to the psychological impact of dementia (Winter, Korchounov, Zhukova, & Bertschi, 2011). A UK study indicates that when the person living with dementia is supported by a family member who is a full-time carer, often the carer themselves is an older person (usually a spouse) who has their own chronic health problems (Health and Social Care Information Centre, 2016).

There are psychological conditions that can develop in later life, such as mild cognitive impairment (MCI) or depression, which can result in memory or concentration problems. Such conditions are sometimes mistaken for the early stages of dementia, but they can be improved through psychological treatments. This sometimes makes the early stages of dementia diagnosis difficult, for example, some people become depressed in later life but have symptoms that mistakenly are thought to be dementia, such as mood changes and loss of concentration. Others become depressed after learning they have dementia. There is increasing evidence that a significant proportion of those with MCI will go on to later develop dementia (Roberts et al., 2014).

Agitation and restlessness in dementia, for example, the increased restlessness in the early evening that occurs with some people living with dementia, historically has often been treated with antipsychotic medication or sedatives. The general use of antipsychotic medication in people who were not psychotic prior to their dementia onset is not viewed as clinically appropriate in the UK (Banerjee, 2009), although it has been argued that the use of atypical antipsychotics in dementia should be considered on a case by case basis by US researchers (Gareri et al., 2014). The risks of sedative use in dementia are being highlighted increasingly (Thompson, 2015). Alternative, non-pharmacological approaches to reducing agitation and restlessness, including distraction or using the calming effect of familiar music, are an increasing focus of research (Millán-Calenti et al., 2016). Sometimes agitated behavior may be a result of pain or discomfort – for example, due to an undetected urine infection – that the person living with dementia has trouble explaining because of their cognitive difficulties.

Memory loss may not be the most evident early symptom of dementia. Other signs include the inability to fulfill activities that involve following a sequence (such as putting on clothes or preparing a meal), mood changes, disinhibited behavior, and inability to concentrate. It is important that people experiencing these symptoms take their concerns to a primary care physician if they find the symptoms are persisting or occurring repeatedly.

While the most common forms of dementia, Alzheimer's disease and vascular dementia, are predominately found in people over the age of 65, dementia can develop earlier, for example, people in their 40s or 50s. There is evidence that for the African-Caribbean community in the UK there is an elevated risk of younger onset vascular dementia (Pham et al., 2018; Stewart, Richards, Brayute, & Mann, 2001). Some studies have indicated that there is a worldwide under-diagnosis of dementia (Lang et al., 2017).

The Impact of Dementia in the Economically Underdeveloped World

The *World Alzheimer Report 2018* (Alzheimer's Disease International, 2018) indicates that by 2050 72% of all those living with dementia will be found in low- and middle-income countries. With global improvements in the quality of life, nutrition, and public health, such as better sanitation and access to clean water, the general increase in longevity experienced by the economically developed world is now extending to the less economically developed areas of the world.

The United Nations' report *World population ageing* (2015) points out that by 2050, 20% of the world's population will be over the age of 80, with the fastest rises in longevity occurring in the economically underdeveloped world. By 2050, about two-thirds of all those over the age of 80 will be living in the economically underdeveloped countries. The United Nations' report indicates that in Latin and Caribbean countries, average lifespan in the first half of the 1950s was 51.2 years. By 2010–2015 this had risen to 74.5 years. More people globally are now living long enough to experience the age-related risks of dementia.

Currently there are no pharmacological treatments that can cure Alzheimer's disease, the most prevalent form of dementia, and generally pharmacology has limited benefits across all forms of dementia (Berk & Sabbagh, 2013). There have been no significant developments in making an effective drug treatment for Alzheimer's disease advancing to the stage of human clinical trials for several years (Cummings, Morstor, & Zhong, 2014). Despite most of the research funding for treatments for dementia being invested in pharmacological treatments, on a day-to-day basis managing the psychological and behavioral challenges of dementia often depends on the support of family carers or paid support workers. In most cases, people living with dementia also have one or more other chronic health problems that affect their quality of life, yet family carers often know little about dementia or any of the other physical illnesses the person living with dementia may be managing (Maidment, Aston, Moutela, Fox, & Hilton, 2017). Paid support workers may be poorly trained or even untrained, and working for a very low wage in a demanding and stressful role (Ross, Strathearn, & Macaskill, 2016). In the economically underdeveloped world, the main physical demands of the role of carer for a person living with dementia are often allocated to the family members with the least family status (Gupta & Pillai, 2012).

In the economically underdeveloped countries, the lack of knowledge about dementia and the cultural stigma associated with illnesses of the mind often lead to families being reluctant to seek help from outside the family. Family members providing care for dementia sufferers may struggle to do so as they lack knowledge about the illness and are reluctant to seek outside help due to a sense of family shame.

Pharmacological research into effective drug treatments for dementia has poor reach into the populations of economically underdeveloped countries and the minority ethnic and migrant communities of economically developed countries. People from these communities are wary of volunteering as research subjects for treatment studies or donating their organs as a source of material in brain banks. Thus, the potential risks of reduced effectiveness or enhanced side effects due to ethnicity or population-level genetic risks are often unknown (Woods, Mentes, Cadogan, & Phillips, 2015). With the emphasis on a pharmacological treatment for dementia underpinned by the need for pharmaceutical companies to make a profit from the mass availability of licensed treatments, the possibility is that a treatment created in the economically developed world may not be affordable in the economically underdeveloped world. If a pharmacological treatment for dementia is developed that is principally effective at the early stages of diagnosis, its utility and impact will be limited for populations where general knowledge about dementia is poor, diagnostic infrastructure is underdeveloped, and people living with dementia tend to present for diagnosis at the later stages of illness.

Supporting education programs for raising awareness about dementia, encouraging early diagnosis, and mobilizing the social resources to support people living with dementia and their carers are more urgent policy priorities across the economically underdeveloped nations (Alzheimer's Disease International, 2015) and for the migrant and minority communities in the economically developed nations than the development of a pharmacological cure for dementia. Even if such a treatment was available in the economically developed world, it is unlikely that it would be available affordably and at scale across the economically underdeveloped nations.

An Overview of Dementia in Minority Ethnic and Migrant Communities in the Economically Developed World

Within national dementia strategies across the developed world, the challenges dementia presents to minority ethnic and migrant communities are often overlooked. For some minority ethnic and migrant communities there are increased risks of Alzheimer's disease and vascular dementia. The cultural issues affecting care provision, such as interpreting needs, cultural stigma about dementia, and cultural expectations regarding intimate personal care, can have a profound impact on the day-to-day arrangements for providing care and support.

As there is limited research literature on the subject, the focus in this chapter will be on the USA and UK literature, where some systematic work has been developing over the past few years. The chapter will also briefly summarize the indications from work in Canada, Australia, and Europe, where there are substantial minority ethnic and migrant communities. Japan, the demographically oldest of the economically developed nations, historically has a very low migrant population, of which the most significant are the Korean communities.

Not all minority ethnic communities are necessarily migrant communities. For example, in the United States, Native Americans are classed as a minority ethnic community, despite being the indigenous natives. The Inuit and Native Indian populations of Canada, and the Aboriginal population of Australia, are similarly classified. A significant proportion of the US African-American population is descended from people brought to the United States from the African continent in the period of chattel slavery. The heterogeneity of the African-American community in the United States is often not considered in those US studies of dementia and ethnicity which often use only broad, census-based ethnic distinctions.

Some migrant communities may identify themselves within the host population through their religious identity rather than their ethnicity, for example, the Orthodox Jewish or Sikh communities. Within these religious identities, however, ethnicity and social–historical issues, including the communities' migration history, may have an impact on customs and practices in everyday life that has an implication for the practicalities of care and support for those living with dementia. Even though many settled families of migrant origin have several generations of residency in the host country, their identification by mainstream services as being of minority ethnic or migrant origin can have significant consequences for their access to information and support for dementia. An older person reliving their early years in the rural community of the country in which they were born and raised before migrating may be communicating about a world completely outside the experience of their children, who are acting as their carers but who have been born and raised in the host country. It should not be assumed that matching the ethnicity or religion of support workers with that of the person living with dementia will itself produce culturally appropriate care (Jutlla & Moreland, 2009; Uppal, Bonas, & Philpott, 2013).

A common assumption within national strategic planning for dementia is that the migrant and minority communities constitute a small and demographically static proportion of the demand for dementia services. It is often assumed that at an individual case level the complexity of the dementia cases in minority ethnic and migrant communities will be roughly equivalent to the complexity found in cases of dementia in the majority host population. It is also assumed that the overall incidence of dementia across the migrant and minority communities will be the same as for the majority population. Finally, since the average age of migrant communities is known to be lower than that of the majority host country population, it is often assumed that the numbers of people from those communities living with dementia will be too low to have a substantial impact on local demand.

At a more granular level, none of the assumptions above holds up and this leads to a significant failure by service planners to understand and plan for the growing scale of dementia and the impact on the healthcare services needed by people in minority ethnic and migrant communities.

In 2015, the UN *International migration report* (United Nations, 2016) indicated that internationally, 13% of the people in the world's migrant populations are aged over 65. This is twice the proportion of those over 65 in the global population generally. As most economic migration involves adults of working age, it would be expected that those migrant communities that are more long-standing or settled in their host communities will be demographically older than the more recently arriving migrant communities. A report on migrant health from the International Organization for Migration (2015) highlights that poor diet, lack of exercise, and smoking are more prevalent in migrant populations. All these factors are increasingly seen as raising the risk of Alzheimer's disease (International Organization for Migration, 2015), or are associated with the increased risk of vascular dementia as a result of stroke (Gorelick, 2004).

Differentiating between settled and newer minority ethnic and migrant communities illustrates that some migrant communities are significantly demographically older than others, and consequently at much higher age-related risk of Alzheimer's disease and vascular dementia than others. Work based on UK census data suggests that the Irish, African-Caribbean, and Indian populations are the largest minority ethnic communities in the UK, with the greatest age-related risks of dementia due to the age structure of those populations (Truswell, 2014).

To date there has been little investigation into lifetime poor health in minority ethnic and migrant populations, and the impact of this on the risk of developing Alzheimer's disease or vascular dementia, but one might expect that in minority ethnic and migrant populations with lifetime poor health, as longevity increases, the risk of Alzheimer's and vascular dementia will increase as people increasingly live long enough to develop these illnesses rather than dying at an earlier age from other causes.

Minority Ethnic and Migrant Communities and Dementia in the United States

An important summary of research on dementia in the United States is collected in a 2006 book, *Ethnicity and the dementias* (Yeo & Gallagher-Thompson, reprinted 2013), which gives an overview across a wide cross section of minority ethnic and migrant communities. There is a gradually building evidence base of the differential risk factors across communities in more recent years. Mayeda et al. (2014) identified Native Americans and African-Americans living with type 2 diabetes as the groups at highest risk of going on to develop dementia. Their study of more than 22,000 people living with diabetes also included those of non-Hispanic white, Asian, and Latino ethnic categorization. Work such as that by

Hohman et al. (2016) starts to look in more detail at possible genetic determinants for the higher risk of late-onset Alzheimer's disease in the African-American community, but pinning down a discrete set of physiological or genetic markers is some way off. Mehta and Yeo (2017), after reviewing 1,215 studies in the United States, concluded that the African-American and Caribbean-Hispanic communities have the highest incidence of dementia, but in their view detailed data are still needed on many communities. They also point out the need to identify the high-risk communities as a national US health policy goal, and to prioritize information and service development work with these high-risk communities.

In a detailed paper on the economic cost of dementia in the African-American community, Gaskin, LaVeist, and Richard (2013) estimate that one-third of the annual cost of Alzheimer's disease and other dementias ($71.6 billion in 2012) is borne by the African-American community. Due in part to the increased prevalence of dementia in the African-Caribbean community, they identify African-Americans as composing 20% of all those diagnosed with dementia. While also paying due regard to the emotional cost of caregiving, in examining the economic cost based on hours of unpaid caregiving they estimate that this amounts to $43.6 billion in annual costs contributed by unpaid care by family members. The US Census Bureau identified in 2016 that 13.4% of the country's population were in the census category "African-American alone" (https://www.census.gov/quickfacts/). The US healthcare system places the onus on people paying for their own health care through insurance. As many of those living with dementia will also be simultaneously treated for other physical comorbidities, this is a significant issue for the African-American community. Gaskin et al.'s work (2013) makes it clear that the main part of the financial burden of dementia will be borne by individuals in the African-American community, at considerable personal economic and emotional cost. It is to be expected that a similar picture could well hold for other minority ethnic communities in the United States.

Significant information gaps regarding dementia incidence across minority ethnic communities in the United States need to be filled, and the lack of information on the Native American population is clearly one priority as risk factors for dementia are increasingly being identified in this population. For instance, type 2 diabetes is known to be of higher prevalence in this community. Regional demographics with high diversity in the United States, such as the state of Hawaii, may present challenges for care and support services in dementia due to the rich diversity of ethnic and cultural history (Suzuki, Goebert, Ahmed, & Lu, 2015).

The risks across the Hispanic population need further elucidation. While Mehta and Yeo (2017) identify higher risk across the Caribbean-Hispanic communities, the origins of the US Hispanic community are as diverse as the Spanish-speaking world itself. Some studies indicate that Hispanic/Latino communities fare no worse than non-Hispanic white communities in the incidence of dementia, while other studies have shown better outcomes on some indices. There could be differential levels of dementia risk within the Hispanic population that need more careful analysis, and this may require a more nuanced approach than printing all dementia information in Spanish as there may be differential levels of risk across the Hispanic communities.

Minority Ethnic and Migrant Communities and Dementia in the UK

All-Party Parliamentary Group on Dementia (APPG, 2013) produced *Dementia does not discriminate*, a significant report highlighting the need to pay more attention to the impact of dementia on minority ethnic and migrant communities in the UK. In a report in 2014 *Black and minority ethnic communities and dementia: Where are we now* (Truswell, 2014) summarized research on the issues over the preceding five years and set this in the context of a detailed analysis of 2011 UK census data on age and ethnicity. This report pointed out that while the APPG report had identified that there would be a sevenfold increase in the incidence of dementia over the next 35 years, this increase would primarily affect the "oldest" of these communities: the Irish, African-Caribbean, and Indian (also called South Asian in the UK census).

Due to the historic pattern of migration into the UK there are several minority ethnic communities that have been in the country for several generations, for example, the Chinese, Orthodox Jewish, and Turkish communities, of whom little is known about the incidence of dementia and care for people living with dementia. In some metropolitan areas, the number of people living with dementia from minority ethnic and migrant communities is significant and requires that services have a substantial understanding of the impact of cultural issues on providing dementia care. While national guidelines for developing culturally sensitive dementia services have been around for some time (Vickers, Craig, & Atkin, 2012), there is little evidence that this guidance is practically implemented in local strategic planning. Research on the impact of dementia on UK minority ethnic and migrant communities is sparse. There is an emerging grassroots movement across not-for-profit community organizations such as the Dementia Alliance for Culture and Ethnicity (www.demace.com) to press for more culturally appropriate provision of information and services.

A growing body of evidence suggests that the UK African-Caribbean community has increased risk of vascular dementia and early onset dementia compared with the country's white majority population (Adelman, Blanchard, Greta Rai, Leavey, & Livingston, 2011; Adelman, Blanchard, & Livingston, 2009). This is linked to the known higher incidence of cardiovascular disease, hypertension, and diabetes in this population. The Indian and Irish populations have similar population-level health risks of these and other diseases that are increasingly thought to raise the risk of vascular dementia developing. There are no national health education programs targeting information to the African-Caribbean population about the raised risk of vascular dementia. Until recently, national campaigns on dementia rarely included images of people of visible migrant or minority ethnic origin. Dementia care personnel are largely untrained in working with the cultural issues that often add a further level of complexity to the diagnosis and development of care plans for people living with dementia from minority ethnic and migrant communities.

While there has been a degree of consistency in national policy statements since 2009 referencing the problems faced by migrant and minority communities living with dementia, this has had limited impact on investment decisions by healthcare and socialcare commissioners at local levels when developing dementia information and services. Similarly, at the national-level, dementia not-for-profit organizations providing information and support for dementia have shown at best a fragmented engagement with the concerns of minority ethnic and migrant communities, supporting a few well-intentioned but isolated brief initiatives but lacking a consistent and effectively resourced strategic program of work for tackling the issues (Jeraj & Butt, 2018).

While there is some research focusing on the experience of particular communities, mainly the African-Caribbean and Indian, there is a notable lack of studies of one of the largest and most long-standing minority communities, the Irish. The development of best practice in delivering cultural-competent dementia care in multiethnic settings – including offering effective information, signposting services, and providing access to appropriate community support, nursing home care, and end-of-life care – is largely under-researched territory. The challenge of providing information, care, and support to minority ethnic and migrant communities living with dementia in rural areas is also unexplored. While national-level dementia research programs constantly refer to the lack of involvement of people from minority ethnic and migrant communities, these research organizations themselves show limited evidence of committing to engagement strategies for targeting these communities where there is increasing evidence of higher risk.

Modest national strategic commitments to respond to some of the issues of living with dementia faced by minority ethnic and migrant communities have not yet been carried through into consistently funded information and service resources on the ground. Often people responsible for funding and developing these resources locally lack the detailed understanding of the ethnic composition of their local older population, or awareness of the population-specific health risks associated with dementia. There is increasing mobilization of local grassroots, not-for-profit community organizations working with people from minority ethnic and migrant communities living with dementia and their family carers that is challenging poor local provision. However, this challenge lacks a national-level infrastructure that could consolidate such local challenges into a national campaign.

Minority Ethnic and Migrant Communities and Dementia in Europe and Other Parts of the Economically Developed World

The picture for minority ethnic and migrant communities across the economically developed world is like that for the USA and the UK, with even less research work to illuminate national issues and localized areas of concern. Dementia has yet to be taken up as an issue by international agencies focused on the health of minority ethnic and migrant communities, but global shifts in longevity will push the issue up the international migrant health agenda as the incidence of dementia rises. Populations at greater risk of dementia within the minority ethnic and migrant communities, such as the African-Caribbean community in the UK and the African-American population in the United States, need to be compared with native Caribbean and

African populations. It is important to understand whether these risk factors are consistent from the point of historical origin and across the diaspora.

While Canada and Australia, like the United States, have indigenous populations identified as minority ethnic communities, a common feature of these populations is poor lifetime health and political and social marginalization. This means that there are likely to be similarities in dementia risk, lack of information and access to services, and family carers bearing the burden of care. As longevity increases, the age-related risk of Alzheimer's disease and vascular dementia as a sequel of stroke in these populations will increase. Poor lifetime health history increases the likelihood that developing dementia in these populations will be accompanied by other physical health comorbidities. International sharing of models and methods of improving information and services would assist in more rapidly developing interventions in an area where painstaking work is needed to develop successful approaches as the costs of dementia globally and to the individual continue to rise.

While there are a growing number of studies of the impact of dementia in migrant communities of across Europe (Rosendahl, Söderman, & Mazaheri, 2016; Sagbakken, Spilker, & Ingebretsen, 2017), patterns of migration have resulted in variable dementia profiles for the various migrant communities. Comparability of academic research can be further restricted when research reports are written in languages other than English. Transnational minority ethnic communities such as Gypsies and Travelers have some of the poorest lifetime health and poorest access to services across Europe, but only in a few countries such as the UK have researchers begun to look at the impact of dementia (Tilki, 2016).

Diagnostic tools for dementia effective across minority ethnic and migrant communities are essential for developing early diagnosis and early intervention in dementia for these communities. This would be a useful area for improved international research and cooperation, with important benefits for improving planning of care and sustaining effective community-based support. Clinicians working in areas where there are proportionally high numbers of service users from migrant and minority communities living with dementia are frequently working in isolation from any dialogue about individual case work with peers or the stimulation of peer review studies that are valuable for clinicians for continuously refining and improving their practice.

Minority Ethnic and Migrant Communities and Healthcare Rights

The World Health Organization (2016) builds on the United Nations' Convention on the Rights of Persons with Disabilities to develop a framework for human rights for people living with dementia. The briefing singles out minority ethnic and migrant communities as a priority concern as people living with dementia from these communities often find that access to the host country's healthcare services is problematic. People living with dementia from minority ethnic and migrant communities often present to diagnostic services at later stages of the illness and are more likely to present with multiple health problems. Cultural issues that impact on the provision of care further complicate the situation as do fears of discrimination from services and lack of cultural understanding within services

In balancing the complexities of these demands, service providers and service commissioners need to recognize their responsibility to enable people living with dementia to secure their human rights. People living with dementia who use services will fluctuate in their ability to advocate for their rights themselves and to recognize the need to have someone advocate on their behalf. Early stage work in the diagnostic setting should include advanced planning to support advocacy and the choice of advocates for a future point when capacity for self-advocacy is severely diminished. Clinical and support staff on a day-to-day basis may be making shifting judgments on the capacity of people living with dementia. These judgments will be affected by cultural stereotypes.

People from minority ethnic and migrant communities may have well-founded fears about access to dementia services because of cultural stigma regarding mental health-related issues and the concern that services will treat them in a discriminatory way. First-generation migrants may well have had lifelong experience of their access to healthcare treatment in the host country always being challenged. They may have had little experience of the assumed right of access to health care that most of the host country's mainstream population have always taken for granted (Truswell, 2018).

It remains to be seen whether the mainstream movement developing internationally for achieving improved human rights across the spectrum for all those living with dementia captures the key significance of the right of access to health care for those from minority ethnic and migrant communities in the economically developed countries.

Mobilizing an International Approach to Dementia in Minority Ethnic and Migrant Health Communities

As there are an increasing number of studies of the impact of dementia on national populations and international conferences sharing work from national studies across the world, it might be assumed that understanding of the impact on minority ethnic and migrant communities is developing at a rapid pace. This is not the case. For example, the experience of an older Chinese person, who has always lived in China, getting old and developing dementia in China is quite different from that of an older Chinese person who has lived in the UK since they were in their 20s getting old and developing dementia in the UK. One might find more commonalities between the latter and a Chinese person who migrated in their youth to France, Canada, or Australia. While there is a generally accepted framework within which health issues common to migrant communities are addressed through international cooperation on migrant health issues, dementia is not seen as a priority concern for international migrant health. This must change.

In a globally interconnected world, psychological and emotional connections to parents and family obligations change yet remain in place, mediated through family connections facilitated increasingly by the internet. This happens not only through text, voice, and video exchanges but also through economic transfers. The global migration of people through economic crisis, war, persecution, economic and career opportunity, relationship building, and simple curiosity is impelled by powerful forces. Many modern minority ethnic and migrant families maintain important psychological links with the family remaining in their country of origin and with family members who may be geographically scattered.

As parents and grandparents live longer, and as the number of people living with dementia increases, interconnectedness with the experience of dementia will become greater for all, young and old. The emotional and economic costs and the repercussions of those costs do not simply impact on the person living with dementia; the reach and impact of the illness extends far beyond the headcount estimate of the number of people living with dementia.

In the same way that international commonalities are recognized in the study of other migrant health issues, dementia needs to be more strongly prioritized as a signature growing minority ethnic and migrant health issue in the twenty-first century. Key populations worldwide, such as the African-Caribbean in the UK and the African-American in the United States, are increasingly being identified as high risk. Do these high-risk profiles hold internationally and at the point of origin of the diaspora for these communities? Some indigenous populations, such as the Native American, have risk indicators that ought to lead to high incidence of dementia, but there is little research to explore this and the impact on preventative measures and services.

The author's experience across a variety of minority ethnic and migrant community organizations in the UK indicates that numerous issues are common to those living with dementia across these communities (Truswell, 2019). These issues include:

- anxiety about stigma in their own community group regarding dementia, which leads them to withdraw from the community;
- a feeling of community isolation by carers;
- a fear of experiencing discrimination or lack of understanding from mainstream dementia services that makes people reluctant to seek help;
- a lack of information on dementia that feels relevant for their personal circumstances;
- a belief that dementia is a natural part of aging and nothing can be done; and
- a fear of losing independence and being seen to be vulnerable.

On the preventative side, there is little other than anecdote to help with understanding why the lower-risk communities such as the Chinese appear to have consistently lower rates of incidence. The possibility that continued social engagement and support could be a factor in slowing the development of dementia in some cultures with strong traditions of elder support and social participation is suggested in recent news reports on work with the Maori population in New Zealand (University of Auckland, 2017), but as yet there are no comparisons with other communities with similar traditions.

A question largely unexplored by research is the quality of unpaid family care given that dementia frequently coexists with other physical health problems and the probability that the family carer has little knowledge about dementia. Family carers can have multiple care burdens, for example, also being a parent of school-age children. These factors can contribute to the risk of carer burnout or an increased risk of elder abuse through frustration on the part of the carer or an increased risk of medication errors by carers due to polypharmacy (Parand, Garfield, Vincent, & Franklin, 2016). Drawing out some international commonalities of experience, including that of accessing services as member of a minority ethnic or migrant community, could provide useful templates for supporting minority ethnic and migrant family carers across the globe.

The overreliance on a primarily pharmacological perspective in the dementia research, and lack of investment in non-pharmacological interventions, must be challenged internationally if it is to have any impact on the pharmacological lobby capturing dementia research investment. Good quality trials at scale need to be conducted on some of the non-pharmacological interventions that seem to show quality of life improvements and a degree of symptom reduction in those small-scale studies done to date. Music-based interventions seem to be one area with positive results over several small studies. Environmental design is another largely underexplored area.

Summary

This chapter has pointed out that over the next 35 years the greatest increase in dementia globally will be in the economically underdeveloped world, while in the economically developed world some minority ethnic and migrant communities are at significantly higher risk of developing dementia than the host majority communities. National policy documents on dementia strategy in the economically developed world may not refer to the vulnerabilities of minority ethnic and migrant communities. Health and socialcare planners rarely take this into consideration in regional or local service planning due to poor understanding of the age structure of local minority ethnic and migrant communities at a granular level and a lack of awareness of population-specific health risks for some of these communities.

A combination of features increases the likelihood that people from minority ethnic and migrant communities living with dementia will delay seeking help until a crisis in either their health or that of a key family carer brings the case to the attention of mainstream dementia services. By this point, existing care arrangements may be at breaking point as the person living with dementia has multiple health issues along with cultural concerns impacting on the provision of care and support. Through the lifetime of the illness the delay in seeking help and poor understanding of how the cultural issues impact on the provision of care make it likely that the person living with dementia and family carers in minority ethnic and migrant communities in the economically developed countries will bear the emotional and economic cost unsupported even by their own community resources.

Internationally, despite the higher risk and routinely more complex case profile that increasingly is being found for some groups, for example, the African-Caribbean and Indian (South Asian) populations in the UK, and the African-American and Caribbean-Hispanic groups in the United States, there is little active attempt to engage these communities in dementia research. Some groups, for example, the Native American in the United States and the Irish in the UK, which have high-risk factors thought to be associated with the main forms of dementia, Alzheimer's disease, and vascular dementia, remain largely unexamined by international and national dementia research.

Minority ethnic and migrant communities are often marginalized within the mainstream debate on human rights and dementia currently in the USA and the UK and indeed many other parts of the developed world. It is important to insist unequivocally on the fundamental priority to secure the right of access to health care for those from minority ethnic and migrant communities living with dementia, as this is an essential gateway to recognition of all their other human rights as people living with dementia.

Grassroots community organizations are increasingly pressing for equitable and appropriate healthcare provision in support of those living with dementia. There needs to be a funded national strategic program to develop diagnostic tools, deliverable information packs, clinical guidance, support, and training for carers, and to refine a culturally informed approach to providing care and support from diagnosis to end-of-life care for those living with dementia from minority ethnic and migrant communities.

References

Adelman, S., Blanchard, M., Greta Rai, G., Leavey, G., & Livingston, G. (2011). Prevalence of dementia in African–Caribbean compared with UK-born White older people: Two-stage cross-sectional study. *The British Journal of Psychiatry*, *198*, 1–7.

Adelman, S., Blanchard, M., & Livingston, G. (2009). A systematic review of the prevalence and covariates of dementia or relative cognitive impairment in the older African-Caribbean population in Britain. *International Journal of Geriatric Psychiatry*, *24*, 657–665.

All-Party Parliamentary Group on Dementia (APPG). (2013, July). *Dementia does not discriminate*. London: HM Government.

Alzheimer's Disease International. (2015, August). *World Alzheimer report 2015: The global impact of dementia: An analysis of prevalence, incidence, cost and trends*. London: Alzheimer's Disease International.

Alzheimer's Disease International World. (2018, September). *Alzheimer Report 2018 The state of the art of dementia research: New frontiers*. London: Alzheimer's Disease International.

Banerjee, S. (2009). *The use of antipsychotic medication for people with dementia: Time for action. A report for the Minister of State for Care Services*. London: Department of Health.

Berk, C., & Sabbagh, M. (2013). Successes and failures for drugs in late-stage development for Alzheimer's disease. *Drugs & Aging*, *30*(10), 783–792.

Bruscoli, M., & Lovestone, S. (2004). Is MCI really just early dementia? A systematic review of conversion studies. *International Psychogeriatrics, 16*(2), 129–140.
Bunn, F., Burn, A.-M., Goodman, C., Rait, G., Norton, S., Robinson, L., Schoeman, J., & Brayne, C. (2014). Comorbidity and dementia: a scoping review of the literature. *BMC Medicine, 12*, 192.
Cahill, S., Pierce, M., Werner, P., Darley, A., & Bobersky, A. (2015, July–September). A systematic review of the public's knowledge and understanding of Alzheimer's disease and dementia. *Alzheimer Disease & Associated Disorders, 29*(3), 255–275.
Cummings, J. L., Morstor, M., & Zhong, K. (2014). Alzheimer's disease drug-development pipeline: Few candidates, frequent failures. *Alzheimer's Research & Therapy, 6*, 37.
Gareri, P., Segura-García, C, Manfredi, V. G., Bruni, A., Ciambrone, P., Cerminara, G., ..., De Fazio, P. (2014, August 16). Use of atypical antipsychotics in the elderly: a clinical review. *Clinical Interventions in Ageing, 9*, 1363–1373.
Gaskin, D., LaVeist, T. A., & Richard, P. (2013, September). The costs of Alzheimer's and other dementia for African Americans. *Us Against Alzheimer's*. Retrieved from http://www.usagainstalzheimers.org/sites/default/files/USA2_AAN_CostsReport.pdf
Global Observatory for Ageing and Dementia Care. (2016, September). *World Alzheimer report 2016: Improving healthcare for people living with dementia: Coverage, quality and costs now and in the future*. London: Alzheimer's Disease International.
Gorelick, P. (2004). Risk factors for vascular dementia and Alzheimer disease. *Stroke, 35*, 2620–2622.
Gupta, R., & Pillai, V. K. (2012). Elder caregiving in South-Asian families in the United States and India. *Social Work and Society, International Online Journal, 10*(2), 1–16. Retrieved from http://www.socwork.net/sws/article/view/339/676
Health and Social Care Information Centre. (2016, January). *Focus on dementia*. Health and Social Care Information Centre. Retrieved from www.hscic.gov.uk/pubs/dem-focusjan16
Hohman, T. J., Cooke-Bailey, J., Reitz, C., Jun, G., Naj, A., Beecham, G., ..., Cuccaro, J. (2016, March). Global and local ancestry in African-Americans: Implications for Alzheimer's disease risk. *Alzheimer's & Dementia, 12*(3), 233–243.
International Organization for Migration. (2015). *World migration report 2015*. Grand-Saconnex: International Organization for Migration.
Jeraj, S., & Butt, J. (2018). *Dementia and Black, Asian and minority ethnic communities: Report of a Health and Wellbeing Alliance project*. London: VCSE Health and Wellbeing Alliance. Retrieved from https://raceequalityfoundation.org.uk/wp-content/uploads/2018/09/Dementia-and-BAME-Communities-report-Final-v2.pdf
Jutlla, K., & Moreland, N. (2009). The personalisation of dementia services and existential realities: Understanding Sikh carers caring for an older person with dementia in Wolverhampton. *Ethnicity and Inequalities in Health and Social Care, 2*(4), 10–21.
Lang, L., Clifford, A., Wei, L., Zhang, D., Leung, D., Augustine, G., ..., Chen, R. (2017). Prevalence and determinants of undetected dementia in the community: A systematic literature review and a meta-analysis. *BMJ Open, 7*, e011146. doi:10.1136/bmjopen-2016-011146
Lock, M. (2013). *The Alzheimer conundrum: Entanglements of dementia and aging*. Princeton, NJ: Princeton University Press.
Maidment, I. D., Aston, L., Moutela, T., Fox, C., & Hilton, A. (2017). A qualitative study exploring medication management in people with dementia living in the community and the potential role of the community pharmacist. *Health Expectations, 20*(5), 929–942. doi:10.1111/hex.12534
Mayeda, E., Karter, A., Huang, E., Haan, M., Moffet, H., & Whitmer, R. (2014, April). Racial/ethnic differences in dementia risk among older type 2 diabetic patients: The diabetes and aging study. *Diabetes Care, 37*, 1009–1015.

Mehta, K., & Yeo, G. (2017, January). Systematic review of dementia prevalence and incidence in United States race/ethnic populations. *Alzheimer's & Dementia, 13*(1), 72–83.

Millán-Calenti, J. C., Lorenzo-López, L., Alonso-Búa, B., de Labra, C., González-Abraldes, I., & Maseda, A. (2016, February 22). Optimal nonpharmacological management of agitation in Alzheimer's disease: Challenges and solutions. *Clinical Interventions in Ageing, 11*, 175–184.

Moriarty, J., Sharif, N., & Robinson, J. (2011, March). *SCIE Research briefing 35: Black and minority ethnic people with dementia and their access to support and services.* London: Social Care Institute for Excellence.

Nielsen, T. R., Vogel, A., Phung, T. K., Gade, A., & Waldemar, G. (2011). Over- and under-diagnosis of dementia in ethnic minorities: A nationwide register-based study. *International Journal of Geriatric Psychiatry, 26*(11), 1128–1135.

Parand, A., Garfield, S., Vincent, C., & Franklin, B. D. (2016, December 1). Carers' medication administration errors in the domiciliary setting: A systematic review. *PLoS One, 11*(12). Retrieved from https://www.ncbi.nlm.nih.gov/pubmed/27907072

Pham, T. M., Petersen, I., Walters, K., Raine, R., Manthorpe, J., Mukadam, N., & Cooper, C. (2018, August 8). Trends in dementia diagnosis rates in UK ethnic groups: Analysis of UK primary care data. *Clinical Epidemiology, 10*, 949–960.

Roberts, R., Knopman, D., Mielke, M., Cha, R., Pankratz, V., Christianson, T., …, Petersen, R. (2014). Higher risk of progression to dementia in mild cognitive impairment cases who revert to normal. *Neurology, 82*(4), 317–325.

Rosendahl, S. P., Söderman, M., & Mazaheri, M. (2016) Immigrants with dementia in Swedish residential care: An exploratory study of the experiences of their family members and Nursing staff. *BMC Geriatrics Open Access, 16*(18), 1–12.

Ross, K., Strathearn, D., & Macaskill, D. (2016). *Voices from the front line: Exploring recruitment & retention of social care support workers.* Scottish Care. Retrieved from http://www.scottishcare.org/wp-content/uploads/2016/06/Voices-from-the-Front-Line.pdf

Sagbakken, M., Spilker, R. S., & Ingebretsen, R. (2017). Dementia and migration: Family care patterns merging with public care services. *Qualitative Health Research, 28*(1), 16–29.

Scrutton, J., & Brancati, C. U. (2016, April). *Dementia and comorbidities: Ensuring parity of care.* London: The International Longevity Centre.

Stewart, R., Richards, M., Brayute, C., & Mann, A. (2001, March). Vascular risk and cognitive impairment in an older, British, African-Caribbean population. *Journal of the American Geriatrics Society, 49*(3), 263–269.

Suzuki, R., Goebert, D., Ahmed, I., & Lu, B. (2015, June). Folk and biological perceptions of dementia among Asian ethnic minorities in Hawaii. *The American Journal of Geriatric Psychiatry, 23*(6), 589–595.

Thompson, K. (2015). *Dementia diagnosis and management : A brief pragmatic resource for general practitioners.* London: NHS England.

Tilki, M. (2016, July/August). Dementia among gypsies and travellers. *Journal of Dementia Care, 24*(4), 12–13.

Truswell, D. (2014). *Black and minority ethnic communities and dementia: Where are we now?* Better Health Briefing 30. London: Race Equality Foundation. Retrieved from http://www.raceequalityfoundation.org.uk/resources/downloads/black-and-minority-ethnic-communities-and-dementia-where-are-we-now

Truswell, D. (2018). Dementia, human rights and BAME communities. *Journal of Dementia Care, 28*(1), 22–23.

Truswell, D. (2019, November). *Supporting people living with dementia from Black, Asian and minority ethnic communities.* London: Jessica Kingsley Publications.

United Nations. (2015). *World population ageing 2015*. Department of Economic and Social Affairs, Population Division.
United Nations. (2016, September). *International migration report 2015*. Department of Economic and Social Affairs, Population Division.
University of Auckland. (2017). Dementia: Supplementary findings from LiLACS NZ for section five, "Service use and common health conditions" in the report "Health, independence and caregiving in advanced age". School of Population Health, Faculty of Medical and Health Sciences. Retrieved from https://www.fmhs.auckland.ac.nz/assets/fmhs/faculty/lilacs/research/docs/Dementia-Supplement-Research-Report.pdf
Uppal, G. K., Bonas, S., & Philpott, H. (2013). Understanding and awareness of dementia in the Sikh community. *Mental Health, Religion & Culture, 17*(4), 400–414.
Vickers, T., Craig, G., & Atkin, K. (2012). *Research with black and minority ethnic people using social care services*. Methods Review 11. National Institute for Health Research: School for Social Care Research. Retrieved from http://www.lse.ac.uk/LSEHealthAndSocialCare/pdf/SSCR_Methods_Review_11_web.pdf
Winter, Y., Korchounov, A., Zhukova, T. V., & Bertschi, N. E. (2011). Depression in elderly patients with Alzheimer dementia or vascular dementia and its influence on their quality of life. *Journal of Neurosciences in Rural Practice, 2*(1), 27–32.
Woods, D. L., Mentes, J. C., Cadogan, M., & Phillips, L. R. (2015). Ageing, genetic variations, and ethnopharmacology. *Journal of Transcultural Nursing, 28*(1), 56–62.
World Health Organization. (2016). Ensuring a human-rights based approach for people living with dementia. Retrieved from http://www.who.int/mental_health/neurology/dementia/dementia_thematicbrief_human_rights.pdf
Yeo, G., & Gallagher-Thompson, D. (2013). *Ethnicity and the dementias* (2nd ed.). New York, NY: Routledge.
Zubair, M., & Norris, M. (2015). Perspectives on ageing, later life and ethnicity: Ageing research in ethnic minority contexts. *Ageing & Society, 35*, 897–916.

Chapter 22

Mental Health/Illness Revisited in People of African-Caribbean Heritage in Britain

Florence Gwendolyn Rose and Tony Leiba

Background to the Hagar Mental Health project

The Hagar project was set up in 1992 with an aim to support African-Caribbean Heritage people with mental health problems. The vision of the project initiators is to (a) empower people to take control of their lives and future; (b) nurture independence; (c) provide education and information to increase awareness of the effect of mental health; (d) challenge the oppression and ignorance that perpetuates stigma, paralyses and interferes with the use of wisdom; and (e) promote respect for the individual's rights, dignity and humanity through caring and affirmation. All names of places, organisations and people mentioned here have been changed for the purpose of confidentiality and data protection.

Definition of Schizophrenia

Schizophrenia is a long-term mental disorder of a type involving a breakdown in the relation between thought, emotion and behaviour, leading to faulty perception, inappropriate actions and feelings, withdrawal from reality and personal relationships into fantasy and delusion, and a sense of mental fragmentation.

A mental disorder that is characterised by disturbances in thought described as delusions, perception which could present as hallucinations, and behaviour which include disorganised speech or catatonic behaviour, by a loss of emotional responsiveness and extreme apathy, and by noticeable deterioration in the level of functioning in everyday life, called also dementia praecox.

Schizophrenia often involves an inability to orient oneself with reality, a withdrawal from social interactions, and a failure to integrate thoughts with emotions so that emotional expression is inappropriate. There are several subtypes of schizophrenia, including paranoid schizophrenia and those types marked by catatonia.

These states of mind could be triggered by stressful situations where the person has one or more traumatic experience in a short space of time. Experiences may include extreme violence as in a war, abuse or bereavement.

Other terms, which may or may not be labelled schizophrenia, are: insanity, insaneness, dementia, mental illness, derangement, dementedness, instability, unsoundness of mind, lunacy, distraction, depression, mania, hysteria, frenzy.

> Gibraltar's schizophrenia continues to be fed by colonial pride.
> (Harper, 2009)

Medical Definition of Personality Disorder

A psychopathological condition or group of conditions in which an individual's entire life pattern is considered deviant or non-adaptive although the individual shows neither neurotic symptoms nor psychotic disorganisation. A diagnosis of personality disorder is often linked with other mental health difficulties such as depression and anxiety, and is often treated by psychiatrists with medication to relieve the symptom rather than non-invasive treatment which addresses the causes which may exacerbate the symptoms. Health promotion education in healthy lifestyles for the individual condition is not often a choice for those with lower education attainment or external cultural norms.

Definition of Depression

There are different theories of depression, which is not yet fully understood by the medical fraternity. It is however described by patients as feelings of severe despondency and dejection, and self-doubt. The term is synonymous with melancholy, misery, sadness, unhappiness, sorrow, woe, gloom and the action of lowering something or pressing something down on the spirit of the person. The biological cause is described as a change in the functioning of the chemistry and neurotransmitters working in the brain. This may be triggered by a major life event such as bereavement, trauma that may be short term but if not treated appropriately could result in long-term illness.

Manic depression according to the respondents (although this has never been explained) is oscillating between a feeling of the need to self-harm during the very low period of depression to period of feeling exhilarated and happy. During the period of low mood there is also self-neglect when family members or nursing staff are required to provide reminders for personal care including the administering of medication.

Other forms of depression are also included in the other forms of mental illnesses such as personality disorder, schizophrenia and post-traumatic stress (PTS).

Gilbert (2009) provides an interesting on overview on depression but does not provide a medical definition. This is an interesting approach as the focus to this text is more on how to treat the condition, which manifest itself in different ways for different people. The styles of depressive thinking and how to use different styles of management provide a comprehensive outline of which can be used by professionals with their client. However, this kind of approach is time consuming and expensive and not often on offer for people in the lower socioeconomic strata.

Observations and Unstructured Interviews with Advocates and Members of the Mental Health Project for African-Caribbean Black and Minority Ethnic (ACBME)

It was difficult to focus on members who have been given a diagnosis as advocates were not sure of the diagnosis of each person who attended the project. Members were not always sure of their diagnosis or they have not been given a diagnosis although they were being treated for a mental illness or psychotic episodes over many years. This is indicative of the difficulties with getting appropriate diagnosis for a mental health condition among the people in this population group.

Respondents 1–3 are members and Respondents 4 and 5 are advocates of the project.

Respondent 1

> I was diagnosed with manic depression and given medication 39 years ago, when I was 19 years old. No one has ever explained what manic depression is. I have attempted suicide on three occasions that I can remember. I have a monthly injection and counselling. The project helps me as this is somewhere I can come to where I am not treated as an outcast.

Respondent 2

> I was diagnosed with schizophrenia when my son was 8 weeks old and there was other traumatic life events such as breakdown of my marriage, social isolation as I had no family in this country. I was told by my GP about the diagnosis after the first hospital admission. During both period of hospitalisation I was heavily medicated. The second hospital was a death house I was lucky to escape alive. Many people who were admitted to this hospital did not come out alive. The experience was horrible. I still hear the voices in my head telling me I am a bad person. I know I am not a bad person. I am a beautiful person and my minister reminds me that God loves me. My ex-husband took my children and although I went to court to get custody, the judge said I was not fit to look after my children because of the mental breakdown.

Respondent 3

> The story of a carer: The consultant described a psychotic episode before he was admitted to hospital. He was medicated during his hospital stay and persuaded to have monthly injections without discussing this with me. I think this is because they could not be bothered to supervise his oral medication and monitor any side effects.

Respondent 4

During one of the interviews there was knock on the door and a member came in and said 'Can I speak with you?' She did not have an appointment to be interviewed but I agreed to speak with her, as she appeared really keen to tell me her story. She was articulate but unable to explain why she wanted to speak with me. On four occasions I asked her what she wanted to speak with me about. She was adamant that she did not have a mental health issue but that she was being persecuted by her neighbour and the housing association or police was not listening to her. She came to the project because the advocates listened to her. She described many incidents of persecution by her neighbour and an incident of acid being thrown outside her front door. She was very frightened to be in her flat or to go to sleep. She was very tired as she has not had a good night's sleep for months. I explained that she seemed anxious and that she should not go back to the flat if she was so frightened. At this point she appeared to calm down but was still not engaging with the conversation. Alarm bells started to ring so I discussed this with the project manager and an advocate who confirmed that this member was experiencing some delusions as she has visited her at home and explained that some of her fears were irrational.

Respondent 5

The project has not achieved its vision or has there been any improvement in the treatment and diagnosis since its inception about 20 years ago. I joined the project about 18 years ago as social worker because it was the only project offering this service at the time. The vision of the then founders has been lost due to lack of ownership, changes over the years, cutbacks in grant and management. Then we had about 22 paid staff. There are now 4 whole time equivalent members of staff. We do not engage volunteers because volunteers could subject the members to abusive situations. Therefore we cannot really meet the needs of the population given the nature and fear surrounding of mental illness so we cannot report any improvement in the diagnosis and treatment since the inception of the project.

Observations and Unstructured Interviews with Advocates and Members of the Mental Health Project for ACBME

From advocates at the project – All mental health issues in the Black community are labelled bipolar so that the same treatment can be given by Psychiatrists. The advocates state that all the patients are misdiagnosed because the model for diagnosis is based on the Eurocentric model and the cultural background of the patient is not taken into consideration. People from the Black community are not offered the more sophisticated treatments such as counselling and CBT (Cognitive Behaviour Therapy) suitable to their cultural background because there are not enough professionals who are trained in this field, and also there is the economic limitations of being in the lower income bracket and social class stratification for the family. Due to the nature of mental illness and its taboo, plus encouragement from the 'Welfare state' in Britain, patients are not encouraged to seek and to maintain gainful employment. Families are not encouraged to support and encourage their relative to seek and to maintain gainful employment. Misdiagnosis, medication and lack of training about their condition and having to resort to self- help are designed to keep the community in the status quo of submissiveness. This is compounded by low self-esteem; fear of authority compounded by the fear of their illness or simply limited mental capacity. Where limited mental capacity could be corrected if it accepted that it is short term, the failure of the system to provide short term solution mean that what may start out as a short term solution results in lifelong mental disability. The medications are designed to keep the patient in a submissive state where it is the consultant Psychiatrist and other health professionals who have the power to decide which treatment is best. The medications are also designed to maintain the financial position of the pharmaceutical companies. The side effects are treated with more medication instead of trying to find a medication that suit the individual and the individual's lifestyle without the side effects.

Analysis

Respondent 2 was tearful at times but really eager to tell her story, although at times her memory appears fragmented. She did not want her name to be changed and she wanted the world to know about what she regards as mis-treatment by her husband and by the system. She lost her family by coming to the UK, then in the UK she lost her marriage, then her health, then her children and now there is no way back and the socioeconomic shackles which are racially defined remain. She regards herself as 'lucky to be alive'. For many the celebration of life and a better after life becomes the accepted norm as it was in the days of African-Caribbean slavery. The barbaric treatment of beatings and being tied in the ships transporting slaves, and then getting similar treatment from slave master has been replaced with drugs and limited understanding of the person who is being given drug therapy.

Respondents 1, 3 and 4 tell a very different story but all allude to the same common factor.

Advocates and members view mental health from differing perspectives as their experiences are of mental health, mental illness and the mental health services as providers and/or receivers of services.

The common factors for both staff and members of the project are a feeling of powerlessness due to their position in society where oppression and human indignity is the normal social position. Other contributory factors to the feeling of powerlessness are unhealthy lifestyles and the subsequent poor management. There is limited understanding of, or the requirement to provide management programmes which are not only drug related but also to lifestyle and culture, and treating other conditions such as obesity, diabetes and other conditions which are prevalent among the population of African-Caribbean people in the UK.

Jean-Baptiste and Wexler's (2007) weight management programme found that a well-designed behavioural programme around diet and vitamins produce lasting effects such as improving metabolic indices and decreasing symptom of schizophrenia. There is a high incidence of diabetes among the African-Caribbean population which is another condition where diet and other lifestyle factors in patients with schizophrenia are not been addressed. There is a scarcity of evidence about the best way to an active lifestyle change in the diagnosis and treatment. Krabble and Pederson (2007) make reference to the prevalence of an unhealthy lifestyle as contributory factor to brain-derived neurotropic function and a predisposing factor to insulin resistance in type 2 diabetes.

The project is limited in what it can offer its members due to limited funding and the low access to education programmes which are designed to change lifestyles. There is also limited opportunity to understand the importance of participating in research which will contribute to a reduced need for inappropriate drug therapy. The scarcity of evidence, the opportunity to understand the importance of research to provide evidence is yet another example of oppression and the maintenance of powerlessness among the African-Caribbean population.

In his book *Crossing the divide* Hylton (2009) make a call to embrace diversity by changing the thinking around mental illness. The stark reality is that mental illness in African-Caribbean people is that this is unlikely to happen due to the double jeopardy of stigmatising mental illness and the stigmatising of Black people. More recently this has become triple jeopardy as the population ages as a result of migration in the late 50s–70s (Rose, 1999).

It is a commonly held view that mental illness is a medical problem, a disease like any other physical disease. This however is not always the case; the history of psychiatry is immersed in falsification, philosophy, politics and social control.

Littlewood and Lipsedge (1988) highlight the fact that patients who are hospitalised and sedated by psychiatrists with the help of nurses who dishonestly promised that they will be allowed home in the morning feel betrayed. Regardless of any future development of trust, this initial betrayal is not usually addressed and continues as an undercurrent for the failure of any future treatment or therapy.

Perhaps the medical illness model is used to justify the psychiatric institutionalisation of the mentally ill and the carrying out of treatments such as: medicalisation, lobotomies and electroconvulsive therapy. People do become mentally ill but the way in which psychiatrists diagnose and treat are not always respectful to the person's rights and wellbeing. It must be remembered that mental illnesses are a complex set of conditions that are incapacitating with physical, psychological, sociological and cultural factors contributing to their manifestations. There are the depressions, bipolar experiences, PTS disorder, schizophrenia, anxiety states, groups of mental illnesses referred to as the neuroses and the psychosis including puerperal psychosis. There are mental illnesses related to organic contributions such as: acute and chronic brain damage, genetic disorders, and the dementias that have aspects of behaviour and experiences that mimics mental illnesses. There are also the various conditions brought on by alcohol and illegal drugs. Furthermore, learning disability and other ability conditions which may the present behaviours require the attention of the psychiatrist. The medical professions with all its specialism do diagnosis, treat and care for the many illnesses and diseases which people endure. The position of this chapter is not to be negative about their contributions to health care, but to attempt to point out their deficiencies with regard to mental illnesses and in particular to the mental health of people of African-Caribbean Heritage.

The *Diagnostic Statistical Manual-fifth edition* (American Psychiatric Association, 2015) and the *International Classification of Diseases-Tenth Edition* manuals (2016) are the psychiatrist's diagnostic tool. Accordingly, the criteria by which schizophrenia is judged and thus diagnosed rests on the decision that the person does not act in a socially acceptable manner, they are social misfits and they suffer from socially unacceptable thoughts. This situation causes problems with the World Health Organisation (2017), because what is socially acceptable varies from culture to culture. Szasz (1970) argued that mental health issues and psychiatry are essentially ethical, moral, legal and political, and that psychiatry is an institution of the state coercive apparatus ensuring the social and political control of peoples. Of concern is the use of sectioning through the Mental Health Act (Department of Health, 2007) that is the voluntary and involuntary incarceration of people in a mental illness facility and treated with drugs, for example, the neuroleptics that have horrendous side effects. Given these overall psychiatric challenges and the issue of racism the people of African Heritage are discriminated against and receive care and treatment that is not always culturally sensitive (Mental Health and Social Control; http://flag.blackened.net/af/org/issue49/mental.html, accessed on May 28, 2014).

The Trans-Atlantic slave trade lasted more than 400 years from the middle 1400 to 1885 when it was abolished in Brazil. The traffic in human cargo represented the greatest forced population transfer ever. It resulted in millions of Africans forced to work on the plantations in North and South America and the Caribbean, with the demand for cheap labour on the plantations pushing up the demand for slaves. Slaves once bought and/or captured were taken to holding forts shackled together in pairs with leg irons and carried to the slave ships. Once on board they were restricted in their movements, they could not change positions and were chained down. They were then branded with their owners' marks with a red-hot iron and their clothes removed.

Shackled in darkness and filth, seasickness and diseases were rife. The heat in the hold could be over 30°C and the slaves would have no access to toilets or washing facilities. So foul was the smell of slave ships that other vessels would steer clear away from them. In such conditions many slaves died and their bodies were thrown overboard. At the end of the outward voyage came the sale where the slaves were auctioned. The battered tired and sick slaves were lined up, the seller starts with a price and the highest bidder takes the bought slave away from family and friends never to be seen again. The males were presented with iron shackles around their necks and the women with ropes around their necks with their frightened children clinging to the ropes (Everett, 1991). In evidence at the slave auctions were handcuffed, whipped, chained and bloodhounds. Once bought the slave owners controlled the slaves by: using brute force such as whippings and beatings; imprisonment and starvation; splitting up family members; selling slaves to other owners, hiring slaves out to other slave holders' plantations; controlling when, where and whom they meet with; requiring passes when leaving and entering the plantation; forbidding literacy and punishing those caught reading and writing; and controlling who and when they marry. The slaves never wanted to marry someone on the same plantation because they would have to endure the continual misery of seeing their spouse flogged and abused without daring to say a word. This knowledge extended the control of the slave owners over slave couples Walvin (1992).

On the plantation they worked around the 24 hours, they had no rights and their families were constantly being broken up as family members and children were sold on. The planters instituted barbaric regimes of repression to prevent revolts. The penalty for any slave resistance was extreme and deadly (Selfa, 2002). In Barbados punishment was executed by nailing resisting slaves down on the ground with sticks and then applying fire to their feet and hands, burning them gradually to the head. With their death the planters could claim a reimbursement of £25 from the British Government (Blackburn, 1997).

Slave resistance and revolts took place constantly, from their capture, transportation and their lives on the plantations in America and the Caribbean. These resistances took place despite the deadly penalties of the Slave Laws instituted by the British Government and the slave owners' control measures. Jamaica had always been a centre of black resistance to slavery. The first slave revolt was in 1673, less than 20 years after the British seized the island from the Spanish. On average there was a slave revolt every five years, the most serious were the 'Tacky's Rebellion' of 1760 which took six months to put down, and the 'Great Slave Revolt' of 1831 after which 344 slaves were executed.

When the British invaded Jamaica in 1665 many Africans who had been enslaved by the Spanish escaped to the mountainous regions, and over time runaway slaves joined them, they were known as the Maroons. The British could not defeat them despite the wars the British waged with the Maroons between 1730 and 1739. The wars ended with an agreement that gave the Maroons large areas of land and some of this land remains Maroon territory today. The Maroons remain today as a symbol of that indomitable desire that will never yield to captivity (Newsinger, 1992).

An Act of Parliament abolished the British Slave Trade in 1807; in 1833 the Emancipation Act was passed becoming law in 1834, stipulating that slaves in the British Empire would become formally free only after a four-year period of apprenticeship. The slave owners were handsomely compensated for the loss of their property, and not the slaves for their years of exploitation, servitude and oppression. In Jamaica the ex-slaves found themselves living in extreme poverty with the country still controlled by the white former slave owners. Wages were cut, people were starving disease and illness rife and the prisons were overflowing, and the ex-slaves were forced to steal to survive. There was bitterness throughout the land and a widespread fear that the former slave owners would reinstate slavery. It was this situation that led Paul Bogle to lead a resistance 'The Morant Bay Rebellion' on the 11 October 1865. Paul Bogle was born before the abolition of slavery, probably between 1815 and 1820 and he lived in Stony Gut in the Parish of St Thomas. One of his neighbours was George William Gordon, an African Heritage landowner and politician; both Bogle and Gordon were Baptists. At this time Edward John Eyre was the Governor of Jamaica, he was born in Hornsea, Yorkshire. Early in 1865 Bogle led a group of people from Stony Gut to Spanish Town to let Governor Eyre know about their plight, but gave up hoping that he would help. On the 11 October 1865 two men from Stony Gut were on trial in the Morant Bay Court House. A man shouted out in the Court House and when the police tried to arrest him Bogle stood between the man and the police and the man ran away. The police then went to Stony Gut to arrest Bogle, the people fought off the police and sent them back to Morant Bay. Bogle and his people then marched to Morant Bay Court House where armed policemen and soldiers were on guard. A fight broke out, the guards fired and people were killed and wounded, the people drove the guards back and set fire to the building. The Government supported by Governor Eyre sent troops into Stony Gut, the troops shot and whipped many people, they destroyed Stony Gut and Bogle's Chapel, Bogle was captured, he was taken to Morant Bay for trial and he was hanged at the Court House. The troops hunted down the poorly armed people and savagely massacred them. The soldiers shot or hanged everyone they came across and burned down over 1,000 houses. According to Edward Underhill of the Baptist Missionary Society 439 people were killed and 354 were executed after trial by lynching and hanging including George William Gordon. Over 600 men, women and children were flogged with cat-o-nine-tails, and the tails were twined with wire to increase the severity of the punishment. Many also received long prison sentences. The rebellion was crushed, but the massacre caused questions to be raised in Britain, but the ruling class rallied to Governor Eyre. When Eyre returned to England in August 1866 a public banquet was held in his honour (Newsinger, 1992; Semmel, 1962, 1969; Stromberg, 1999).

It is important to point out that because of the profit generated by the British Trans-Atlantic Slave Trade, the State, the established church the Church of England, academics in Universities particularly in elite institutions and philosophers, all agreed with and supported slavery as a worthwhile enterprise. There were dissenting voices but it took them hundreds of years to complain effectively and only after many revolts by the slaves and after many massacres of the slaves by the slave owners and their agents of social control. Such treatments during the whole slave trade, slavery institution and the resultant sufferings have left a heritage and knowledge that haunts African-Caribbean people today and leaves unanswered questions in how they deal with today's world. Furthermore, the relevance of the conditions of slavery and the examples of how the slaves fought back must be engaged with. Much of the negative attitudes and covert and overt behaviours towards African-Caribbean by Europeans and other racial and ethnic groups developed out of slavery and continue today. African-Caribbean are seen as less than human to be exploited and when they resist, they are imprisoned, deemed mentally ill, killed or massacred. These situations adds to the stresses of living, therefore, engaging with these issues will enable African-Caribbean peoples to be resilient and to continue to work for their civil rights. All of our lives matter and positive mental health is a necessity.

No thought was given to the slaves' mental health, actually more thought was given to analysing the so called mental illness 'drapetomania' which was used to describe, when slaves wanted to flee from being exploited, abused and oppressed (Cartwright, 1851). Because the slaves were brutalised constantly, they would have suffered from what we today consider to be PTS disorder. Other mental illnesses would include depression, suicidal behaviour, suicide, hyper-vigilance and anxiety. The legacy of slavery is still experienced today through racism and discrimination. This legacy results in constant humiliation, which is evident in the institutions and is exemplified in sports and the media. For example, the media deals with immigration in a most ahistorical, offensive and inaccurate manner, and the crux of the immigration debate is the notion that there are too many people of African Heritage in the UK. Must the nation be reminded that African Heritage people are here because of 'Empire' and the 'Trans-Atlantic Slave Trade' of which the British population is proud? Furthermore, it can be argued that the peoples of the British Isles have populated and continue to populate, Canada, USA, New Zealand, Australia and South Africa, to mention but some countries they emigrate to, and when they colonised these countries they did not live with the people there but set about to steal, exploit, abuse and massacre them. These racists practices are not random but are involved in psychological and sociological hostilities, intimidation and jingoism, which are aimed at reducing the self-worth and devaluing the lives of people of African Heritage and other First Nation peoples.

Racism has many forms, direct attack is present but less common than perceived discrimination and exclusion in interpersonal communications and relationships. Racism can be considered as a stressor, where the individual's perception is of the society as racist and discriminatory (Bhugra & Cochrane, 2001).

Research by Krieger, Berkman, and Kawachi (2000) presented the argument that interpersonal discrimination and racism has been associated with increased rates of hypertension, depression and stress after racist murders and attacks, particularly if such killings and attacks occurs in the health, social and or justice services. Furthermore, individuals might react by being generally more suspicious. However, it must be noted that such suspiciousness may represent a healthy coping strategy in a continuous discriminatory and racist societal environment (Sharpley, Hutchinson, & Murray, 2001).

An example of the appalling racism in the mental health system is in the treatment of black men that have resulted in their deaths. Carvel (2004) presented the case of Mr David 'Rocky' Bennett who died at a unit in Norwich on 30 October

1998. As a result of David Bennett who after racist taunts and being moved to another ward became resistant and non-compliant. Four nurses held him down as he struggled trying to break free. The nurses did not release him until he stopped moving and was quiet. The injuries he sustained resulted in his death due to excessive pressure. The inquest into his death opened on the 3 May 2001, nearly two and a half years after he died. The inquiry reported that the nursing staff ordered Mr Bennett about with little regard for the destructive effect of racist abuse upon a black person. The ward was inadequate in resuscitation equipment, and the doctor took more than an hour to arrive on the scene. Of concern is the fact that Mr Bennett is not an isolated case, Michael Martin, Joseph Watts and Orville Blackwood all died in Broadmoor Hospital. All the reports on these deaths comments on the presence of organisational racism, and that the staff and management do not appear to appreciate how this subtle form of racism operates (Inquest, 2004).

Much mental health research runs the risk of medicalising social struggles and distress. Such research by focussing on the discriminated against group, may serve to maintain the medical institution's power over the victimised group. Fernando (1991) has argued that European Psychiatry developed when racist doctrines were rife in western culture, and the racist ideology became incorporated into psychiatry as a discipline. Furthermore, psychiatry with its emphasis on pathology, with insufficient attention paid to social pressures due to race, ethnicity and culture renders psychiatry a racist institution.

If racial harmony is considered the aim of a civilised society, then mental healthcare teams and their practitioners need to develop a competence in understanding and working with these issues.

Bell (2004) argued that some psychiatrists have advocated making racism a psychiatric disorder. Others have maintained that doing so would medicalise a social and psychological problem. However, the practice of covert and overt racial discrimination, race hate in the media, persecution, exclusion, institutional racism and domination on the basis of racial superiority are all social and psychological learning processes. Therefore psychiatry is the medicalisation of social and psychological problems. Is it too far-fetched to suggest that racism is a mental disorder, which resides in the racists? For example, it is known in psychiatric theory that people with a paranoid disorder projects their unacceptable feelings and ideas on to other people and groups. So is it not possible for these people if they are racists, to project their unacceptable feelings and ideas on to different ethnic and racial individuals and groups?

Because behaviour is multidimensional racism and discrimination is also multidimensional. However, psychiatry has been reluctant to consider whether or not some forms of racism are manifestations of psychiatric disorder. Maybe the question of racism as a mental illness is so contentious that it precludes consideration of the issue at all. Furthermore, along with racism, the psychiatric classification of mental illnesses should include other extreme prejudices such as sexism, ageism and heterosexism.

If racism can be a factor in mental disorders in African Heritage people, if racists can be considered as suffering from a mental disorder, then a theoretical approach in psychiatry such as that of Franz Fanon could prove useful.

Franz Fanon was born in 1928, in his books *Black Skin White Mask* (1967) and *The Wretched of the Earth* (1968); he explores the psychological impact of racism on both coloniser and colonised. Born in Martinique, he received a conventional colonist education. He went to France to train as a psychiatrist and later he fought in the French Resistance. His assimilationist illusions were shattered by the racism he experienced in France. Fanon regard people as social beings and factors such as political conflict, social tension and economic stress can affect their mental health. He pays attention to those factors and concludes that alienation, oppression, unemployment, and tyrannical rulers exist, and as we all know they exist today too. Furthermore, he argued that mental illness couldn't be solved by drugs alone but by changes in the political and social order, where all human problems can be seen in their historical and cultural context.

Psychiatry has largely been an uninterested bystander in the history of racism and so has neglected the effects of social and political oppression on the mental health of peoples of African Heritage.

Fanon as a psychiatrist and political activist was and is still ignored by Western Psychiatry, which considers his views to be too political. An important concept in Fanon's theory is alienation in the individual. This he argued is due to the processes of oppression, racism and discrimination.

The alienation of the individual or group from the society may manifest itself as follows:

From oneself, one's body and personal identity; from significant other resulting in estrangement from family, language, cultural and personal groups; and from others because of the tensions between different racial and ethnic groups.

Mental health service providers must make themselves available to users and their carers.

Although users and their carers are involved in care planning, they are still not receiving adequate communication and explanation. Also users have reported that they were only aware of their keyworker when a problem situation occurred. Users continue to report not understanding the contents of documents given to them. Users and their carers must be involved in all aspects of the care and treatment provided. Written, verbal and visual communications must take place and it might be necessary to provide an interpreter. Advocacy must be a part of everyday care. Users must be enabled to: exert a measure of control over their lives; express their views and have options and choice. Users must be empowered through: an awareness and understanding of their rights, able to build their self-esteem; and explore the consequences of their behaviour and take responsibility for their outcomes.

Healthcare providers must acknowledge the presence of institutional racism in mental health services. There is a need to change the heavy prescription of medicines as the primary form of treatment and to offer more psychotherapy 'talking therapies'. Care professionals must break the negative perception they have of African Heritage peoples, to develop a culturally competent workforce. Cultural competence is defined, as the ability of providers and organisations to effectively deliver healthcare services that meet the social, cultural and linguistic needs of service users. A culturally competent healthcare system can improve health outcomes and quality of care, and can contribute to the elimination of racial and ethnic health disparities. Examples of strategies to move healthcare systems towards these goals include: providing relevant training on cultural competence and cross-cultural issues to health professionals and creating policies that reduce administrative and linguistic barriers to service user care, and to understand the institutional processes and practices that discriminate against African Heritage people, and to challenge these (Hooper & Zaagman, 2002). Care staff must: talk and reflect about race and mental illness, inequality, discrimination, oppression, power, powerlessness and social divisions, this must take place during training and as continued professional development; assist African Heritage people to talk about their experiences of racism in their everyday life; provide care and treatment with respect and dignity and to tease out differences due to race, ethnicity, culture, gender, sexuality, disability and religion. The growing service user movement and their efforts to improve services should be supported. Finally, staff must support African Heritage mentally ill people to define their recovery, by reclaiming power and control and empowering themselves, because taking this power back is crucial to resilience and recovery.

If racism can affect the mental health of the perpetrators and the victims, there is a need to acknowledge this and to take on the ideas of Franz Fanon into mainstream psychiatric education. In order to provide effective care and treatment it must be remembered that excluded, stigmatised and marginalised people require positive relationships.

Furthermore, psychiatry must pursue and eradicate racism and other prejudices such as ageism, sexism and heterosexism. Actions and processes are required to challenge the history written by the oppressors, academics, historians, scientists and philosophers who have misrepresented the facts. Parents, educational institutions and the teaching by religious organisations must be aware of the racism and other prejudices which they imbue in the young of every generation and so maintain racism and oppression.

References

American Psychiatric Association. (2015). *Diagnostic statistical manual* (5th ed.). Washington, DC: American Psychiatric Association.
Bell, C. (2004). *Racism: A mental illness: Taking issue.* Arlington, VA: American Psychiatric Association Publishing INC.
Bhugra, D., & Cochrane, R. (2001). *Psychiatry in multicultural Britain.* London: Gaskell.
Blackburn, R. (1997). *The making of the new world slavery.* New York, NY: Verso.
Cartwright, S. A. (1851, May). Report on the disease and physical peculiarities of the Negro Race. *New Orleans Medical and Surgical Journal,* May, 619–715.
Carvel, J. (2004). How the death of one black patient treated as a 'lesser being' showed up race bias. *Guardian,* February 6.
Department of Health. (2007). *Mental Health Act.* London: HMSO.
Everett, S. (1991). *History of slavery.* Secaucus, NJ: Brompton Books.
Fanon, F. (1967). *Black skin white black mask.* New York, NY: Grove.
Fanon, F. (1968). *The wretched of the earth.* New York, NY: Grove.

Fernando, S. (1991). *Racism as a cause of depression*. London: Macmillan Mind.
Gilbert, P. (2009). *Overcoming depression*. London: Robinson.
Hooper, M., & Zaagman, P. (2002). Culturally competent health care: Equipping our students. In C. Cox (Ed.), *Enhancing the practice experience* (pp. 32–45). Chichester: Nursing Practice International.
Hylton, O. (2009). *Crossing the divide: A call to embrace diversity*. Nottingham: Inter-Varity Press.
Inquest. (2004, February 5). Working for truth justice and accountability. Inquest briefing. The restraint related to the death of 'Rocky' Bennett. Retrieved from http://www.inquest.org.uk/pdf/rocky_bennett_briefing.0204.pdf
International Classification of Diseases-Tenth Edition Manual. (2016). Geneva: World Health Organization.
Jean-Baptiste, T. M., & Wexler, B. E. (2007). A pilot study of a weight management programs with food provision in schizophrenia. *Journal of Schizophrenia Research*, *96*(1–3), 198–205.
Krabble, K. S., & Pederson, B. K. (2007). Brain derived neutrophic factor (BDNF). *British Journal of Psychiatry*, *184*(47), S102–S105.
Krieger, N., Berkman, L., & Kawachi, I. (2000). *Discrimination and health in social epidemiology* (pp. 36–75). Oxford: Oxford University Press.
Leiba, T. (2012, October 3). Mental scars of racism. *Nursing Standard*, *27*(5), 22–23.
Littlewood, R., & Lipsedge, M. (1988). Psychiatric Illnesses among British Afro-Caribbeans. *British Medical Journal*, *296*, 950–951.
Newsinger, J. (1992, December). Jamaica rebellion, slave revolt against White Man's law. *Socialist Review*, *225*. Retrieved from http://pubs.socialistreviewindex.org.uk/sr225/newsinger.htm. Accessed on December 8, 2005.
Rose, F. G. (1999). Ethnic minority elders! Who cares? Health and social care of needs of black and ethnic minority elders by statutory services. *Journal of Managing Clinical Nursing*, *1*, 111–115.
Royal College of Psychiatrists. (2015). Personality disorder. Retrieved from http:/www.psych.ac.uk/healthadvice/personality disorder
Selfa, L. (2002). Slavery and the origins of racism. *International Socialist Review*, *26*(November–December). Retrieved from http://www.isreview.org/issues/26/roots_of_racism.shmtl. Accessed on June 9, 2011.
Semmel, B. (1962, October). The issue of 'race', in the British reaction to the Morant Bay Uprising of 1865. *Caribbean Studies*, *2*(3), 3–15.
Semmel, B. (1969). *Democracy versus empire: The Jamaican Riots of 1865 and the Governor Eyre controversy*. New York, NY: Garden City.
Sharpley, M., Hutchinson, G., & Murray, R. (2001). Understanding the excesses of psychosis among African Caribbean in England: Review of current hypotheses. *Journal of Psychiatry*, *178*(Suppl. 40), 60–68.
Stromberg, J. (1999). A policeman's lot is not a happy one – At home and abroad: Governor Edward Eyre and the Joys and Sorrows of Empire. Retrieved from http://www.antiwar.com/stomberg/s112399/html. Accessed on February 27, 2006.
Szasz, T. (1970). *The manufacture of madness*. New York, NY: Dell.
Walvin, J. (1992). *Black ivory: A history of British slavery*. London: Harper Collins.
World Health Organisation. (2017). *Mental health-definition of depression*. Geneva: WHO.

Chapter 23

Researching African-Caribbean Mental Health in the UK: An Assets-based Approach to Developing Psychosocial Interventions for Schizophrenia and Related Psychoses

Dawn Edge, Amy Degnan and Sonya Rafiq

The injustice of Black people's inferior access, experience and outcomes in the United Kingdom's (UK) equity-based National Health Service (NHS) was the primary motivation for undertaking research in this area. Membership of voluntary sector and NHS management boards highlighted the urgent need to address the crisis in Black schizophrenia care. Dialoguing with service users and their families, community members, policy makers, healthcare commissioners and service providers, it became apparent that novel approaches were required. Previous and current approaches were not working, resulting in sub-optimal care in general and for people of African-Caribbean origin in particular.

This chapter focusses on partnership work with African-Caribbean service users (patients) diagnosed with schizophrenia, their families, healthcare professionals and members of the wider community to develop a clinically and culturally appropriate talking treatment. The explicit purpose of this endeavour is to improve access to evidence-based psychological care for members of this community. We focus on schizophrenia and related psychoses because of the disproportionate number of people from African-Caribbean backgrounds with these diagnoses in the UK's mental health system (Tortelli et al., 2015).

A note on terminology, 'African-Caribbean' refers to people of African ancestry with family origins in the Caribbean. This includes people who self-identify as 'Black British', 'Mixed' heritage or 'Black Caribbean'. We use 'service user' versus 'patients' because this is the term preferred by the people who have received psychiatric labels (diagnoses) with whom this work was undertaken. Whilst acknowledging that Black, Asian and other groups equate to a 'global majority', the terms 'ethnic minorities'/'minority ethnic'/'minority groups' are used to reflect the nomenclature in contemporary research and academia.

Overarching Takeaway

Minority communities are often labelled 'hard-to-reach'. We suggest they are 'seldom heard'. Findings from our Community-partnered Participatory Research (CPPR) confirms that, given the opportunity, individuals (including those diagnosed with serious mental illnesses) are keen to participate in solution-focussed approaches to co-producing culturally acceptable and more accessible interventions.

Introduction

African-Caribbean Mental Health in the UK

One of the most consistent epidemiological findings from over 50 years of mental health research in the UK is that Black people of Caribbean origin or 'African-Caribbeans' are significantly more likely than other ethnic minorities or the White majority to be diagnosed with schizophrenia and related psychoses (Harrison, Owens, Holton, Neilson, & Boot, 1988; Morgan et al., 2006, 2017; Sugarman & Craufurd, 1994). For example, the Aetiology and Ethnicity in Schizophrenia and Other Psychoses (AESOP) study reported that, compared to White British people, African-Caribbeans' risk of being diagnosed with 'narrowly defined' schizophrenia (American Psychiatric Association, 2000) is nine times greater (Fearon et al., 2006).

Potential explanations for increased rates of diagnosis are contested and equivocal. Whilst some commentators suggest psychological explanations such as attributional style (Sharpley, Hutchinson, Murray, & McKenzie, 2001), childhood and adulthood trauma (Morgan et al., 2017), and the impact of racism, stigma and discrimination (Karlsen, Nazroo, McKenzie, Bhui, & Weich, 2005; Veling, Hoek, & Mackenbach, 2008); others emphasise biosocial factors. These include 'migration hypotheses' (Bhugra & Bhui, 2001), which theorise that high rates of schizophrenia in migrant communities could arise because (i) there are high rates in the host counties, (ii) individuals predisposed to schizophrenia are most likely to migrate or (iii) that the stressful nature of the migration process itself might trigger schizophrenia and other psychoses. It has also been noted that migrants' concentration in urban, often socio-economically deprived, communities is associated with elevated rates of schizophrenia diagnosis (Bhugra & Jones, 2001).

However, some scholars believe that the higher rates of schizophrenia diagnosis are artefactual. People like Suman Fernando (Fernando, 1989) posit that elevated rates of schizophrenia diagnosis are not indicative of actual levels of morbidity in these communities but rather reflect unconscious bias and institutional racism in diagnostic practice. In this context, it has been suggested that culturally informed expressions of distress and coping strategies are misinterpreted by predominantly White and South Asian psychiatrists, resulting in Caribbeans being labelled 'Big, Black & Dangerous', which might partly explain disproportionate use of coercive care and the number of deaths in service (Crichton, 1994). Findings of significantly lower levels of diagnosis in the Caribbean – specifically Trinidad (Bhugra et al., 1996, 2000), Barbados (Mahy, Mallett, Leff, & Bhugra, 1999) and Jamaica (Hickling & Rodgers-Johnson, 1995), lend credence to this perspective. However, the recently-published 10-year follow-up to the AESOP study reported that baseline social disadvantage contributed to disparities in clinical, social and service use between the UK's African-Caribbean population and White British peers (Morgan et al., 2017).

Irrespective of what gives rise to the elevated prevalence and incidence rates amongst Black people who have their origins in the Caribbean, what is not in doubt is that such diagnoses are associated with inferior access, experiences, and outcomes of psychiatric care compared with both the White British majority population and other minority sub-populations (Bhui et al., 2003; Healthcare Commission, 2010; Morgan et al., 2005; Morgan, Mallett, Hutchinson, & Leff, 2004). People of African-Caribbean heritage are more likely to come into psychiatric care via the Mental Health Act (Mental Health Taskforce, 2016), police, and criminal justice system versus the more benign route of general practice and the family physician (Morgan et al., 2005; Morgan et al., 2002). As psychiatric inpatients, African-Caribbeans experience more coercive care, including higher rates of seclusion, control and restraint techniques and use of injected antipsychotic medications (Morgan et al., 2005). On average, African-Caribbeans stay more than twice as long in psychiatric hospitals as their White British peers and are more likely to have restrictions imposed following discharge (National Institute for Health & Care Excellence, 2009). They are also significantly less likely to receive psychological therapy or 'talking treatments' (Mental Health Taskforce, 2016; National Institute for Health & Care Excellence, 2014). Highlighting a 'systematic failure' to provide mental healthcare for people of African and Caribbean heritage (Mental Health Taskforce, 2016).

Negative reports about psychiatric care are common in African-Caribbean communities, generating a great deal of fear and mistrust (Keating, Robertson, McCulloch, & Francis, 2002). African-Caribbeans' fear of the deleterious consequences of engaging with services has been cited in partial explanation for delays in receiving specialist care, resulting in their being labelled 'hard-to-reach' by mental health services (Keating et al., 2002). However, there is evidence that, far from being reluctant to engage with statutory mental health services, African-Caribbeans often overcome their mistrust making multiple attempt to get help and support but are impeded by structural barriers, particularly in primary care (Morgan et al., 2005).

Delays in receiving diagnosis, care, and treatment are stressful for the individual experiencing symptoms of psychosis. Additionally, in a population where symptoms of mental illness are sometimes attributed to demonic possession and/or deviance (Arthur et al., 2010), those experiencing symptoms are at an increased risk of social ostracism and isolation, which is associated with higher rates of relapse and re-hospitalisation (Del Vecchio et al., 2015). Family members in general and primary carers, in particular, can come under tremendous strain when living with someone experiencing symptoms of psychosis, especially in the absence of a diagnosis, lack of understanding of the condition and/or limited coping strategies (Onwumere, Smith, & Kuipers, 2010). In other words, schizophrenia and other psychoses can adversely affect both the physical and mental health of not only the individuals experiencing symptoms but also of those who live with and care for them. Shame, stigma and a lack of awareness within these communities mean that families commonly find it difficult to recognise the nature and significance of the problems, often seeking help and support only when in crisis (Mantovani, Pizzolati, & Edge, 2016).

Seeking Solutions: An Assets-based, Community-centred Approach

There have been numerous policy and practice initiatives aimed at reducing ethnically based inequalities in mental healthcare, most notably the Department of Health's flagship 'Delivering Race Equality' (DRE) (Department of Health, 2005) programme. A key aspect of DRE was employing Community Development Workers to work with the African-Caribbean and other minority communities to reduce the fear of mainstream services and promote more timely engagement with mental health services. Evidence suggests this approach had limited success as there has been little improvement of African-Caribbean people's experiences or relationship with UK mental health services (Care Quality Commission, 2011). In consequence, the National Institute for Health and Care Excellence (NICE) concluded that there was a crisis in schizophrenia care as experienced by African-Caribbeans and that novel solutions were urgently required (National Institute for Health & Care Excellence, 2014).

This 'call to arms' by NICE was timely. It endorsed findings from a series of community mental health conferences and engagement activities between members of the African-Caribbean community, policy makers, healthcare commissioners, service providers and academic researchers (Edge & Grey, 2018). The overwhelming message from African-Caribbean service users, their families and advocates who attended these conferences was that two main things were urgently needed. First, access to 'talking treatments' specifically designed to be culturally relevant. Second, more information about 'schizophrenia', including: the nature and presentation of the mental health problem, different approaches to care and treatment and how 'The System' works. Furthermore, people signalled their willingness to engage in making this happen.

In light of the longstanding history of mistrust of mental health services and lack of research 'giving voice' to African-Caribbean community perspectives on the most appropriate interventions for managing schizophrenia, we sought to establish an authentic partnership between the community, health providers and academics (Jones & Wells, 2007). Our CPPR approach was based on that developed by US-based NGO Healthy African American Families and Charles R Drew Medical Centre in Los Angeles, California (Jones & Wells, 2007). CPPR adopts an explicitly assets-based (vs deficits) approach, acknowledging and mobilising community strengths and building capacity to engage in future research and other solutions-focussed endeavours (Wells & Jones, 2009). Importantly, capacity-building is considered a two-way process in which academics and healthcare professionals acknowledge the need to learn alongside supporting community members to acquire and enhance knowledge, skills and experiences.

Central to our model of CPPR was building trust by actively seeking to flatten hierarchies, fostering equality between partners in identifying problems and creating solutions (Edge & Grey, 2018). This model underpinned our approach to developing research *with* or *by* members of the African-Caribbean community versus *for* or *about* them (INVOLVE, 2012). Accordingly, via post-conference follow-up community events including: radio 'phone-ins', articles in community newspapers and presentations in 'Black-Majority-Churches', we sought to engage former and current service users, their families and wider the African-Caribbean community to partner with healthcare professionals and academics in co-producing a new culturally-appropriate talking treatment. Given the aforementioned pressures on the family associated with untreated psychosis, it was mutually agreed that a talking treatment that involved the family versus the service user only was required. Mindful that only evidence-based interventions would be considered commissionable, it was agreed that we would take a standard model of Family Intervention (FI) (Barrowclough & Tarrier, 1992) as our starting point and change it into a form that members of the African-Caribbean community would find acceptable.

FI 'Talking Treatment'

FI is a well-established 'talking treatment' with a strong evidence-base for being effective in the management of schizophrenia and related psychoses, especially when combined with properly titrated medication (Pharoah, Mari, Rathbone, & Wong, 2010; Pilling et al., 2002). Although there are a several approaches to FI in psychosis, fundamental principles and practice include: establishing effective ways or working with, acknowledging and addressing family conflict and tension, setting reasonable and achievable goals, and developing strategies to maintain gains achieved in therapy by embedding them in everyday life.

Reported benefits of FI include better self-care, problem-solving and coping for both service users and carers, which reduces the risk of relapse and re-hospitalisation (Barrowclough & Tarrier, 1992; Bird et al., 2010). Families who have received FI report better general health and wellbeing and reduced burden of care (Lobban et al., 2013). Whilst there is no reason to believe that these benefits would not be obtained by African-Caribbean people, there is little empirical evidence to support the implementation of current FI models in a community in which members often operate by the maxim "*you don't talk your business*" in relation to personal and family challenges (Edge & Rogers, 2005). Nevertheless, galvanised by the need to address the lack of access to psychological therapy and perceived over-reliance on antipsychotic medication, African-Caribbean community members (including a former service user and a mother of a service user) partnered with academics to successfully bid for funding from the UK's National Institute for Health Research (NIHR) to undertake research to develop Culturally adapted FI (CaFI) (Edge et al., 2018).

What Does CaFI for Schizophrenia Look Like?

The process of culturally adapting, implementing and evaluating CaFI with African-Caribbean community members has been detailed elsewhere (Edge et al., 2016, Edge & Grey, 2018). Here, we provide an overview of the intervention, in particular, the features that make it uniquely African-Caribbean.

We culturally adapted Barrowclough and Tarrier's model of FI (Barrowclough & Tarrier, 1992) which comprises: (i) Service user assessment, (ii) Family and carer assessment, (iii) Psycho-education, (iv) Stress management and coping strategies and (v) Problem-solving and setting achievable goals. When presented with this model, stakeholders (e.g. service users, carers and healthcare professionals) concluded that the constituent parts were all relevant. However, the consensus was that, as it had been developed by *"middle-class" White Europeans who don't really know the Black agenda* (African-Caribbean Male Service User, Focus Group 1) (Edge & Grey, 2018), important modifications were required to ensure that the emergent therapy was capable of meeting the specific needs of African-Caribbean service users and their families.

In relation to the *Service User Assessment* component of the existing model, stakeholders stated that two main additional topics were needed. These were racism and discrimination (including explicit reference to institutional racism and racialization) and alternative conceptualizations of mental health and illness such as beliefs about the role of spiritual/supernatural forces in the genesis of and recovery from mental illness. These elements were integral to the CaFI model alongside greater emphasis on resilience, recovery and hope for the future.

To improve the cultural-specificity of *Family Assessment*, it was suggested that the new therapy should focus on meaningfully exploring family structures and dynamics (such the role of age and gender) in African-Caribbean families. Understanding how these dynamics coupled with ongoing family tension and conflict, resulting from delayed access to care and lack of understanding of the symptoms of psychosis, was regarded as particularly salient for African-Caribbeans. Additionally, who counts as *'family'* was an important consideration. Stakeholders highlighted the tendency of mental health services and other governmental agencies to pathologise Black families and adopt a seemingly arbitrary and inflexible stance when dealing with service users' networks, in which friends and extended family members may feature as or more prominently than biological kin (Edge & Rogers, 2005). Refusal to acknowledge the significance of these ties risked further alienating African-Caribbean service users and their families as well as reducing the likelihood of receiving family-based therapy, especially when biological families were estranged or absent, for example, due to migratory patterns. In the CaFI approach, service users nominated significant others (such as friends, youth or key workers, community or religious leaders) to participate in therapy with them as Family Support Members. In the study to test CaFI (Edge et al., In Press), community volunteers were also recruited to 'come alongside' service users who wanted to participate in therapy but were unable to nominate family or significant others. This is a prime example of the CPPR philosophy of drawing on community assets.

Psycho-education is arguably the core element of FI. Stakeholders found the term highly stigmatising, concluding that it should be changed to reflect the new way of working espoused by the model. In this context, it was agreed that this component of the CaFI therapy should be renamed *Shared Learning*. Whilst maintaining a focus on understanding schizophrenia and psychosis, and exploring beliefs and models of health and illness, greater emphasis is placed on related factors that particularly affect Black people such as the role of the police and the (over)use of The Mental Health Act (Mental Health Taskforce, 2016) in accessing mental healthcare. Understanding and being sensitive to working with different explanatory models of mental health difficulties such as the associations between deviant behaviours and onset of psychosis (Arthur et al., 2010) and beliefs that service users could but chose not to control symptoms were regarded as important additions to ensure CaFI's relevance for African-Caribbean families. Additionally, sensitivity to religion and belief systems and how such explanatory models might affect help-seeking behaviours, coping strategies, and wellbeing were perceived as fundamental to fostering collaborative working and therapeutic alliance.

In the FI model that we culturally adapted (Barrowclough & Tarrier, 1992), *Stress Management, Problem-solving & Coping* emphasises examining stresses within the family, focussing particularly on elements of the service user's experiences that families find especially challenging. These include 'negative symptoms' of psychosis such as lack of motivation, social withdrawal and poor self-care as well as other difficult behaviours, including overt aggression and suicidal tendencies. It was agreed that an important aspect of culturally-adapted therapy would be enabling family members to first acknowledge the mental health problem in order to evaluate its impact on their wellbeing and develop effective coping strategies. This was regarded as particularly significant given reluctance to talk openly about mental illness within this community (Edge & MacKian, 2010; Edge & Rogers, 2005).

Stakeholders welcomed the approach to *Problem-solving and goal setting* that emphasises a solutions-based persective by breaking down goals into small, achievable steps and rewarding progress versus focussing on failure. Opportunities to celebrate successes were regarded as particularly helpful in changing family dynamics to create less conflict-fuelled interactions and promoting more benign home environments. Furthermore, it was believed that these approaches would encourage family members to focus on service users' strengths and to work more collaboratively to foster harmony and plan for how best to deal with future challenges and difficulties, including relapse.

In our CaFI model, we incorporated two new elements: *Communication* and *Staying well and maintaining gains*. *Communication* was deemed important as African-Caribbean families reported difficulties communicating with mental health services, due to deep-seated fear and mistrust; arguably reinforced by difficulties in successfully negotiating timely access to appropriate mental health care (Morgan et al., 2005). CaFI therefore includes work to build communication and advocacy skills and enhance confidence in communicating with mental health professionals in the context of adversarial relationships, negative experiences and power imbalance. As families reported being excluded from decision-making and being unable to express their needs and/or those of service users to professionals, opportunities to practice effective communication in 'a safe space' was an important aspect of meeting service users' and families' needs. Additionally, exploring unhelpful ways of communicating within the family such as criticising and blaming and developing more helpful alternatives such as practicing active listening skills, assertiveness, and ways of expressing positive and negative feelings were also regarded as integral to improving service users' and families' sense of control. Improved communication was thus inextricably linked to developing effective problem-solving and coping strategies, including planning for crises.

The final component of CaFI is *Staying well and maintaining gains*. In these sessions, service users and families work with therapists to consolidate the material from preceding sessions to develop individualised plans for staying well as a family and reducing the risk of further relapse. For this to be effective, it is important to develop a clear understanding of what recovery means for each family and to help them develop realistic expectations.

Each family develops a *relapse prevention action plan* (or *action plan* for short) designed to help them identify early warning signs that the service user is becoming unwell (also known as a *relapse signature*) in order to initiate their own individualised step-by-step guide to getting the right support from others. This includes knowing what actions to take and who to contact if early signs occur.

Stakeholders arrived at consensus that what would truly make CaFI *African-Caribbean specific* was placing its content within a different *ethos of delivery* as embodied by the rejection of *psycho-education* in favour of the less stigmatising *shared learning*. This approach advocates an explicitly collaborative, three-way approach, which acknowledges that therapists have as much to learn from service users and families as they could 'teach' about psychosis. In addition, therapists should always respect the language and terminology used by each family to describe their experiences, including seeking to understand unfamiliar terminology. An important aspect of working with African-Caribbean people is developing awareness cultural heterogeneity (*there's no such thing as African-Caribbean culture*) and not reinforcing misconceptions and stereotypes such as the automatic association of Caribbean people with illicit drug (specifically, marijuana) misuse. These issues were stated by stakeholders as being essential for building trust which underpins engagement in therapy and therapeutic alliance without which therapy will not be effective.

This approach requires a significant shift in some therapists' thinking and practice. This might include, for example, more openly acknowledging the magnifying effect of race or ethnicity on the power imbalance inherent in therapy when White therapists work with Black service users. Additionally, therapists' willingness and genuine interest to understand African-Caribbean cultures and their ability to be open to dealing with 'uncomfortable truths' such as 'White privilege' was regarded as key to trust building. This is crucial in developing the therapeutic alliance needed for successful outcomes, especially when racism and discrimination are central to service users' and families' explanatory models and help-seeking practices.

This highlights an important issue that emerged from qualitative work with healthcare professionals. Namely, therapists' self-reported lack of confidence to work with people of different cultural background for the fear of being insensitive and/or judged as racist. Despite bespoke training, some therapists in our study reported that, whilst the training significantly improved their insight and understanding of how to work with people who are culturally different from themselves, they often lacked the confidence to explore issues such as ethno-cultural beliefs and experiences of personal and institutional racism.

Testing CaFI

To test CaFI (Edge et al., 2016), we recruited 31 family units comprising service users diagnosed with schizophrenia and their families or Family Support Members where biological family members were not available. In all, 26 family units took part in CaFI, and 24 of the 26 family units completed all 10 sessions of CaFI therapy.

Importantly, half of the family units involved Family Support Members who were either nominated by service users or recruited by the study team. Ratings and qualitative findings of therapy sessions by key stakeholders found CaFI to be a positive experience. From service users' perspectives, benefits included improved: confidence, self-esteem, coping skills, communication, insight and knowledge of mental health problems and services. Additionally, service users, family members, therapists and key workers of the service users involved all stated that they would recommend CaFI to others, highlighting the success of the intervention to others. Given the long history of African-Caribbean people's negative experiences of mental health services, this is an important step in addressing the community's desire to develop culturally-appropriate talking treatments.

Discussion and Conclusion

In response to the National Institute for Health and Excellence's (NICE) (2014) call for novel interventions to address the crisis in schizophrenia care for African-Caribbeans and research by our team highlighting the importance of adapting evidence-based interventions in schizophrenia (Degnan et al., 2018), we partnered with service users, their families, community members, and healthcare professionals to: (i) determine whether a culturally-adapted version of FI was desirable and (ii) identify modifications of an extant evidence-based model of FI (Barrowclough & Tarrier, 1992) to co-produce a more culturally-appropriate version thereof. Given historically adversarial relationships between African-Caribbeans and mental health services (Department of Health, 2005; Keating et al., 2002; Morgan et al., 2005), using CPPR principles to achieve meaningful engagement with members of this so called 'hard-to-reach' community was an important achievement.

Applying CPPR principles (Jones & Wells, 2007) meant, for example, that African-Caribbean service users, their families, and members of the wider community were actively involved in every stage of the research process. Shared leadership within the partnership is evidenced by the various service users and carer roles as members and chairs of the study's Research Management and Research Advisory Groups (Edge & Grey, 2018).

In-keeping with CPPR, two-way capacity-building was also integral to this assets-based approach. This included, for example, embedding academics and clinicians within the community to enhance their learning from and understanding of African-Caribbean people's cultures and perspectives and community members being part of the research team. Service users, carers and community members who wished to do so received honorary university contracts, thus facilitating access to academic resources. We also provided tailor-made research methods training to enhance capacity-building and support development of future research for the benefit the community.

Our experience suggests that a community frequently labelled 'hard-to-reach' are, in practice, 'seldom heard' (Redwood, Gale, & Greenfield, 2012). We found that members of the African-Caribbean community were highly motivated to engage in solutions-focussed research to improve the community's experiences and outcomes of engaging with mainstream mental health services (Chung et al., 2010; Wells & Jones, 2009). In this context, their involvement in co-producing a culturally-appropriate 'talking treatment' for schizophrenia (a highly stigmatising and contested condition) might have important implications beyond mental health. For example, more meaningful collaboration with African-Caribbeans and other minority groups might result in health promotion initiatives and interventions to improve physical health outcomes for conditions which disproportionately affect these groups such as diabetes, hypertension and stroke.

Implications

In our study (Edge et al., 2016), CaFI was able to meet the needs of a 'seldom heard' service user group, indicating the possibility of developing similar interventions for other ethnic groups. We also successfully delivered CaFI in acute hospital and community settings with biological family members and Family Support Members. This is important because, according to NICE guidelines, FI should be offered to service users in regular contact with their families.

Had we adopted this approach, half the people in our study (Edge et al., 2018) would not have been eligible to receive CaFI. This underscores the UK's Mental Health Task Force's (Mental Health Taskforce, 2016, 2017) that new ways of working are required to reduce the apparently intractable inequalities faced by African-Caribbean service users and other ethnic minority users in accessing mental health care in general and psychological therapy in particular.

Wider Context of CaFI

According to the World Health Organization (WHO) (2016), there is a 75% mental health 'treatment gap' in Low and Middle-Income Countries (LAMICs), including many countries in the Caribbean and African diasporas.

The WHO (Dua et al., 2011) recommends antipsychotics and psychosocial interventions such as Cognitive Behavioural Therapy and FI for the treatment and management of schizophrenia and related psychoses. However, given the scarcity of resources, such as the shortage of professional staff, to meet the needs of populations in LAMICs; psychosocial interventions, delivered via non-specialist providers, offer potential solutions. Recent studies in LAMICs have demonstrated the beneficial effects of such interventions (Singla et al., 2017; Weobong et al., 2017).

Currently, most of the evidence of the clinical and cost-effectiveness of psychosocial interventions is from high-income countries (Patel et al., 2007). Our findings suggest that CaFI has the potential to be applied in LAMICs. However, further work is needed to test its clinical and cost-effectiveness compared with usual care and adaptability for non-UK contexts alongside more culturally valid outcome measures (Degnan, Berry, Jenkins, & Edge, 2018).

Acknowledgments and Compliance with Ethical Standards

- Disclosure of potential conflicts of interest
  DE – None
  AD – None
  SR – None
- Research involving Human Participants
  The study involved only human participants. Ethical approval was given by Greater Manchester East National Research Ethics Service (NRES) Ethics Committee (13/NW/0571). All procedures followed were in accordance with the ethical standards of the Independent Review Board (IRB) and the Helsinki Declaration of 1975, as revised in 2000.
- Informed consent
  All participants gave written informed consent to being included in the study. For current service users to participate, they were deemed well enough and had capacity to consent (as assessed by care coordinators/clinical teams).

Funding

The CaFI study was funded by the NIHR, Health Service and Delivery Research Programme (HS&DR) (12/5001/62).

Disclaimer

This chapter presents independent research funded by the NIHR. The views and opinions expressed therein are those of the authors and do not necessarily reflect those of the HS&DR Programme, NIHR, NHS or the Department of Health. The study sponsor is The University of Manchester and the host NHS Trust Greater Manchester Mental Health NHS Foundation Trust (formerly Manchester Mental Health & Social Care Trust).

References

American Psychiatric Association. (2000). *Diagnostic and statistical manual of mental disorders: DSM-IV-TR®* (4th ed.). Washington, DC: American Psychiatric Association.

Arthur, C. M., Hickling, F. W., Robertson-Hickling, H., Haynes-Robinson, T., Abel, W., & Whitley, R. (2010). "Mad, Sick, Head Nuh Good": Mental illness stigma in Jamaican communities. *Transcultural Psychiatry, 47*, 252–275. doi:10.1177/1363461510368912

Barrowclough, C., & Tarrier, N. (1992). *Families of schizophrenic patients: Cognitive behavioural interventions*. London: Chapman & Hall.

Bhugra, D., & Bhui, K. (2001). African-Caribbeans and schizophrenia: Contributing factors. *Advances in Psychiatric Treatment, 7*, 283–291. doi:10.1192/apt.7.4.283

Bhugra, D., Hilwig, M., Hossein, B., Marceau, H., Neehall, J., Leff, J., ... Der, G. (1996). First-contact incidence rates of schizophrenia in Trinidad and one-year follow-up. *The British Journal of Psychiatry, 169*, 587–592. doi:10.1192/bjp.169.5.587

Bhugra, D., Hilwig, M., Mallett, R., Corridan, B., Leff, J., Neehall, J., & Rudge, S. (2000). Factors in the onset of schizophrenia: A comparison between London and Trinidad samples. *Acta Psychiatrica Scandinavica, 101*, 135–141. doi:10.1034/j.1600-0447.2000.90049.x

Bhugra, D., & Jones, P. (2001). Migration and mental illness. *Advances in Psychiatric Treatment, 7*, 216–223. doi:10.1192/apt.7.3.216

Bhui, K., Stansfeld, S., Hull, S., Priebe, S., Mole, F., & Feder, G. (2003). Ethnic variations in pathways to and use of specialist mental health services in the UK: Systematic review. *The British Journal of Psychiatry, 182*, 105–116. doi:10.1192/bjp.182.2.105

Bird, V., Premkumar, P., Kendall, T., Whittington, C., Mitchell, J., & Kuipers, E. (2010). Early intervention services, cognitive-behavioural therapy and family intervention in early psychosis: Systematic review. *The British Journal of Psychiatry, 197*, 350–356. doi:10.1192/bjp.bp.109.074526

Care Quality Commission. (2011). *Count me in 2010: Results of the 2010 national census of inpatients and patients on supervised community treatment in mental health and learning disability services in England and Wales*. London: Care Quality Commission.

Chung, B., Jones, L., Dixon, E. L., Miranda, J., Wells, K., & Community Partners in Care Steering Council. (2010). Using a community partnered participatory research approach to implement a randomized controlled trial: Planning the design of community partners in care. *Journal of Health Care for the Poor and Underserved, 21*, 780–795. doi:10.1353/hpu.0.0345

Crichton, J. (1994). Comments on the Blackwood Inquiry. *Psychiatric Bulletin, 18*, 236–237. doi:10.1192/pb.18.4.236

Degnan, A., Baker, S., Edge, D., Husain, N., Nottidge, W., Press, C., ... Drake, R. (2018). The nature and efficacy of culturally-adapted psychosocial interventions for schizophrenia: A systematic review and meta-analysis. *Psychological Medicine, 48*, 714–727. doi:10.1017/S0033291717002264

Degnan, A., Berry, K., Jenkins, S., & Edge, D. (2018). Development, validation and cultural-adaptation of the knowledge about psychosis questionnaire for African-Caribbean people in the UK. *Psychiatry Research, 263*, 199–206. doi:10.1016/j.psychres.2018.03.013

Del Vecchio, V., Luciano, M., Sampogna, G., De Rosa, C., Giacco, D., Tarricone, I., ... Fiorillo, A. (2015). The role of relatives in pathways to care of patients with a first episode of psychosis. *International Journal of Social Psychiatry, 61*, 631–637. doi:10.1177/0020764014568129

Department of Health. (2005). *Delivering race equality in mental health care: An action plan for reform inside and outside services and the Government's response to the Independent inquiry into the death of David Bennett*. London: Department of Health.

Dua, T., Barbui, C., Clark, N., Fleischmann, A., Poznyak, V., van Ommeren, M., ... Saxena, S. (2011). Evidence-based guidelines for mental, neurological, and substance use disorders in low- and middle-income countries: Summary of WHO recommendations. *PLoS Medicine, 8*. doi:10.1371/journal.pmed.1001122

Edge, D., Degnan, A., Cotterill, S., Berry, K., Baker, J., & Abel, K. (2018). Culturally-adapted Family Intervention (CaFI) for African Caribbeans with schizophrenia and their families: A feasibility study of implementation and acceptability. *Health Service & Delivery Research (NIHR Journals), 6*(32), 1. doi:10.3310/hsdr06320.

Edge, D., Degnan, A., Cotterill, S., Berry, K., Drake, R., Baker, J., ... Abel, K. (2016). Culturally-adapted Family Intervention (CaFI) for African-Caribbeans diagnosed with schizophrenia and their families: A feasibility study protocol of implementation and acceptability. *Pilot and Feasibility Studies, 2*, 1–14. doi:10.1186/s40814-016-0070-2

Edge, D., & Grey, P. (2018). An assets-based approach to co-producing a culturally adapted family intervention (CaFI) with African Caribbeans diagnosed with schizophrenia and their families. *Ethnicity and Disease, 28*(Suppl 2), 485–492. doi:10.18865/ed.28. S2.485.

Edge, D., & MacKian, S. C. (2010). Ethnicity and mental health encounters in primary care: Help-seeking and help-giving for perinatal depression among Black Caribbean women in the UK. *Ethnicity & Health, 15*, 93–111. doi:10.1080/13557850903418836

Edge, D., & Rogers, A. (2005). Dealing with it: Black Caribbean women's response to adversity and psychological distress associated with pregnancy, childbirth, and early motherhood. *Social Science & Medicine, 61*, 15–25. doi:10.1016/j.socscimed.2004.11.047

Fearon, P., Kirkbride, J., Morgan, C., Dazzan, P., Morgan, K., Lloyd, T., ... Murray, R. (2006). Incidence of schizophrenia and other psychoses in ethnic minority groups: Results from the MRC AESOP Study. *Psychological Medicine, 36*, 1541–1550. doi:10.1017/S0033291706008774

Fernando, S. (1989). *Race and culture in psychiatry*. Hove: Routledge.

Harrison, G., Owens, D., Holton, A., Neilson, D., & Boot, D. (1988). A prospective study of severe mental disorder in Afro-Caribbean patients. *Psychological Medicine, 18*, 643–657. doi:10.1017/S0033291700008321

Healthcare Commission. (2010). *Count me in: National mental health and learning disability ethnicity census 2010*. London: Healthcare commission.

Hickling, F. W., & Rodgers-Johnson, P. (1995). The incidence of first contact schizophrenia in Jamaica. *The British Journal of Psychiatry, 167*, 193–196. doi:10.1192/bjp.167.2.193

INVOLVE. (2012). *Briefing notes for researchers: Involving the public in NHS, public health and social care research*. Eastleigh: INVOLVE.

Jones, L., & Wells, K. (2007). Strategies for academic and clinician engagement in community-participatory partnered research. *JAMA, 297*, 407–410. doi:10.1001/jama.297.4.407

Karlsen, S., Nazroo, J. Y., McKenzie, K., Bhui, K., & Weich, S. (2005). Racism, psychosis and common mental disorder among ethnic minority groups in England. *Psychological Medicine, 35*, 1795–1803. doi:10.1017/s0033291705005830

Keating, F., Robertson, D., McCulloch, A., & Francis, E. (2002). *Breaking the circles of fear: A review of the relationship between mental health services and African and Caribbean communities*. London: Sainsbury Centre for Mental Health.

Lobban, F., Postlethwaite, A., Glentworth, D., Pinfold, V., Wainwright, L., Dunn, G., ... Haddock, G. (2013). A systematic review of randomised controlled trials of interventions reporting outcomes for relatives of people with psychosis. *Clinical Psychology Review, 33*, 372–382. doi:10.1016/j.cpr.2012.12.004

Mahy, G. E., Mallett, R., Leff, J., & Bhugra, D. (1999). First-contact incidence rate of schizophrenia on Barbados. *The British Journal of Psychiatry, 175*, 28–33. doi:10.1192/Bjp.175.1.28

Mantovani, N., Pizzolati, M., & Edge, D. (2016). Exploring the relationship between stigma and help-seeking for mental illness in African-descended faith communities in the UK. *Health Expectations, 20*, 373–384. doi:10.1111/hex.12464

Mental Health Taskforce. (2016). *The five year forward view for mental health*. London: The Mental Health Taskforce.

Mental Health Taskforce. (2017). *Five year forward view for mental health: One year on*. London: The Mental Health Taskforce.

Morgan, C., Dazzan, P., Morgan, K., Jones, P., Harrison, G., Leff, J., ... Fearon, P. (2006). First episode psychosis and ethnicity: Initial findings from the AESOP study. *World Psychiatry, 5*, 40–46.

Morgan, C., Fearon, P., Lappin, J., Heslin, M., Donoghue, K., Lomas, B., ... Dazzan, P. (2017). Ethnicity and long-term course and outcome of psychotic disorders in a UK sample: The ÆSOP-10 study. *The British Journal of Psychiatry, 211*, 88–94. doi:10.1192/bjp.bp.116.193342

Morgan, C., Hutchinson, G., Bagalkote, H., Morgan, K., Dazzan, P., Samele, C., ... Leff, J. (2002). GP referral and ethnicity in the AESOP (Aetiology and Ethnicity in Schizophrenia and Other Psychoses) first onset study. *Schizophrenia Research, 53*(3), 49–49.

Morgan, C., Kirkbride, J., Mallett, R., Hutchinson, G., Fearon, P., Morgan, K., ... Leff, J. (2005). Social isolation, ethnicity, and psychosis: Findings from the AESOP first onset psychosis study. *Schizophrenia Bulletin, 31*, 232–232.

Morgan, C., Mallett, R., Hutchinson, G., & Leff, J. (2004). Negative pathways to psychiatric care and ethnicity: The bridge between social science and psychiatry. *Social Science & Medicine, 58*, 739–752. doi:10.1016/S0277-9536(03)00233-8

Morgan, C., Mallett, R., Hutchinson, G., Bagalkote, H., Morgan, K., Fearon, P., ... Group, A. S. (2005). Pathways to care and ethnicity. 2: Source of referral and help-seeking: Report from the AESOP study. *The British Journal of Psychiatry, 186*, 290–296. doi:10.1192/bjp.186.4.290

National Institute for Health and Care Excellence. (2009). *Schizophrenia: Core interventions in the treatment and management of schizophrenia in adults in primary and secondary care (update)*. London: The British Psychological Society and the Royal College of Psychiatrists.

National Institute for Health and Care Excellence. (2014). *Psychosis and schizophrenia in adults: Treatment and management. NICE clinical guidelines*. London: Department of Health.

Onwumere, J., Smith, B., & Kuipers, E. (2010). Families and psychosis. In D. Bhugra & C. Morgan (Eds.), *Principles of social psychiatry* (2nd ed., pp. 103–116). Chichester: John Wiley & Sons Ltd.

Patel, V., Araya, R., Chatterjee, S., Chisholm, D., Cohen, A., De Silva, M., ... van Ommeren, M. (2007). Treatment and prevention of mental disorders in low-income and middle-income countries. *Lancet, 370*, 991–1005. doi:10.1016/s0140-6736(07)61240-9

Pharoah, F., Mari, J., Rathbone, J., & Wong, W. (2010). Family intervention for schizophrenia. *Cochrane Database of Systematic Reviews, 12*. doi:10.1002/14651858.CD000088.pub2

Pilling, S., Bebbington, P., Kuipers, E., Garety, P., Geddes, J., Orbach, G., & Morgan, C. (2002). Psychological treatments in schizophrenia: I. Meta-analysis of family intervention and cognitive behaviour therapy. *Psychological Medicine, 32*, 763–782. doi:10.1017/S0033291702005895

Redwood, S., Gale, N. K., & Greenfield, S. (2012). 'You give us rangoli, we give you talk': using an art-based activity to elicit data from a seldom heard group. *BMC Medical Research Methodology, 12*, 7. doi:10.1186/1471-2288-12-7

Sharpley, M. S., Hutchinson, G., Murray, R. M., & McKenzie, K. (2001). Understanding the excess of psychosis among the African-Caribbean population in England: Review of current hypotheses. *The British Journal of Psychiatry, 178*, 60–68. doi:10.1192/bjp.178.40.s60

Singla, D. R., Kohrt, B. A., Murray, L. K., Anand, A., Chorpita, B. F., & Patel, V. (2017). Psychological treatments for the world: Lessons from low- and middle-income countries. *Annual Review of Clinical Psychology, 13*, 149–181. doi:10.1146/annurev-clinpsy-032816-045217

Sugarman, P. A., & Craufurd, D. (1994). Schizophrenia in the Afro-Caribbean community. *British Journal of Psychiatry, 164*, 474–480. doi:10.1192/bjp.164.4.474

Tortelli, A., Errazuriz, A., Croudace, T., Morgan, C., Murray, R. M., Jones, P. B., ... Kirkbride, J. B. (2015). Schizophrenia and other psychotic disorders in Caribbean-born migrants and their descendants in England: Systematic review and meta-analysis of incidence rates, 1950–2013. *Social Psychiatry and Psychiatric Epidemiology, 50*, 1039–1055. doi:10.1007/s00127-015-1021-6

Veling, W., Hoek, H. W., & Mackenbach, J. P. (2008). Perceived discrimination and the risk of schizophrenia in ethnic minorities: A case-control study. *Social Psychiatry Psychiatric Epidemiology, 43*, 953–959. doi:10.1007/s00127-008-0381-6

Wells, K., & Jones, L. (2009). "Research" in community-partnered, participatory research. *JAMA, 302*, 320–321. doi:10.1001/jama.2009.1033

Weobong, B., Weiss, H. A., McDaid, D., Singla, D. R., Hollon, S. D., Nadkarni, A., ... Patel, V. (2017). Sustained effectiveness and cost-effectiveness of the Healthy Activity Programme, a brief psychological treatment for depression delivered by lay counsellors in primary care: 12-month follow-up of a randomised controlled trial. *PLoS Medicine, 14*. doi:10.1371/journal.pmed.1002385

World Health Organization (WHO). (2016). *mhGAP intervention guide for mental, neurological and substance use disorders in non-specialized health settings: Mental health gap action programme (mhGAP): Version 2.0*. Geneva: World Health Organization.

Chapter 24

'Lone Wolf' Case Study Considerations of Terrorist Radicalisation from the Black Experience

Nicholas Banks

This chapter uses two case studies of individuals who converted to Islam, became radicalised and carried out terrorist acts: in the UK, Richard Reid, and in the US, Carlos Bledsoe. Issues of religion, mental health and radicalisation are explored from the black experience. Attachment related principles are applied to the case study examples at the end of the chapter to explore the psychological and social vulnerability of the case study individuals.

There is no likely single encompassing explanation for terrorism or for the psychology or those who perpetuate such acts. Some theories contribute to an understanding of some forms of terrorism, but do not explain all. Many of the theories of terrorism are conceptually, not empirically, grounded. Defining terrorism is difficult due to there being an overwhelming number of definitions (Schmid, 2011), with no overall definition agreed upon. Horgan (2017) suggests that terrorism may be a convenient label to categorise acts which are disagreed with by mainstream government and thinking, when 'they do it to us'; however, 'if we do it to others' it may then be conceptualised as a justifiable act involving collateral damage. The semantics of labelling is therefore in operation as a psychological tool of conceptualising terrorism and associated acts. As Horgan (2017) identifies, although terrorism is often seen as a political action, there is much evidence identifying that terrorists rarely achieve their claimed goals (English, 2016). Thus, one may need to consider that there is much more political motivation behind individual acts of terrorism, particularly when these involve what are typically seen as 'lone wolf' type attacks.

Brannan, Esler, and Strindberg (2001) have argued that Western notions of terrorism tended to make a number of fundamental errors in their limited conceptions for understanding the triggers for terrorism. One of these errors is a tendency for a condescending and antagonistic view of terrorists that does not accurately reflect their motives and goals. Thus, there is a culturally encapsulated error of not understanding the actions of terrorists from their own perspective (Alonso et al., 2008). This error can be seen in the early explanations of terrorism acts being committed by those perceived as having a mental illness and the assumption that most terrorists had mental health concerns, encouraging attempts at linking all terrorism to psychopathology (Hurlow, Wilson, & James, 2016). There appear distinctions between lone wolf terrorists and 'network based' terrorists. Greunewald, Chermak, and Freilich (2013) found some 40% of lone wolf terrorists had mental illness relative to 7.6% of network based terrorists. Similarly Gill, Horgan, and Deckert (2013), in a review of 119 lone wolf terrorists, found 31% had a history of mental illness. Similar results were found by Spaaij (2012). Psychologists appear to recognise that motives for terrorism can be varied (Horgan, 2017). In extending this view, this chapter considers that the motivation may not always be about achieving clear political goals, but in some individuals, who convert to Islam, an expression of psychological disturbance, through extreme actions, when moving through a psychological process of identity disruption. Difficulties are likely to develop if one takes a single, narrow perspective of seeing terrorism as an indication of clinical mental ill health. This is likely to misunderstand the personal and social contexts in which individuals who carry out such acts come from. Similarly, some have taken the view that there are no clearly defined personality characteristics that distinguish those engaging in terrorism from those who do not (Lester, Yang, & Lindsay, 2008; Moghaddam, 2006). Common in many of the lone wolf terrorists' experience is that of expressing outrage, anger and a sense of humiliation. This would appear to be a common factor driving action. Anger and a sense of grievance and injustice may be the more likely driving forces for extreme action, than those of earlier suggested theories of mental illness as a single factor (Gill & Corner, 2017). Individually acting, or lone wolf terrorists, however, may have increased mental disturbance compared to those other terrorists with clear organised group affiliations (Gill et al., 2013; Hewitt, 2003; Simon, 2013; Spaaij, 2010, 2012). Also, in considering mental disorder, psychopathy (Victoroff, 2005) and narcissism (Pearlstein, 1991) have been suggested as likely contributors to individual terrorist action. However, other 'conditions' such as autism, particularly Asperger's Syndrome, and mild intellectual impairment with a tendency for a high level of suggestibility and gullibility, have not been well considered in the literature as potential drivers for groups to attract those who may adhere to ordered actions with little question. Post (2010) suggests that those with mental disorders would be too emotionally unstable and be seen as too high a risk to the group's functioning. This would assume that discrete cells and firewalls of communication are not in place.

Identity, too, has been identified as a significant notion in terrorism (Huntington, 1996). Schwartz, Dunkel, and Waterman (2009) identify that terrorists may not be searching for an identity, but rather they may carry out terrorist activity as a direct expression of an existing identity. Identity has elements relating to cultural identity, social identity and personal identity. Cultural identity relates to the particular cultural values incorporated into a person's world view for principles of behaviour involving collectivism, absolutism in belief and family based practices (Schwartz, Montgomery, & Briones, 2006). Social identity, on the other hand, relates to the significance associated with social groups to which one belongs and where one draws one's sense of self (Tajfel & Turner, 1986). Identity, much like attachment, tends to be associated with beliefs and feelings about one's connectedness to what one sees as one's own group. Personal identity relates to the individual's chosen values and beliefs and the individual perspectives a person holds in making sense of the world.

Curiously, Schwartz et al. (2006) argue that a prerequisite for terrorism is that of collectivism, prioritising the group over the individual. This, from the present writer's perspective, appears questionable in that many individuals, from those of a European ethnic background who commit right-wing acts of terrorism, may not have strong elements of collectivism central to their culture and may prioritise their individual perspectives over group perspectives. Schwarz et al.'s (2006) perspective also may lead to the view that terrorism is a collective, rather than individual act. Such a notion does not well explain 'lone wolf' type terrorist behaviour. Indeed, the view that collectivism is a prerequisite for terrorism appears to pathologise collectivism.

Closely linked to notions of terrorism are the associated processes of radicalisation. There are many unagreed definitions of radicalisation (Della Porta & LaFree, 2012). One definition of radicalisation adopted by the European Commission (2008) is that of 'socialization to extremism which manifests itself in terrorism' (p. 7). A further definition of the term 'radicalisation' is one of a process of radical ideas being accompanied by the willingness to directly support or engage in violent acts (Dalgaard-Nielsen, 2010). There are difficulties in accepting either definition, as radical ideas may not always lead to action. As Milla and Faturochman (2013) note, radicalisation is an important path which may lead to terrorism, although not all radicals become involved in terrorism, and may maintain distance from groups involved in acts of terrorism even when radical views continue to be advocated. Therefore, a distinction from those who become radicalised, and use violence, needs to be maintained between those who become radicalised and communicate this through non-violent means. A distinction may need to be made as to whether individuals are 'activists', 'radicals' or 'terrorists'. Activists, as the term implies, would be actively involved in promoting ideas that may be seen as radicalised, but nonetheless are legal and non-violent. Radicals may be seen as having more of a tendency towards promoting violent actions, where terrorists would be active in carrying out illegal and violent actions (Moskalenko & McCauley, 2009). There are further problems of conceptualisation here, in that what are labelled as 'extremist ideologies and beliefs' may not achieve international consensus. What is extreme today may achieve, through radical political action, mainstream acceptance tomorrow. One only has to look at the historical political struggles of black people in the Civil Rights Movement in the US or South Africa as examples.

Many models of the process of radicalisation exist. Difficulties in theorising these may be that individuals are not so much radicalised by specific formal processes, but are radicalised through life experience and achieve, what they may see as 'enlightenment' as a means of expressing frustration and anger towards those who are seen as the cause of frustration and oppression. Personal grievances and frustrations may trigger what are seen as subgroup acceptable means of grievance expression which receives reinforcement and subgroup confirmation.

Two case study examples will now be used in this chapter to explore the process of radicalisation: that of a UK citizen, Richard Reid, also known in the British media, as the 'Shoe Bomber' and Carlos Bledsoe in the USA.

The UK Case Study: Richard Reid

Richard Reid was a mixed 'race' British national with a white English mother and a black Jamaican father. His mother was a librarian and his father had been, when not frequently incarcerated, a railway worker. Reid boarded an American Airlines flight from Paris to Miami in 2001 and attempted to use explosives hidden in his shoes to destroy the aircraft. Reid's father is described as a career criminal with Richard Reid himself spending many years as a petty criminal and converting to Islam while in prison. Reid is described as becoming radicalised while in prison and travelling to Pakistan and Afghanistan in 1999 and 2000 for Jihadi training. Reid's early crimes involved graffiti and then accumulating 10 convictions for crimes against the person and property and serving sentences at a young offenders' institution and then prison. Reid received a three year prison sentence in 1992 for street robberies. When released from prison in 1995, he is said to have joined a South London mosque and later attended Finsbury Park mosque which was presided over by the infamous Abu Hamza Al-Masri. In a letter sent to Reid's mother by email, Reid explained his rationale for his terrorist actions:

> [...]. What I am doing is part of the ongoing war between Islam and disbelief ... I know you will find many Muslims very quick to condemn the war between us and the US and ... I have sent you a copy of my will .... The reason for me sending you it is so that you can see that I didn't do this act out of ignorance nor did I do it just because I want to die, but rather because I see it as a duty upon me to help remove the oppressive American forces from the Muslim lands, and that is the only way for us to do so as we do not have other means to fight them. I hope that what I have done will not decur while you are, from looking into Islam or even calls you to hate the religion as the method of Islam is the truth, this is why we are ready to die defending the true Islam rather than to just sit back and allow the American government to dictate to us what we should believe and how we should behave, it is clear that this is a war between truth and falsehood .... This is a war between Islam and democracy .... I ask HIM that HE guide me to the truth and cause you to understand why I've done what I've done. Forgive me for all the problems I have caused you both in life and in death and don't be angry for what I've done.

Here one sees that Reid saw himself as both deeply connected with and committed to fighting for a cause he saw as just and honourable.

Reid's father is reported to have spent almost 20 years in prison in total and described himself as 'I was no great example to my son'. In the *Daily Telegraph* article, interviews with family identify his aunt describing him as a 'lonely lad with the empty life who found solace with his Muslim brothers'. Background material claims to suggest that Reid was:

> vulnerable, easily manipulated misfit with a grudge against, what he saw as, a cold and unjust society: a young man who latched onto a faith he believed would give him the identity he lacked and the revenge he sought against the society in which he was raised. (*Daily Telegraph*, 2001)

Further insight is given by Reid's mother when describing him as:

> He was so lonely, his life was so empty. He found solace with his Muslim brothers, with him it became much more than a religion, they became his family.

and:

> I don't believe for a second, from my conversations with him, that he was burning with hatred against the West. I believe he was very vulnerable and they asked him to do something. He called them brothers and he believed he owed them loyalty. They had become his family. Wouldn't you be prepared to die for your family? Most people would. I believe he thought he was in a holy war.

Further information from people who attended Reid's school identify that he was a marginal figure making few friends:

> He made it difficult to like him. He was always a bit weird and not very good at anything. He always tried to act tough, to play the hard man. Frankly, he didn't come to school much. He bunked off with the kids he met on the streets.

A close friend of Reid at school made the claim that Reid was "Trying to sort out where he was from, his roots. He wanted to find out an identity – but he's got two white parents."

A further friend at Reid's school said that Reid had difficulties identifying with both black and white peers, where his black peers:

> didn't seem accepting of him. He always walked behind – bringing up the rear. I don't think he had attitude. He didn't have the edge. He just didn't belong.
>
> Reid was also said to be "quick to follow the crowd if it would give him status."

These descriptions suggest an insecure attachment profile. Further interview detail from *The Guardian* newspaper, 2001, reports the father saying Richard Reid's attempt to bring down the plane was a cry for help:

> It's a shout for help. I know my son is determined enough to do it if he wanted to. All he had to do was go to the toilet, sit in there and then boom! Why do it in front of passengers if it's not a cry for help?

Reid's father also shared his guilt about his poor relationship with his son in the same interview saying:

> Of course I feel responsible. I couldn't give him the love he wanted. I wasn't there – I know I wasn't – but I could have been. A part of me said he can deal with it, take care of himself .... That's not good enough. If I thought killing myself would appease people, I would – to say, leave my son alone, but I know it won't do no good.

Reid's father left home within a year after Reid's birth and he had little further contact with Richard Reid, except during a chance meeting in a shopping precinct. Richard Reid's father was imprisoned for burglary when Richard Reid was born, with his mother beginning divorce proceedings within weeks. Reid was said to be then brought up by his white mother and her new white partner (*The Guardian*, September 2001).

A primary theme that arises in Reid's background is one of him searching for a grounded identity, sense of purpose and belonging and an emotional connection with a father figure.

An article in the *Daily Telegraph* (2001) identifies Richard Reid's father as telling Richard Reid when seeing him by chance in a shopping mall:

> I told Richard I had converted because of racism. I said to him "Why don't you become a Muslim, they have treated me alright. I certainly don't feel guilty about encouraging him because the sort of Islam I encountered was about loving mankind – it wasn't about blowing up planes.

Reid is said not to have seen his father for a further six years. It was in 1995, when released from a further prison sentence, that Reid remembered the conversation with his father and began attending the Brixton mosque. Reid was described as questioning issues of world-wide oppression, particularly as they related to Africa and the Middle East, and the lack of support from Western governments. Reid was described as being an eager pupil of the Qu'ran and beginning to learn Arabic and on religious conversion changed his name to Abdel Rahim. Changes with Reid were noticed when he met Zacarias Moussaoui, a French Moroccan, who was said to be an outspoken radical who was later convicted of conspiracy over the 9/11 events. It was at this point that Reid was said to have become more confrontational, argumentative and angry, challenging the more moderate teachings of the South London mosque. His history of social experience, from an attachment perspective, suggests a lack of empathy and low concern for others. Some 10 years after his conviction, in 2011, Richard Reid was said to have little remorse, telling researchers 'I do believe my actions to have been permissible in Islamic law, although I admit many people would dispute that and disagree with me on that point'.

One can see that as a result of marginalisation and separation from family and, importantly, bereft of a black father role model, Reid was searching for a sense of self and connection with an identity. Islam appears to have provided him this identity and sense of family group based connection. His motivation appeared not one of anger, but a need for acceptance and belonging achieved through deference to religious mentors.

The US Case: Carlos Bledsoe

Gartenstein-Ross (2014) provides an insightful US case study of Carlos Bledsoe, an African-American who, in June 2009, killed people in a military recruiting centre in Arkansas, US. Despite having a middle-class background with his parents involved in their own business in Memphis, Tennessee, Bledsoe became involved in gang activities and later received a conviction for drug possession and possession of a firearm. The case study details suggest that despite his family's description of him as a 'fun loving kid', Bledsoe was an emotionally needy young man and involved in several incidents of violence before attending college. A conviction appears to have unnerved Bledsoe who was then described as seeking out religion for the purposes of what can be seen as an existential crisis requiring support. A journalist who Bledsoe wrote to while in prison after the killing of individuals at the recruitment centre described Bledsoe as having grown increasingly disillusioned with Christianity, due to his view that the doctrine of the Holy Trinity did not describe a monotheistic religion. From a psychological perspective, this appears somewhat of an autistic preoccupation and indicates little tolerance for ambiguity. Kruglanski (2004) posits similar notions with the psychology of terrorists, where those who distort Islamic ideology discuss this in clear-cut terms, which is appealing to individuals who have little tolerance of ambiguity. Before finding Islam, Bledsoe moved on to an interest in Judaism, but was said to have been rejected by orthodox synagogues because he was black. Bledsoe took the view that Judaism excluded him because of his ethnicity. Bledsoe then explored Islam and when visiting a mosque in Nashville, Tennessee, was attracted by the 'salah' or group prayer. When attempting to participate, it became obvious that he was unfamiliar with the required ritual movements. When later asked about this, Bledsoe declared that he had an interest in Islam, but was not a Muslim. The mosque was described as responding with enthusiasm, with Bledsoe writing of his experience of this as 'embraced me like I was a long lost brother' (Gartenstein-Ross, 2014), achieving acceptance and belonging, with this acting as a process of validation and confirmation in deep contrast to his experience of rejection and personal invalidation from Judaism. This became a significant emotional connection for Bledsoe and also a welcoming in to Islam, and what would have most likely been experienced as unconditional positive regard, similarly described in the British case study of Richard Reid in his welcoming in to Islam in the UK.

Although Bledsoe is reported to have given a cognitive rationale for his rejection of Christianity, this being dissatisfaction with its 'lack of 'monotheism', one must look beyond this rationalisation, to the expressed acceptance and kinship that Bledsoe experienced when he attended a mosque. This appears more of a convincing explanation for the attraction to Islam; his immediate acceptance appears the prime motivator. From this, and his personal study, it appears that Bledsoe then embraced Islam at the age of 19. It is important to question whether Bledsoe was attracted to religion, or whether he was looking for something to fill a gap or void in his identity and bolster a low self-esteem and lack of emotional relationship support.

Potential Explanations for the Terrorist Inclinations of Reid and Bledsoe

Both Reid, in the UK, and Bledsoe in the US appeared to experience an extreme sense of alienation and depersonalisation through their intra-personal difficulties in relating to others and perceived non-acceptance from both black and white society. Turning to Islam appeared to achieve Bledsoe's need for belonging, but does not explain why he turned to terrorist activities. Not all believe that religious belief is significant in psychological radicalisation of all individuals (McCauley & Moskalenko, 2011; Mueller, 2012; Pape & Feldman, 2010). Some cases may be more related to the psychological profile of particular terrorists acting as 'lone wolf' individuals.

One model which attempts to use a psychological perspective in individual terrorist radicalisation processes is that of Silber and Bhatt (2007). This model considers, what it sees to be, a staged process of radicalisation. Silber and Bhatt (2007) suggest that rather than being seen as a unified, planned and coordinated threat of terrorism from a single organised source such as Al Qaeda, or DAISH (aka Islamic State), such large-scale organisations may only be an inspiring ideological reference point impacting on an individual terrorist's sense of self. Silber and Bhatt (2007) describe a four stage radicalisation process, that of: Stage One, or pre-radicalisation, Stage Two, or self-identification, Self Three, or indoctrination and the final Stage Four of jahadization. Each of these stages is said to be unique, with not all individuals who begin the process of radicalisation necessarily passing through all the stages. There is the potential to cease the process at different points. Regardless, Silber and Bhatt (2007) believed that those who do follow through each of the four stages 'are quite likely to be involved in the planning or implementation of a terrorist act'. This model has some utility in the conceptualisation of the individual psychology of those who may become radicalised. What appears remarkable in the analysis of Silber and Bhatt (2007) is their view "the majority of the individuals involved in these plots began as 'unremarkable' – they had 'ordinary' jobs, had lived 'ordinary' lives and had little, if any, criminal history" (p. 6). This description is neither true of Reid or Bledsoe.

What is missing from the model are the 'drivers' or the motivation for what are described as 'unremarkable individuals', such as Reid and Bledsoe, to plan, engage and commit acts of terrorism. As identified by Silber and Bhatt (2007), in the stage of pre-radicalisation, there is an assumption that such 'unremarkable' individuals become exposed to, and adopt, jihadi-Salafi Islam. Silber and Bhatt (2007) appear to demonise or denigrate Salafi Islam, without considering the wider social political influences, for example, racism that these 'unremarkable' individuals are exposed to. Importantly, Silber and Bhatt do not well consider the early backgrounds of the 'unremarkable' individuals and their early personal and social experiences. Although conceptually useful, the model, particularly at the pre-radicalisation stage, appears to identify the adoption of jihadi-Salafi Islam as the trigger, without any consideration of the psychological motivation, or initial predisposition, of individuals who convert to initially develop an interest in Islam. In contrast, Liu and Woodward (2013) believe that attempts to locate the blame for terrorist violence in religious beliefs are a form of scapegoating, as Salafi-ism or Wahhabi-ism are no more inclined towards violence than other religious groups (Woodward, Amin, & Rohmaniyah, 2010). It may be that the inclination towards violence comes from the individual's personal psychology rather than religious roots, but is expressed and enabled through religious cloaking.

The next stage of self-identification is said to be a phase where individuals, influenced by both internal and external factors, begin to explore Salafi Islam. However, again the influences of these internal and external factors are not described or well considered as, if such undescribed factors are having such significant influence and impact, surely it is here, in the early stages, that one would want to intervene as a means of circumventing the dangerous behaviours that will later come about. Silber and Bhatt (2007) go on to say that radicalised individuals in this self-identification phase will gradually move away from their old identity and increasingly associate themselves with 'like-minded individuals and adopt this ideology as their own'. Silber and Bhatt attempt some consideration of what the motivation for this huge shift in preference and identity might be, which is described as a 'cognitive opening, or crisis, which shakes one's certitude in previously held beliefs, and opens an individual to be receptive to new world views'. Silber and Bhatt (2007) suggest other types of triggers which may serve to create this cognitive shift, including losing a job, blocked mobility, alienation, discrimination, racism – real or perceived, international conflicts involving Muslims, or a death in the close family. What is missing from the analysis is the degree to which these economic, social, political or personal triggers actually feature in the radicalisation process. The experience of alienation through discrimination and racism, along with poor early family relationships, may have featured more in the psychology of Reid and Bledsoe than can be given credence in the Silber and Bhatt model.

The next stage of indoctrination is one where an individual becomes progressively radicalised with intensities in their beliefs and 'wholly adopts jahadi-Salafi ideology and comes to believe that militant action is required to support and further the cause'. Silber and Bhatt (2007) believe that this phase is enabled and driven by a religious mentor type figure. Silber and Bhatt (2007) argue that the initial self-identification process may be through an individual's motivational processes, but the association with similar believing individuals is an important influence in enabling and facilitating the development and maintenance of radical views. This intensification of beliefs would be so with both Reid and Bledsoe.

The final stage is that termed jahadization, where individuals become part of what is termed a cluster, with a belief and acceptance of individual duty to participate in jihad, and come to see themselves as religious warriors. Silber and Bhatt (2007) also suggest timings for this process, with the final stage of jihadization being a rapid process, only taking a few months or even weeks, with the earlier processes taking place gradually over two to three years. Although Reid may have had connections with 'a cluster' in his early training and equipping for his attack, this is not obviously so with Bledsoe. In further considering the social triggers to radicalisation, Silber and Bhatt (2007) argue that, in contrast to oppressed Arab populations, 'The transformation of a Western based individual to a terrorist, is not triggered by oppression, suffering, revenge or desperation' (p.7). Silber and Bhatt (2007) argue that it is a phenomenon 'that occurs as the individual is looking for an identity and a cause and unfortunately, often finds them in the extremist Islam'. This latter argument lacks 'black experience credibility' and appears to stem from the Silber and Bhatt's belief that such oppression or desperation could not exist in the west. A further flaw in the paper by Silber and Bhatt is that it does not address differences related to those who were born in to the Muslim faith, as opposed to those who convert to Islam.

Importantly, Silber and Bhatt (2007) did not identify why individuals seek religious connections rather than the readily available ideologies, such as socialism or nationalism (McCauley & Moskalenko, 2011). Alienated individuals, however, tend to search for an identity potentially separate from that of an identity in which they feel alienated (Mazarr, 2004). This may be due to other ideologies tending to be white or Eurocentric in their view and not allowing for a perceived connection with black issues and identity in contrast to what is perceived when visiting a mosque with its high black visibility in apparent order, synchronisation and harmony through prayer. This is more likely to give an immediate emotional connection to someone searching for belonging and acceptance. This was so for both Reid and Bledsoe. For example, Bledsoe was rejected by white Jews in his initial attempts at forming a relationship. This experience did not offer him the important ethnic identity connection and is likely to have increased a sense of hurt and rejection, making him even more emotionally needy in his search for acceptance. One attractive factor in becoming a Muslim may be due to its international ethnic diversity, having less of a focus on issues of 'race' and being experienced as more open and embracing of ethnic diversity. This too can be said of Christianity, although for some reason, black churches, as would have been readily available in New Orleans for Bledsoe, and also in the UK for Reid, were not seen as satisfactory or offering the connection Bledsoe or Reid required. As Gartenstein-Ross and Grossman (2009) argue, political radicalisation, with a small 'p', not religious belief alone, may be the strongest motivation. It may be that what facilitates the radicalisation and the motivators, is that of struggling to overcome personal oppression in a manner that is ill-conceived, with no other avenues or alternatives being considered, or importantly, provided.

An important influence is the role of the religious or ideological mentor who becomes the interpreter of the Qu'ran for the convert. This may not always be given the influential significance it deserves even by government research in the UK (MI5, 2008). Without an ideological mentor with high status motivational credibility, there can be no guidance or mis-interpretation of the Qu'ran. Direct interpretative access to the Qu'ran presents difficulties with those who convert to Islam, as they tend not to be Arabic speaking where their access to the Qu'ran may be processed through the misguided interpretations applied by 'radicalisers' in a distorted way. Therefore, justifications for violence become misapplied to current situations with uncritical acceptance or radicalisation by the individual as a form of deference or level of uncritical trust and emotional connection to the religious mentor (Jenkins, 2010; Pantucci, 2008). It will not be lost on individuals who are familiar with psychological notions of attachment, to see the depth of connection here with what is a trusted father figure often lacking in the convert's history. The radicalised individual's sense of self is not one of personal identity and increased understanding, with personal identity becoming subordinated to group identity based on distorted Islamic principles (Milla & Faturochman, 2013) to continue with a sense of belonging and achievement of the group goals. The mentor serves as a model whose standards and ideals need to be met to continue to connect with the source of psychological support and nurturing. Crenshaw (2011) identifies a key role here of the religious mentor needing to develop and maintain a collective belief system and linking this to the actions of the group. Crenshaw (2011) also suggests that the authority of such leaders tends to be based on factors of intellectual authority, military authority or personal authority, but related to charisma and those who are charismatic, tend to further enable and strengthen their influence. Reicher, Hopkins, Levine, and Rath (2005) discuss influences in the process of conversion, where individuals act on the basis of group identity or goals, not because they are overwhelmed by the power of their leaders, but more because the group ideology and its interpretation through their leaders, comes to define and determine who they are.

Other theorists (Moghaddam, 2006, 2010) have proposed, what is termed as a 'staircase metaphor', in explaining the process of global radicalisation, which emphasises identity, perceived injustice and a moral shift, as central components. Thus, radicalisation is associated with not only an identity crisis, but also a perception of unjust treatment with a moral shift occurring where terrorism becomes morally justified, moving individuals from passive cognising, to active terrorist behaviours. Fundamentalist religious principles and a sense of injustice or unfairness appear as clear influencing factors (Moghaddam, 2008; Rogers et al., 2007). Such views give ideological and social context explanations of terrorist activities. There is, therefore, a perceived interaction and dynamic involved in the two processes (Muluk, Sumaktoyo, & Ruth, 2013). Both Reid and Bledsoe share the significance of perceptions of injustice and unfair treatment. From this, there is likely to be a connection at an interpersonal level, with this connected with prejudice, discrimination and racism in the British and US context. Moghaddam

(2006) and Krueger and Maleckova (2003), however, emphasised perceptions of injustice, and thus subjectivity, and argued that terrorism had little to do with real treatment or disadvantaged economic and social status. These views may dismiss the lived black life experiences of Reid and Bledsoe in not allowing an interaction between the perception of injustice and personal, more psychological factors at play in becoming radicalised.

At a similar time to Moghaddam (2006) and Silber and Bhatt (2007), Wiktorowicz (2005) studying a Muslim activist group, Al-Muhajirioun, in the UK, suggested a four stage model of radicalisation being that of the first stage of a cognitive opening (this term comes from social movement theory which identifies an individual becoming available and open to influence) that comes about after an experience of personal disconnection giving rise to a personal grievance, perhaps through discrimination or that of a group grievance, seen as oppression and group discrimination. This appears relevant to both Bledsoe and Reid. In the next stage, the individual was seen as connecting with the extremist group through personal social connections either through friendship or kinship or attending study groups or demonstrations. Again, this appears relevant to both Bledsoe and Reid. In the third stage, the individual came to accept the leader of Al-Muhajirioun, Omar Bakri Mohammed, as a rightful authority for interpreting Islam and activity that should take place. From this, the fourth stage is one of the developments of a belief as interpreted by the legitimate authority, Omar Bakri Miohammed, that the 'right way' is through supporting radical or terrorist action. The connecting feature in the various theories, appears to be that of the experience or perception of discrimination, oppression and anger and perceiving personal, emotional acceptance or bond to an important, influential attachment figure, most often an ideological or religious mentor. This process described by Wiktorowicz, as summarised, appears to better explain the radicalisation experiences of both Bledsoe and Reid than the aforementioned notions.

Application of Aspects of Attachment Theory to Reid and Bledsoe

Using Attachment Theory, one could argue that both Reid and Bledsoe had attachment related difficulties in that there is a clear sense of them having dependency type characteristics, a feeling a lack of mastery and control, not having satisfactory inter-connectedness with others, including their family and wider groups. Bowlby's (1982) early notions of the psychological states associated with the disturbance and disruption of early attachments are 'acute distress or protest', 'despair', involving preoccupation, 'withdrawal and hopelessness'. These actions/psychological states can be seen with Reid and Bledsoe searching for connectedness, not achieving/receiving this, and moving on in their continued search for acceptance. Neither appears to perceive this as coming from earlier, long-term social connections involving either groups or individuals. This then leads them onto Bowlby's third state of 'detachment', where Reid and Bledsoe appear to recover from protest and despair, but with no attempts to reconnect with their early attachment objects. Similar to Bowlby's observations of infants in the detachment phase, Bledsoe and Reid become apathetic towards their historical attachment figures, with such apathy negating earlier bonding. This results in a high level of self-absorption and superficial sociability. Fonagy et al. (1997) and Meloy and Yakeley (2014) have argued that disrupted and disturbed attachment systems may be involved in both instrumental or emotionally based acts of violence with instrumental cases involving an individual seeking out an object with the primary motivation of being destructive, whereas in emotionally based or impulsive acts of violence, an intense defensive reaction of a violent nature is involved. Similarly, Bowlby (1982) took the view that violence and crime were primarily disorders of the attachment system effected by a deficit of emotional connection with others, and distorted views on the nature and process of social engagement. Although the information on Bledsoe's emotional connection with his family is sketchy, for Reid, the journalists provide information which appears to indicate considerable potential for disruption of primary bonds and emotional struggle in the relationship between Reid, his mother and stepfather. One may speculate that Bledsoe had considerable compromised secure attachment development as shown by a history of antisocial behaviour. Insecure attachments can display themselves in a lowered sense of control over the personal and physical environment, reducing/negating attachments to communities and groups and result in individuals who have difficulty in committing to historical emotional connections. For both Reid and Bledsoe, Islam appeared to provide them with an attachment base fulfilling lost historical needs of connection and belonging. One sees the process of bonding beginning with the acceptance that both found in contrast to the rejection Reid and Bledsoe both experienced from other groups which they attempted to connect with. Importantly, attachment serves as a haven of safety at times of threat or danger, to enable protection. Bowlby (1982) discussed situations which could activate the attachment system, effecting attachment behaviours, with one of these situations being frightening or alarming environmental situations. If the black individual is experiencing racism, then this may impact their emotional connections through a sense of powerlessness, hopelessness and despair. Where historical attachment figures have not met the individual's need for protection and emotional support, alternatives may be sought. Religion is likely to offer a secure attachment base, particularly when considering Bledsoe's need for a monotheistic model. Religious belief allows attachment to an attachment figure who is ever-present, and perceived as omnipotent, to provide a safe, comforting, reassuring and secure base. As Bowlby (1973) argued:

> When an individual is confident that an attachment figure will be available to him whenever he desires it, that person will be much less prone to either intense or chronic fear than will an individual who, for any reason, has no such confidence. (p. 202)

Attachment Theory is, however, not without its contradictions in offering a comfortable explanation for terrorism. Attachment Theory would predict that for individuals who achieve acceptance and can later form bonds with others, resolution would result in appropriate, more normalised, less angry, social and emotional connections being made. However, it is the deviant path provided by a radical, ideological mentor which appears to distort and inhibit the individual from normalising in their attachment development. In explaining why not all become radicalised, the answer may be that with those who do, there is a predisposition and willingness to respond with aggression and violence, with the voice of a radicalised mentor having more attraction than the voice of a moderate mentor. For example, Reid rejected the more moderate teaching of one ideological mentor. Thus, the radicalised mentor may serve to reinforce the prospective terrorist's historical predisposition to violence, with anger and aggression serving as a mediating factor in the bonding process through a sharing of maladaptive beliefs along with predetermined ways of interpreting and responding to others. Fonagy et al. (1997) argued the point that 'violence is a solution to psychological conflict because meta-cognitive capacity is limited and ideas and feelings are experienced in physical, often bodily terms' (p. 256). Greater consideration of the lived black experience is necessary from qualitative case study approaches to explore the different reality of vulnerable converts to Islam and their attachment styles, which may yield important predictive and explanatory information about those who are most vulnerable to radicalisation and acts of violence in 'lone wolf' actions.

References

Alonso, R., Björgo, T., DellaPorta, D., Coolsaet, R., Khosrokhavar, F., Lohelker, R., ... De Vries, G. (2008). Radicalisation processes leading to acts of terrorism. A concise report prepared by the European Commission's Expert Group on violent radicalisation. Submitted to the European Commission on 15 May 2008.

Bowlby, J. (1973). *Attachment and loss: Vol. 2. Separation: Anxiety and anger*. New York, NY: Basic Books.

Bowlby, J. (1982). *Attachment and loss: Vol. 1. Attachment*. New York, NY: Basic Books.

Brannan, D. W., Esler, P. F., & Strindberg, N. T. (2001). Talking to terrorists: Towards an independent analytic framework for the study of violent sub-state activism. *Studies in Conflict and Terrorism*, *24*, 3–24.

Crenshaw, M. (2011). *Explaining terrorism: Causes, process and consequences*. London: Routledge.

Daily Telegraph. (2001, December 30). Retrieved from www.telegraph.co.uk/news/uknews/1366666/from-tearaway-2-terrorist-thestory-of-richard-reid.html

Dalgaard-Nielsen, A. (2010). Violent radicalisation in Europe: What we know and what we do not know. *Studies in Conflict and Terrorism*, *33*(9), 797–814.

Della Porta, D., & LaFree, G. (2012). Guest editorial: 'Processes of radicalisation and de-radicalisation'. *International Journal of Conflict and Violence*, *6*(1), 4–10.

English, R. (2016). *Does terrorism work? A history*. London: Oxford University Press.

European Commission. (2008). Expert Group, Radicalisation processes leading to acts of terrorism: A concise report prepared by the European Commission's Expert Group on violent radicalisation. Submitted to the European Commission on 15 May 2008.

Fonagy, P., Target, M., Steele, M., Steele, H., Leigh, T., Levinson, A., & Kennedy, R. (1997). Morality, disruptive behaviour, borderline personality disorder, crime, and their relationship to security of attachment. In L. Atkinson & K. J. Zuker (Eds.), *Attachment and psychopathology* (pp. 223–276). New York, NY: Guilford Press.

Gartenstein-Ross, D. (2014). Lone Wolf Islamic terrorism: Abdulhakim Mujahid Muhammad (Carlos Bledsoe) case study. *Terrorism and Political Violence, 26*(1), 110–128.

Gartenstein-Ross, D., & Grossman, L. (2009). *Home grown terrorists in the US and the UK: An empirical examination of the radicalisation process.* Washington, DC: Foundation for the Defense of Democracy.

Gill, P., & Corner, E. (2017). Their and back again: The study of mental disorder and terrorist involvement. *American Psychologist, 72*(3), 231–241.

Gill, P., Horgan, J., & Deckert, P. (2013). Bombing alone: Tracing the motivations and antecedent behaviors of lone-actor terrorists. *Journal of Forensic Sciences, 59*(2), 425–435.

Greunewald, J., Chermak, S., & Freilich, J. D. (2013). Distinguishing loner attacks from other domestic extremist violence: A comparison of far right homicide incident and offender characteristics. *Criminology in Public Policy, 12*(1), 65–91.

Hewitt, C. (2003). *Understanding terrorism in America: From the Klan to al Qaeda.* London: Routledge.

Horgan, J. G. (2017). Psychology of terrorism: Introduction to the special issue. *American Psychologist, 72*(3), 199–204.

Huntington, S. P. (1996). *A clash of civilisations and the remaking of world order.* New York, NY: Touchstone.

Hurlow, J., Wilson, S., & James, D. V. (2016). Protesting loudly about prevent is popular but is it informed and sensible? *British Journal of Psychiatry Bulletin, 40,* 162–163.

Jenkins, B. M. (2010). *Would be warriors: Incidents of Jihadist terrorist radicalisation (in the United States) since September 11, 2001.* Santa Monica: Rand Corporation.

Krueger, A. B., & Maleckova, J. (2003). Education, poverty and terrorism: Is there a causal connection? *Journal of Economic Perspectives, 17*(4), 119–144.

Kruglanski, A. W. (2004). *The psychology of closed mindedness.* New York, NY: Psychology Press.

Lester, D., Yang, B., & Lindsay, M. (2008). Suicide bombers. Are psychological profiles possible? *Studies in Conflict and Terrorism, 27*(4), 283–295.

Liu, J. H., & Woodward, M. (2013). Towards an indigenous psychology of religious terrorism, with global implications: Introduction to AJSP Special Issue on Islamic terrorism in Indonesia. *Asian Journal of Social Psychology, 16*(2), 79–82.

Mazarr, M. J. (2004). The psychological sources of Islamic terrorism: Alienation and identity in the Arab world. *Policy Review, 125*(125), 39–60.

McCauley, C., & Moskalenko, S. (2011). *Friction: How radicalisation happens to them and us.* Oxford: Oxford University Press.

Meloy, J. R., & Yakeley, J. (2014). The violent true believer as a "lone wolf": Psychoanalytic perspectives on terrorism. *Behavioral Sciences and the Law, 32*(3), 347–365.

MI5. (2008, June 12). *Behavioural Science Unit operational briefing note: Understanding radicalisation and violent extremism in the UK.* Report No. BSU 02/008. MI5 Security Services, UK

Milla, M. N., & Faturochman, D. A. (2013). The impact of leader–follower interactions on the radicalisation of terrorists: A case study of the Bali bombers. *Asian Journal of Social Psychology, 16*(2), 92–100.

Moghaddam, F. F. (2008). *How globalisation spurs terrorism.* Westport, CT: Praeger Security International.

Moghaddam, F. M. (2006). *From the terrorists' point of view: What they experience and why they come to destroy.* Westport, CT: Praeger Security International.

Moghaddam, F. M. (2010). *The new global insecurity.* Santa Barbara, CA: Praeger Security International.

Moskalenko, S., & McCauley, C. (2009). Measuring political mobilisation: The distinction between activism and radicalism. *Terrorism and Political Violence, 21*, 239–260.

Mueller, J. (2012). *Terrorism since 9/11: The American cases*. Columbus, OH: Ohio State University.

Muluk, H., Sumaktoyo, N. G., & Ruth, D. M. (2013). Jihad as justification: National survey evidence of belief in violent jihad as a mediating factor for sacred violence among Muslims in Indonesia. *Asian Journal of Social Psychology, 16*(2), 101–111.

Pantucci, R. (2008). Britain's prison dilemma: Issues and concerns in Islamic radicalisation. *Terrorism Monitor, 6*(6), 628.

Pape, R. A., & Feldman, J. K. (2010). *Cutting the fuse: The exposure of verbal suicide and terrorism and how to stop it*. Chicago, IL: University of Chicago Press.

Pearlstein, R. M. (1991). *The mind of the political terrorist*. Wilmington: Scholarly Resources.

Post, J. M. (2010). When hatred is bred in the bone: The social psychology of terrorism. *Annals of New York, Academy of Sciences, 1208*, 15–23.

Reicher, S., Hopkins, N., Levine, M., & Rath, R. (2005). Entrepreneurs of hate and entrepreneurs of solidarity: Social identify as a basis for mass communication. *International Review of the Red Cross, 87*(860), 621–637.

Rogers, M. B., Loewenthal, K. M., Lewis, C. A., Amlott, R., Cinnirella, M., & Ansari, H. (2007). The role of religious fundamentalism in terrorist violence: The social psychological analysis. *International Review of Psychiatry, 19*(3), 253–262.

Schmid, A. P. (Ed.). (2011). *The Routledge handbook of terrorism research*. London: Routledge.

Schwartz, S. J., Dunkel, C. S., & Waterman, A. S. (2009). Terrorism: An identity theory perspective. *Studies in Conflict and Terrorism, 32*, 537–559.

Schwartz, S. J., Montgomery, M. J., & Briones, E. (2006). The role of identity in acculturation among immigrant people: Theoretical propositions, empirical questions and applied recommendations. *Human Development, 49*, 1–30.

Silber, M. D., & Bhatt, A. (2007). *Radicalisation in the West: The home grown threat*. City of New York Police Department. Retrieved from www.brennancentre.org

Simon, J. D. (2013). *Lone wolf terrorism*. Amherst, NY: Prometheus Books.

Spaaij, R. (2010). The enigma of lone wolf terrorism: an assessment. *Studies in Conflict & Terrorism, 33*, 854–870.

Spaaij, R. (2012). *Understanding lone wolf terrorism: Global patterns, motivations, and prevention*. New York, NY: Springer

Tajfel, H., & Turner, J. C. (1986). The social identity theory of intergroup behavior. In S. Worchel & W. G. Austin (Eds.), *The psychology of intergroup behavior* (pp. 7–24). Chicago, IL: Nelson Hall.

The Guardian. (2001, September). Retrieved from content.time.com/time/world/article0,8599203478-2,00.html

Victoroff, J. (2005). The mind of the terrorist: A review and critique of psychological approaches. *The Journal of Conflict Resolution, 49*, 3–42.

Wiktorowicz, Q. (2005). *Radical Islam rising: Muslim extremism in the west*. Oxford: Rowman & Littlefield.

Woodward, M., Amin, A., & Rohmaniyah, I. (2010). Muslim education, celebrating Islam and having fun as counter radicalisation stages in Indonesia. *Perspectives on Terrorism, 4*(4), 28–50.

Part V

Clinical Practice

Chapter 25

Spotlight on Sensory Processing Difficulties

Lisa Prior and Tiffany Howl

What Is Sensory Processing and Why Is It Important?

Sensory processing is the mechanism by which our bodies take in sensory messages (touch, taste, smell, sight, hearing and movement/balance) from our environment, organise, interpret and respond to them (Champagne, 2009). If we are lucky we are born with fully functioning sense organs: eyes, ears, nose, skin and tongues. Then our early experiences of sights, sounds, noises, smells, textures, movement, touch, temperatures and tastes help our immature nervous systems develop (Kutz, 2003). The inputs we receive are processed by our brains and help us decide on appropriate responses and to develop skills to include coordinated movements, awareness of our own body positions, good balance, language, visual perceptual skills and control over our bodies and emotions (Blyth, 2013). Williamson and Anzalone (1996, cited in Yack, Sutton and Aquilla, 2002) stipulate five steps for successfully processing sensory information:

1. Registration.
2. Orientation.
3. Interpretation.
4. Organisation of response.
5. Execution of response.

Example 1 of Sensory Processing Expected Response

Imagine you are eating an ice cream on a hot day and some drips down your hand. You may see and feel it drip (sensory registration), locate where on your body it is (orientation), make sense of what has happened (interpretation), think about how you will respond (organisation of response) then respond (execute) lick it, wipe it and wash your hands.

Example 2 of Under Responsive Sensory Processing

Imagine you are eating an ice cream on a hot day and some drips down your hand. You do not notice (underactive sensory registration, you don't orientate the sensation as it is not noticed). You do nothing (no interpretation or plans are made or response executed).

Example 3 of Over Responsive Sensory Processing

Imagine you are eating an ice cream on a hot day and some drips down your hand. The sensation is unbearable (overactive sensory registration). You can't locate where the unbearable sensation is on your body (difficulties with orientation). You don't know what caused this sensation or how to make it stop (sensation is aversive). You have no idea how to respond (difficulties organising an appropriate response). You respond unpredictably perhaps burst into tears, run off and hide, throw the ice cream and lash out at yourself or others. You may have a meltdown. You may feel angry, anxious and scared but you may not understand these emotions or be able to let others know. (You respond in fight and flight mode and ride it out until the sensation stops.) You may never want to eat ice cream again, go out in the sun again and so on and so on ....

Irrespective of culture in a young child whose neurological systems are immature, as parents and adults we would generally be quick to help the individual make sense of their difficulty. Perhaps saying to the child with under responsive sensory processing 'Your ice cream has dripped onto your hand, its cold and yucky, shall we wipe it off?' Or to the child with over responsive sensory processing 'Has your ice cream dripped on your hand? Is it cold and yucky? Shall we wipe it off?'

Yet in older individuals there is an expectation that they will learn to interpret and manage such difficulties themselves. Thus such responses are less likely to be put down to the 'neurological traffic jam' sensory processing disorder (Ayres, 2005) causes and more likely to be considered abnormal, oppositional or naughty behaviours (Rodd, 1996). In the context of African Caribbean families these behaviours may furthermore be seen as a mark of disrespect and as failings on behalf of the parents to persevere with discipline and teach appropriate behaviours (Beishon, Modood, & Virdee, 1998). Indeed in her experience with the African Caribbean Community Initiative in Wolverhampton, Howl found those accessing services were reluctant to do so, mistrusting mainstream National Health Service (NHS) services which they found to be euro centric (McKenzie, 1999) and even more reluctant to readily accept diagnoses or labels.

Sensory Processing Disorder (SPD)

Children are often measured in terms of age-related developmental norms for growth, abilities in everyday tasks, management of emotions, reasoning, academic achievement, social development and indeed sensory responsiveness

(Pathways, 2017). If an individual's nervous system is thought to be under or over responsive to any form of sensory input it can be understood as inadequately processing sensory information and the individual is referred to as having SPD (Kranowitz, 2005).

SPD it is a widely documented and diverse phenomenon (Tomchek & Dunn, 2007) and there was a recent unsuccessful application to have SPD as a standalone diagnosis within DSM-V. Zimmer and Desch (2012) currently hold a view that SPD is a collection of symptoms best understood as features within other diagnoses to include, Autistic Spectrum Disorders (ASD), Attention Deficit Hyperactivity Disorder (ADHD), Attention Deficit Disorder (ADD), developmental coordination disorders and childhood anxiety. Thus diagnosing SPD alone might mean other more complex presentations are not fully assessed (Zimmer and Desch, 2012). A further cause for debate is the fact that no two individuals with SPD are alike. It is usual for an individual to have some over, under and typical patterns of responsiveness when compared to peers (Dunn, 2001).

Sensory Integration

Ayres (2005) and her followers have documented in their practice that for decades individuals lack the ability to organise sensations for use. An ability she refers to as sensory integration. Ayres is known as the founder of Sensory Integration Theory and since its introduction to numerous networks and specialist training now exist for those professionals and individuals pursuing better understanding, treatments and management of SPD (Williams & Shellenberger, 2001; Sensory Integration Network, 2017; STAR Institute, 2017). Miller (2014) is among those driving forward the SPD agenda recognising in her practice the numbers of individuals whom would not meet criteria for alternate diagnoses but nevertheless experience significant difficulties which impact on their abilities to fulfil functional activities and roles, like accessing school and maintaining friendships due to SPD.

Whether you favour the caution of APA or advocate the Sensory Integration communities' beliefs that SPD should be given the standing of a separate diagnosis, with the implications of more funding for research, assessment, diagnosis and treatment, the debate goes on as the current time access to evidence-based treatment remains inequitable.

Occupational Therapists

As an occupational therapist, I understand mental and physical health as directly related to an individual's ability to successfully engage in their chosen roles and activities. When problems arise (alongside diagnostic screening) occupational therapists use activity analysis to break down tasks into the internal and external factors which might be causing the problem (Royal College of Occupational Therapists, 2017). As such in my experience SPD is a common feature in those young people who present at CAMHS and must be considered to avoid inappropriate diagnoses or treatment.

Example 4: SPD versus Social Anxiety

In the clinic, I came across a 15-year-old boy referred for cognitive behaviour therapy (CBT) for social anxiety. He had been attending an educational diversity setting and was managing well in the smaller environment. So school arranged for him to return for a visit to mainstream. On arriving at the school he experienced, racing heart and thoughts, a hot flush and uncharacteristic of his usual demeanour appeared to the support teacher in an agitated state and ran off and was missing for a few hours much to the distress of teachers and parents. It was assumed that he had experienced an anxiety attack brought on due to concern over the social situation he was about to access.

However, in formulating his own interpretation of the situation, with exploration of his history and thoughts about returning to mainstream, it became apparent that he was unconcerned about the social aspect of the visit. He had always preferred 1:1 friendships but was ambivalent about the opinions or judgements of his peers. He had however always hated crowds, struggling with the noise and movement and often found symptoms of fight and flight in these situations and reported feeling overwhelmed. By leaving the situation, he found the symptoms rapidly receded and indeed had not experienced these difficulties in the smaller school setting. As such an SPD assessment was completed and it was concluded in his case that rather than viewing the educational diversity setting as no longer needed as his anxiety appeared to have gone, he would benefit from remaining in the educational diversity setting in order to avoid becoming overwhelmed by the sensory demands of the busy mainstream school.

Sensory Profile

In the face of the complexity of SPD presentations, the ongoing controversy around its diagnosis and treatment and having limited time, training and resources to commit to its assessment, it would be easy to shy away. However, akin to many occupational therapists working in CAMHS, I have endeavoured to utilise: observational skills, developmental history taking, liaising with carers and schools, the sensory profile (Dunn, 2001) standardised assessment questionnaires and attended training in Alert Programme (Williams & Shellenberger, 2001) in order to screen for SPD, highlighting the triggering areas of difficulty to young people. Carers and teachers were able to suggest common-sense ideas to help compensate for and in some cases improve self-regulation skills in those with SPD presentations. However, I remain a strong advocate for referral on to a more comprehensive sensory integration therapy input where this is available.

Dunn (2001) created the sensory profile assessment tools, of which there are various versions to include the infant, caregiver, adolescent/adult and school companion measures. These standardised assessment questions describe behavioural responses to every day sensory events and the caregivers, teachers or individuals themselves score the frequency with which they engage in these behaviours. When scored it is possible to compare these behaviours to typically developing peers and indicates four patterns of behaviour:

1. Sensory seeking behaviours.
2. Sensation avoiding behaviours.
3. Sensory sensitivities.
4. Low registration.

These patterns are thought to relate to the individuals neurological thresholds and self-regulation strategies. Dunn (2001) proposes that individuals with strong processing patterns in each of these areas have unique patterns of nervous system needs and habituation, which impact on temperament and personality. Thus thinking back to Example 4, continuing with CBT for anxiety and expecting the young person to learn to habituate, through behavioural experimentation aimed to overcome his anxiety like state, may have been unrealistic and was more importantly not his goal. He preferred to avoid crowds and noisy environments as a personality choice, perhaps shaped in some part by his SPD. Thus in this case helping him and those around him understand the trigger for his difficulty and adapting his educational environment was a more acceptable intervention.

Self-regulation

The Alert Programme (Williams & Shellenberger, 2001) is designed to be used on a 1:1 or group basis in order to teach people to better understand and improve self-regulation of their arousal levels through use of sensory interventions and activities sometimes referred to as sensory diets. The programme is unique, in that it uses an analogy where people are asked to view their bodies like car engines that sometimes run on high (hyperactive), sometimes run low (lethargic) and sometimes run just right (alert and focussed). The programme acknowledges that everyone experiences these changes in engine speed. In fact, in the average day we may need to use all states for differing activities, such as needing our engines high when playing football, needing to be alert and focussed when in class writing and needing to be running lower when it is time to go to sleep. The full programme works through activities to help people notice the engine levels in themselves and others with help from adults, then alone. Then further teaches that five options can be experimented with in order to bring about changes in our engine levels.

1. Put something in the mouth.
2. Move.
3. Touch.
4. Look.
5. Listen.

Example 5: Alert Programme Strategies

It is all about trial and error and finding the right strategies and coming up with new ones if things stop working. However, we might predict that an individual who is struggling to wake in the morning may find eating breakfast (put something in the mouth) will help them wake. The same individual might be struggling towards the end of the first lesson to concentrate and be seen fidgeting, they might try moving (running around in the playground at break) and this activity might increase how alert they feel. Then after school they might have done homework and been out playing again and look hyperactive and feel they can't settle to sleep, so might try: touch look and listen (choosing to take a bath and listen to some slow calming music or visualisation script).

Helping people develop tools that work for them and recording the impact of trying different sensory interventions is really important in individuals with SPD. Think back to the ice cream examples, things that seem obvious to us may not be clear at all to those with SPD.

Sensory Modulation Programmes

Whilst the Alert principles apply to people of all ages the engine analogy in my experience appeals best to younger individuals. There are lots of other interventions out there with a growing evidence base such as Champagne's (2009) recent study, which advocated the use of sensory modulation programmes involving CBT, sensory processing screening, increased self-awareness, development and modulation of sensory diet and kits. These interventions help people learn how to increase alertness or grounding through sensory modulation and or environmental modification to support sensory processing needs. Champagne (2009) trailed these interventions to help individuals with Post-Traumatic Stress Disorder, depression and trauma histories whom she found to also have had SPD.

SPD and African Caribbean Community

There is little in the way of specific African Caribbean Community studies around prevalence of SPD. Mentions can be found in the context of ASD and ADHD (Waltz, 2011). Due to the continued controversy around SPD as a diagnosis, it is easy to see why this area of research evidence is currently sparse.

There are areas of good practice, such as the African Caribbean Community Initiative in Wolverhampton, which is set up in a community resource centre, away from medical centres, adopting a more relaxed approach providing a hot drink in a non-clinical setting and listening and responding to the clients wishes around anonymity. The resource centre's use of language in formulating difficulties (e.g. using the wording 'low in spirits' rather than 'depressed') adopts respect for client beliefs around the roles of religion and spirituality in healing (Rabiee & Smith, 2014).

Drawing on Howl's experiences of how best to approach mental health difficulties with this community, and in the absence of robust research guidance or consistent treatment for SPD, the remainder of this chapter will provide experiential-based advice for use by clinicians working with those with SPD. It is not exhaustive but is provided to help clinicians identify behaviours that may indicate SPD, how SPD difficulties might be simply explained and basic ideas around what might help.

Behaviours That Might Indicate SPD

Although indicators are common with other diagnoses, it is useful to consider behaviours that may indicate an underlying SPD and sensory approaches in managing these behaviours. Individuals with SPD are sometimes identified through recurrent unwanted behaviours, avoidance of crowds, struggling to cope with change, struggling to organise self, fussy eating, unexplained meltdowns and temper tantrums, unusually high or low activity levels, emotional dysregulation – difficulty in regulating and recognising emotions in self and others, crying easily, being over or under affectionate or over or under sensitivity to touch, sights, sounds, smells, tastes or movement (Table 1).

Table 1. Indicators of SPD.

Sensory Input	Over Responsive Sensory Processing	Under Responsive Sensory Processing
Touch	Avoid hugs, aversion to labels, scratchy fabrics or wearing clothes in general, react negatively to even light touch or lashes out when nudged such as in ques by peers. May sit stiffly and unusually still. Avoids messy play. Dislikes splashing water on skin or feel of sand, grass beneath toes. Avoid certain textures of food. Dislike having hair brushed or cut, dislike water on face, dislike, toothbrush, gags when using cutlery	May not cry when hurt. May seek tight hugs. May prefer tight clothing or crave certain fabrics. Play too rough with others. Not know their own strength. Not notice dirt on skin, need prompting with personal hygiene. Constantly fidgeting or touching things and people. Loves splashing water on skin or feel of sand, grass under toes
Taste	'Fussy-eaters', may avoid strong and unknown flavours and have a few preferred foods. Gags on certain textures and cutlery in mouth. Dislike toothpaste	Eat strong tasting, hot or spicy foods without a problem. Chewing clothes, mouth none food items and biting nails
Smell	Dislike strong smelling foods, washing powders and perfumes, notice smells before others and feel nausea due to them	Wear lots of spray, enjoy strong smelling perfumes, not notice or be bothered by strong odours

Table 1. Continued.

Sensory Input	Over Responsive Sensory Processing	Under Responsive Sensory Processing
Sound	May loud noises overwhelming, can be seen holding hands over ears or avoiding crowds, may struggle to hear instructions or name being called when there are competing sounds such as in classrooms, may complain of people or teachers shouting when they deny this. Easily startled by loud and unpredictable noises	May prefer loud music, may not respond to name being called or not hear instructions. May make own sounds to get feedback
Sight	May struggle to find things or people in busy environments, may keep things ordered to cope with this difficulty, may be easily distracted by visual stimuli in their environments. May complain lights are too bright and cover eyes	May have a tendency to miss visual clues, difficulty finding things, people in busy environments, get lost easily, miss direction signs, not notice when others are upset or angry. May stare at things or people intensely
Movement/ balance	May avoid excessive movement, dislike bouncing, feet being off the ground, play equipment, car journeys, struggle to master balance-related activities such as riding a bike. May seem lethargic	May be hyperactive, seek out movement of all kinds, twirls, spins, rocks, tendency to struggle to sit still, may be seen rocking on chair, drumming fingers, climbing. Loves heavy work tasks pulling, pushing, and bouncing where there is lots of feedback from movement activity. Seeks movement. Bumps into things. Poor coordination. Prop self on objects

Explaining SPD to Young People, Parents and Teachers

How our bodies interpret sensory input that varies from person to person. In fact, we all have sensory preferences but for some people these preferences are the result of heightened or lowered sensitivities and result in them not being able to function in their everyday tasks, environments and roles. In practice, I never cease to be surprised by the impact of showing an interest in atypical age-related behavioural responses to sensory stimuli. Then being able to offer possible explanations for these behaviours in terms of under and over responsiveness patterns and helping individuals come up with common-sense ideas to manage these experiences (Table 2).

Table 2. Ways to Explain SPD to Others.

Sensory input	Over Responsive Sensory Processing	Under Responsive Sensory Processing
Touch	Imagine the slightest tap on the shoulder feels like someone poking you with a sharp pencil this is how it can feel for someone overly sensitive to touch	Imagine a hard poke in the arm, to get your attention, feels as soft as a feather touch this is how it can feel for someone under sensitive to touch
Taste	Imagine someone replaced your glass of water with fresh squeezed lemon juice this is how intense things can taste for someone overly sensitive to taste	Imagine someone replaced the lemon in your lemonade with water this is how it can taste for someone under sensitive to taste
Smell	Imagine you washed your clothes with fresh cut onions, when you open your wardrobe and put them on your nose and throat might itch and your eyes might water. This is how strong fragrances can impact on someone overly sensitive to smells	Imagine your body spray was replace with water, you may spray it lots and still not smell anything whilst others are overpowered by the scent. This is how it can be for people under sensitive to smells
Sound	Imagine you turn on the radio and its stuck on full volume, you cover your ears with your hands whilst you dash around heart racing trying to find the remote to turn down the volume, whilst you friend tries to tell you something, you can't hear them and when you find the remote you turn it off and calm down and ask the friend to stop shouting. This is how crowds, the playground and even the average classroom can feel for people over sensitive to sound	Imagine you turn on the radio but hear nothing, you turn it up higher and higher but can barely hear it and when you finally get fed up of trying to hear it you turn it off and notice your friend stood next to you complaining you have been ignoring them. This is how it can be for someone under sensitive to sound

Table 2. Continued.

Sensory input	Over Responsive Sensory Processing	Under Responsive Sensory Processing
Sight	Imagine you are in a busy crowded subway station, people and trains are coming and going, the lights are blinding, there are numerous signs and screens everyone seems to be moving in fast forward and the screens are changing rapidly with information. You are trying to find your way, buy a ticket and get on the right train but you can't seem to see the things you need. This is what it can feel like for someone overly sensitive to sights when, for example, trying to get on with their work in a classroom	Imagine you are in a busy subway station and are aware of the people, trains, movements and know you need to buy a ticket and get on a train but the lights are turned down and try as you might you can't orientate yourself or see the information you need. This is how it can be for someone under sensitive to visual stimuli
Movement/ balance	Imagine the car journey to school feels like a roller coaster ride. This is how it can be for someone over sensitive to movement	Imagine you have lots of energy and are struggling to feel the chair or notice the position of your limbs. Before you know it you are rocking on the back too legs and in trouble again with the teacher. This is how it can be for someone under sensitive to movement

What Can We Do Try To Help?

No two people's sensory sensitivities are exactly the same but signposting them to sources of further information or Occupational and where available Sensory Integration Therapists is highly recommended. Where that is not possible or individuals do not wish to access such services do not be afraid to adopt a problem solving approach perhaps using the Alert Programme (Williams & Shellenberger, 2001) resources and engine analogy to help them self-regulate their arousal levels. Other recommendations that might help are presented in Table 3.

Spotlight on Sensory Processing Difficulties 499

Table 3. Strategies to Try.

Sensory Input	Over Sensitive Suggestions	Under Sensitive Suggestions
Touch	Ask and prepare them before touching them such as having hair brushed or cut. Soft hairbrushes and scissor cuts over clippers. Cut out scratchy labels in clothes, consider letting them try on fabrics for clothes and socks. Think about soft natural sponges for bath time, letting them wear goggles or wash hair with a jug of water over the sink or in baths rather than showers. Consider experimenting with use of brushed cotton sheets for bedtime. Soft bristle toothbrushes. Let them stand at the back of ques and crowds where possible. Be mindful of food textures and experiment together with different textures touching with hands and feeling them in their mouths. Allow avoidance of certain textures of food if still good range. Try soft cutlery, textured pen and pencil holders	May like firm touch and hugs. May prefer cloths to be tight. May settle to sleep better with heavy blankets tucked in tight. May need to be prompted not to play too rough and practice using graded strength tasks. May benefit from prompts to wash when messy
Taste	Encourage them to experiment testing new foods in raw, cooked, and mashed forms where appropriate to try and widen choices of food. Where practical they may prefer to have food separate on plate. Try to involve in shopping, food handling and preparation as there can be a tendency to avoid a whole food group just from one overwhelming food experiment. Remind them that taste buds change overtime and so encourage them to experiment again from time to time	They tend to eat a good variety, general encouragement to them to eat a balanced diet and not add too much sugar or salt. May have a tendency to eat rapidly and large amounts. Practice slowing down eating. Serve food items one at a time. Get then to try mindful eating spending time to look at, smell, feel and taste food

Table 3. Continued.

Sensory Input	Over Sensitive Suggestions	Under Sensitive Suggestions
Smell	Consider washing products with little or natural scents. Let them come along and smell things when shopping and those in close proximity may want to give more personal space or limit use of strong scents where practical. Opening or closing windows can help limit odours. If they find one particular scent soothing carrying a tissue or item smelling of this around that be helpful	Are generally not bothered by strong odours but might need encouragement to shower or air sweaty trainers or bedrooms. Might benefit from use of roll on deodorants so the sensation on the skin may be detected where the scent is not
Sound	May benefit from use of ear defenders or shutting doors and windows and turning off tv's and radios to reduce sound stimuli when trying to concentrate. Others concentrate better with earphones with white noise or predictable sounds in order to block out distracting unpredictable sounds and reduce becoming startled by sudden loud noises which can make them feel overwhelmed such as in class or shopping. May prefer to access quieter activities away from crowds and, for example, loud music. May benefit from sitting away from sources of noise such as away from speakers, doors and windows in class and furthest from the tv at home. Encourage them to let people know politely if they are speaking to fast or loud and ask to be given instruction one at a time or even written instructions. Adults should get the individual to repeat back instructions to check the message has been received. Some individuals with this difficulty benefit from smaller classes or small group working opportunities	May benefit from use of earphones and rhythmic music to get stimulated to work. People should try to make eye contact before giving verbal instructions and ask that they repeat these instructions back to ensure they have been heard. May need prompts to stay on task and benefit from smaller class settings and paired working

Sensory Input	Over Sensitive Suggestions	Under Sensitive Suggestions
Sight	May benefit from things being placed in the same place after use and tidy surroundings. May benefit from lower lights such as lamps instead of overhead lighting. May benefit from provision of written instructions and sitting in good line of sight with the board in class. May need prompts with directions and in locating things. May benefit from smaller school settings	May benefit from prompts, working on computers which provide adequate stimuli to keep them on task and smaller class room settings with reduced distracting visual stimuli
Movement/ balance	May benefit from opportunities to experiment with less demanding physical activities like walking. May struggle in PE and benefit from small groups for these activities. May benefit from referral to paediatric occupational therapists to explore movement activities in a graded manner. May be better in cars than on school buses. May benefit from treatment for travel sickness	Generally love and seek out all movement activities and PE. May be thrill seekers. Movement activities and heavy work tasks such as carrying, pushing and tug of war activities can help give the input they seek. Allowing use of balance cushions, fidget toys and such may help them stay seated and concentrate to get on with work

Conclusion

When we reflect on common interpretations of SPD-related behaviours, without raised awareness of this condition, individuals may remain misunderstood, struggle in educational environments and in their relationships with peers, parents and their communities. There are implications for delivery of mental health interventions in terms of the role SPD has as a feature of other presentations (ADHD, ADD, ASD and anxiety) and as a coexisting difficulty for many individuals. Whilst the assessment and treatment of SPD remains lacking in many areas and robust research evidence around SPD and prevalence in African Caribbean communities is needed in the future, we as clinicians can do our part to raise awareness of this difficulty and its implications on delivery of existing evidence-based practice modalities such as CBT. Do not be afraid to be curious about behaviours that might indicate SPD and talk to families about it and then encourage them to experiment for themselves with ways of managing these difficulties. They may have been using these strategies for years without understanding why they needed them. Being curious together and passing the problem solving over to the families and teachers is always an empowering experience.

References

Ayres, J. (2005). *Sensory integration and the child. Understanding hidden sensory challenges.* Torrance, CA: Western Psychological Services.

Beishon, S., Modood, T., & Virdee, S. (1998). *Ethnic minority families.* London: Policy Studies Institute.

Blyth, S. (2013). *Enable me programme.* Chichester: Therapy for Independence Group.

Champagne, T. (2009). *The influence of posttraumatic stress disorder, depression and sensory processing patterns on occupational engagement: A case study.* Amsterdam: IOS Press.

Dunn, W. (2001). The sensations of everyday life: Empirical, theoretical and pragmatic considerations. The 2001 Eleanor Clarke Slagel Lecture. *American Journal of Occupational Therapy, 55*, 608–620.

Kranowitz, C. (2005). *Introduction to the out-of-sync child: Recognizing and coping with sensory processing disorder* (2nd ed.). New York, NY: Perigee Books.

Kutz, L. (2003). *How to help a clumsy child: Strategies for young children with developmental motor concerns.* London: Jessica Kingsley Publishers.

McKenzie, K. (1999). Something borrowed from the blues. *BMJ, 318*, 616.

Miller, L. (2014). Identification of SPD. *Star Institute Quebec.* Retrieved from https://www.spdstar.org/basic/identification-of-spd

Pathways. (2017). *All developmental milestones.* Chicago Pathways Org. Retrieved from https://pathways.org/topics-of-development/milestones/

Rabiee, F., & Smith, P. (2014). Understanding mental health and experience of accessing services among African and African Caribbean service users and carers in Birmingham, UK. *Diversity and Equality in Health Care, 11*(2), 125–134.

Rodd, J. (1996). *Understanding young children's behaviour: A guide for early childhood.* Crows Nest: Allen & Urwin.

Royal College of Occupational Therapists. (2017). *Occupational therapy terminology. Supporting occupation centred practice.* London: Royal College of Occupational Therapists.

Sensory Integration Network. (2017). Ayres' sensory integration therapy. Retrieved from https://www.sensoryintegration.org.uk/
STAR Institute. (2017). What does treatment for SPD look like? Retrieved from https://www.spdstar.org/
Tomchek, S., & Dunn, W. (2007). Sensory processing in children with and without Autism: A comparative study using the short sensory profile. *American Journal of Occupational Therapy*, *61*, 190–200.
Waltz, M. (2011). Identifying Autism in children from ethnic minorities. Retrieved from http://www.communitycare.co.uk/2011/02/24/identifying-autism-in-children-from-ethnic-minorities/
Yack, E., Sutton, S., & Aquilla, P. (2002). *Building bridges through Sensory integration: Therapy for children with Autism and other Pervasive Developmental Disorders* (p. 22). Arlington, TX: Future Horizons.
Zimmer, M., & Desch, L. (2012). Sensory Integration Therapies for Children With Developmental and Behavioral Disorders. *Pediatrics*, *129*(6), 1186–1189. doi:10.1542/peds.2012-0876.

Bibliography

Ayres, J. (2017). Ayres sensory integration therapy. Retrieved from https://www.sensoryintegration.org.uk/What-is-SI
Bharadwaj, S. V., Daniel, L. L., & Matzke, P. L. (2009). Sensory-processing disorder in children with cochlear implants. *The American Journal of Occupational Therapy*, *63*(2), 208–213. Retrieved from https://search.proquest.com/docview/231968891?accountid=48180
Brout, J., & Miller, L. (2015). DSM-V application for sensory processing disorder (Appendix A). Retrieved from https://www.researchgate.net/project/DSM-5-SPD-Proposal
Dunn, W. (1999). *Sensory profile: User manual*. Harcourt Assessment.
Gavin, W. J., Dotseth, A., Roush, K. K., Smith, C. A., Spain, H. D., & Davies, P. L. (2011). Electroencephalography in children with and without sensory processing disorders during auditory perception. *The American Journal of Occupational Therapy*, *65*(4), 370–377. Retrieved from https://search.proquest.com/docview/875961564?accountid=48180
Wallis, C. (2007). Is this disorder for real? *Time*, *170*(24), 62–66.
Williams, M. S., & Shellenberger, S. (1996). How does your engine run? *A leader's guide to the alert program for self-regulation*. Albuquerque, NM: Therapyworks Inc.
Williams, M. S., & Shellenberger, S. (2001). *The Alert Program. Self-regulation made easy*. Albuquerque, NM: Therapy Works Inc. Retrieved from https://www.alertprogram.com/new-to-alert-program/

Chapter 26

Forced Marriage as a Representation of a Belief System in the UK and its Psychological Impact on Well-being

Doreen Robinson and Reenee Singh

Introduction

South Asian people originate from the Indian subcontinent and include Hindus, Muslims, and Sikhs. (In the US, the term "Asian" may also mean people of Chinese or Filipino origin.) Following Indian independence from the British in 1949, many South Asians emigrated from Bihar, Northern India to the Caribbean islands of Grenada (Sookram, 2009), Jamaica, Trinidad, and Guyana, known as the West Indies, as well as to the US, Canada, the UK, and South Africa. However, prior to 1949, many South Asians went to the Caribbean as part of indentured service to work on the sugar plantations after the emancipation of African slaves on August 1, 1838. In Grenada, they arrived between 1857 and 1885 (Sookram, 2009).

The United States Census (2010) reported that the Asian Indian population grew from 0.6% of the US population in 2000 to 0.9% in 2010. In the UK, the 2011 Census recorded 2.3% of the total population as Indian; the 2001 Census figure was 1.8%. South Asians emigrated from Punjab, Gujarat, Pakistan, Bangladesh, and Sri Lanka due to civil unrest following partition into Muslim and Hindu states after Indian independence. In the 1970s, South Asians who had settled in Uganda were expelled by President Idi Amin on the grounds of their ethnicity and economic success. They moved to the UK. Many South Asians emigrated to the UK as British Commonwealth citizens, in the same way that many African-Caribbeans emigrated to the UK at its request to help reconstruct the country following the Second World War in the 1940s and 1950s.

The South Asians and African-Caribbeans have established communities which have transitioned between assimilation and integration into the UK culture throughout the communities' history of emigration. In the UK in the mid-1980s:

> The terms class, race and sex have broadened to include culture, faith and gender, wherein lay the opportunity to consider poverty and economic difference. (Robinson, 2008, p. 35)

For African, black African, and South Asian communities, there exists a hierarchy of a class or caste system, based upon economic status and physical appearance. Colonization, slavery, and plantocracy societies have constructed and reinforced inequalities based upon difference in wealth and skin color. In India, the Dalits are the "Untouchables" caste, who perform menial outdoor tasks and whose skin becomes darkened by the sun. They are placed at the bottom of society in a similar way to black African slaves. Darker-skinned people are not accorded status of intelligence and desirability.

In the Caribbean, an ethnic group was created through plantocracy, which elevated mixed-race or biracial people (known as Creoles), with usually a white father. They were the administrators of the plantation system. In India, Anglo Indians were a similar administrative group of civil servants under British rule before independence.

Thus a hierarchy based upon skin color, class, and caste was reinforced which to this day has a strong influence.

Structure of This Chapter

In this chapter, we will describe the belief system of Izzat, which is central among South Asian families. The idea of forced marriage is based upon the concept of Izzat, or honor, which is a cornerstone of family life in South Asian communities.

Thiara and Breslin (2006) suggest that South Asian community members are deeply affected by what others say about them. The closest English translations to Izzat and Sharam are honor and shame, respectively. The authors argue that Izzat and Sharam are mechanisms that safeguard patriarchal customs, such as arranged marriage, which are familiar to us from our backgrounds as two Asian women. It is our belief that Izzat is the highest "context marker" (Pearce & Cronen, 1980) for forced marriages.

We will illustrate the concept of Izzat through two vignettes and explicate theoretical ideas, based on Izzat, to include Boszormenyi-Nagy's ideas about belief systems.

Research by Ryan Brown (2016) at the University of Oklahoma on "honor cultures" in the US draws some parallels in gendered discourses about the power of men over women. He suggests that high levels of murder rates as well as reluctance to address mental health issues are present in honor cultures. These ideas resonate with the strong influence of Izzat upon South Asian family and community systems, which we have met in our practice. The development of our practice was in response to issues arising from our clinical work in these communities (Robinson, 2016).

We will explore the continuum of marriage to include forced, arranged, and consensual marriage within the context of Izzat.

We will also consider issues of cultural competence and expertness and how these interplay with strongly held belief systems such as Izzat. We will end with some clinical implications and pointers for practice.

Honor

Narratives in films, and particularly Asian films, can deliver subliminal messages on themes of life including struggles between good and bad, falling in love, searching for happiness, and avenging wrongdoing.

Recently, I (DR) saw a thought-provoking film called *Honour* (Khan, 2014). A scene from the film shows a young Muslim woman talking to her younger brother at his workplace. Set in the UK, *Honour* is the story of a young Muslim woman who was felt to have brought dishonor, Sharam, to her family name by having a relationship with a Muslim man from a different caste or class, with whom she planned to elope. In order to maintain the family honor, the young woman's boyfriend was frightened off by her mother and brothers. The mother then hired a bounty hunter (from an extremist white supremacy group) to kill the daughter. Fortunately, she managed to escape and keep her life.

Izzat and Sharam

The film put me in mind of the clinical issues and the concepts of Izzat and Sharam that we, as two South Asian family systemic psychotherapists, work with in a London Child and Adolescent Mental Health Service (CAMHS) team.

Gangoli, Razak, and McCarry (2006) suggest that South Asian community members are deeply affected by what others in their communities say about them. The closest English translations to Izzat and Sharam are honor and shame, respectively (Gangoli et al., 2006). There is also an argument that Izzat and Sharam are mechanisms that safeguard patriarchal customs such as arranged marriage which are familiar to us from our backgrounds as two Asian women. It is our belief that Izzat is the highest "context marker" (Pearce & Cronen, 1980) for forced marriages, by which we mean that communities in which forced marriages take place are so intent on protecting family honor that they do not consider the young person's happiness.

Research on "honor cultures" in the US by Ryan Brown (2016) of the University of Oklahoma draws some parallels in gendered discourses about power of men over women. Brown suggests that high levels of murder rates as well as reluctance to address mental health issues are present in honor cultures.

The beliefs of Izzat and Sharam (written about by authors such as Gangoli et al., 2006; Gardner, 1995; Lau, 1995; Krause, 1995, 1998, 2012; and Malik & Krause, 2005) were also culturally familiar to us. However, in our clinical practice, we experienced a growing awareness of the dilemma between arranged (culturally normative) and forced marriages for women and the impact upon the children with whom we worked.

Belief Systems Within South Asian Families

Another idea that we draw on in our work is that of belief systems. A belief system as described by Boszormenyi-Nagy (Boszormenyi-Nagy & Framo, 1965) is a framework of philosophy and established codes of thought which shapes belief and action. Boszormenyi-Nagy used the term "legacy" to explain "indebtedness" with families:

> The roots of the individual's very existence become a source of systemic legacies that affect his or her personal entitlements and indebtedness. The origins are multigenerational; there is a chain of destiny anchored in every generative relationship. (Boszormenyi-Nagy, Grunebaum, & Ulrich, 1991, p. 163)

Systemic psychotherapy holds at its core the principle of how belief and behavior are recursively related. Belief systems are born from societal codes such as Izzat.

An external representation is maintained which places Izzat at the highest context. There can be a struggle to maintain the external expectation of adhering to Izzat within the South Asian culture.

The effort to hold on to this belief system at all costs can create huge pressure and create a double bind for women who go into a marriage which is forced or coerced but adhere to the idea that it has been mutually arranged. For a woman to draw attention to the pressure and abuse she is experiencing would bring Sharam upon the marriage and family. A breakdown of the marriage would also bring Sharam. The concept of Izzat would demand that marriage is to be maintained at all costs and this can often result in women and their children being severely emotionally and physically abused. We believe that the expression of this belief system at its most rigid allows for forced marriage.

This belief system of Izzat is not unique to South Asian families. For example, Greek and Middle Eastern communities arriving in Australia between the 1950s and the 1980s had similar familial experiences. We are also aware of the same for Gypsy and Traveler communities across Europe. We can see how the understanding of Izzat as explained here can be seen in other cultural groups across the UK, the US, Canada, Africa, Australia, Europe, and the Caribbean. Muslim and Hindu communities in Guyana, South America adhere strictly to the concept of Izzat. Marriage between Africans and Asians within the Caribbean can create huge conflict on both sides if the implicit rule of "marrying out," that is marrying out of class, caste, culture, is broken. Such transgression can lead to disownment or "putting out," that is ostracization of the person (usually a woman) from their community.

We see this as a manifestation of Izzat, where the unspoken code of behavior is broken, Izzat is not adhered to, and Sharam is brought upon both families of different cultures and classes.

Marrying out of caste or tribe for Africans also contravenes Izzat. An example of this is between the Yoruba and Igbo peoples in southern Nigeria. There is a political and economic context to how, in northern Nigeria, economic developments required peaceful communications, and many interethnic and interfaith marriages took place pre-1990. However, in southern Nigeria, Yoruba–Igbo marriages were far less common and marriages were subject to ethnic endogamy; that is, limitation of marriage to members within one group, community, or tribe.

For example, I (RS) am working with an orthodox Jewish family, where family relationships were disrupted because one of the adult sons married a Catholic woman. He chose to get married on the Sabbath (Saturday), which his father and father's families observed strictly as a religious day.

The belief system of Izzat can help clinicians use a theoretical framework from which to approach familial situations which can appear to be intractable. Boszormenyi-Nagy et al.'s (1991) idea about legacy and indebtedness fits very closely to Izzat, which requires maintaining certain codes of behavior with unspoken but clearly understood boundaries and taboos.

Clinical Practice

Our clinical experience of working with children in South Asian communities involved behavioral problems among the children and difficulties regarding parenting of children (Robinson, 2016). There were also high levels of depression among the mothers, self-harm among mothers and daughters, and suicidal ideation for girls and young women.

They seemed to experience higher levels of stress and domestic violence than other communities with whom we worked, and the situations seemed intractable as the mothers felt they would bring Sharam upon their families should they leave their marriages.

Sanghera's Sanghera (2007) work describes such situations and has been helpful to us in understanding how Izzat organizes a family system.

There was a connection between the experiences of the families we worked with and her description of her own family.

Sanghera's experiences, which she has described eloquently in her books (Sanghera, 2007, 2009, 2011), led us to consider how there can be a continuum of marriage among certain communities, including South Asian communities, where forced marriages are represented at one end of the continuum, arranged marriages are in the middle, and love marriages are at the other end. Considering the notion of forced marriage, on a continuum, Gangoli talks about "slippage" (Gangoli et al., 2006, p. 10) between arranged and forced marriage. Slippage is when a marriage can be described as consensual but coercion moves it into a forced marriage.

It is also helpful to consider the dilemmas of the South Asian families with whom we worked in their adherence to Izzat, how this positioned them with regard to how marriages were made, and the resulting effects upon their children. We became curious about how Izzat and Sharam intersected with the continuum of marriage. We began to see through our clinical work how forced marriage had become a representation of a belief system.

We present two vignettes to illustrate how clinicians can work with these beliefs and practices.

Vignette 1

Nadira and Raj had married across faiths – she was Muslim, he was Hindu. Raj became violent toward Nadira, and due to their love marriage (with three children, Mandeep, Mona, and Meera), which was outside of their family conventions, they were unsupported by both of their families (see Fig. 1)

Nadira became clinically depressed. Their daughter, Mandeep, disclosed sexual abuse from her father. At this point, Nadira took her children, left Raj and instigated divorce proceedings, and sought family therapy.

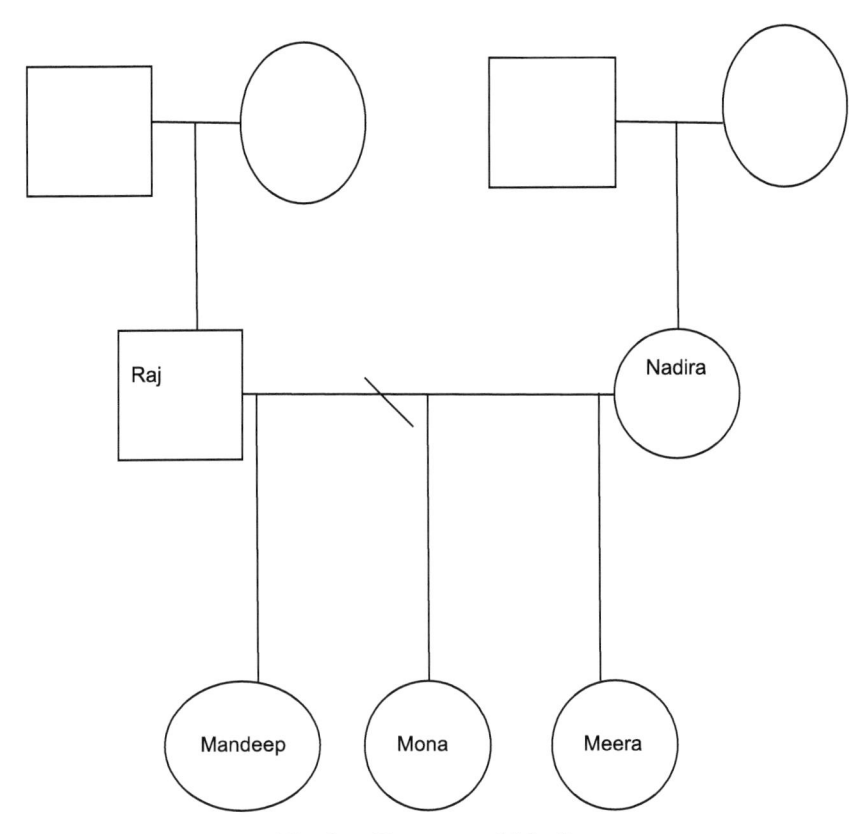

Fig. 1. Genogram 1 Nadira.

Nadira felt that she had broken Izzat by having a love marriage, which meant that she could not seek help from her family when the marriage broke down. Nevertheless, over time she regained contact with her family and she and the children were welcomed back.

Process of the Work

I (DR) began with a family session to include Nadira and her children. It soon became very clear that Mandeep, who had disclosed the sexual abuse, was extremely angry with her mother, partly because she had remained with Raj through a violent marriage. She was also confused and hurt about the sexual abuse. At first, Nadira found it difficult to engage in the sessions with her children. We agreed to have two or three individual sessions for Mandeep and also some sibling sessions alongside individual sessions for Nadira.

I conducted the individual sessions and a male colleague joined me for the sibling and subsequent family sessions. This enabled us to focus upon each child's needs and expressions of feelings regarding the abuse and the father's absence from the family. My female colleagues and I deliberated at length about a male colleague joining me in the work. We were sensitive to the impact upon the family, and especially Mandeep. However, we found that this allowed us to explore issues of gender, power, and control, and for the family to have a different experience of a male person within the system. It emerged from the sibling sessions that Meera had a learning disability, and we encouraged Nadira to find and use the appropriate resources for her.

My sessions with Nadira helped her to understand how depression had insulated her from fully meeting her children's needs. After three sessions, we were able to focus upon the development of the relationships with her children. The children became more responsive to Nadira's more playful side when we used play techniques as a way to enhance communication between them. Mona, who had been quieter than the others, found her voice and often suggested activities for them to complete as a family, which were supported by an increasingly confident Meera. The children became curious about Nadira's younger self at the ages of Mandeep, Mona, and Meera. I was able to move position myself to join each child in their curiosity about their mother when she was their own age. I then moved to position myself alongside Nadira in her curiosity about herself when she was the age of each of her children. This helped her to connect to aspects of her past life as well as to relationships which she could renew.

This curiosity opened up conversations about Nadira's family of origin (who lived elsewhere in the UK) and Nadira's relationships with them. This seemed to be a turning point for the children as they could appreciate Nadira differently than the abused and depressed person they had known in the recent past, and could feel confident in her ability to create a more positive future. Contact with Raj had been reconsidered but none of the children wished to have contact. Raj did not contest this.

During individual sessions with me, Nadira talked about her childhood, emerging sexuality, and parental expectations of her regarding marriage. As a

South Asian woman, I connected with her about the strong expectations upon us as young women to ensure Izzat by safeguarding our own and our family's reputations by not inviting Sharam in our behaviors. Nadira met and fell in love with Raj, who was Hindu and completely outside of her family's culture. She felt strongly enough about their love for each other to position herself away from her family and to break Izzat. This was both a brave and a lonely position to maintain, especially when violence entered the marriage and Mandeep was abused. By choosing to have a love marriage, Nadira positioned herself outside of her family and community. This had the effect of isolation and no supporting resource in the face of abuse. Nadira's belief that she had broken Izzat led her to feel that she was responsible for bad things happening to her, and what began as a consensual love marriage became a coercive marriage due to Raj's violence toward Nadira.

Raj may have felt able to move to an abusive position himself in the context of a love marriage which had positioned Nadira outside of the protection of her family. This also initially prevented her from seeking help for herself, but she did so when Mandeep was abused.

Mandeep regained her status as the valued older sibling and highly regarded daughter, and the family began to take on a new identity as a single-parent family with abuse in its past.

Family sessions had the children at the focal point to think about the narrative of hurt and distrust. It is possible that these narratives were present in the parents' own families, which may have led them to choose a love marriage. The impact upon the children was isolation from protective extended family members and blame for parental conflict. The therapy helped the children to understand that the responsibility for Mandeep's abuse was her father's. Nadira intensified her role as the protective and loving parent, and she renewed relationships with her estranged family. They, in turn, became substantial emotional and practical supports, which helped Nadira take up her position as a single parent.

Faced with the complexities presented in the above vignette, we were curious about the fit between belief systems, the families' and our own, and how we and the families could be positioned differently. It seems important at this point to consider theoretical ideas we draw upon as well as beliefs held within South Asian cultures. We will explicate the ideas we drew on after discussing the next vignette.

Vignette 2

Kavitha and her family, who were from a Sikh background, were referred to the CAMHS by Children and Family Court Advisory and Support Service (CAFCASS) for an intractable contact dispute. Kavitha had been married to Kulwinder for 15 years. Although Kavitha described her marriage as one that was arranged by her parents, as the marriage progressed, elements of coercion emerged. This is consistent with other cases in our experience, where the boundaries between arranged and forced marriage can sometimes be blurred (Gangoli et al., 2006, p. 10).

The couple had three daughters together. Kavitha had conceived only one male child, who had died of a congenital heart condition when he was a few months old (see Fig. 2).

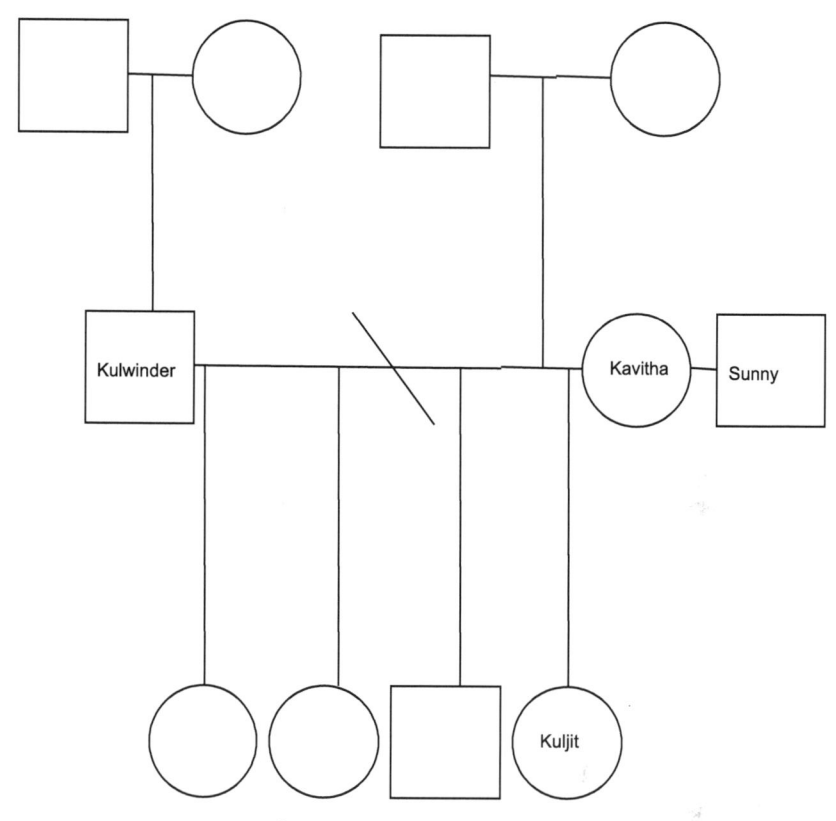

Fig. 2. Genogram Kavitha.

Kavitha and Kulwinder lived in her in-laws' home with their daughters. Following the death of their son, things began to deteriorate between Kavitha and her husband's family. They accused her of having an affair and being physically abusive toward her daughters.

One day, Kavitha came home to find that the locks on the front door had been changed and her possessions were lying outside. She was asked to leave for bringing Bezti (dishonor) to the family. Her two older daughters refused to have contact with her. Although she was allowed contact with Kuljit, the youngest, Kuljit would not allow her mother to hug her and was forced by her grandmother to wash her face and change her clothes as soon as she returned home from contact visits with her mother.

Soon after Kavitha was asked to leave the house, Kulwinder instigated divorce proceedings and his parents found him a new bride. The two older girls referred to her as "Mum" and used derogatory words when they spoke about Kavitha.

In this patriarchal family, the grandparents claimed that Kavitha was having an affair, but she was sure that her inability to bear a son, a male heir, was the reason why she was thrown out of her husband's home and lost contact with two of her daughters.

Process of the Work

As a number of different professionals had been involved with helping Kavitha try to gain access to her two older daughters, I (RS) realized early on that it would be futile to go down the route of insisting that the two older girls have a relationship with their mother. It felt important to bring an aspect of difference to the therapeutic work by respecting the older girls' wishes to focus upon a possible area of change for the family.

My first session was with the parents and Kuljit, who was eight at the time. The session coincided with the day before the birthday of their only son/brother. He would have been 10 if he had lived. I explored rituals of mourning and grieving in this family, and how Kavitha could write to her two older daughters, marking this solemn occasion. It was important that the older daughters' grief for the loss of their sibling was acknowledged.

I arranged for the next session to be with the grandparents and father as I thought it was culturally important to respect the hierarchies in the family. For this family in particular it was important to respect the patriarchal hierarchy in view of the death of the first son and grandson. Understanding how Izzat operates helped us work with the family's belief systems even in the way we dressed, greeted the family, and observed the family hierarchy (Malik & Krause, 2005, p. 96).

The grandparents talked about their Bezti because of Kavitha's actions and I explored the role of forgiveness in their religion. The grandparents and father were adamant that it was the two older girls' decision not to have contact with their mother and that there was nothing they could do to facilitate this.

Just when I had decided to close the case, I received a phone call from the father. Kuljit had requested a session with CAFCASS (she meant me) as she wanted to discuss the fact that she did not like her mother's new boyfriend, Sunny.

Sunny came from India, was a Bollywood actor/dancer, and was 28. Not surprisingly, the entire extended family considered him to be unsuitable for Kavitha. Kuljit was scared that Kavitha's involvement with him would mean that she would lose her mother's love and attention, while Kavitha was terrified that she would lose contact with her daughter.

In the year that followed, I met with the family for a total of 12 sessions. I worked mostly with Kavitha and Kuljit, meeting with both parents occasionally, and with Kavitha and Sunny as a couple twice. On two other occasions, I included Sunny in my sessions with Kavitha and Kuljit.

My work was child focused and I asked Kuljit to keep a diary in which she could draw and write both "good and bad things" about the periods between our sessions. She would bring her diaries to the sessions and I would use them as a way to help her communicate with her parents. I facilitated the parents to enable Kuljit to make a transition between her two homes, allowing her to bring toys and clothes between one home and another. As her mother's home was considered contaminated, this had not been possible before my work with the family.

During my sessions with the different subsystems of the family, I was able to work respectfully and privately with the grandparents in their role as parents and grandparents. I invited both the grandparents to the second session but Kulwinder attended with only his father. I would have liked further sessions with the grandparents but they did not attend. The session with Kulwinder and the grandfather had the effect of helping the grandparents to reposition themselves toward Kavitha, not only as a former daughter-in-law but as mother of their grandchildren. This then allowed Kulwinder to reposition himself in relation to Kavitha as an ex-wife and also as the mother of his children. The hierarchy of the family was respected, which allowed for the fluidity of positioning of the grandparents and Kulwinder, resulting in Kuljit having contact with her mother and Sunny.

I encouraged Kavitha and Kuljit to have time spent exclusively together, with other times being put aside to spend as a threesome, with Sunny. Slowly, Kulwinder and his family began to feel less anxious about Kuljit's weekends as she began to be happier and more settled with her mother. Sunny and Kavitha grew closer and decided to get married. The act of getting married helped Kavitha attain a more respectable status in the eyes of the extended family and community. Izzat was restored to the wider family. It further helped Kuljit to feel comfortable moving between both her homes. The relationship between Kavitha and her ex-husband improved and they were able to communicate about the older two daughters' schooling and well-being.

Just as abruptly as Kuljit had requested that I meet with her, she announced that she no longer needed to see me. I met with Kavitha on her own for one session to review the work. She was keen to tell me her entire story in a way that she hadn't been able to before. Perhaps she felt Izzat had been restored and her position as mother had been reinstated partly due to her renewed status as a wife. This was in keeping with Izzat, a culturally accepted belief.

As I worked in a CAMHS setting, and Kavitha wanted help in her own right, I referred her to a counselor in a local general practitioner (doctor's surgery).

Although this case could be referred to as one of parental alienation, which is increasingly common (Gardner, 1998), it is different, first because of the intergenerational nature of the family structure, and second because of familial/cultural beliefs of patriarchy and Izzat.

Reflections

Faced with the complexities presented in the above vignettes, we were curious about the fit between belief systems, the families' and our own, and how we – and the families we worked with – could be positioned differently. It seems important at this point to consider theoretical ideas we draw upon as well as beliefs held within South Asian cultures.

Positioning Theory – Professionals and Families

When working with families, positioning theory is helpful, and especially so when working with firm beliefs such as Izzat, which is the one we are concerned with in this chapter. Campbell and Groenback's view is:

> A position is a cluster of duties and rights, with various associated psychological matters such as emotions and relevant skills. Positions are available in micro-cultures, the members of which can come to take up positions, reject or abandon positions, contest positions and so on. Positions appear as much in talk as in action. In either mode, unravelling them depends on the meanings, not only of what is said, but also what is done. (Campbell & Groenback, 2006, p. 17)

Hence, we could position ourselves as very similar to or different from our clients, who could simultaneously be positioning us as middle-class, Western professionals, working in a predominantly white institution. Our positions and those of our clients are fluid rather than fixed and this lends considerable flexibility to our approach. In addition to how we position ourselves vis-à-vis our clients, we think about our position in relation to other professionals in the system. As South Asian professionals, we might be positioned by our colleagues as cultural insiders, that is, our lived experience as women growing up in South Asian cultures and our understanding of how Izzat affects family life. In some instances, this may be an advantage, such as appreciating why children and young people may be reluctant to be critical of parents and older people in their families as this would be considered disrespectful or rude. Izzat also requires that personal family matters are not to be shared outside of the family with professionals as this would draw attention to possible problems which the family cannot resolve and would indicate a level of failure to manage the family.

In other situations, an alliance with our Western colleagues may give us more leverage to effect change, as South Asian families may draw us to collude with them to keep family difficulties private. In this way, we are positioned and position ourselves on a number of different constructs or dimensions, such as physical chastisement. Within the discourse of physical chastisement, for example, we could position ourselves, on the one hand, as believing that one should never hit a child, and on the other hand, as identifying with the position of "spare the rod and spoil the child." Our personal experiences of being parented and parenting within South Asian cultures led us to position ourselves between these polarities. For example, physical chastisement toward us as children was extremely rare, so we experienced it as extraordinary and used only in response to very bad behavior. The effect was that we learned the point at which we crossed the line from naughty to unacceptable behavior. I (DR) do know of friends from my community where there was regular physical chastisement of the children. So as a cultural insider, I am aware of the variance in use of physical chastisement within South Asian communities and can understand how it can be used. Our clinical training added to our values and ethics regarding safeguarding, and so as South Asian clinicians we are able to appreciate the position of a parent who may wish to follow cultural ways of chastisement and can offer a different position to take.

A cultural outsider, for example a clinician trained in Western practice, may see only the act of chastisement and not appreciate why a parent behaves in that way. Professional training may not be culturally sensitive enough to appreciate the shame or Sharam that the parent may experience should a child be naughty, as their view is that child-rearing is wholly their responsibility and the child's behavior reflects upon the whole family. This of course should never prevent clinical safeguarding of children and young people, despite cultural differences between clinician and family.

The children in the clinical examples were positioned by grandparents and parents as well as by their siblings. The overriding belief system which influenced them was Izzat. They may not have been able to reject or abandon their positions until grandparents and parents did so themselves. We, as clinicians, through our systemic training, can hold differing positions with the micro-cultures or subsystem overriding of the family, until they are ready to reposition. This can involve a difference of pace and we often align ourselves alongside the children and young people who feel the constraining effects of adhering to Izzat. This can put them in a double bind as they like and respect their culture but can feel restricted to behave in ways that adhere to Izzat and not bring Sharam upon their families. We can also align ourselves alongside parents (from more than one generation in the family). Hence, our positions as South Asian professionals can involve mediating between the belief systems of the different generations.

A clinician's ability to maintain curiosity can help them to understand why it is so important for families to maintain Izzat. This can allow for family members to feel that Izzat has been acknowledged. A clinician can then work within the family system to help family members take different positions without feeling that their authority has been diminished. This can then lead to willingness to reposition relationships within a context where Izzat is recognized.

In cases where there is risk, safety becomes the highest context marker before therapy can commence and the clinician should refer to a specialist service such as Karma Nirvana in the UK (founded by Jasvinder Sanghera), which offers emergency advice and support to young people.

The Effect of Migration and the Diaspora on Belief Systems

Krause (2012) talks about the self-agency of individuals:

> We therefore need to consider culture as a more complicated process which allows room for an appreciation of individuals actively participating in reproducing, reconstituting and changing their own cultural contexts. (Krause, 2012, p. 364)

An explanation for the preservation of Izzat can include the values that South Asian communities hold with regard to cultural beliefs and the importance of family life. These values are not limited to these particular communities but are universal (Aponte, 1985).

Diasporas are spreading out of cultures away from where that particular culture originated, for example, UK Nigerians from southern Nigeria. Nigeria is the emotionally secure base of the diaspora. The establishment of a South Asian diaspora needs a secure base, which is the country of origin. This becomes the reference point to which South Asians can adhere or move away from in their cultural identity. A sense of identity may be distilled into an ancestral belief system, which is Izzat. While this can be seen as a continuity in pattern from a cultural point of view (Krause, 2012), when countries of origin are damaged due to war and invasion, what is left to those who have migrated is their belief system and Izzat.

Brown (2016, p. 32) describes honor cultures as "ones characterised by a deep concern for reputation and a sense of being duty-bound to retaliate against anything perceived as a slight." Therefore, the way in which the belief of Izzat is maintained may become intensified and possibly more rigid within the South Asian diaspora, especially where forced marriage is a practice in the country of origin (Sanghera, 2011).

Maintaining the Concept of Honor

Looking through a feminist lens and considering how power and gender affect families (Burck, 1995), one can view many South Asian communities as patriarchal. Children are raised to be respectful of Izzat and Sharam is not tolerated. Mothers, aunts, and grandmothers may be charged with ensuring the maintenance of the honor of their daughters and to encourage behaviors to preserve Izzat, as portrayed in the film *Honour*.

Brown (2016) notes that in 2015, Donald Trump, now the US president, drew attention to the fallen reputation of (his) country and his shame about this. As clinicians, we are aware that patriarchal extended families are constructed differently from Western "nuclear" families, and that we should be careful not to impose our own constructions of family life on the clients we work with (Gabb & Singh, 2015; Singh, 2009).

The Asian community in both Asia and the diaspora is quick to employ surveillance and rapidly report upon any hints of shameful behavior. Gurinder Chadha, director of the movie *Bend It Like Beckham* (Chadha, 2002), tells of restrictions upon a Sikh girl, who dares to play football secretly, and who explores her sexuality by meeting and bringing home a white boy. The eyes and ears of the community are everywhere. The parents' feelings of restriction by the community and elders to whom they are answerable can influence how rigid a stance they take against their own children. Kavitha's older children were subject to the rigid stance that their grandparents took by not allowing them to see Kavitha when she was put out of the home. The grandparents would have felt that they were answerable to their community and elders by allowing the children to have contact with Kavitha. This would have been viewed as condoning Kavitha's behavior of bringing Sharam.

Marriage

We can consider how the concept of marriage is positioned in the minds of communities. Marriage holds great prominence in order to maintain Izzat. This is partly to maintain the honor of young women of the community and to continue the role of family as central to the harmony of the community.

Sanghera (2007) would argue that what was initially presented as an arranged marriage within her family had a high degree of coercion to marry and remain in an abusive marriage in order to maintain Izzat in her family's community. Gangoli et al. (2006) and Chantler and Gangoli (2011) have written about the link between forced marriage and violence against women where this is a practice. In some cases, forced marriage is used to prevent a love marriage taking place if the family and community consider that the young people are from backgrounds which are too dissimilar.

Discussion and Clinical Implications

Psychological Effects Upon Children and Young People

While domestic violence is not unique to cases where forced marriage is an issue, the strong adherence to Izzat adds another layer of pressure upon children to keep the problems secret. The wider community may often be aware of abusive behavior within families but feel unable to challenge it as there is the fear that Sharam would be brought upon the community. We would argue that the community's maintenance of forced marriage depletes the family by creating a false sense of well-being, placing the family in a double bind. The psychological stress upon such children can be enormous and may only come to light in their presentation at school or when they self-harm as a way to release stress (Husain, Waheed, & Husain, 2006).

The psychological struggle for young women (and some young men) to maintain Izzat can result in a range of self-harm. Emile Durkheim (1858–1917) was a French sociologist who developed theories about suicide. Gill talks about Durkheim's idea that suicide is related directly to the larger social context:

> So that in some Asian cultures, suicide may be viewed as a better alternative to remaining alive if it protects the family from shame, exposure or embarrassment. (Gill, 2004, p. 38)

Often, parents are constrained by their own parents or older siblings as well as elders in the community who feel that they bear the responsibility for maintaining Izzat. This is connected to Boszormenyi-Nagy and Framo's (1965) idea about ledgers and indebtedness across generations, so while elders may feel that they are doing their protective duty, they may, in their rigid enforcement of Izzat, inadvertently push their children to bring Sharam. Young people may feel they have no choice but to run away or go into a forced marriage where abusive pressures may lead to self-harm, depression, or suicide. Their children may also be at risk of harm.

Positioning and Curiosity

> The power of the polarities model is that it's respectful and it's egalitarian. (Barratt, 2013, p. 177)

When a therapist is faced with a rigid belief system, she may feel positioned to take a less rigid position alongside the family, or to take a position in opposition to the family, which may create feelings of confusion and of being overwhelmed. This may be dependent upon her lived experience (White & Epston, 1990) and her understanding of Izzat. She may feel positioned alongside the one who has been disowned. The therapist may have a view about power, control, and gender (Burck, 1995) and how these interplay in the clinical situation she is faced with. One therapist may feel able to acknowledge the family's belief system in a respectful way and another may feel moved to challenge the belief system from a position of a duty of care to the children and to the one who has been disowned. Barratt (2013, p. 176) talks about how positioning theory can help people step back. For Nadira and her children, their circumstances had led to them stepping back. Nadira, having stayed in an abusive relationship, had stepped out of the marriage on discovering her daughter had been abused. She may have believed that she had chosen a love marriage and that decision positioned her life choices. Her belief in Izzat would mean that she needed to stay in the marriage, especially because she had married out of her culture and faith. However, her position as mother, in contrast to her position as wife, took precedence when her daughter was harmed. Nadira's capacity to hold a different position regarding arranged marriage, that is to make her own choice for a love marriage, may have enabled her to reposition to choose no marriage.

This could add another position on the continuum of marriage, thus creating:

> Forced marriage ... arranged marriage ... love marriage ... no marriage

One could consider how "no marriage" shows itself in the Caribbean, where often couples have relationships and families outside of the convention of marriage. Is that the ultimate Sharam or a product of the colonial experience in the Caribbean?

Self-reflexivity: The Self of the Therapist

How did the therapist position herself in the first case example?

Like her Western colleagues, she (DR) felt sadness and anger at Nadira's plight. At the same time, she understood the family's values of Izzat and Sharam and knew that Nadira's transgression could not be taken lightly or forgiven. She worked with her insider cultural knowledge and decided to focus on the relationships where change was possible, namely between Nadira and her children and subsequently Nadira's parents. She thus positioned herself and was positioned by the family as cultural insider and outsider – insider as she was connected to the family by cultural knowledge, and outsider as a professional clinician working within the CAMHS.

How did the therapist position herself in the second case example?

RS, when meeting Kavitha's family for the first time, took a position of stepping back. Kavitha's older children were initially positioned as distant from her. The girls were themselves positioned by their grandparents and possibly by their own views about their mother. RS, by stepping back at this time, created some space, which later allowed the grandparents to step back themselves. This resulted in the grandparents later feeling able to give Kuljit permission to visit her mother's home.

Kuljit, through the process of therapy, became positioned nearer to her mother. This opened up the possibility of a different and more positive kind of relationship for the older children with Kavitha in the future.

The grandfather and his family were repositioned when Kavitha and Sunny made the decision to marry. This restored Izzat to the wider family, which made it more acceptable for Kavitha's ex-husband to talk to Kavitha about her older children.

Another turning point in the therapy for the children would have been when Kavitha's home became viewed as less "contaminating" to enable Kuljit to visit. Here, the sessions with the grandparents were invaluable as all of the children were highly influenced by their view of Kavitha.

Systemic psychotherapy can allow for consideration of polarities, continuums, and positioning within the context of strongly held belief systems. It is possible to hold the concept of Izzat and to explore degrees of difference which do not annihilate or intensify belief systems but which serve to rebalance positioning and positioning of others along the continuum.

Understanding how Izzat operates can help us work with the family's belief systems even in the way we dress, greet the family, and observe the family hierarchy (Malik & Krause, 2005, p. 96). This work can take place when families and communities feel secure within themselves to allow this exploration to take place.

Indeed, there are happy and enduring arranged marriages, which involve extended families and tradition among modern lifestyles across continents. Perhaps, these are the families who have repositioned themselves on the marriage continuum, having a less rigid grasp on the need to maintain Izzat, and who are less fearful of the impact of Sharam. An example of repositioning around Izzat can be found in a film, *Monsoon Wedding* (Nair, 2001). The father of a bride supports a young woman, Ria, who has grown up in his family as his own daughter. The father remains indebted to Tej, a respected elder male accorded high status because he had continued to help the family after partition in India. It is a family wedding. Ria sees Tej approach a girl in the family with a view to abuse her and she challenges him about his sexual abuse of her when she was a child. The father of the bride tells Ria that his hands are tied over challenging Tej, but he later agonizes over his position and refuses to let Tej and his wife take any further part in the wedding ceremony. He asks them to leave his home and his family.

For us, as clinicians, our work with Nadira and Kavitha and innumerable other Asian women brings up some important questions. Is the concept of Izzat a renewed orthodoxy in the face of powerless communities? Does breaking Izzat mean that an Asian woman is shunned, disowned, becomes a nonperson to the family, and is seen as "dead in our eyes" (Sanghera, 2011, p. 60)?

Or is the concept of Izzat a potent tool of patriarchy, which is the dominance of the male lineage?

The influence of Izzat in families can bring about overwhelming emotions for families as well as for clinicians. Appropriate supervision can help to position clinicians to neither over- nor underreact. Consultation with specialist organizations such as Karma Nirvana can also be helpful.

Parental Alienation

In considering disownment, we can draw parallels to parental alienation (Gardner, 1998; O'Brien, 2012), as in the case of Kavitha. Both Gardner and O'Brien state that parental alienation exists as an issue in divorce or child custody litigation.

Kavitha's husband's family alienated her and attempted to prevent contact between her and her children. The rationale that they used for this behavior was that Kavitha had brought Sharam to the family by ostensibly having an affair. The unsaid reason was that she had not produced a living male child, which was important for the patriarchal lineage. What allowed for Kavitha's disownment was the family's firm positioning in the belief that Izzat had been broken. Our understanding of parental alienation is that it usually happens in divorce proceedings where one parent can prevent the children from having contact with the other parent. The difference in this case was that it was not only one parent alienating the other but the paternal family's belief that Kavitha had broken Izzat, which meant Sharam. Sharam justified disowning Kavitha.

Conclusion

In exploring forced marriage as a representation of a belief system we have used two clinical examples and four theoretical ideas linked to clinical examples where children have been at the forefront of the work. We have also used our self-reflexivity when working with the belief of Izzat as cultural insiders. Our perspective is that Izzat as the highest context marker allows for the conditions where forced marriage and coercion within marriage can occur.

We have used positioning theory as well as ideas about ledgers and indebtedness to explain how Izzat can be so organizing and how positioning theory can help clinicians to intervene in and create some change in family systems where Izzat is so influential. Respectful curiosity can be extended to discover how patriarchy organizes families, and especially women and girls, in the culture in which clinicians are working.

We acknowledge that the belief in Izzat is not confined only to South Asian communities but also has resonance for many different cultural groups, both at home and in the diaspora. Through the clinical vignettes we have shown the rigid manifestations of Izzat and Sharam, which we feel are also present within African and African Caribbean communities. We contend that Izzat as a representation of a belief system is central to the practice of forced marriage.

A deconstruction of the practice of arranged marriages leads us to consider the complexity of the practice of marriage within South Asian cultures. It is important to remain open to the idea that arranged marriages are culturally normative, and it is the abuse of arranged marriage by strict adherence to Izzat which is pathological.

Pointers for Practice

1. For systemic practitioners, used to working with the entire family, there may be a pull to invite all members when a young woman presents with an "Izzat" issue, such as wanting a divorce or to avoid an arranged/forced marriage. In the first instance, the practitioner needs to establish whether it is safe to work with the entire family. It may be that initially the practitioner can work with some members of the family, and this can then be extended to other family members, as in Kavitha's case.
2. When the professional has established what kind of marriage a young woman may be entering into (on a continuum of love and arranged), it is important that they remain open to the idea that arranged marriages are not pathological. Where there is or has been little or no knowledge about arranged marriage, there can be a negative view of its practice, seeing it as dangerous and possibly pathological. However, a deconstruction of the practice leads us to consider the complexity of the practice of marriage within South Asian cultures. As more understanding has developed about arranged marriage as a normative cultural practice, instances have been uncovered where what has been described as arranged marriage has indeed been found to be forced marriage.

    Where there has been a reluctance to challenge cultural ideas of marriage, clinicians may have felt that they could not differentiate between consensual arranged marriage and what has come to be described as forced marriage. This can leave clinicians feeling helpless and possibly overwhelmed by the complexity of the practice of marriage in South Asian cultures. We are aware that there are other cultures where values, family hierarchy, and moral codes also follow closely delineated practices for marriage. The themes which arise in these cultures can be the same as in South Asian cultures.
3. Be respectfully curious. Extend your curiosity to ask about women and girls in the culture in which you are working. How may they feel about growing up? Are there ceremonies or markers for their transition into adolescence from girlhood? Examine how their status changes and what they anticipate may change or stay the same for them. This may open up ideas about relationships and marriage.

References

Aponte, H. (1985). The negotiation of values in family therapy. *Family Process*, 24(3), 328–338.

Barratt, S. (2013). Evolving applications of systemic ideas. Towards positioning and polarities: David Campbell in interview with Charlotte Burck. In C. Burck, S. Barratt,

& E. Kavner (Eds.), *Positions and polarities in contemporary systemic practice. The legacy of David Campbell* (pp. 171–183). London: Karnac.

Boszormenyi-Nagy, I., & Framo, J. L. (1965). *Intensive family therapy: Theoretical and practical aspects* (pp. 33–87). New York, NY: Harper & Row.

Boszormenyi-Nagy, I., Grunebaum, J., & Ulrich, D. (1991). Contextual therapy. In A. Gurman & D. Kniskern (Eds.), *Handbook of family therapy* (Vol. 2). New York, NY: Brunner/Mazel.

Brown, R. P. (2016). *Honor bound: How a cultural ideal has shaped the American psyche*. New York, NY: Oxford University Press.

Burck, C. (1995). *Gender and family therapy*. London: Karnac.

Campbell, D., & Groenback, M. (2006). *Taking positions in the organisation* (pp. 13–33). London: Karnac.

Chadha, G. (2002). *Bend it like Beckham [movie]*. Los Angeles, CA: Kintop Pictures.

Chantler, K., & Gangoli, G. (2011). Violence against women in minoritised communities: Cultural norm or cultural anomaly? In R. Thiara, M. Shroettle, & S. Condon (Eds.), *Violence against women and ethnicity: Commonalities and differences across Europe* (pp. 353–366). Leverkusen: Barbara Budrich Publishers.

Gabb, J., & Singh, R. (2015). Reflections on the challenges of understanding racial, cultural and sexual differences in couple relationship research. *Journal of Family Therapy*, *37*(2), 210–227.

Gangoli, G., Razak, A., & McCarry, M. (2006). *Forced marriage and domestic violence among South Asian communities in North East England*. Bristol: University of Bristol and Northern Rock Foundation.

Gardner, K. (1995). *Global migrants, local lives. Travel and transformation in rural Bangladesh*. Oxford: Clarendon Press.

Gardner, R. A. (1998). *The parental alienation syndrome. A guide for mental health and legal professionals*. Cresskill, NJ: Creative Therapeutics.

Gill, A. (2004, October). A lethal code of honour. *Community Care*, *28*, 38–40.

Husain, M. I., Waheed, W., & Husain, N. (2006). Self-harm in British South Asian women: Psychosocial correlates and strategies for prevention. *Annals of General Psychiatry*, *5*(7), 1–7.

Khan, S. (2014). *Honour [movie]. Isle of Man Films*. London: Film Production Company.

Krause, I.-B. (1995). Personhood, culture and family therapy. *Journal of Family Therapy*, *17*(4), 363–382.

Krause, I.-B. (1998). *Therapy across culture*. London: Sage.

Krause, I.-B. (2012). Culture and the reflexive subject in systemic psychotherapy. In I.-B. Krause (Ed.), *Culture and reflexivity in systemic psychotherapy: Mutual perspectives* (pp. 1–39). London: Karnac.

Lau, A. (1995). Gender, power and relationships: Ethno-cultural and religious issues. In C. Burk & B. Speed (Eds.), *Gender, power and relationships* (pp. 110–117). London: Routledge.

Malik, R., & Krause, I.-B. (2005). Before and beyond words: Embodiment and intercultural therapeutic relationships in family therapy. In C. Flaskas, B. Mason, & A. Perlesz (Eds.), *The space between* (pp. 95–109). London: Karnac.

Nair, M. (2001). *Monsoon wedding [movie]*. New York, NY: Mirabai Films Inc.

O'Brien, L. (2012). *Essay: An examination of the debate around parental alienation*. NUI Maynooth.

Pearce, W. B., & Cronen, V. E. (1980). *Communication, action and meaning*. New York, NY: Praeger.

Robinson, D. (2008). Working in a multicultural context: Implications for systemic practice. *Context*, *96*, 34–35.

Robinson, D. (2016). A systemic approach to community in family: Working with family mental health. In T. Afuape & I.-B. Krause (Eds.), *Urban Cahms* (pp. 145–156). New York, NY: Routledge.
Sanghera, J. (2007). *Shame*. London: Hodder & Stoughton.
Sanghera, J. (2009). *Daughters of shame*. London: Hodder & Stoughton.
Sanghera, J. (2011). *Shame travels*. London: Hodder & Stoughton.
Singh, R. (2009). Constructing "the family" across culture. *Journal of Family Therapy*, *31*(4), 359–383.
Sookram, R. (2009). *Challenges and achievements: The history of Indians in Grenada: Understanding the Indian experience in a small colonial state, 1857–1950*. London: VDM Verlag Dr Müller.
Thiara, R., & Breslin, R. (2006). *A look at domestic violence among families from ethnic minorities* (pp. 32–33). Retrieved from http://www.communitycare.co.uk/2006/11/01a-look-at-domestic-violence-among-families-from-ethnic-minorities/
United States Census. (2010). Retrieved from http://factfinder2.census.gov
White, M., & Epston, D. (1990). *Narrative means to therapeutic ends*. New York, NY: W. W. Norton.

Chapter 27

Systemic Family Therapy with Transgenerational Communities in Haiti and the Dominican Republic

Karen Carberry, Jean Gerald Lafleur and Genel Jean-Claude

Introduction

The Haitian indigenous community is an under-researched population, and there is a scarcity of information and literature on the black Haitian families' experience of family therapy or parenting programmes (Bibb & Casimir, 1996; Carberry, 2016; Gopaul-McNicol, 1993).

Elsewhere, researchers have been active in community family therapy, offering extensive models for the profession to step further out of the paradigms which are somewhat limiting (Kasiram & Thaver, 2013). Extending across national boundaries, crafting skills and knowledge through collaborative partnership work, will provide multiple families with a better quality of life (Asen, 2002; Doherty & Beaton, 2000).

What we do know is that there are long-held and traditional values regarding preserving community networks, and supporting neighbouring families who find themselves in need. This chapter will illustrate how systemic family therapy has begun to take shape in its own form, following the impact on indigenous communities in the wake of the 2010 earthquake.

A brief history of the social and political context of Haiti, provides a backdrop to the landscape in which we were able to develop a collaborative model of therapy across communities. Cultural pride is an important aspect of the Haitian belief system. As an 'outsider' looking like an 'insider', the first author, a black British woman in her 50s of Jamaican ancestry, alongside the second and third authors – black male Haitian pastors in their early 40s – will recount, the development of a community family therapy intervention, as a process of transgenerational healing following the Haiti earthquake in 2010, together with a series of concurrent community interventions delivered within the Dominican Republic.

The International Handbook of Black Community Mental Health, 527–555
Copyright © 2020 by Emerald Publishing Limited
All rights of reproduction in any form reserved
doi:10.1108/978-1-83909-964-920201033

The voice of the family therapist, pastors as translators and co-facilitators, together with feedback from participants is presented, followed by a discussion on the importance of developing cultural competence in working cross-culturally to ensure an authentic experience in therapy.

History

The history of the Caribbean is multi-faceted, with a rich colonial background in European oppression, via the transatlantic slave trade. Hayti, or Haiti as it is known, was not an exception. In 1492, the original inhabitants, the Taino Indians, encountered Columbus, who left some of his Spanish comrades to infiltrate the population. What appeared initially to be a process of friendship over several years eventually led to indigenous disappearance through Spanish repopulation, smallpox, slavery and the brutal dissemination of the Taino.

Then, up to 10 million blacks made up of children, men and women over 400 years were transported to the country. The enslaved people were made up of several races, 'Bantus from the Congo and Angola formed the majority. Guineans of the Gold Coast and Coast of Slaves … Senegalese were less common' (Heinl & Heinl, 2005, p. 22). The transatlantic slave trade was responsible for enormous riches for Europe and the Americas, and mass genocide of black people, together with generations of traumatic loss and separation of the black family system.

Class Structure

The attempted destruction of the black family structure left a legacy of transgenerational and intergenerational trauma (Lagos & Chaura, 2015). Importing white female prostitutes from the jails in Europe, sailors subsequently married them and set up an upper class system that the ruling class from the countries which these women had travelled from, would have objected to, due to their extremely low social standing in their countries of origin.

In Haiti, the new ruling class ensured that there were strict rules for blacks, and those of a lighter skin 'Mulatre', with laws prohibiting education for 'the blacks' who were kept illiterate and Creole speaking, juxtaposed with the light-skinned Mulatre, literate and French speaking. With strict rules about intercourse between 'the blacks' and through rape, the Mulatre, revealed a new class of 'homme de coleur' who were mixed or multi-racial people of colour, who did not have the same rights as the Mulatre.

'A basic 170 classifications of racial coloration ensued, … which might result from the mating of whites, noires (blacks) mulatres, [*mixed or multiracial*] or those with Carib Indian strains' (Heinl & Heinl, 2005, p. 34) [first author emphasis]. Therefore, the white population delivered an inconsistency of rules throughout the nation. This class structure remained endemic within the future ruling class of the nation and throughout the Caribbean.

Due to Taino, Spanish and French influences, the whole island was often called Haiti, Hayti, Santo Domingo, Saint-Domingue or San Domingo. The colonial terms Saint-Domingue and Santo Domingo are often and sometimes applied to the whole island, with latterly The Dominican Republic on one side of the island and the Republic of Haiti on the other.

The Dominican Republic

1630–1659 Spanish, French and English Treaties

On the other side of the island known as La Torgue, 130 years of French rule prevailed over the area known as Saint-Domingue. There are incredible stories of rebellion, with family groups living in the mountainous terrain, and records show that generations of people were born and lived outside of enslavement, sometimes living up to the age of 64. These types of Haitian family systems, known as 'lakou', remain today, although life expectancy is much reduced.

Haiti

1859–1870 Establishment of the First Black Republic

A slave rebellion in Saint-Domingue in 1791 sparked off the Haitian revolution, led by Toussaint L'Ouverture with an army of former slaves. The revolution eventually led to Saint-Domingue becoming independent in 1804, and on January 1 of that year, Saint-Domingue was declared the Republic of Haiti, the first independent black state outside Africa.

However, France desired compensation for the loss of capital and revenue from plantations, slave labour and sugar exports as a result of the establishment of the new republic. Fear of threatened re-enslavement impacted the development of the country's infrastructure, and Haiti took a whole century to repay the required fee. Plans for free national education and healthcare service were put on hold and abandoned. Embargos imposed by France, Britain and the United States relegated Haiti from the richest colony to one of the poorest nations in the western hemisphere (Dubois, 2013; Heinl & Heinl, 2005).

Political Unrest

During 1915–1934, Haiti underwent occupation by the United States; the United States intervened in the nation's elections, stating:

> The Government of the United States considers its duty to support a constitutional government. It means to assist in the establishment of such a government and to support it as long as necessity might require. (Heinl & Heinl, 2005)

The message to the Haitian nationals inferred that if they proceeded to elect their preferred president rather than the person the United States desired, then the election would not be permitted to go ahead. As a result, US occupation began and many lost their lives in battles with the Marines on the streets of Haiti. The following narrative is a succinct chronology of the key political systems and natural disasters which have affected Haiti to date:

1934–1957: Dictatorships, coups and civil unrest.
1957–1971: François Duvalier (Papa Doc) elected president despite numerous attempts to overthrow him. Stories abound of the executions and horrors he presided over (Heinl & Heinl, 2005).
1971–1986: Jean-Claude Duvalier (Baby Doc) takes over as president and survives three attempts to overthrow him.
1986: Jean-Claude Duvalier flees Haiti.
1986–1988: Henri Namphy became president of the interim government.
1988: Leslie Manigat becomes Haiti's president. Removed by military coup.
1988: Henri Namphy overthrew Magniat and becomes president until Sept, then deposed.
1988–1990: Prosper Avril president until March 1990 – went into exile following riots.
1988: From 10 to 13 March Herard Abraham – Acting President for three days.
1990: From 13 March 1990 to 7 February 1991, Ertha Pascal Trouillot – Acting President.
1991–1991 February–September: Democratic election of Jean-Bertrand Aristide. Catholic priest, favoured for his compassion to the poor. Presidency ended by military coup.
1991–1991: From 29 September to October 8, Raoul Cedras – De Factor Leader of Haiti.
1991–1992: From 8 October to 19 June 1992, Joseph Nerette – Provisional President.
1992–1993: From 19 June 1992 to 15 June 1993, Marc Louis Bazin – Provisional President.
1993–1994: From 15 June 1993 to 12 October 12 1994, Emile Jonassaint – Provisional President.
1994–1996: Aristide returns to power with assistance of the United Nations (UN) and the United States.
1996 February–2001: Rene Preval – Elected President.
2001–2004: Aristide elected as the president for the second time.
2003: Voodoo recognised as a religion.
2004: Assignations abound with President Clinton about to visit the nation. The US army is dissolved and the UN peacekeepers take command. Vice president Al Gore helps to celebrate the Haitian presidency election.
2004: Severe storms and floods. Aristide forced into exile. UN peacekeepers arrive in Haiti.
2004–2006: Gerard Latortue – Elected President.
2006–2011: Preval elected as the president for the second time.
12 January 2010: Earthquake of 7.0 magnitude hits Port-au-Prince, the capital, and surrounding towns – Hundreds of thousands died.

2010 October: Outbreak of cholera brought in by the UN peacekeepers. Thousands died.
2010 November: Hurricane Thomas.
2011: Michael Martelly – Elected President of Haiti.
2016: Hurricane Matthew.
2017: Jovenel Moïse elected to presidency.

The history of Haiti has been tumultuous, with centuries of adverse political activity from key players from Europe and the United States, appearing to have some influence on the nation's leadership and fiscal security.

The racial divide emulates the division between the rich and poor. Ninety per cent of Haiti's population are black, described as 'noirs', and 10 per cent are mixed with Caucasian blood and are known as 'jaunes' or 'Mulatre'. This racial division – Haitians call it exactly that, and speak of 'two races' – which is the most important fact of life in Haiti as it dominates the country's whole existence (Heinl & Heinl, 2005, p. 4).

Clearly, the transgenerational effects of the nation's economic and political history culminated in the catastrophic effects of the 2010 earthquake. Some Haitian nationals sought refuge in the United States and the Dominican Republic. However, some Haitians in the Dominican Republic have had to return due to recent legislation regarding nationalism. Repatriated from the Dominican Republic and hidden from the world's cameras, tented communities still exist, cheek by jowl. The new Haitian president and his government, together with international non-governmental organisations (NGOs) and charities, continue to support the healing of people affected by the 2010 devastation. Unfortunately, not having a joined up approach the NGOs contributed to the confusion, as they were 'unfamiliar with local conditions and resources. They squandered millions of dollars in ill-conceived and poorly executed projects that actually made life worse for the Haitian people (Patterson, 2018). Although there were allegations of unaccountability and corruption, both political and within some of the larger NGOs where donations meant for disaster relief were siphoned off and/or retained, millions in potential revenue remain (Farmer, 2011; Gerard, 2010).

Mental Health Services

According to the Pan American Health Organisation (2003), the country's mental health system has been stymied by Haiti's economics. As a result, there are four strands for providing support across the country:

- Public institutions administered by the Ministry of Public Health and Population.
- The private non-profit sector, composed of NGOs and religious organisations.
- The mixed non-profit sector, where staff are paid by the government but management is carried out by the private sector.
- The private for-profit sector, which includes physicians, dentists, nurses and other specialists working in the private sector or in clinics in urban centres.

Fifty per cent of the population are aged 20 and below and, as previously discussed, families live together in three or more generations. Elders within the family are highly respected, and pastors and ministers in the community are looked to for local and wider leadership and solutions. Thus, the stage was set for an innovative systemic practice.

Mission as a Vehicle for Delivering Family Therapy within the Community

During the aftermath of the earthquake, the second author was contacted by a mutual acquaintance of Pastor Christie John-Baptiste, founder of the British charity Support A Nation (SAN), who had offered to provide support to the small community in Morne Oge in Jacmel, Haiti, with a social work team in 2011. SAN provided play and creative arts activities with the children, and teaching on behaviour management within the school, juxtaposed with the provision of clothes and toiletries. The following year, Pastor John-Baptiste was invited to speak at the annual crusade of 10,000 people to celebrate lives saved in 2010. Therefore, in January 2012, the first author travelled from the United Kingdom to Haiti with Pastor Jean-Baptiste, a light-skinned British woman of St Lucian descent. We travelled and represented SAN as part of a church humanitarian aid team, which we call a 'mission trip'.

Airport Experience – Witnessing Oppression

In Miami, and while in transit, the first author observed how the Haitian men were treated. There were two queues formed to board the plane to Haiti. My colleague and I tucked behind the Haitian men and saw that the other line comprised mainly white Europeans or white Americans. That line with the white people went through quickly, while our line remained static.

The white airline attendant proceeded to walk up and down our line of black men and shouted at them to 'move up' and 'move' [along]. Onwards he continued to shout, while peering over at the other diminishing line. The black men in our line shuffled forward, heads down – oppressed. The first author and colleague stopped the airline attendant as he walked past us and queried his attitude. Upon hearing British accents, he stopped in his tracks and asked to see our passports. When we showed him these, his tone softened as he said 'We will board you soon' and then he invited us to join the other queue. We declined and stood resolutely with the Haitian men. We engaged in conversation with the men, some of whom were returning to Haiti for the first time in over 30 years in order to find/see their families after the tragedy of the earthquake.

When we approached the desk for our boarding passes, we complained about how these men were treated. The ground crew asked what they could do to help and we asked for an upgrade for all of us. We were promptly given business-class tickets and we settled into our seats on the plane, only to be dismayed as our 'comrades' in line continued on into economy class.

I (the first author) felt duped, and it made me reflect upon the wealth of information that I as a black woman, black daughter to a black father, black sister to black brothers, black auntie to black nephews and black mother-in-law to a black son-in-law sometimes take for granted of my own visibility as a woman, and unconsciously misunderstood all the deficit ways in which black men are not viewed positively. I reflected on the incident and wondered, had I not used my voice to express my disquiet, how my inaction could have made me complicit in rendering these black men as 'invisible' (Boyd-Franklin, 1989; Ellison, 1952; Munroe, 2001).

Upon disembarkment, I shared this episode with the second author, who agreed that this experience was a frequent occurrence and said this feedback was helpful in formulating multi-systemic concepts for delivering family therapy from a community achievement position, being mindful of deficit models of black family and community functioning that feed into linear feelings of shame and indignation.

Haitian Family Life

Contrary to what is often published in the international press or shown in the media, Haiti is a beautiful country, with glorious beaches, parks and countryside, yet it has communities in which the poor live cheek by jowl across the class system. The first author has travelled to Haiti annually over the past six years, staying at a beautiful local hotel Leviya within the Morne Oge community. The hotel is owned by a Haitian man, who, through this venture, provides opportunities for local employment and is active in both friendship and partnership with the second author, providing support for the community in times of trauma and economic need. Haitian people are proud, hardworking and, in the first author's experience, reflective and generous, going out of their way to show their appreciation, even in times of hardship, disappointment and trauma.

Studies exploring the Haitian lakou system reveal a model of family life in which extended and multi-generational families live together, providing financial and other forms of care, including supporting struggling mothers and families to alleviate parental stress. Lakou is thus defined as:

> [...] clusters of homes in which Haitian families reside, as well as to the extended and multiple-generation family form that is prominent in Haitian culture. Initially, the members of a lakou worked cooperatively and provided for each other with financial and other forms of support. (Edmond, Randolph, & Richard, 2007)

As a result of this model, it is suggested that family conflicts are few and far between, and the latest findings of 'mothering' in Haiti suggest that family programmes still need to be implemented to build on the strengths of the lakou system, and to address psychological consequences of poverty and stress attributed to mothers' and others' perceptions of poor parenting, which allegedly result in the failure of children to thrive (Edmond et al., 2007; LaRose, 1975). This is a country where extreme poverty can be found, and yet the literature rests children's failure to thrive at their parents' door rather than looking at the wider ramifications of the social political system, and the history behind the West's determination to keep Haiti in a subjugated state, coupled with foreign aid agencies working independently of the Haitian government.

Working with Fathers

Village fathers' clubs in rural Haiti, aimed at improving children's health, conducted research on the practice and beliefs about parenting among fathers of young children. In addition, the research sought to explore the role of fathers' clubs in the lives of fathers, mothers, children and communities. Findings revealed that fathers were very involved in the care of their children and that they worked co-jointly with the children's mother regarding childcare, as well as being responsible for others in the community. Fathers also viewed the fathers' clubs as a strategic element in terms of community survival (Sloand, Gebrian, & Astone, 2012). When we look at Maslow's hierarchy of needs, having a home to live in coupled with food, self-esteem and company appears to be a universal construct (Maslow, 2013). However, in terms of Haitian families, a wider organising focus is on a community, transgenerational ethos with a core sense of spirituality.

Incorporating Spirituality in Systemic Family Therapy in Communities

Spirituality is an organising construct across many cultures. In a recent conference, Dr Rabia Malik enthused about the importance of integrating religious, spiritual and cultural beliefs in working systemically with Muslim families, in order to explore challenges and use techniques to rework emerging themes. We concur that although systemic therapy is well placed to address cultural and religious contexts, it is dominated by an ethnocentric viewpoint based on Euro-American cultural contexts which historically have split therapy from religion. Integrating religious and cultural contexts of interventions which are meaningful to clients, help to facilitate change, and provide systemic therapy with opportunities to ethically engage in an authentic way, together with 'providing religious practitioners with an opportunity to engage with lived human experiences' (Malik, 2016).

Haitians concept of the world encompasses metaphors to describe low mood, and it draws on not only the visible, but also the invisible spiritual world to express their distress (Rahill, Jean-Gilles, Thomlison, & Pinto-Lopez, 2011; Desrosiers & St Fleurose, 2002). The third author is a Pastor in the Dominican Republic and passionately feels that pastors should have a genuine interest in children's spiritual development, and attests that childhood is a priority within the formation of the human being. It is the stage of life that constitutes a wonderful opportunity for the transmission of faith and values. It is urgent and necessary to guide, accompany, educate and train children in their human spiritual development, which in the case of this Haitian community is a human–Christian development. Children in the Dominican Republic between the ages of 6 and

10 are found to be a fragile, vulnerable population, exposed to dangers such as, abandonment, indigence, intra-family violence, sexual abuse and high-risk diseases, pornography and prostitution, real and virtual, affecting non-formation in spiritual life and in human values (Jean-Claude, De los Santos, & Popa, 2016).

Thus, in the Children's Pastoral Ministry, it is believed that the religious education of the child must start from the moment they try to take their first steps in life, because to delay it until the child reaches adulthood would deprive them of the knowledge of God. The work of the Children's Pastoral Ministry executes its work through an interdisciplinary team that accompanies different children's initiatives of the community, and it is intended to articulate all the processes in strengthening the faith of all children.

The pastoral care of children means being aware of their reality, and valuing the steps that have taken place in the family and in the community, to generate spaces for articulation in children's initiatives through a coordinated work in favour of a healthy childhood. Thus an integral pastoral approach, with those – such as the Evangelical Child Ministry Pastoral in Mira Cielo Sector in the Dominican Republic, who are centrally located within the community – can assess according to the needs and information derived, through to eventual distribution of resources to the children.

To educate children in the faith takes a lot of ingenuity and a deep knowledge of the child's soul. Offering the message of love with art and pedagogical sense, is fundamental in the bases of education that are used in the Children's Pastoral Ministry. To achieve these goals, education must be gradual, accommodating to their tender souls, sensitivity, age and level of understanding. In this way, the objectives of the Children's Pastoral Ministry are to teach the children to know and love God, to initiate them in the mysteries of the faith, to educate their hearts, to bring them closer to Jesus, and to instil values and behaviours like those of Jesus in his childhood. All this is valuable work and a great blessing; however, it is an arduous job (Jean-Claude et al., 2016).

Recent literature has highlighted the concerns regarding the possible high burnout for ministers in pastoral ministry (Dance, 2016), although a survey of 1,500 pastors in evangelical and historical black churches cites that less than 13 per cent left the ministry within 10 years, and some of this data relate to natural endings such as death or retirement (CBN News, 2016; Lifeway Research, 2015). Ministry work is hard – pastors have an extremely heavy workload, and are liable to undergo stress in relation to looking for creative approaches to provide support and to relieve community financial hardship. Partnership work with others who value and understand the culture of the community can provide essential assistance and encouragement to the pastor.

Family Therapy in the Context of Community Following Transgenerational Trauma and Earthquake Survival

The first author has found that the key tool for delivering family therapy with black families is through using the multi-systems approach which emerged in the 1980s (Boyd-Franklin, 1989). This has widened the opportunities for black and multi-racial families to receive therapeutic support incorporating a non-European perspective, tailored by both the practitioner and the family to discover a more culturally competent approach.

All theories of change can be described as 'stories' as we introduce new information, including psycho-education that makes a difference (Coker, Williams, Hayes, Hartmann, & Harvey, 2016). Family therapists are skilled to punctuate family members' perceptions of reality and discern different patterns of functioning in order to develop healthy and healing relationships. Experienced family therapists are taught through an accredited level teaching of several core systemic models in order to understand the process required for change and how to apply them to practice (Cecchin, 1987; Dallos & Draper, 2005; Hoffman, 1991; Mandanes, 1991; Minuchin & Fishman, 1981). In summary:

- A structural therapist will look for organisational patterns (and rules for behaviour which underpin them), which may be repeated over time. Change at the level of family organisation is believed to lead to difference in an individual's experience.
- Strategic therapists are interested in patterns of interaction around behaviours defined as problematic and the attempted solutions to the problem. They intervene with tasks and directives to help change patterns, and identify exceptions to the problem. Change takes place outside of the session.
- Milan/post-Milan therapists explore patterns of beliefs in families and between families and agencies. They are interested in how these beliefs may be affecting family interactions. They intervene by challenging beliefs and enabling family members to see different patterns emerging. Change is expected to be unpredictable.

The multi-systems approach takes into consideration the composite of all of these models (and often others), the extended family systems culture and belief system, rather than a more westernised nuclear family approach. In addition, the success in which the systemic therapist 'joined' with the black families is often interpreted by the embodiment of a concept of 'vibes', which describe the way in which trust between practitioner and family was measured by a tacit sense of inner feeling about the professional working with the family. Black families tend to imbue a 'healthy cultural suspicion when working with White practitioners' (Boyd-Franklin, 1989; McDowell, 2004), and black therapists are not exempt from being tested, especially as the black therapist is usually a graduate of a predominantly white therapeutic institution, and families may feel that the therapist may have 'sold out' or compromised their 'cultural identity' in order to gain their qualification. Having the right balance to focus on the strengths of black families, and challenge unhealthy relationship patterns is a good skill for culturally competent practice (Goode-Cross, 2011).

In private practice the first author, in her work with black clients and families, often experienced the 'shelf test' where black clients will look on the black therapist's book shelf in order to ascertain what reading material or DVDs are displayed as a quick appraisal of whether the therapist is 'woke', which is a concept of self-awareness and cultural pride in their racial and ethnic heritage. It is important to be aware and open to new tests when working cross-culturally and internationally. Internationally, one way trust is earned is through frequent visits and personal investment in terms of service and authentic relationship with the community, particularly in times of trauma.

There is limited empirical evidence which supports using systemic approaches in trauma treatment – there is also a need to generate more research to emphasise systemic interventions as a core consideration in treatment. However, notwithstanding the dearth, Lopez-Zeron and Blow (2017) suggest the following key points for practitioners:

- Trauma should be treated as an event that affects everyone in the family and is nested in societal and cultural contexts.
- Close relationships can maintain or exacerbate problems, but they can also be a powerful source of healing.
- Systemic protocols that not only address interpersonal difficulties but also focus on survivors' relationships are critical for healing in the aftermath of trauma.

Although Haiti does not have a national health system, and a limited primary health care system, the country has been helped by many NGOs and charities. These organisations send global humanitarian aid teams, some with clinical and trauma experience and expertise, others without. Working in the trauma field, it is imperative that family therapists and systemic practitioners have extensive training and experience in debriefing survivors, and knowledge of the experience of mission teams/aid workers (Bennett & Eberts, 2015; Lacet, 2012). The process is not a one-time occurrence during therapy. Working with larger family systems, team members and interpreters, one has to be attuned to the various levels of possible over-identification and areas of disassociation that could take place, together with the various stages of debriefing and the techniques required to safely wind down (Davis, 2014).

During the mission trip to Haiti in 2012, community workshop seminars were used to deliver family therapy to process the effects of transgenerational trauma to 200 parents. Between 2012 and 2017, systemic family therapy continued to be delivered to over 1,000 participants in Haiti and the Dominican Republic (see Table 1).

Attendees included pastors, community leaders, young people, teachers, parents and extended families. Community family therapy helped families understand and process the impact of trauma, family conflict, identity and shadism (skin colour issues), parenting and life cycle issues. This helped to develop collaborative community intervention and solutions to help multi-generational families in crisis, and to develop strategies for community happiness and well-being (Boyd-Franklin & Bry, 2000; Carberry, 2016, 2017; O'Grady & Orton, 2016; Preston-Shoot, 2007; Thomas, 2013).

Review of parenting programmes in developing countries found few studies that evaluated parenting studies to prevent psychological difficulties in children, and only 8 studies out of 44 had a follow-up. Gaps in research highlighted that less was done to prevent or manage emotional and behavioural problems (Mejia,

Table 1. The Timeline Below Illustrates an Overview of Systemic Family Therapy with Communities of Transgenerational Families in Haiti and the Dominican Republic Between 2012 and 2017.

		Previous Therapeutic Work				
2012	2013	2014	2015	2016	2017	2017
Location	Location	Location	Location	Location	Location	Location
Haiti	Haiti	Haiti	Haiti	Haiti	Haiti	The Dominican Republic
Theme	Theme	Theme	Theme	Theme	Theme	Theme
Impact of transgenerational trauma to 200 parents/carers	Managing troubled teenagers to 50 parents and their adolescents	Parenting skills, review and vision to 50 parents and children	A vision for transgenerational success to 118 parents/carers	Activate the vision. Parenting across generations to 100 teachers/parents and carers	Managing conflict in the home to 200 parents	Family Life cycle learning how to love cross-generationally to 160	Mental and emotional wellbeing in the family to 200 parents
Enhancing self-esteem to 65 young people			Certificated	Certificated	Certificated	Certificated

Calam, & Sanders, 2012) or explore how the therapist addresses parents' requests to process family conflict in a community setting.

Parenting programmes have been found to use effective tools and strategies in managing children's behaviour and emotions in order to prevent further difficulties. However, efficacy of these programmes tend to be carried out in high-income countries in the West, rather than in developing countries. Therefore, there is a need for collaboration with indigenous communities to use culturally appropriate measures for evaluation and implementation of evidence-based parenting interventions (Jean-Claude et al., 2016; Mejia et al., 2012).

Becoming culturally competent in delivering family therapy and parenting programmes in developing countries, drawing on extended family members and clergy, is a useful transformative model (Bean, Perry, & Bedell, 2002; Boyd-Franklin, 1989; Rose, 2012; Smith, 1997).Through the 'mission' model, the protocol of receiving an invitation through the pastor as 'gatekeeper' is a respectful way to gain access to work with the Haitian community, and allows an iterative process to begin. Engaging the gatekeepers in therapeutic work is key to culture and customs (Dash, 2001). These opportunities to work in partnership with elder members of the community through their skills as community protectors, cultural brokers, translators and 'para-professionals' assist in delivering therapy and parenting programmes, and provide collaboration and local ownership of learning, tailoring the method to meet the cultural values and spiritual beliefs of the community (Carberry, 2017; Dash, 2001; Desrosiers & St Fleurose, 2002).

The second and third authors are gatekeepers – both have participated as members of the community in receiving 'teaching' – and are translators/interpreters and co-facilitators with the first author. Pastor David Badio (centre) (Fig. 1) has also participated in this role in Haiti and the Dominican Republic. Pastor Jean Gerald Lafleur (left) and Pastor Genel Jean-Claude (right) who are second and third authors, respectfully, are pictured with him. The concept of 'teaching' appears to be the way in which understanding systemic family therapy processes and its effects are learned, experienced and understood. The recursive process of active 'in the moment' therapy is an ongoing emerging process linked to the participant's voicing of intervention and desired outcomes.

Expanding the Psycho-educative Approach

We are acutely aware of Haiti's history that the 'debt' paid to France for the loss of revenue due to Haiti's independent state led to a cessation of the development of free education, social advancement, health and well-being. To this end, it has been important to restore that which has been lost through joined up work and collaboration without fees. The church community is likened to a hospital in which people can encounter opportunities for healing, whether emotional, physical, financial and familial. The second author established the Restoration Christian Academy (Haiti) in 2010 to provide quality teaching initially to pre-school children in the local area of Morne Oge. This establishment has now increased its class sizes, bringing together the much-needed vision for a holistic approach to

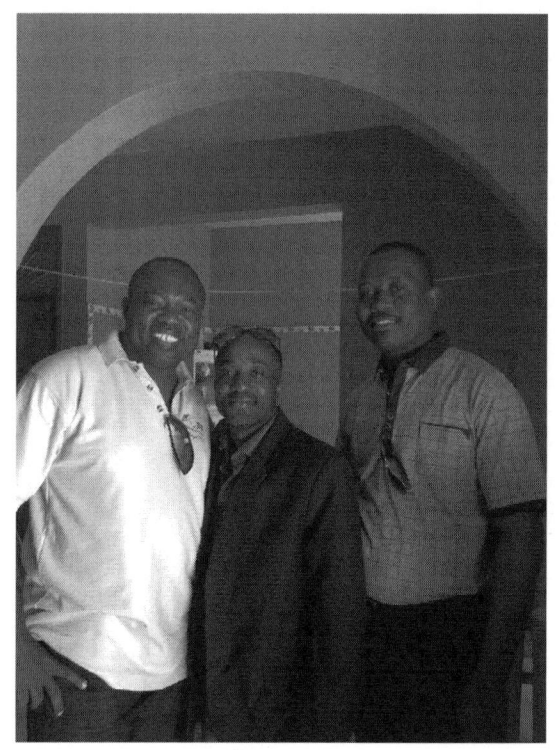

Fig. 1. Pastor Jean Gerald Lafleur (left); Pastor David Badio (centre); and Pastor Genel Jean-Claude (right). Haitian Pastors - Community Elders and Gatekeepers.

provide education for all within the community, encompassing emotional and physical well-being.

Over many years, utilising a collaborative approach with partners across the globe has proved successful and has secured sponsorship for children's education. There is a clinic established where medical services and dentistry is provided, and a child feeding programme in which local people also contribute to. Working under a culture of 'helping yourself', the local people invest their time and money into the education of their children, seeing their children as champions being groomed as future leaders of Haiti (Lafleur, 2013, 2017). With such a vision for political and social advancement, a community strategy and technique for managing and encouraging children's good behaviour and enhancing family dynamics is a key (Coker et al., 2016). Building on therapeutic work over several years and widening the scope of this work, in January 2016, the local schools were closed for 2 days while over 60 parents and 50 teachers attended the therapeutic sessions on 'activating the vision: parenting across generations' (Table 1).

It was at this session that the first author was introduced to the third author (by the second author) who attended on the second day and subsequently invited the first author to bring the 'teaching' to his congregation in the Dominican Republic in October 2016.

The Intervention

The purpose of the therapeutic work is to equip constellations of black Haitian families with strength-based strategies, utilising an approach of family therapy and systemic practice, and cultural awareness of the communities' values and beliefs, including spirituality, to illuminate 'resilience' – a subject of national pride – as a key component in Haitians' cultural beliefs, to stymie the impact of trauma, relocation and reconstruction of family and community life (Lacet, 2012; O'Grady & Orton, 2016).

It was this innate resilience that American social workers who worked with the 'tented communities' encountered after this tragic disaster in 2010, in which over 230,000 people died and more than 1.5 million people were displaced (Pan American Health Organisation, 2003). In attempting to be of service three months after the incident, they noticed that 'concepts such as family therapy, cognitive behavioural therapy, and posttraumatic stress disorder and school social work have never been heard of in Haiti by the ordinary citizen', suggesting these types of treatment would be invaluable to emotional and mental recovery (Reardon, 2010, p. 1).

In conjunction with our mission team (Fig. 2), we prepared by reflecting on the historical, political and our therapeutic approach. We also kept in mind our very first sessions in Haiti as participants streamed in to attend the systemic community family therapy sessions.

Use of Curiosity

As a mission team and collaborative team of facilitators we thought about our past memories and whether the plans for the day would be prejudiced by these past experiences. We used our systemic curiosity (Cecchin, 1987) when we talked about prejudices, meaning in therapy terms the set of fantasies, ideals, accepted historical facts, accepted truths, hunches, biases, personal feelings, moods, unrecognised loyalties, and pre-existing thoughts that contributed to our views. We used our tool of 'curiosity' to help keep an open mind, to allow the work and process to unfold. The second author in his co-facilitative role always gave permission for participants to be aware of any western influences that jarred with their Haitian values, and to take what they felt comfortable with, and open up areas for discussion.

Over the years, and in each country in which we have worked, whether Haiti or the Dominican Republic, we have wondered how many people would attend our sessions. We were curious then about the families' creation and beliefs, and in what way the families were similar to or different from each other and our own, as 'getting to know another culture allows a curiosity' (Cecchin, 1987). How had religion and class influenced the family systems? More importantly, how would the families know the sessions had been helpful?

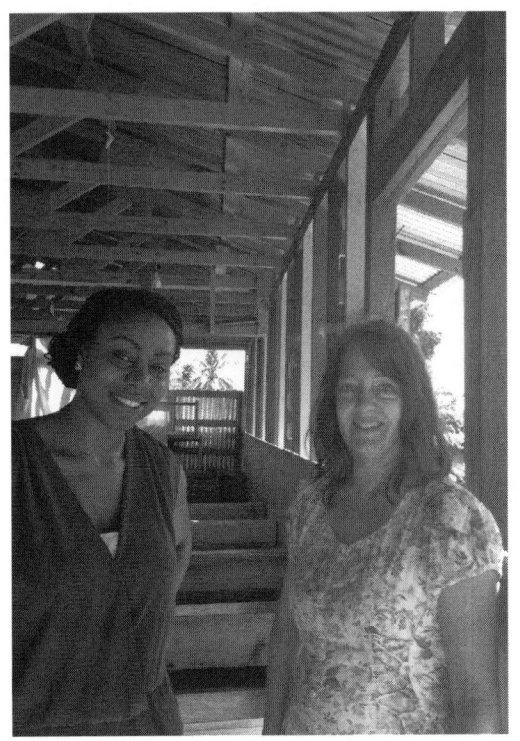

Fig. 2. Abisola Ifasawo and Alison Greenaway - UK Haiti Mission Team 2015.

Joining: Eye Contact and Safe Touch (Handshake)

It is important for family therapists to connect and engage, through a structural intervention called 'joining' (Minuchin & Fishman, 1981). In larger community settings making a non-verbal connection with participants, coupled with a verbal greeting – 'Bonjour' (Hello) or 'Bonsoir' (Good evening) – is the team's first task of engagement. In Haiti, whether the sessions were situated within the school or the church, the UK mission team stood at the entrance of the building and engaged with the participants. In the Dominican Republic, the host church team provided the welcome for participants and the visiting team found other ways to connect, whether shaking hands with the seated participants or being 'hands on' by facilitating the children's ministry while the parents attended the sessions. Making contact through 'soft eye' and 'warm handshake' is the way in which we liked to join with the families to make our interactions feel as though they all mattered. Often, if I (first author) missed a participant entering the room, I could be sure to be able to rely on a member of the community to point out that person out to me, so that we could 'join' with that person – such was the level of mutual community care.

Eye contact in many cultures can be problematic, and culturally we used this introduction to explore and talk about secure attachment. The second author as translator often used humour and cultural proverbs to talk further about eye contact and its meaning and manifestation in the Haiti culture, as eye contact on a continual basis could be seen as threatening (Gopaul-McNicol, 1993). To empower the community, in particular in the cross-cultural interactions and migration experience, we took this task further – often the community were encouraged to greet one another at the start of the session to ease the joining process and assist in alleviating shyness.

Although many of the participants may not have had the opportunity to attend school, through these sessions we were all involved in the school of life. Through the lens of this therapeutic experience, we are taught about some of the cultural norms and differences of family life and their extended systems via the route of friendships. We shared the myriad ways families define and celebrate and honour special events through rituals such as birthdays, marriages, graduation, grief and celebration of lives.

Brief Thematic Overview of the Work

In order to ascertain how the families would know the sessions had been helpful, we used inquiry and circular questioning to ask, draw and write down what they would like to have covered, and developed our conversations and tasks around these requests. Requests regarding parenting tended to include the following areas:

- How to speak with their children (with authority and care)?
- How to manage children (behaviour)?
- How to show affection/love?
- Showing good manners (in the family).
- How to discipline with love.?

To cover all these areas would be outside the scope of this chapter, so we will concentrate on the first inquiry 'How to speak to children' (with authority and care).

Attachment

Mary Ainsworth, in her book *Infancy in Uganda: Infant Care and the Growth of Love* (1967), demonstrated that in her observations, African women were so in tune with their babies, they knew the precise moment the child wanted to relieve themselves. Thus began Ainsworth's tripartite classification of 'avoidant', 'secure' and 'ambivalent' infant-mother attachment relationships. Ainsworth found that out of a sample of 28, 16 babies cried infrequently and were deemed to be 'securely' attached, using their mothers as a 'safe and secure base' juxtaposed with 7 babies, who cried frequently when either alone or in company and deemed 'ambivalent'. The remainder were babies who not perturbed when left alone, or responded to their mother when she returned and were classed as 'insecure'. When Ainsworth developed the laboratory 'strange situation', where a child is separated from their mother and observed on the reaction to separation, she assessed the attachment between low-risk (no child welfare involvement) white mothers and white babies, and compared their attachment patterns to those of low-risk African-American mothers and African-American babies. When the mothers left, a larger number of African-American babies explored the room and engaged with the 'stranger' in the room without distress than did white babies. The African-American babies appeared to be assessed as insecure-avoidant when the mother who had left the room returned (Jackson, 1996). Presumably, not unlike the African children in Ainsworth's first study, the study did not take into account that African-American babies from a collective community in which children were exposed to more caregivers as part of their socialisation process and were thus simply divergent, developing in a different way.

The Lakou system in Haiti utilises community-based parenting to support and strengthen family functioning. Many children are alone, orphaned and taken in within the community, as part of the extended family. Informal adoption in Caribbean is a normative occurrence. Likewise, many adults in Haiti and the Caribbean may have had childhood experience of maltreatment that may have influenced their well-being and parenting style (Martsoff, 2004). Hence, strengthening a sense of attachment with children and adolescents in learning how to show love is the framework for our work with Haitian families using systemic processes, cultural stories, enactments, and psycho-education, where black family therapists can draw on knowledge of mutual cultural generational history to sensitively learn and mentor therapy work in this area (Bell-Tolliver, Burgess, & Brock, 2009).

Community Tasks

We used various materials to look at attachment patterns and development in toddlers (small child) in order to address deficit parenting and 'good enough' parenting patterns. We used pens, paper, toddlers' clothes, toddlers' shoes, soaps, moisturising cream, and other items to illustrate some of the articles required to look after children. Utilising a working hypothesis of child development, and curiosity from a cultural and spiritual perspective, we began with looking at children from 0 to 18 months, and explored what a baby/toddler needs to know, to understand that they are loved, and the skills parents wanted to 'speak to children with authority and care'.

Looking at some of the bible verses, for example, *Jeremiah 1 verse 5*, '*Before I formed you in the womb I knew you, before you were born I set you apart; I appointed you as a prophet to the nations*' are useful tools. We talked about the developing child in the womb, and how talking with children can begin before they were born. As they develop, babies are attuned to sounds and their mother's and father's voices. In skills building we then began to move on to talking to babies/toddlers once born and learning to respond to a different cry – which is the baby/toddler's way of communicating their needs. Augmenting the therapeutic process with psycho-education has been a good way to engage multiple generations of families who come along together, where they can share stories along the continuum of pregnancy, including loss. We also looked at the impact of, and on parents who are unable to meet the needs of the child due to many reasons, and these were identified by the families, and community; such as trauma following a natural disaster, abandonment, addiction, not being taught by anyone, isolation, ill health. We normalised the impact of trauma on personality and behaviour, sensitively made drawings, walked these drawings around the room to see parents nodding in agreement, or seeking clarification from another parent who added to or intervened with a response which 'thickened' the conversations.

In Haiti, the second author responded to requests to sometimes use 'French' rather than 'creole', citing that certain words or phrases provided a softer translation. This sensitive 'checking in' recursively with the families was skilfully processed, utilising 'observation' to any type of distress that may require additional support by the team. This may come in the form of 'a light touch on the arm to show support'. The second author also deepened the level of translation and interpretation with Haitian metaphors, stories and fables to compare, contrast and embed into the local culture, without colonising participants' minds.

Often parents would stand up and share a personal dilemma pertaining to the subject matter, and due to the transparency of the community and church system, there appeared to be no stigma encountered.

At the end of the sessions, the community shared refreshments, picked up children from nursery and joined together in prayer and song, closing the session until the following day. On the second day, certificates of attendance were promised and subsequently issued and collected from the school office. It was important to be a witness to these parents collecting their certificates, particularly as for many, they had not received education or had their name written on an official document. It is always a very moving moment.

Managing Challenging Teenagers

One year we had a session with teenagers and their parents (Table 1) who were given the task of being participants in enactments, which in this context was to perform the solution to the dilemma of parenting 'challenging teenagers'. The young people worked in groups of three, symbolising two parents and a child, and asked the following question: Can you get into Groups of 3.... 'If you could be your own parent(s) how would you show love?'

Although extensive summation of these sessions are outside the scope of this chapter, it is pertinent to share that the children used enactment to display their desire for 'hugs', and enacted a desire for verbal affirmation with statements (while acting as the parent) such as 'son I'm so proud of you'. This was well received by their parents and caregivers, expressing lots of positive connotation from the parents in the form of humour, lots of laughter and soft smiles.

As a family therapist (first author), I found that working with multiple families requires a wide repertoire of skills, experienced preparation of the skill 'in acting moment by moment' and checking visually on body language and tone for authenticity and gentle challenge.

The child/parent relationship in this session had the opportunity to deliver the 'learning from the ground up' approach, in relation to the power dynamic of the parental subset. Systemically, ideas of 'showing how to talk to children' and 'showing how to love' used a recursive model through enactments with good outcomes.

With multiple family and transgenerational systems in attendance, the sharing of the teenagers' collective desires and knowledge, spread across the community, enhancing attachments and change. One of the mothers who attended both teenagers session, and the community sessions, wanted to share something of her experience through testimony about how these systemic family therapy community sessions had impacted her family. This is shared in the following vignette.

Vignette

Mothering – Testimony

Testimonies are often verbalised following the sessions; it is sometimes the only way in which you are aware of the impact of the work. I (first author) am always surprised at what I hear, and humbled that these wonderful people would take what they have learned in therapy back into their family lives. One mother, we shall call her Maria, offered me a letter at the end of the session and speaking in French Creole directed me to ask the second author, in his pastoral/counsellor role (Billings, 2000) to read it to me. She has given written permission to share her story in this chapter. Her testimony is reproduced and written in her verbal vernacular.

> Friday 8th January, 2016
>
> > I want to thank the staff because you do a lot for my family, for my household. I did not know how to live well with the children. … But since I've been taking these trainings, I have been coming to this workshop, my life has changed. Especially with my husband and the children. These teachings are so good for my family. If I am cooking for example, [*and*] is grating the coconut, so we work together. I want to say thanks to Karen very much because when I was younger I didn't get a chance to receive these types of teaching. My brother used to beat me a lot. Hence I thought beating [*was normal*], that's what has got changed. Please always come to help other people who have not yet [*have had*] explained that change in their life in that way. I don't have money to give you but I am very grateful for this training. May this work continue for others to explain the same change? Thank you, thank you very much. May God bless you, sister

In reading Maria's letter, I was struck by the number of people who are impacted by this intervention of systemic family therapy in transgenerational communities of families. Maria talks about being able to put into words the way her life has changed, and 'explain' to others that the difficulties experienced in childhood, can be overcome in adulthood with the right treatment and support (Martsoff, 2004).

It is not just the attendee affected, but often their mother/father/grandfather or adult children, and other family members and friends we do not see. When we look at the numbers of people who attend, we often find there is a core number of around 35–40 people who come each year. It is staggering that there are substantial numbers of people attending for the first time. This then provides us with a new starting point for each session to embed some of the 'old ground' and seek information from new participants about what they would like to focus on, incorporating their views and collectively listing the themes and dovetailing the sessions to meet their needs. We find that the themes are similar each year in terms of managing conflict and wanting to find different ways to show love and affection to their children and family members. Some of these themes are also requested by the Haitian congregation in the Dominican Republic, whose upbringing are similar, but have the added issue of migration, and racism, which affects employment, and laws on naturalisation. We find that the systemic work is very intensive, and the issue of identity and belonging within the political system can be far reaching in terms of collective stress and trauma.

Working with Families in the Dominican Republic – Dealing with Rejection

The third author asked for sessions on dealing with and 'managing family conflict' with the families in his community. We looked at the 'attachment model' and explored the area of parental 'rejection' and whether healing can truly come about. As discussed before, stories are a very powerful tool to share within the Haitian communities; it dissolves the taboo of shame, and opens up conversations that are not usually spoken about. It calls for courage, and when shared by an elder in an authentic way, opens up the channel for the possibility of healing. Below is a vignette from the third author's personal story shared with his congregation during one of the systemic community sessions in the Dominican Republic, in response to questions about attachment and whether one can heal from paternal rejection.

> *Pastor Genel Jean-Claude's testimony given in 2017 in the Dominican Republic*
>
> I was born into a Christian family, a very humble family. The name of my father is Dieuné Jean-Claude and my mother's name is Julita Petit-Frère.
>
> Both were members of the Baptist Church of l'Azile, a town in the department of Nippes, Haiti.
>
> When my mother gave birth to me, a cousin of my dad came saying 'that child is not my cousin's son, look at the shape of his mouth, the shape of his cheek, his colour', etc. ... The problem was that my father was almost white and my mother was a black woman.

Then there came the conflict, the contempt, the discrimination, among others. Also my father said that the child was not his son. I started to develop and grow; thanks to God I was very smart in school.

My dad stopped telling me that I am not his son when his father came one day to visit the family. Upon entering the house my grandfather saw me and said 'Look, this child looks just like my brother Celou' (uncle of my father), then my mother looked my dad in his eyes, and said, 'Is it true?' Then he said, 'Hmm!'

Even so, he continued to despise me because of my colour.

When I did something bad in the house, he said, 'Certainly this boy is not my son, I do not know where this boy is coming from, and he is really not my son.'

At this time of my life I felt humiliated, I was 15 years old. I said when I was 18 years old I'll change my name and my last name, when my mother heard that, she said, 'Never do that because your father knows very well that you are his son, it's because he let himself be carried away by his mother and his cousin, your father is very close to his relatives. Do not listen to him, my son'.

At the age of 19 they sent me to Port-au-Prince, the capital of Haiti, to continue my classical studies. From there the Most High God began to use me in the preaching and I began to travel within the country on missionary trips. In a vacation period I went to spend the holidays with them [family]. After greeting my beloved ones, my dad told me, 'I have information that you are taking the gospel in the village. Then, my son, continue to preach the word of God, because I did not show you another way than this, continue like that, my son. I am happy to know that you are preaching the Word of God.' One day I went out with him. When he arrived at the place, he was telling his people, this is my second son, he was very happy saying that.

Thank God because he saved my dad from that resentment. After all that, my dad loved me as his own eyes. In the same way God gave me a lot of love for my dad and I did not change my name. With the love that God has given me for him, I felt proud to be the son of my dad and bring his last name.

I continue to thank God that he has helped us overcome and resolve this family conflict.

Systemic Family Therapy with Transgenerational Communities **549**

As a Christian, in this process that I was, I learned that we must submit our hearts to the Holy Spirit.

Whatever the level of the conflict, whatever the scope, we must let God enlighten us (Jean-Claude, 2017).

The process of a shared testimony is that in retelling the story of the episode, stories unheard become part of the patchwork of undiscovered narratives which can and do give meaning to another's story in which tools for overcoming challenges are shared. In addition, being a witness to another person's struggle gives credence to another person's journey and shows them that they are not alone and can approach others for support. The preservation of the family against distress and conflict may be the highest context marker for Haitian families in seeking therapeutic help through systemic community sessions, in order to simply ameliorate family dynamics and conflict in intergenerational relationships.

Separation, loss and collective trauma, from disasters such as the earthquake of 2010 and Hurricane Matthew in 2016, provided an impetus for the community to seek a sense of solidarity for transgenerational healing. However, a longer-term vision appears to have been sought, embraced, and is ongoing as families encourage each other and testify of how they use these processes to consult with one another in a reflective and reflexive process, sharing skills, techniques and strategies.

Pastors as Counsellors and Translators

Haiti is a patriarchal society and working alongside male pastors who were able to use aspects of themselves in both the translation and expanding upon their

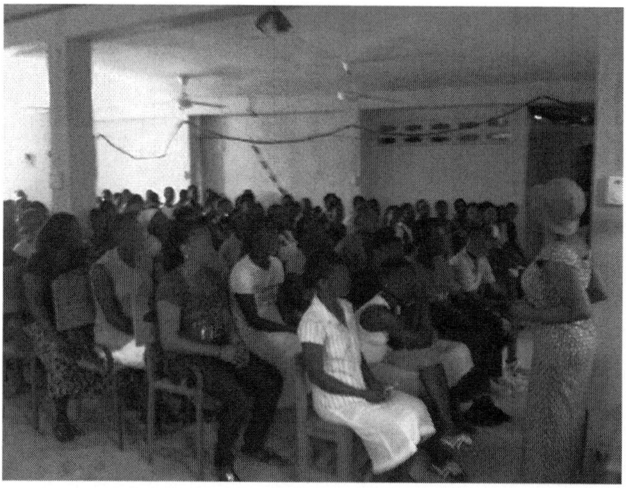

Fig. 3. Karen Carberry (left) delivering Community based transgenerational Systemic Family Therapy with Pastor Jean Gerald Lefleur (out of picture shot).

personal experience is reminiscent of 'in the moment' reflective and reflexive practice. They have drawn on their strong pastoral training and experience of addressing large groups of community members, and are sensitive to the impact of racism, social and political aspects of life which affect their members, and wider community. They are able to draw on their cultural beliefs and customs regarding low mood, and the metaphors and cultural meanings around this. They are aware that:

> Existing theories and interventions for depression are constructed by specific groups, namely middle-class white professionals working primarily with middle-class white clients in post-industrial urban Western settings. These theories and interventions tend to be uncritically transferred to other affected groups without the benefit of cultural translation. (Falicov, 2003)

Therefore, during our work, the Pastors at the start of the sessions give permission for members not to take on European thinking over Haitian custom through this therapeutic process, while at the same time allow descriptions for patterns of feelings with explanations that resonate with participants. To confirm purity of translation, the second author utilises impromptu reverse translations with the first author. That is the second author speaks in Creole and the first author translates it into English. This has happened in Haiti and the Dominican Republic. In addition, where participants were fluent in Spanish and not Creole, the third Pastor will translate the English into Creole and Spanish when necessary. Thus, the role of Pastors as translators has a wide ranging responsibility, as elders within the community, with a 'Fathering' role, and gatekeeper and counsellor.

Although a more extensive discussion on fathering and fatherhood in the context of the pastors as fathers of a community is outside the scope of this chapter, we are aware that the experience of fatherhood and being fathered in the black community is a sensitive subject. The first author has witnessed over the years, how both the second and third co-authors have comprehensively shared their experiences of being fathered, with their communities, and as elders who spiritually oversee and father communities. Their testimonies have been imperative in detoxifying the taboo subject of fatherlessness, together with strategies for hope and healing.

We looked at the attachment cycle of children of secure and insecure attachment, together with the impact of trauma and transgenerational loss. The role of the facilitator is key in shaping emerging patterns of communication so that multiple voices and perspectives are honoured and the tension is worked with. Having worked extensively over 20 years with translators in therapy in her role as manager of family centres and child contact centres in the UK, the first author is attuned in her practice to the emotional resilience of translators 'moment by moment', and will come alongside translators to draw them back from moving on from translation, into interpretation, particularly if the therapeutic process in which the family therapist is leading comes to a premature end; the first author will ask the translator to 'pause' and wait. Burck (2005) encapsulates this well in that:

> The insight from examining what a therapist represents to the other and how the other feels and so reacts provides a way to accept and resolve ambiguous or conflicted reactions from insiders

Or, in this case, co-facilitators who are translating. We may need to wait for a spiritual movement or change in atmosphere within the community, that elicits more information or an utterance of insight from one or others within the room preparing to speak. Therefore, although the therapeutic process may look as if it has come to an end, it may just be beginning to move to another level of revelation or complete the ending of the process in a more measured way, with the translator attuned to this movement, or ending the session within the acceptable cultural norms.

Likewise in the collaboration with translators these situations have to be respectfully managed, framed and understood differently, taking account of prejudices, for example western thought process versus the preferred indigenous values, so that professional co-working relationship is progressive. This entails the family therapist stepping back, reflecting internally (Rober, 1999) and recognising that consequences of the represented identity in the local environment and tacitly gaining a fresh perspective on what might otherwise be a disrupting experience for the outsider therapist. Cultural theory then provides complementary approaches to cultural meaning and cuts across theoretical borders, and requires acute cultural competency in the therapists' approach when working with translators (Tribe & Lane, 2009).

Through our vignettes, we can see that the historical and generational impact of skin colour issues prevails, together with the sensitive topics of paternity, belonging and existence. Likewise, the impact of migration in mental health and wellbeing must be noted. It is to this end that I (first author) learned that not only are these toxic subjects hurtful, there is also the reality that many people do not have a sense of belonging because they do not have a birth certificate to prove that they exist. If you do not exist, you cannot get married, or travel out of the country. This therapeutic work not only gives an understanding of the reason behind pain and trauma, but by hearing stories through testimony, there presents a space for an isomorphic process of a collective witness As a person attending, others witness another's presence, that one exists, irrespective of one's legal status.

To take this notion of existence further, in 2015, the first and second author felt that having a certificate with one's name on it, proves that they exist. The third author also acted on this same notion. The certificate as an external object gave validity to those who attended that they had received training. Participants could share this learned knowledge with each other, and also be 'teachers' and part of a whole community group of recursive inter-relational educators. That one is important, and matters. This phenomenon is a concept that the first author has coined 'isomorphic mattering' – everyone learning together, everyone in existence, and witnessed as existing, and enabled to learn and teach others, whether Pastors, family therapists, children, or the adults in the wider community transgenerational system. New theories in cultural competence are essential for therapeutic healing (Chu, Leino, Pflum, & Sue, 2016), and 'isomorphic mattering' is a new component in the essential development of new theories of cultural competency in family therapy and psychotherapy.

Summary and Conclusion

This work is rich in systemic experiences, and with a dearth of literature on Haitian families in family therapy, and black family therapists working with black multi-generational families; this model of family therapy, facilitated within a different cultural environment, will contribute to a reconstruction of theory building based on the current models of systemic practice. This collaborative work will also contribute towards the body of work on family therapy with transgenerational communities as a healing intervention.

Ethical Considerations

In recent years, the international press has exposed some disturbing information regarding the conduct of some employees working for NGOs who have taken advantage sexually of the poor and destitute. NGOs have been accused of coming to Haiti and setting up their own projects without ascertaining from the government what is required. Responsible Pastors or elders as gatekeepers are imperative to safeguard vulnerable communities and avoid mental and emotional colonisation. Gatekeepers are aware of what support is required within their communities, and are able to galvanise services that are suitable for their communities. As family therapists and missionaries ministering in non-western cultures, one must be sensitive to the issue of vulnerability. As therapists we must relearn how to manage conflict with families and, when necessary just as we exhort our clients towards a theory of change, we must learn to use shared values, mediation or prayer effectively to build the bonds of love, fellowship, and to develop discernment for safety, starting in our own clinical and training institutions. (Lingenfelter & Mayers, 2003).

Each year the Haitian communities illustrate their strong survival mechanism by having an annual 'celebration of lives saved' on the annual anniversary of the 2010 earthquake. Tens of thousands of people march around the city, stopping to pray at each strategic point, for example, the Banking Centre. What a difference in memorial meetings from the West! The development of cultural competence in the family therapist and family therapy training must be addressed and incorporated seamlessly in training and supervision in order to have maximum impact on the lives of the families we work with, nationally and internationally, moving out of our clinics and into the community.

References

Ainsworth, M. (1967). *Infancy in Uganda: Infant care and the growth of love*. Baltimore, MD: The Johns Hopkins Press.

Asen, A. (2002). Multiple family therapy: An overview. *Journal of Family Therapy, 24,* 3–10.

Bean, R. A., Perry, B. J., & Bedell, T. M. (2002). Developing culturally competent marriage and family therapists: Treatment guidelines for non-African-American therapists working with African-American families. *Journal of Marital and Family Therapy, 28*(2), 153–164.

Bell-Tolliver, L., Burgess, R., & Brock, J. L. (2009). African American therapists working with African American families: An exploration of the strengths perspective in treatment. *Journal of Marital & Family Therapy, 35*(3), 293–307.

Bennett, M. M., & Eberts, S. (2015). The experience of short-term humanitarian aid workers in Haiti. *Mental Health, Religion & Culture, 18*(5), 319–329.

Bibb, A., & Casimir, G. J. (1996). Haitian families. In M. McGoldrick, J. Giordano, & J. K. Pearce (Eds.), *Ethnicity & family therapy* (pp. 97–111). New York, NY: The Guilford Press.

Billings, A. (2000). Pastors or counsellors. In D. Willows & J. Swinton (Eds.), *Spiritual dimensions of pastoral care: Practical theology in a multidisciplinary context.* London: Jessica Kingsley.

Boyd-Franklin, N. (1989). *Black families in therapy: A multi-systems approach.* New York, NY: The Guilford Press.

Boyd-Franklin, N., & Bry, B. H. (2000). *Reaching out in family therapy: Home-based, school and community interventions.* New York, NY: The Guilford Press.

Burck, C. (2005). Living in several languages: Implications for therapy. *Journal of Family Therapy, 26,* 314–318.

Carberry, K. (2016, October 18–19). Haiti after the earthquake: Humanitarian family therapy via workshop in a community setting. *Bridging & humanifying family therapy practice conference,* Crowne Plaza Hotel, Chani Airport, Singapore. PPIS FTI [PDF document]. Retrieved from http://fticonferencesg.wixsite.com/ppisfti/workshop-info-1

Carberry, K. (2017, April 26–28). *Black masculinity and fathering. Who fathers the father?* Ambleside: The 3rd Bedfordshire International Systemic Spring School, Luton: University of Bedfordshire.

Carberry, K. (2017, February 1). Workshop certificate in parenting: Haitian families of the Caribbean and isomorphic mattering. Creativity in research. *Research Graduate School Annual Conference,* University of Bedfordshire, England.

CBN News. (2016). Why so many pastors are leaving the church. Retrieved from http://www1.cbn.com/cbnnews/us/2016/January/Why-So-Many-Pastors-Are-Leaving-the-Church

Cecchin, G. (1987). Hypothesising-circularity-neutrality revisited: An invitation to curiosity. *Family Process, 26,* 405–413.

Chu, J., Leino, A., Pflum, S., & Sue, S. (2016). A Model for the theoretical basis of cultural competency to guide psychotherapy. *Professional Psychology, Research and Practice, 47*(1), 18–29.

Coker, F., Williams, A., Hayes, L., Hartmann, J., & Harvey, C. (2016). Exploring the needs of diverse consumers experiencing mental illness and their families through family psychoeducation. *Journal of Mental Health, 25*(3), 197–203.

Dallos, R., & Draper, R. (2005). *An introduction to family therapy: Systems theory and practice.* New York, NY: McGraw-Hill.

Dance, M. (2016). *Pastors are not quitting in droves.* Lifeway. Retrieved from https://www.lifeway.com/pastors/2016/09/28/pastors-are-not-quitting-in-droves/

Dash, J. M. (2001). *Culture and customs of Haiti.* Westport, CT: Greenwood Press.

Davis, W. (2014). *Debriefing survivors of major incidents. Course Workbook.* Leicester: The APT Press.

Desroisiers, A., & St Fleurose, S. (2002). Treating Haitian patients: Key cultural aspects. *American Journal of Psychotherapy*, *56*(4), 508–521.
Doherty, W. J., & Beaton, J. M. (2000). Family therapists, community and civil renewal. *Family Process*, *39*(2), 149–161.
Dubois, L. (2013). *Haiti: The aftershocks of history*. London: Picador.
Edmond, Y. M., Randolph, S. M., & Richard, G. L. (2007). The lakou system: A cultural, ecological analysis of mothering in rural Haiti. *Journal of Pan African Studies*, *2*(1), 1–9.
Ellison, R. (1952). *The invisible man*. New York, NY: Random House.
Falicov, C. (2003). Culture, society and gender in depression. *Journal of Family Therapy*, *25*(4), 371–387.
Farmer, P. (2011). *Haiti after the earthquake*. New York, NY: Public Affairs.
Gerard, P. (2010). *Haiti: The tumultuous history – From pearl of the Caribbean to broken nation*. Basingstoke: Palgrave Macmillian.
Goode-Cross, D. T. (2011). Same difference: Black therapists' experience of same-race therapeutic dyads. *Professional Psychology: Research and Practice*, *42*(5), 368–374.
Gopaul-McNicol, S. A. (1993). *Working with West Indian families*. New York, NY: The Guildford Press.
Heinl, R. D., & Heinl, N. G. (2005). *Written in blood: The story of the Haitian people, 1492–1995*. Lanham, MD: University Press of America.
Hoffman, L. (1991). A reflexive stance family therapy. *Journal of Strategic and Systemic Therapies*, *10*, 4–17.
Jackson, J. F. (1996). An Experimental procedure and scales for assessing relationships in African-American infants – Alternatives to Ainswooth models. In *Handbook of tests ad measurements for black populations*. Oakland, CA: Cobb & Henry Publishers.
Jean-Claude, G. (2017, October 28). *Testimony during community family therapy session on Sunday at Tesliogos Church, Santo Domingo, Dominican Republic*.
Jean-Claude, G., De los Santos, E., & Popa, N. (2016). *Incidence of the Evangelical Pastoral of children from 6 to 10 years in socio-spiritual development in the community of Mira Cielo, San Cristóbal, Dominican Republic*. Unpublished thesis.
Kasiram, M., & Thaver, W. (2013). Community family therapy: A model for family and community problem solving and development in South America. *Journal of Family Psychotherapy*, *24*(2), 155–172.
Lacet, C. E. (2012). *Trauma and resilience: The relocation experience of Haitian women earthquake survivors*. Boston, MA: College University Libraries. Retrieved from http://hdl.handle.net/2345/2744
Lafleur, J. G. (2013, January 18). Restore Haiti message. [Video File]. Retrieved from https://www.youtube.com/watch?v=HXqkTjM6Twg. Accessed on June 6, 2018.
Lafleur, J. G. (2017). *Address to parents and community during 7th annual xonference Restoration Christian Academy at Restoration Ministries, Morne Oge, Jacmel, Haiti*.
Lafleur, J. G. (2017, October 11). *Testimony during community family therapy session Thursday at Restoration Ministries, Restoration Ministries, Morne Oge, Jacmel, Haiti*.
Lagos, C., & Chaura. (2015). Working with transgenerational/international trauma: The implication of epigenetic considerations and transcultural perspectives in psychotherapy. *The Psychotherapist*, *59*, 23–25.
LaRose, S. (1975). The Haitian lacou, land, family and ritual. In A. Marks & R. Romer (Eds.), *Family and kinship in Middle America and the Caribbean* (pp. 482–501). Willemstadt: Institute of Higher Studies in Curacao.
Lifeway Research. (2015). Despite stresses few pastors give up on ministry. Retrieved from https://lifewayresearch.com/2015/09/01/despite-stresses-few-pastors-give-up-on-ministry/. Accessed on September 15, 2015.
Lingenfelter, S. G., & Mayers, M. K. (2003). *Ministering cross-culturally: An incarnational model for personal relationships*. Grand Rapids, MI: Baker Academic.

Lopez-Zeron, G., & Blow, A. (2017). The role of relationships and families in healing from trauma. *Journal of Family Therapy, 39*, 580–597.

Malik, R. (2016). Incorporating spirituality in systemic family therapy in communities. *Bridging & humanifying family therapy practice conference*, PPIS Family Therapy Institute, Singapore.

Mandanes, C. (1991). Strategic family therapy. In A. S. Gurman & P. David (Eds.), *Handbook of family therapy*. Philadelphia, PA: Bruner/Mazel.

Martsoff, M. (2004). Childhood maltreatment and mental and physical health in Haitian Adults. *Journal of Nursing Scholarship, 36*(4), 293–299.

Maslow, A. H. (2013). *A Theory of Human Motivation*. Floyd, VA: Wilder Publications.

McDowell, T. (2004). Exploring the racial experience of therapists in training: A critical race theory perspective. *The American Journal of Family Therapy, 32*(4), 305–324.

Mejia, A., Calam, R., & Sanders, M. (2012). A review of parenting programs in developing countries: Opportunities and challenges for preventing emotional behavioral difficulties in children. *Clinical Child Family Psychological Review, 15*, 163–175.

Minuchin, S., & Fishman, H. (1981). *Family therapy techniques*. Cambridge, MA: Harvard University Press.

Munroe, M. (2001). *Understanding the purpose and power of prayer. Earthly licence for heavenly interference*. Nassau: Faith Ministries International.

O'Grady, A. O., & Orton, J. D. (2016). Resilience processes during cosmology episodes during cosmology episodes: Lessons learned from the Haiti earthquake. *Journal of Psychology & Theology, 44*(2), 109–123.

Pan American Health Organisation. (2003). *Haiti: Profile of the health services system* (pp. 1–19). Retrieved from http://new.paho.org/hq/dmdocuments/2010/Health_System_Profile-Haiti_2003.pdf.

Patterson, M. (2018). Are NGO's in Haiti doing more harm than good. In *America The Jesuit Review*. Retrieved from https://www.americamagazine.org/politics-society/2018/02/22/are-ngos-haiti-doing-more-harm-good. Accessed on February 22, 2020.

Preston-Shoot, M. (2007). *Effective group work*. London: Palgrave Macmillan.

Rahill, G., Jean-Gilles, M., Thomlison, B., & Pinto-Lopez, E. (2011). Metaphors as contextual evidence for engaging Haitian clients in practice: A case study. *American Journal of Psychotherapy, 65*(2), 133–149.

Reardon, C. (2010, August 6). Service on a global stage: –Social workers' response to Haiti earthquake. *Social Work Today*. Retrieved from http://www.socialworktoday.com/archive/exc_061810.shtml. Accessed on February 20, 2020.

Rober, P. (1999). The therapist's inner conversation in family therapy practice: Some ideas about the self of the therapist, therapuetic impasse, and some of the processes of reflection. *Family Process, 38*, 209–228.

Rose, G. (2012). *Health promotion –: Spiritual healing*. Bloomington, IN: AuthorHouse.

Sloand, E., Gebrian, B., & Astone, N. A. (2012). Fathers' belief about parenting and father's clubs to promote child health in rural Haiti'. *Qualitative Health Research, 22*(4), 488–498.

Smith, A. (1997). *Navigating the deep river: Spirituality in African American families*. Cleveland, OH: United Church Press.

Thomas, D. F. (2013). *H is for happiness. Choose Life International Publications*. Kingston: Xpress Litho Limited.

Tribe, R., & Lane, P. (2009). Working with interpreters across language and culture in mental health. *Journal of Mental Health, 18*(3), 233–241.

Chapter 28

Engaging with Racialized Process in Clinical Supervision: Political or Personal

Isha Mckenzie-Mavinga

Introduction

Racialized process manifests from the microinjection of racism and the ways that it becomes embedded in behavioral and psychological patterns. It embodies both conscious and unconscious responses to racism. This process is impacted by the intergenerational and socio-cultural contexts of racism, passed on via families, systematic institutional racism and individual internalized racism.

Racialized process that occurs in therapeutic work and clinical supervision shows up in the ways that therapist and supervisor acknowledge and address, or deny the impact of racism in the therapeutic space. It is an element of the dynamic process between therapist clients and supervisor. It is political and personal and therefore an important occurrence in the psychological, physical and emotional process of therapeutic triads.

The cause of actively addressing the impact of racism in mental health and psychological support is often seen as political rather than psychological. Needless to say, this cause straddles on both sides of the coin, and in the Western world, it is unlikely that one aspect of this socio-cultural dichotomy can be facilitated without attention to the other. Attempts to divide these two vital elements can distract from the traumatic nature of racism and hinder empathic connection.

Until the late twentieth century, ideas about working with the impact of racism and its contribution to black psychology and low self-esteem were excluded in mainstream traditional theories about how humans cope with trauma, hurt, loss and oppression. Previously, political discourses that considered women's oppression and oppressive views on homosexuality dominated the reflective process of literature and training institutions and efforts to engage with black mental health were marginalized.

Training courses in the UK did not specifically place attention on the phenomenon of racism and its contribution to anxiety and mental ill health (Howitt & Owusu Bempah, 1994). Instead, patterned responses about competing oppressions were projected into the center of training spaces and these responses filtered into therapeutic spaces. Individuals argued that discussing racism would place this oppression in a hierarchical position over and above other important oppressions. A kind of a political bartering was applied rather than a willingness to address racism. This outcry was a form of denial and silenced students who wanted to redress the imbalance. This important concern was denied adequate reflection in training groups due to fear, naiveté and the guilt of white students and lecturers. Silence and shutdowness seemed to remain on the surface of the educational system.

Concerned groups wanted to examine ways to draw attention to providing appropriate mental health services for black people, which considered the impact of racism, disempowerment and disenfranchisement.

Dalal (2002) addressed the racism in psychology. Burke (1984), Fletchman Smith (2011) and others produced literature about transforming attitudes to black people and mental health.

This chapter will also address this theme and I shall share some useful concepts to provide a framework for addressing racialized process in supervisory and clinical settings. I have called these concepts: "black Western archetype," "recognition trauma" and "a black empathic approach" (Mckenzie-Mavinga, 2009, 2016). Examples of casework will be used with the permission of contributing therapists.

Moving on from neo-liberalist responses seems to suggest that institutional racism has been dealt with, this chapter will address the ethical and socio-cultural context of actively attending to this divide that has often not been fully addressed when supporting clinical work.

Using some examples, I shall reflect on how this feature has been experienced by black women of African and Caribbean heritage who have attended Transcultural supervision. Black women have a particular cultural disposition with regards to the intersection of racism, sexism and systematic oppression. Often the black Western Archetype that mitigates against her, pushes her into oppression burn out. The intersection of these oppressions cause her low self-esteem and unrecognized efforts to work harder to prove her worth. The accumulation of these factors can result in unethical practice and care negligence toward the black woman.

In the UK, day-to-day racism still takes place, police brutality to black men continues to occur and

> Past and recent research suggests that some groups – notably black Caribbean, black African and other black groups – are over-represented in psychiatric hospitals. [7] The high number of African Caribbean people being diagnosed with schizophrenia is well documented, with some studies reporting between two to eight times higher rates of diagnosis compared to the White population. [8]

Secondary to black men' Women from the black and mixed White/black groups were two or more times likely than the general population to be admitted to psychiatric hospitals' (MIND Mental Health Facts and Statistics, 2010. Retrieved from www.mind.org.uk/mental_health_a-z/8105_mental_health_facts_and_statistics).

More recent data show that in comparison with the data produced in 2010 there has been little change in the presentation of black people in the mental health system.

Proportion of people in contact with secondary mental health and learning disability services on March 31, 2016 who were subject to the Mental Health Act:

White: 1.2%
Mixed: 2.5%
Asian or Asian British: 1.9%
Black or Black British: 4.8%
Other Ethnic Groups: 1.3%.

Proportion of inpatients in secondary mental health and learning disability services on March 31, 2016 who were detained under the Mental Health Act:

White: 54.7%
Mixed: 68.8%
Asian or Asian British: 64.4%
Black or Black British: 69.6%
Other Ethnic Groups: 50.8%.

Uses of the Mental Health Act and Ethnicity REF

Certain traumas linked to the evolution of white supremacy and systematic oppression to the black community contribute to the inflation of these statistics.

Oppression in the workplace, racism in the education system and the impact of internalized racism harbored within black families and individuals, continue to take a toll on the psychology of black people, causing physical and psychological illness.

The victims and survivors of racism generally address challenges to racism themselves, consequently black people have been the educators of others in this scenario that often denies their own learning. These efforts can exacerbate trauma caused by racism.

White females have dominated psychotherapy in the UK, yet ironically the traditional theories they inherit are mainly from white males of the early twentieth century. Consequently an inbuilt white patriotic, phallocentric stance has perpetrated the denial of racism in the profession. The backlash to this was white feminism that has not fully taken on board black women's needs. Accountability for the impact of this discourse must be recognized for transformation to take place.

Politics have always been a key motivator for mental well-being, peace and equilibrium; therefore, one cannot deny the close relationship between the couch and the campaigner. I work with a supervisee who often feels the urge to liberate and educate her clients about the impact of racism. This manifests in her recognition of powerful feelings associated with the mention of racism or related experiences. I call this area of racialized process, recognition trauma (Mckenzie-Mavinga, 2009). She feels an urge to cheer on the client who observes micro oppressions. She wants to save the client who is immersed in internalized racism. This brings out the campaigner in her and suppresses her empathy for the client's situation. As a black woman with a black client, the intense connection of their experiences causes her to behave toward the client's experience as though it were her own, thus projecting her powerful feelings of rage and pursuance of liberation into the racialized process, before offering an opportunity to work through the client's experience.

Embodied within a cause to model, healing and transforming the scars of history and heritage and the impact of colonialism slavery and racism on generations lie a stubbornness alongside willingness to participate in such a volatile theme (Ackbar 1996). This contradiction causes fear, guilt, rage and denial that can fester under a layer of shame.

Attending to racialized process has been inhibited by the idea that addressing racism is solely a political stance imposing on a psychological discourse, or viewed as educating clients and therefore non-therapeutic. Therefore, it is often deemed inappropriate to explicitly mention racism. Following this stance can create unethical practice that denies the opportunity to process racism. Interestingly, this response is not applied when feminist discourse influences psychotherapy. Although primarily advocating women's empowerment, feminist theory in its early stages whitewashed women's experiences, thus further excluding the intersection of racialized process on black women. Inadvertently, racism was operating within this discourse. Black feminists such as bell hooks challenged this exclusion in the book *Ain't I a Woman?* (hooks, 1987)

Although feminist discourse helped to challenge male domination and female subservience, the assumption that a feminist approach can be applied to all women was an error. In thinking about the cultural implications of assimilation and racism on black people and people of color, this approach needed to be challenged. This challenge breaks open the assumption that understanding the pain of sexism also means understanding the pain of racism. While appropriately useful for women's oppression, feminist understanding is not directly transferable to the experience of racism. Therefore, a discourse that evokes action on the impact of racism has become necessary.

Developing discourses brought to light the intersectionality of oppressions influenced by institutional racism. Micro experiences of racism and attitudes of professionals working in Mental Health services were highlighted. A spotlight shined on deaths in police custody and mental health institutions (IPCC for England & Wales, 2015/2016).

Many of these were black men. A new phenomenon of listening to the voices of mental health users was activated. Projects that supported the role of therapy and befriending black mental health evolved.

History, heritage, cultural influences and the impact of racism were some of the key concerns for professionals working with individuals in this group and therefore the role of training and appropriate supervision also needed to be scrutinized. Accreditation processes dodged specific examination of the therapist and supervisor's ability to work with aspects of diversity where racialized process was present. A study carried out. Mckenzie-Mavinga (2005) demonstrated that students in training experienced the least support for exploring black issues on their placements. This response forms institutional denial and serves to perpetuate racism in clinical settings. De Grury (2005) describes this phenomenon as "Cognitive dissonance."

Some therapists fear the consequences of being with clients in a racialized process. Reasons for this can vary, depending on personal experience and awareness and supervisory approaches. They may fear the client's rage about the injustice of racism. Often rage in this context is interpreted as madness. Some therapists feel unsupported and silenced due to institutional neglect and supervisors burying their heads in the sand and remaining silent and inactive. This leads to confusion and hopelessness and perpetuates racism. I have known therapists who do not share their experience of black clients with their white supervisors. So what gets transferred into supervision and the therapeutic space?

I have also known supervises who work actively with racialized process in client work and supervision. In the following scenario, it is clear that the acknowledgment of racism and internalized racism are integral features of the work between therapist, supervisor and client.

> PM (a black African Caribbean Therapist) worked with a black female client who was a social work trainee on placement. The client's work was located in a very white area. Within the predominantly white organization she worked in, she was being accused of being aggressive when she disagreed with certain things. PM wondered if as a black woman in this context, she was experiencing racism.
>
> Drawing on her own experiences of institutionalized racism and her awareness of feeling silenced, PM took a risk to ask the client directly if she felt she was experiencing racism. The client did not answer directly, but she shared that her placement supervisor had also mentioned to her about the possibility of racism. The client had not specifically mentioned racism, but by having it pointed out to her she became aware that there was an opportunity to talk about it if she wanted to. This example demonstrates that once the therapist feels supported enough to address racism, silence about racism can be broken. Insertion of

the term "racism" into the therapeutic dialogue can be seen as both political and personal. On the one hand bringing to consciousness and naming a socio-cultural concept that is generally used to underpin the scenario described by the client. On the other hand embracing the client's personal experience empathically by drawing on the therapist's knowledge and experience of racism. I call this a black empathic approach, because it explicitly addresses the racialized process.

PM also worked with a white supervise who did not have black people in her social circle. The supervisee was sharing something about a client. She was being quite detrimental and using negative language like the client was "difficult," "defensive." PM noticed that this supervise was not usually judgmental about clients. It transpired that the client being discussed was a young Muslim woman.

PM used an educational stance by pointing out aspects of Islamophobia such as stereotyping and attacks on Muslims and the socio-cultural negativism towards them. As a supervisory tool, this helped the therapist who seemed to be naive about this area of oppression. At the following supervision meeting the therapist had become more empathic towards her Muslim client. In this situation PM challenged the supervisee's racism by using her knowledge of Muslim oppression, to inform and enlighten her about her own attitude towards this client.

The approach to racialized process in this scenario may be viewed as both political and therapeutic, because it served to open the therapist's naiveté and conduct, resulting in reflective practice and personal development, which can in the long run foster greater empathy for the client.

PM recalled that she had attended a transcultural supervision group, where she presented a situation about a young African woman struggling with intercultural and intergenerational influences from family heritage and being at university in the UK. She feels that she now has a much better understanding and acceptance that "this is a norm, their reality." "I recognize that my stereotype of how 'normal' families are supposed to be needed to be challenged because I felt judgmental of the parents putting stress on their young people", She said. It was important that I should be aware of cultural heritage of African women and not judge. She feels supported by her black male supervisor who acknowledges and names racism and she also appreciates the opportunity to discuss these things in the group supervision.

The parallels in these scenarios highlight an essential contribution to working with racialized process. PM's shared experience shows that if openness about racism in the therapeutic space is integrated into the supervisory setting, the therapeutic triad can assist progression of the relationship with the client in this area.

In both situations, internalized oppression is attended to and supported. In the first situation, PM draws the client's attention to racism that she seems unable to name, whether she is aware of it or not. This was the second time that the client had received feedback that named the possibility of racism. This client's unawareness or inability to name and address without prompt and support is a significant feature of racialized process. A culturally appropriate gaze was offered to enlighten and encourage the client to use the therapeutic space to explore the impact of racism. Here an institutional intergenerational discourse that addressed racism via supervision, between senior practitioner, therapist and with clients becomes reinforced and eliminates the possibility of unethical practice.

In the second scenario, the therapist as supervisor to a white therapist presents an attitude of challenge rather than collusion. She demonstrates anti-oppressive practice that therefore works against perpetuating racism. This is where anti-racism as a political tool weaves itself into the therapeutic relationship. A necessary interruption to the impingement of racism on the black person's psyche and an expectation that white therapists will engage with this process in their personal development and therapeutic practice. This therapist's sincerity in modeling an empowering black consciousness in therapeutic discourse assists the white therapist to reflect on her attitude toward her black Muslim clients. If the political outlet was missing in this scenario, the attitude of the therapist might fall foul to collusion and lack of congruent facilitation in a racialized process.

Institutionalized neglect in this area must come under scrutiny. Therefore, attention to racialized process in the training of psychotherapists, psychologists and counselors is important. One major concern is the accreditation of both newly qualified and senior practitioners that leaks a certain lethargy into mainstream training with regards to addressing racialized process in practice.

Guidelines for ethical training and practice need to be explicit about addressing trauma imposed by oppression and more specifically trauma due to the impact of racism. Silence and denial of racism lead to the perpetuation of racism on training courses and in the consulting room, and yes this is political.

Just as male therapists would need to have worked on their own sexism to facilitate women and other men through the impact of sexism. Likewise, white therapists would need to work on their racism to facilitate racialized process. However white guilt, internalized racism, causing denial and fear of being labeled racist sometimes gets in the way.

Denial is a form of silence. It is a secret with an unconscious intention to withhold, usually due to fear of humiliation and persecution.

In some situations, individuals feel silenced by institutions and uninformed lecturers, creating taboo and denial. Shame and humiliation play a significant role in holding this discourse in place. In the following example, KS, a black therapist, describes how she felt shut down and immobilized in her work as a therapist in a school.

> KS. A few things come to mind when I think about the ways in which I have increasingly noticed racism impacting on my therapeutic work. The setting in which I work is an all girls secondary school. The school student population is predominantly white British and white European and there are very few black staff of which I am one.
>
> I have noticed the descriptive language used by staff when talking about black girls falls into stereotyping. They make references to behavior being "aggressive" or black students having a "gang mentality" with some staff feeling threatened. I don't believe students are taken seriously if they express they or their parents are being subject to racism. This has been viewed as pulling out the "race card." Cultural norms regarding presentation of hair and hairstyles are deemed not appropriate – some of which I agree, but not all.

In sessions I have had a student openly talk about her daily experience of racism both in and out of school. She didn't support Black History Month as she felt the school didn't teach her anything about her history at least nothing she would feel proud of.

> Some of these issues have been both discussed and explored in my transcultural supervision group only, so far, but not in my work supervision at the school. Acknowledgement and support are given within this safe environment. Both to be heard and understood is important but also being challenged to take action in some shape or form is where I grow personally and professionally, and although it can feel uncomfortable it's also empowering. In all honesty only in these supervision groups do I feel fully supported regarding concerns about the impact of racism in my therapeutic work. This is because it is talked about, thought about and validated. This enables me to step back from my concerns and view them from different angles without criticism or judgment.
>
> I am being supported to find my professional and personal voice amongst my peers in team meetings. I struggle to assert myself and speak confidently. I want to be able to challenge certain viewpoints and assumptions without feeling I need to do so apologetically and to express exactly what I feel without censoring or filtering. I'm still on that journey but simply being in the group is affirming and I know I am not alone.

KS is clear that she is experiencing racism in the organization that she works in. She is also clear that some of the black students she counsels are experiencing racism within the school and in their daily lives. I call this every day racism. In a sanctuary separate from boyhood sexism, racism appears to be rampant. The students are not silent about racism, but there is a silence that reinforces KS's internalized racism. I use the concept black Western archetypes to describe the attitude of the teachers when they are stereotyping the students. These archetypes are based on generalized thought processes about black females, for example, the "aggressive black woman." Her hurt is not seen as she expresses her anger at injustice. So where do black women get a space to express their feelings about intersecting oppressions such as racism and sexism.

To resolve this matter, care and consideration about institutional racism and its impact on clients, therapists and the supervision process must be given. KS is one of a few black staff members and the black girls are in the minority. The students and the therapist are oppressed by the racism of the staff and a black female therapist struggles to find her voice. I call this situation of psychological disintegration and silence, being "gagged." A psychological gagging DeGrury (2005) uses the term "cognitive dissonance" to describe how this type of fragmentation can affect black people. To over stand this phenomenon, it is necessary to reflect on theories about the development of black psychology (Helms, 1990).

It is difficult to practice under these oppressive racialized conditions, KS finds her regular supervision, within the institution inadequate, as she is aware of the institutional racism and feels gagged. This therapist is subject to direct and vicarious trauma from the impact of racism in her work situation. Alleyne (2005) discusses the impact of "workplace racism." She uses the term "grinding" to explain this process.

KS gains comfort and an appropriate black gaze from an external supervision group that validates her experiences and the experiences of her clients. This forum facilitates her empowerment, so that she can gain confidence to find her voice and bring her concerns into her work situation. Within the workplace, KS does not feel validated and some of her clients do not feel validated.

It is likely that the students are angry about their experiences of racism and being shut down. I call this rage about racism "black rage." Institutional racism creates a racialized process designed to make individuals deny their experiences and it is therefore likely that they feel bad about themselves due to being labeled aggressive and accused of "pulling out the race card."

These acts against the liberation of black people are political and personal and a cause for great concern. They impact the psyche causing internalized racism and therefore appropriate supportive consideration is needed in the therapeutic arena. To counteract this, the client and therapist's experience must be validated and elements of racism must be acknowledged and explored, so that the therapy can do its work as a tool of liberation and empowerment.

This next scenario demonstrates internalized racism, a key element of trauma caused by racialized process. For both therapist and clients, shame, guilt and humiliation connected to racism and denial can accumulate and manifest in behaviors that indicate internalized racism and cause inaction.

CM

I was reluctant to start private practice because there was a belief that no one would come to see a black therapist. It was not about my ability but how I would be perceived as a black woman with dreadlocks. I was reluctant for a long time because of my internal racism. When I actually set up private practice, I crossed that bridge. I noticed that a lot of my clients were of different colors, however they all had differences in common. I only have a couple of classically English people. Even though the difference is not the same as my difference. There is something about it being beneficial that there is a difference. Their difference is not evident in the same way as mine but they experience difference, which may be what attracts them to work with a black therapist. Because maybe on an intuitive level there is an understanding that as a black woman I have lived with difference so I would understand what that is like for them too.

I haven't experienced any racist comments from clients. I think that if they were explicitly racist they would not come. They may be unconsciously racist but I have not experienced that yet.

When I worked in an organization, I was given a client who was covertly racist. A white English male. He said that he was Ku klux clan to me. It was really offensive. I reported it and nothing was done about it. I wanted him out of my group. If I knew that management would have supported me I would have asked him to leave and said I would discuss it with him later. I felt that if I told this client to leave I would have been in trouble. In the end it was me that got into trouble because when I reported it to my manager. My manager said we would have a three-way meeting. I said what! This client violated the therapy agreement; the manager left me to conduct the meeting. He was silent and I could not believe it. The guy continued to come to the group and he continued to be abusive. He refused to leave when I asked him to. I was so angry and I wish that I had threatened to stop the group and not carried on working with him. We had a supervisor who was placid. She was pro-management and was not someone that we could speak openly to about what was going on in the groups. We were in shock and the support system was not good.

Now I have chosen a black supervisor who specializes in this stuff and this has been a good support. My awareness about racism is very limited and I'm not educated about the nuances of racism. I know what it feels like, but I am not intellectually on par with it and this helps. In the Transcultural supervision group some of the experiences are shared, therefore it is more supportive.

I went to a very supportive group in Brixton. It was very supportive. I was really surprised about what I learned about myself that I never used to stand up for myself like other people. I have done it, but not in my workplace, where I felt disempowered. I had to own that I didn't do that. What came to mind was Maya Angelou's poem about the woman who smiled. The Mask (1987) I thought okay I am sometimes the woman who smiles because I'm trying to survive. Sometimes I don't stand up, I just smile as a way of coping and I had to find forgiveness for myself about that and acknowledge that it was a way of coping. I do find it very helpful to hear other people and how they deal with the impact of racism and their struggle with racism. It really brings to light how difficult it is and how universal it is. Even though I have become a therapist and I have a good deal of awareness, it is very difficult sometimes and it is hard to remember not to internalize this. When you have heard other people talking about racism, it helps you to remember that it is not happening to me, it's happening to my skin. There is a way of understanding it that makes it bearable. It makes you feel more resourceful.

CM. Found that she needed a safe reflective space to share her encounters with racism and her difficulty in standing up for herself. These intersecting oppressions contributed to her internalized racism. She was able to identify racialized process and acknowledge her internalized racism in supervision. This was the beginning of her journey to understanding how internalized racism and racialized process Dalal (2002) may impact her relationships with clients and her reluctance to overtly address diversity and oppression.

To conclude, we are left with the question of supervisory support for racialized process. Is it political, psychological, radical or just necessary? Taking action on racialized process means restoring a positive black gaze and integrating a black empathic approach as a feature of anti-oppressive practice. Dhillon-Stevens (2005) suggests that we need to practice in such a way that we do not perpetuate the oppression. This means: that in addition to other oppressions, taking individual and institutional action to voice fears and concerns about addressing racialized process and work through them. In supervision, therapists can acknowledge their naivety and reflect on where they are with addressing racialized process and the challenge of racism. Denial needs to be challenged. Rage must be processed and support to maintain openness about addressing the impact of racism and internalized racism provided. This process can include evaluation of history, heritage, institutional racism, cultural heritage and personal influences.

To develop an appropriate gaze robust enough to cope with racialized process, culturally empathic facilitation is necessary. Therapists need anti-oppressive supervision that can model ways of explicitly addressing racialized process and holding the trauma and powerful feelings associated with this.

I leave readers with a question. Are you allowed to be upset about racism in your training, personal development or supervision?

References

Akbar, N. (1996). *Breaking the chains of psychological slavery*. Tallahassee, FL: Mind Productions.

Alleyne, A. (2005). Invisible injuries and silent witnesses: The shadow of racial oppression in workplace contexts. *Psychodynamic Practice, 11*(3), 283–299.

Angelou, M. (1987). *The mask*. Caged Bird Legacy, LLC. Retrieved from Maya Angelou.com

Browne, D., Francis, E., & Crowe, I. (1993). *Black people mental health and the criminal justice system in the mentally disordered offender in an era of community care*. Cambridge: Cambridge University Press.

Burke, A. (1984, March 1). *Racism and psychological disturbance among West Indians in Britain*. London: Sage Journals.

Dalal, F. (2002). *Race, colour and the process of Racialization*. Brunner: Routledge.

DeGrury, J. (2005). *Post traumatic slave syndrome*. Portland, OR: Joy DeGrury Publications Inc.

Dhillon-Stevens, H. (2005). Personal and professional integration of anti-oppressive practice and the multiple oppression model in psychotherapeutic education. *The British Journal of Psychotherapy Integration, 1*(2), 47–62.

Fanon, F. (1986). *Black skin, white mask*. London: Pluto Press.

Fernando, S. (1984, March 1). Racism as a cause of depression. *International Journal of Social Psychiatry*.

Fernando, S. (1991). *Mental health, race and culture*. London: Palgrave Macmillan.

Fletchman Smith, B. (2011). *Transcending the legacy of slavery*. London: Karnac.

Fletchman Smith, B. (1999). *Mental slavery*. London: Rebus.

Helms, J. (1990). Counselling attitudinal & behavioural pre-dispositions: The Black/White interaction model. In J. E. Helms (Ed.), *Black and white racial identity: Theory research and practice* (pp. 135–143). Westport, CT: Greenwood.

hooks, b. (1987). *Ain't I a woman?: Black women and feminism*. London: Pluto Classics.

hooks, b. (1992). *Black looks*. Boston, MA: South End Press.

Howitt, D., & Owusu Bempa, J. (1994). *The racism in psychology*. London: Harvester Wheatsheaf.

IPCC for England & Wales. (2015/2016). Deaths of BAME people in police custody. Published on 5th August 2016, Full Fact Team.

Kareem, J., & Littlewood, R. (1992). *Intercultural therapy*. Oxford: Blackwell.

Lago, C. (2006). *Race, culture and counselling*. Buckingham: Open University Press.

Lago, C. (2011). *The handbook of transcultural counselling & psychotherapy*. Berkshire, NY: Open University Press.

Lago, C., & Thompson, J. (1982). *Race & culture in counselling*. Buckingham: Open University Press.

Mckenzie-Mavinga, I. (2009). *Black issues in the therapeutic process*. London: Palgrave Macmillan.

Mckenzie-Mavinga, I. (2016). *The challenge of racism in therapeutic practice*. London: Palgrave Macmillan.

Mckenzie-Mavinga, I. (2005). Understanding black issues in postgraduate counsellor training. *Counselling and Psychotherapy Research, 5*(4), 295–300.

MIND Mental Health Facts and Statistics. (2010, May 24). *Ethnicity and use of the Mental Health Act*. London. Retrieved from www.mind.org.uk/mental_health_facts_and_statistics. Accessed on May 24, 2010.

Tuckwell, G. (2002). *Racial identity white counsellors & therapists*. Buckingham: Open University Press.

Part VI

Recommendations

Chapter 29

Recommendations

Patrick Vernon

The *International Handbook of Black Community Mental Health* has critically illuminated distinct areas within the black community, which indiscriminately affects the mental health of people of colour of all ages, and across the family life cycle. The contributions of black women, and women of colour clinicians and professionals within this Handbook, include not only contributions to scholarship, but incorporate narratives associated with the emotional and physical costs to women working in the mental health and education profession. The levels of stress and how it is manifested is far reaching for black women. Working and non-working women of colour continue to be at high risk for developing physiological symptoms such as strokes, the re-occurrence of breast cancer, heart disease, hypertension known as high blood pressure, heart attacks, and death in birth. While the recommendations provided below are for the UK, the topics covered in the examples will be relevant to a global audience.

Since 2017, there have been a number of policy developments around Race Disapirty Audit, review of the Mental Health Act, establishment by National Health Service (NHS) England Equality Taskforce for Mental Health, and the Mental Health Use of Force Act (Seni's Law) which have the potential of tackling some aspects of racism in the mental health system for the black community (for more details, see the chapter "Thirty Years of Black History Month and Thirty Years of Overrepresentation in The Mental Health System" by Patrick Vernon).

However, despite these changes, we still require a fundamental shift in policy and commissioning. We need recommendations for a 10-point action plan for change for the next decade, especially if we want to reverse overrepresentation in the mental health system of black men and to have better recovery outcomes, so they can thrive and have a better quality of life compared to the rest of the population.

1. Many black men have lost trust in services due to experiences of racism and cultural differences that is why Community Treatment Orders needs to be abolished and ensuring places of safety under section 136 of the Mental

Health Act are not police stations as they reinforce lack of trust and human rights of black men with NHS and the Police.
2. Stigma around mental health still exists, making it difficult for black men to talk about problems and to seek early help for fear of being given a diagnosis. We need to more dedicate culturally specific counselling services for black men with more support to promote and extend the role of black therapists, counsellors, clinical psychologist and psychiatrists. We also want more African centric perspectives in counselling training and commissioning of services which the current Cognitive Behavioral Therapy (CBT) and Improving Access to Psychological Therapies (IAPT) services provided by the NHS do not address.
3. The ingrained prejudice and stigma against that all black men as seen and perceived by society as 'Mad, Bad, Dangerous' presents a massive challenge to men who are trying to engage with mental health professionals and the police. We need to have a dedicated national social media campaign led and developed by black men with lived experience working with black media professionals. We also need the current workforce in the NHS and those providers from the private and third sector to have training around cultural competency, cultural heritage of the black community and the impact of racism in how services are delivered. Work of Time to Change and other social media campaigns in health and related sectors.
4. Inequality and discrimination of black communities can lead to increased risk of psychosis particularly for black men. We need to develop a national prevention strategy from early years supporting young black boys to teenagers around mental wellbeing and cultural identity. More work is required to look at schools treatment of black boys around exclusions. We need Black History more embedded in the national curriculum and the promotion of role models to improve self-esteem and confidence.
5. There is a lack of black representation in decision making within the NHS, as well as amongst employees of mental health services. We need NHS England's Workforce Race Equality Scheme (WRES) to be created on a statutory footing to ensure all NHS trusts have a clear and systematic promotion strategy of all BAME staff especially from African and Caribbean community working in senior clinical and managerial roles (including Non-Executives) around the development of mental health services and policy development. In emerging networks such as Association of Black Social Workers (ABSW), BME Voices, KCL African-Caribbean Medical Association, BYP, BAME in Psychiatry and Psychology (BIPP) and Black Aspiring Clinical Psychologists Network (BACPN) need support and funding to widen the profession so young people can access to role models as part of a future mental health workforce.
6. There is a lack of capacity and resources in the black voluntary sector, grass roots and faith groups to develop and deliver mental health interventions for black men. We need a capacity building fund to develop and sustain black led community mental health services which support black men which are safe spaces for support and community connections. We also require more resources and space in academic and community settings to develop new models and thinking around solution on cultural an Afrocentric perspective.

7. Commissioning and development of a network of Black Women Empowerment Groups to collaborate and share good practice in identifying triggers around long-term conditions (stroke, diabetes and cancer) which has an impact on depression provide much needed training in primary care, hospitals and churches/mosques and community groups which will provide peer support for working black female professionals. Stress management courses for young girls from aged 11-15, and Peer support networks to reduce the prevalence of high blood pressure and share strength based techniques and strategies within school and home is needed to process and strengthen the inner person when racism is at work, rather than the CBT type treatment, which would treat racism as an internal construct that needs to be externalised.
8. Most health spending is tied up in acute rather than preventative services. There needs to be a fundamental shift in the commissioning of services where a large proportion of black men are in the special hospitals, medium secure units, forensic wards. Many of these facilities are not appropriate and often is seen as a warehouse to keep black men away from society and the community. The commissioning of Out of Areas lucrative contracts to the private sector providers by NHS England and the Clinical Commissioning Groups further reinforces the lack of commitment and the over use of risk management. We need a national strategy and campaign to create more places of recovery and prevention in community settings so black men feel that there are connected to their communities with a clear plan of recovery.
9. We need to develop new approaches on public mental health around community trauma as a result of knife crime, stop and search. Grenfell and the Windrush Scandal is leading more black people to suffer from PTSD, depression and impact on their physical health. Further work is required to explore current on mental health and wellbeing around intersectionality, experiences of LGBTQ, migration/immigration status, domestic violence and learning disabilities.
10. The NHS and wider government needs to review and acknowledge the impact of structural racism and over representation of black men in mental health services and adopt the definition of Afriphobia as part of the UK's government commitment to The UN Decade of African Descent.

Glossary

We the contributors of *The International Handbook of Black Community Mental Health* confess that we have a preference for people of colour. The authors also acknowledge that there are varied ways in which people of colour self-define themselves across the diaspora. However, the reader will encounter a myriad of descriptions within the chapters they read. Therefore, we include a brief and accessible glossary will help ground both the academic and non-academic audience of the *Handbook* with meanings and terms that are newly introduced, specialised, and/ or uncommon. Race and culture are socially constructed terms. As such, we learn about ourselves by socialising with one another. Providing the reader with the following may enable the reader to have a deeper understanding of the social dynamics related to mental health.

African American: Is a term that refers to people of African heritage in part or in full and typically applies to slave ancestry.

Afrophobia: Is a perceived fear of the culture and people of African descent regardless of origin. Afrophobia is a specific form of racism that results in discrimination, oppression, and other inequitable opportunities including employment, housing, and education.

BAME: Black Asian Minority Ethnic (BAME) is an acronym for people of Black, Black British, Bi-racial, Caribbean multi-racial, the Black Asian, South Asian, and West Indian descent who live in the United Kingdom, that is, British Isles.

Colour: Colour, also correctly spelled as colour, is the British spelling of the word.

Coloured: In the United Kingdom coloured refers to a person of European and non-European heritage, while in the United States, coloured is an antiquated term that has been used to refer to a person who is mixed with European and or Black/African ancestry and sometimes East Asian heritage.

In South Africa the term 'coloured' was used to describe mixed race people.

Coloured was also a term used by some white people (and black elders) to describe black people from the Caribbean.

Critical literacy: Examining who made the message, who sent the message, and from whom the message intended.

Critical race theory: Critical race theory is a lens that examines historical, economic, and equity issues based on legal implications of race.

Cultural competence: The mindful acknowledgement of diversity in beliefs and behaviours that impact communication, while seeking to promote positive and ethical outcomes.

Deconstruction: Understanding the relationship between text and meaning.

Diaspora: Defined by the African Union (AU), the diaspora consists of people of African origin living outside of the continent, irrespective of citizenship and nationality. The AU is divided into five regions of the continent of African Northern, Central, Eastern, Western, and Central. In 2003, the AU recognised the people of the diaspora are the sixth region. There is a common and fractured collective identity of the people of the diaspora based on common experiences due to colonialism, oppression, and perseverance. *The term diaspora can also refer to the displacement of other groups including Jewish people and South Asia.*

Doctrine: Religious beliefs, teachings, and text upon which Christians (and other religious groups) practice their faith.

East Asian: Includes people with China, Hong Kong, Macau, Japan, North Korea, South Korea, Mongolia, and Taiwanese heritage.

Embodiment: The physical and visual manifestation or representation of an idea, spirituality, or faith.

Gender identity: A strongly held belief that you are either male or female based on biological and social influences.

Minoritised: Is a term that signifies the fact that term minority is not a voluntary one and that people who are designated as a minority have that term enforced on them by another group and is not reflective of their humanity or potential. Minoritised people can often be the majority of the population but regulated to minority status by others.

People of colour: Refers to persons who are not of 'White' or European descent.

Reflexivity/Reflexive practice: Used in systemic practice to showcase how the practitioner shapes practice and practice in turn shapes the practitioner and the lens through which decision-making occurs. Adding a spiritual component to this considers the third dimension to the reflexive process.

Reverential power: A deep (and sacred) respect and admiration for deity that honours the spiritual nature of the relationship.

Shadeism: Social, political, and economic discrimination based on the perception of race and the darkness of skin tone. Shadeism is common in Asia, Latin America, the United States, and the West Indies.

Social construction: The joint creation of meaning through language, discourse, and associated power as a social theory.

South Asian: Includes people with Afghanistan, Bangladesh, Bhutan, Sri Lanka, India, the Maldives, Nepal, and Pakistani heritage.

South East Asian: Includes people with Brunei, Burma (Myanmar), Cambodia, Timor-Leste, Indonesia, Laos, Malaysia, the Philippines, Singapore, Thailand, and Vietnamese heritage.

Index

Abuse, categories of, 155–156
Academia, racism in
    changing research topic, 98–99
    competence, 97–98
    conceptualisation of 'ivory tower' of academia, 90–91
    dysconscious racism, 94
    endings, 100–104
    lens, 95–96
    mental health within ivory tower, 93
    misunderstandings, 99–100
    new beginning, 104
    outsiders in ivory tower, 92–93
    under representation of black people on journey to ivory tower, 91–92
    shift in supervisory relationships, 96–97
    stories, 94–95
Academic achievement, 194
Academic disidentification, 194–195
Academic racism (*see also* Institutional racism; Systemic racism), 58
    advocacy in case of discrimination, 64–65
    critical knowledge in multi-layered society, 70–71
    leadership, 60–64
    orchestrating multi-dimensional identities, 65–70
Access to 'Divine Capital', 286
Access to mental health services, 4
    for African Americans, 12
    barriers to, 12, 113
Access to mental health services for African Americans, barriers to, 113
Accreditation process, 553

Activists, 463
Adoption and Children Act (2002), 396
Advocacy, 442
    in discrimination case, 64–65
Aetiology and Ethnicity in Schizophrenia and Other Psychoses (AESOP), 446
African Americans
    and employment, 266–268
    and mental health, 265–266
    VR services for African American with mental health diagnoses, 269–272
African Caribbean Community Initiative (ACCI), 137
African Jubilee Year Declaration, 137
African-Caribbean Black and Minority Ethnic (ACBME), 433–434
African-Caribbean Mental Health in UK, 446–448
    assets-based, community-centred approach, 448–449
    CaFI, 454–455
    CaFI for schizophrenia, 450–453
    compliance with ethical standards, 455
    FI 'talking treatment', 449–450
    implications, 454
    testing CaFI, 453
African-Caribbeans, 177–178, 335, 445
Afriphobia, 143
Afro Caribbean Community, SPD and, 486–487
Afrocentric psychology, 123
Airport experience, 524–525
Al Qaeda, 468
Alert Programme strategies, 485–486
Alzheimer's disease, 413, 415

American Psychiatric Association (APA), 3, 186
Americans with Disabilities Act, 268
Analytical cross-cultural therapy, 370
Anger, 168, 288, 407, 462
Anti-Black racial misandry, 84
Anti-oppressive supervision, 559
Anti-racism, 555
'Anti-racist' education, 352
Anxiety, 168, 242, 370, 432
Arranged marriage, 19, 498, 511
Asian culture, 237, 497
Asperger's Syndrome, 462
Assets-based approach, 448–449
Assimilation, 397
Asylums to community care, 146–147
Attachment theory, 535–536
  to Reid and Bledsoe, 472–474
Attention Deficit Disorder (ADD), 483
Attention Deficit Hyperactivity Disorder (ADHD), 483
Autism, 462
  race problem, 238
Autism diagnostic observation schedule (ADOS), 236
Autism spectrum disorders (ASD), 233–234, 483
  achieving cultural competency in ASD assessment, 239–241
  impact of changes to diagnostic criteria, 235–237
  diagnostic failings in ASD assessment in BME population, 237–238
  multicultural treatment-led model, 233
  tackling inequalities, 241
  therapeutic interventions for, 242–244

'Backdoor' exclusions, 352
BAME clients' and families' value system, 9
Barriers to mental health in Black/African American Community, 113

Battered race syndrome, 6 (*see also* racial battle fatigue)
Behaviour, 357, 441
Behavioural therapies, 2–3
Behaviours indicating SPD, 487–488
Belief systems within South Asian families, 500–501
Bennett Inquiry, 44–45
Bethlem Royal Hospital, 146
Big, bad, mad and dangerous stereotype, 2, 4, 11, 37–52, 135, 137, 143, 447
Black, Asian and Minority Ethnic groups (BAME groups), 7, 40–41, 145, 321, 324
Black and Minority Ethnic communities (BME communities), 1, 38–39, 58, 91–92, 134, 159–160
Black boys
  challenges affecting black boys in schools in UK, 283–286
  comments and recommendations, 202
  cultural competence model for teachers and Black boys, 193
  EL, 195–202
  Excell3's Black Boys Can Intervention Programmes, 286–292
  impact of targeted intervention for disadvantaged pupils, 292–294
  underachievement, 283
Black Boys Can Project, 15, 284, 286–292
Black Boys Empowerment Programme, 287
Black Britain, 133, 445
Black churches, 286, 470, 527
Black community, 8, 177, 563
  stigmas within, 256
Black empathic approach, 550
Black excellence movement, 66
Black experience credibility, 470

Black families, 369–370
Black Health and Wellbeing Commission, 140
Black History Month, 137, 142
Black identity, 329
Black male
  self-actualising, 289
  self-concept, 288
Black males of color (BMOC), 3, 255
Black Mental Health, 133–135, 140
"Black on black" violence, 139
Black patients, 40, 43–44, 134, 178, 335
Black people, 3, 37–38, 445
Black psychology/Afro-centric psychology, 4
Black racial identity status, 372, 390–391
Black therapists, 370
  authors' therapeutic experience, 374–375
  black racial identity status, 372, 390–391
  Caribbean migration and acculturation, 369
  cultural perception study design choice, 371
  impact of curiosity, 382
  demographic characteristics, 375–377
  design, 378
  ethical issues, 378
  eye contact, 382
  findings, 379–381
  limitations and future directions, 384–385
  materials, 375
  method, 375
  participants, 375
  procedure, 378
  questionnaire, 393–394
  reflexivity working within insider/outsider position, 382–383
  research questions, 380–381
  second generation socialisation, 369–371
  status of clients and therapists' own racial identity, 383–384
  white racial identity status, 372–374, 391–392
  working with 'not knowing' position, 384
Black Thrive, 140
Black Western Archetype, 550
Black women
  and cultural disposition, 550
  discrimination, 86
  hyper-policing of, 84
  identities, 92
  as leaders, 16
  leadership experiences of, 319–331
  self-definition and self-valuation, 326
  in UK, 7
Black youth, 256
Black/African American Community, 113
  barriers to mental health in, 113
  community engagement with, 121–124
  cultural competence and humility in, 124
  cultural responses to implicit provider bias, 120
  implicit provider bias and, 110–112
  mental health, 109
  psychosocial issues affecting, 118–120
  review of literature, 114–118
  social determinants of health and, 112–113
  strategies to reducing implicit bias, 124–125
Black/African Americanness, 119
Black/African-American psychology, 5
Black/Afro-centric psychology, 8
Boys 2 Men, 169
Bradford riots, 324
British Association for Counselling and Psychotherapy (BACP), 186, 190

British Nationality Act, 50
British Psychological Society (BPS), 186, 346
British West Indies Regiment (BWIR), 49–50
Burden of acting white, 194–195
Business incubators, 275–276, 278

Care Act (2014), 154–155
Care Program Approach (CPA), 152
Care Quality Commission (CQC), 39, 134
Caretaking whites, 406–407
Caribbean, 497–498, 520
  migration and acculturation, 369
Carlos Bledsoe case study, 467–468
  potential explanations for terrorist inclinations of, 468–474
Celebrating diversity, 406
Centers for Disease Control and Prevention (CDC), 238, 248
Chester M. Pierce, 79, 82, 86
Chicago Add Us In Initiative (AUI Initiative), 276
Child and Adolescent Mental Health Services (CAMHS), 159, 162, 499, 504
Child sexual abuse, 319
Child sexual exploitation (CSE), 319–321
Children, 159, 162
  commissioning services, 164
  lack of data, 161–162
  policy and strategic landscape, 162–164
  impact of race and ethnicity terminology, 160–161
  voluntary and community sector, 164–165
Children Act (1989), 396
Children and Family Court Advisory and Support Service (CAFCASS), 504
Children and Young People, 159–172
  psychological effects upon, 511–512

Choose Life International, 3
Civil Rights Movement, 463
Class, 61, 498
  of community activists, 137
  faces discrimination on, 345
  mental health professional, 181
  structure, 520
  working class feminist, 324
  young people at, 168
Clients' racial identity status, 383–384
Client–therapist racial/ethnic matching, 187
Clinical Psychology, 323, 325, 329, 346
Cognitive behavioral therapy (CBT), 242–243, 455, 484
Cognitive dissonance, 557
Cognitive divide in education, 198
Cognitive frames, 405
Cognitive opening, 469
Cognitive therapies, 2–3
Colonisation, 49–50, 498
Color-blind approach, 139, 300
Colour-blind racial attitudes, 186
Commissioning services, 164
Committee on the Elimination of Racial Discrimination (CERD), 139
Commonwealth and Immigration Act (1962), 50
Communication, 408, 451
Community
  church environment, 310
  community-based parenting, 536
  community-based research approach, 123
  community-based therapeutic service, 326
  community-centred approach, 448–449
  engagement with Black/African American Community, 121–124
  family therapy, 519, 529
  mental health, 448, 564
  tasks, 536–537
  violence, 194

Index **581**

Community Treatment Orders (CTOs), 134, 138–139
Community-partnered Participatory Research (CPPR), 446, 451
Compassion, 208
Competence, 97–98, 183
Compulsion, 152, 244
Conformity, 372
   stage of racial identity statuses, 390
Connection to God, 311
Conscious perpetrators, 94
Constructive conversations, 201
Continuous traumatic stress (CTS), 6
Conventional practice, 185
'Cool Pose' theory, 5
Cooperatives, 276–277
Counselling theories, 179
Count Me In Census, 163
County Asylum Act, 146
Criminal justice system (CJS), 37, 40
Crisis time/non-crisis time interactions, 217–219
Critical knowledge in multi-layered society, 70–71
Critical race theory, 185, 300
Cultural/culturally/culture, 8–9, 133, 187, 239–240
   adapted therapy, 451
   appropriate services, 9, 123, 346
   in ASD assessment, 239–241
   awareness, 240
   baggage, 200
   competence, 8–10, 197, 442
   and competency, 164
   competent healthcare system, 442–443
   cultural-specificity of family assessment, 450
   culture-based treatment, 123–124
   'culture-specific' behaviours, 352
   in delivering counselling and psychotherapy services, 177
   determinism, 181
   evidence for MCC efficacy, 182–183
   focused groups, 122
   gaze, 555
   and humility in Black/African American Mental Health, 124
   identity, 462
   individual and professional practice issues effecting MCC, 187–190
   insider, 171, 382–383, 512, 514
   mental health services, 121
   misconceptions, 194
   mistrust, 4–5
   need for targeted therapy services and training, 183–187
   notions of culture, 178–182
   outsider, 171, 382–383, 509
   paranoia, 4–5
   perception study design choice, 371
   pride, 519
   responses to implicit provider bias, 120
   talking treatment, 445, 454
   theory, 384, 543
   training of GPs, 185
   trauma, 6–8
Culturally adapted FI (CaFI), 450
   for schizophrenia, 450–453
   testing, 453
Cure the NHS, 150–151, 157
Curiosity, 512–514, 533

DAISH, 468
Data, lack of, 161–162
De-colonising approaches, 168
Death, 43, 48, 304, 527
   of Cumberbatch, 37
   in forensic setting, 11
   likelihood of, 41
   in psychiatric system, 334
Deficit psychology, 8
Delivering Race Equality (DRE), 138, 448
   in Mental Health Care, 163
   strategy, 139

Dementia, 17–18, 413–415
  impact in economically underdeveloped world, 415–416
  in minority ethnic and migrant communities, 416–423
  mobilizing international approach to dementia in, 423–425
Denial of racism, 555
Department for Children, Schools and Families, 284
Department for Education (DFe), 283
Department of Health, 184–185
Department of Health and Social Care (DHSC), 152
Depression, 117, 414, 432
Deprivation, 135
Detachment, 472
Developmental coordination disorders, 483
Diaspora effect on belief systems, 509–511
Disabled Business Persons Association (DBA), 274
Disadvantaged pupils, impact of targeted intervention for, 292–294
Discourse, 303–304
Discrimination, 81, 85, 156, 450
  advocacy in, 64–65
  of black communities, 564
  institutional, 85
  interpersonal, 440
  through unwitting prejudice, 47
Disparities, 85, 110, 112, 262, 270, 272, 447
Dissonance, 372, 390
Distorted lens, 96
Diverse leadership deficit, 321–322
Diversity, 155, 186
Dominican Republic, 521
  working with families in, 539–541
Drapetomania, 4, 440
DSM-5, 235–236
Dysconscious racism, 94

Early Start Denver Model (ESDM), 243
Earthquake, 541
  survival, 527–531
Economics, 252–253
Educational achievement, 284–287, 292
Educational institutions, 194, 252
Effective evidence-based strategies, 125
Emancipation Act, 438
Embodiment, 311–312
Emersion, 372
  stage of racial identity statuses, 390
  status, 373
Emotional literacy (EL), 195–202
Emotional Literacy Reflective Interactive Tool (ELRIT), 205, 220–229
Emotional/emotions, 351, 353
  analysis, 220, 222–223
  intelligence, 195
  in learning, 199
  literacy, 205–212
  recognition, 220–221
  regulation, 220, 223–229
  resilience, 195
  understanding, 220, 222
  wellness, 196–197
Empathy, 188–189, 199
Employment
  African Americans and, 266–268
  outcomes, 267, 271–273
Employment assistance providers (EAPs), 73
Employment Intervention Demonstration Program, 267
Enlightened perpetrators/activists, 94
Entrepreneurship (*see also* Self-employment), 274–276, 278
Environmental racial microaggression, 83
Epidemiologic Catchment Area Study, 118
Equality, 186

Ethnic(ity), 40, 69, 187, 238
  identity, 396
  minorities, 446
  REF, 551–560
  socialisation, 402
  studies, 71
  of terminology impact, 160–161
Eurocentric mental health services, 4
European Commission against Racism and Intolerance Report (ECRI Report), 40, 42
Everyday racism, 1–3, 6
Excell3's Black Boys Can Intervention Programmes, 286–292
Exclusion, 42, 70, 72, 134, 162
Eye contact and safe touch, 382, 534–535

Faith, 299, 307
Family
  assessment, 450
  family-based therapy, 450
  instability, 194
  therapy in context of community, 527–531
Family Intervention (FI), 449
  talking treatment, 449–450
Family/community, 254–255
Fight and flight mode, 482, 484
Financial abuse, 156
First Black Republic establishment, 521
Fixed-term exclusions, 352
Forced marriage, 498
  clinical practice, 501
  honor, 499–501
  effect of migration and diaspora on belief systems, 509–511
  parental alienation, 514
  positioning and curiosity, 512–514
  positioning theory, 508–509
  psychological effects upon children and young people, 511
  South Asian families, 501–502
  structure, 498–499
  Vignette 1, 502–504
  Vignette 2, 504–507

Francis Report, 150–151
Fundamentalist religious principles, 471

Ganja psychosis, 136–137
Gatekeeper, 531, 544
Gender, 16, 38, 58, 60–61, 63, 65, 67, 70, 79, 81
  microaggressions, 64, 80
General counselling competence, 188
Girl Talk, 168
Global radicalisation process, 471
God Positioning System (GPS), 304
  metaphor of, 304–305
  staying connected and repositioning practice with, 307–308
Government, 253–254
'Ground up' approach, 538
Grounded spiritual visions, 311–312
Gun crime, 139

Hagar (African-Caribbean mental health project), 18, 431
Haiti, 19, 521
Haiti earthquake (2010), 519
Haitian belief system, 519
Haitian family life, 525–526
Haitian indigenous community, 519
Handshake, 534–535
'Hard-to-reach' communities, 446–447, 453
Health
  disparities, 112
  inequity, 112
  racial disparities in, 85–86
  racism and, 85
Health Complaint Commission (HCC), 150
Healthcare, 112
  providers, 442
  and public health, 253
  rights, 422–423
Helms racial identity interaction model, 371
Help-seeking, 451, 453

Higher Education Statistics Agency (HESA), 58, 93
Honor, 499
   belief systems within South Asian families, 500–501
   Izzat and Sharam, 499–500
   maintaining concept of, 510
Honor cultures, 510
   in USA, 498–499
Honour (film), 499
Hospital, 2–3, 37, 39, 146, 153, 531
Humiliation, 555
Hyper-toxic environments, 81

Identity, 133, 462
   disruption, 462
Illinois Vocational Rehabilitation Agency, 276
Illness model, 436
Immersion stage, 372
   of racial identity statuses, 390
Implicit Association Test, 115
Implicit bias, 47, 81
   strategies to reducing, 124–125
Implicit provider bias, 110–112, 114
   cultural responses to, 120
Inculturation, 179
Indebtedness, 500–501
Independent Review of the Mental Health Act, 147
Individual terrorist radicalisation processes, 468
Indoctrination, 469
Inequality, 2, 352
   of black communities, 564
Inertia following inquires, 43–46
Infant Start, 243
Informal exclusions, 352
INQUEST, 151
Institute of Race Relations, The, 44–45
Institutional discrimination, 85
Institutional racism (*see also* Academic racism; Systemic racism), 2, 46–48, 50, 119, 557
Institutional trauma, 253

Integral pastoral approach, 527
Integrative Awareness, 372
Integrative awareness, 390–391
Intellectual authority, 471
Interactional model, 374
Interethnic Adoptions Provisions (1996), 397
Internalisation, 372, 390
Internalised culture, 180
Internalised racism, 85, 91, 557
International Labour Organization (ILO), 276
Interpersonal discrimination, 440
Intersectionality, 160–161
Islamic State (*see* DAISH)
Islamophobia, 554
"Ivory tower" of academia, 89
   conceptualisation, 90–91
   mental health within, 93
   outsiders in, 92–93
   under representation of black people on journey to, 91–92
Izzat, 19

Jahadization, 470
Jamaica, 49–50, 51, 335, 340, 396, 438–439, 447
Jaunes, 523
Job creation for people with disabilities, 277
Joint Commission, 114, 121
Judaism, 467

Knowledge and attitudes about mental health programs and services, 256

Labeling, 147, 461
Lakou system, 521, 536
Lambeth Black Health and Wellbeing Commission, 45–46
Lambeth Local Authority, 283
Leadership, 60, 321–322
   understanding and solidarity, 62–64
Learning coach, 359

Legacy, 500–501
Lens, 95–96
Local authority, 149, 154, 320–321, 398
London borough of Lambeth, 140
'Lone wolf' type attacks, 461, 462
Loss experiences, 339–340
Low and Middle-Income Countries (LAMICs), 454
Low-income black communities, 261

Madhouse Act, 146
Manic depression, 432
Marginalisation, 467
Marijuana, 452
Maroons, 438
Marriage, 501, 511
Mass media, 254
Meaningful employment, 266
Medical illness model, 436
Medical professionals, 116, 178
Medicalisation, 2, 441
MEE Eight Variables Model, 250–255
Mega church, 306
Meltdown, 19, 482, 487
Memory loss, 415
Mental Capacity Act (2005), 153
Mental disorder, 431, 462
Mental health, 109, 303–304
 administrators and providers, 114
 African Americans and, 265–266
 analysis, 435–443
 black mental health matters, 133–135
 children in UK, 401–409
 depression, 432
 disorders, 284–285, 440
 Hagar mental health project, 431
 within ivory tower, 93
 knowledge and attitudes about mental health programs and services, 256
 medical definition of personality disorder, 432
 Mental Health Project for ACBME, 433–435
 MHA and CTOs, 138–139
 mistrust of mental health treatment services, 256–257
 project for ACBME, 433–434
 providers, 124
 schizophrenia, 431–432
 services, 523–524
 stigmas within black community, 256
 stressors, 118
 from striving to thriving, 139–143
 treatment system, 255
 uprising and riots in 1980s to millennials, 136–138
 and wellbeing, 133, 159
Mental Health Act (MHA), 2, 38, 134, 138–139, 145, 152–153, 343–344, 447, 451, 551–560, 563
Mental health professional (AMHP), 152
Mental Health Task Force (2015), 45
Mental Health Use of Force Act, 141, 563
Mentally ordered offenders, 136
Micro-assaults, 83, 185
Micro-insults, 83, 185
Micro-invalidations, 185
Microaggressions, 81, 84, 185–186
 in mental health, 5–6
Microinvalidation, 83
Migrant communities
 dementia in, 416–418
 in Europe and parts of economically developed world, 421–422
 and healthcare rights, 422–423
 in UK, 420–421
 in United States, 418–419
Migration, 340
 effect on belief systems, 509–511
 hypotheses, 446
Mild cognitive impairment (MCI), 414
Mindfulness, 188–189
Mini-communications, 217–219

Ministerial Advisory Group on Mental Health Strategy, The, 45
Minority ethnic, 446
  dementia in, 416–418
  in Europe and parts of economically developed world, 421–422
  and healthcare rights, 422–423
  mobilizing international approach to dementia in, 423–425
  in UK, 420–421
  in United States, 418–419
Misconception of self, 94
Mission
  model, 531
  trip, 524
Mistrust
  of mental health treatment services, 256–257
  roots of, 4–6
Mixed non-profit sector, 523
'Mixed' heritage, 445
Monotheism, 468
Monsoon Wedding (film), 513
Mothering, 525, 538
Mulatre, 520, 523
Mulberry Bush Outreach organisation, 285
Multi-cultural competencies (MCC) (*see also* Cultural competencies), 14, 177, 179
  evidence for MCC efficacy, 182–183
  individual and professional practice issues effecting, 187–190
Multi-dimensional identities, orchestrating, 65–70
Multi-stakeholder cooperatives, 277
Multi-systemic concepts, 525, 528
Multicultural counselling competence, 188
Multicultural education, 352
Multiethnic Placement Act (1994), 397

Narcissism, 462
National Approved Mental Health Professional Conference, 152
National Education Association (NEA), 293
National Health Service (NHS), 1, 44, 147, 445
  England's Independent Mental Health Taskforce, 139–140
  hospital, 147
  principles, 445
  staffing, 147–148
National Institute for Health and Care Excellence (NICE), 448, 453
National Institute for Health Research (NIHR), 449–450
National Institute of Health (NIH), 239
National Research Ethics Service (NRES), 455
National Service Framework, 162–163
Neglect, 156
Neo-liberalist responses, 550
'Network based' terrorists, 462
Neuroses, 437
New Horizons, 138
No Health Without Mental Health, 138
Non-cognitive divide in education, 198
Non-crisis time interaction exercise, 219
Non-governmental organisations (NGOs), 523
Non-pharmacological approaches, 414–415
Normative implicit provider bias, 111
Notion in terrorism, 462–463

Obsessive-compulsive disorder (OCD) (*see also* Autism spectrum disorders (ASD)), 243
Occupational therapists, 483
Off the Record (OTR), 167, 170–172

Office of Disability Employment Policy (ODEP), 275
Oppression, 524–525, 551
Over responsive sensory processing, 482
Over-/misdiagnosis of schizophrenia, 3
Over-representation
  in mental Ill health and custody, 39–41
  reasons for, 41–42

Paranoid ideation, 136
Paranoid schizophrenia, 431
Parental alienation, 507, 514
Parenting programmes, 531
Parents, explaining SPD to, 488–490
Parkinson's disease, 413
Pastors as counsellors and translators, 541–544
Paths cross, 323–324
Patriarchy, 514
People of colour, 9–10
Persecutory framework development, 340–341
Persecutory system, 336–339
Person-centered care, 147
Personal authority, 471
Personal construct psychology (PCP), 351–358
  derived approach, 17
Personal construct theory (*see* Personal construct psychology (PCP))
Personal identity, 463
Personal perceptions, 351, 353
Personality, 462
  disorder, 432
Perspective-taking strategy, 125
Pictorial Autism Assessment Schedule (PAAS), 241
Place and train (*see* Supported employment)
Plantocracy societies, 498
Policy, 162–164
Political unrest, 521–523
Population health, 260–261

Population needs assessments, 164
"Population-based" study, 274
Positioned/positioning, 93, 96, 346, 512–514
  theory, 508–509
Post colonization, 498
Post-colonial theory, 50
Post-traumatic slave syndrome (PTSS), 6–7
Post-traumatic stress (PTS), 432
Post-traumatic stress disorder (PTSD), 6
Poverty, 194
Power, 209, 303–304
  dynamics, 147
Pre-school Autism Communication Trial (PACT), 242
Prevention-oriented approach, 256
Principles, 123, 148, 358
Private for-profit sector, 523
Private non-profit sector, 523
Protective factor interventions, 15
Protective factors for mental health, 247
  experts, 248
  failure, 250–255
  mental health treatment system, 255–257
  resiliency, 257–262
Provider bias, 115
Pseudo-independence stage, 373
Pseudo-leadership, 330
Psychiatric
  care, 447
  disorders, 112
  labels, 445
Psychiatrists, 43
Psychiatry, 441–443
Psycho-education, 450, 452, 528
  expanding psycho-educative approach, 531–533
Psychological
  interventions, 198
  strengths, 257
Psychopathology, 118
Psychopathy, 462

588 Index

Psychosis, 437, 451
Psychosocial issues affecting Black/African American Mental Health, 118–120
Psychotherapy, 2
Puerperal psychosis, 437
Purnell Model for Cultural Confidence, 240
Purpose, Strategy, Outcome, Review model (PSOR model), 359–365
Pyramid technique, 355

Quality teaching, 531
Questionnaire, 371, 378, 384, 393–394

Race, 38, 69, 187, 395
    critical theory, 61
    lessons, 405–406
    of terminology impact, 160–161
Race Disparity Audit, 46, 139, 563
Race Equality Patient Charter, 140
Race Equality Survey, 91
Race Relations Amendment Act (2001), 138
Racial battle fatigue, 6, 79–83
Racial coloration, 520
Racial connectedness, 289–290
Racial disparities
    in disability diagnosis, 267
    in employment, 85
    in health, 85–86
    in service delivery, 85
    in vocational rehabilitation services, 272
Racial equilibrium vs. racial disequilibrium, 82
Racial harmony, 441
Racial identity theory, 373
Racial inequality, 352
Racial macroaggressions, 80, 82
Racial microaggressions, 1-2, 5–7, 10, 80–83
Racial misogyny, 84
Racial stereotyping, 4, 43
Racial trauma, 6–8

Racial-/cultural-specific trauma model, 6
Racialized process, 549
    day-to-day racism, 550–551
    Mental Health Act and ethnicity REF, 551–560
Racism, 2, 38, 79, 83, 94, 117–118, 266, 339, 351–352, 440, 450, 549–550, 554
    denial of, 555
    and health, 85
    in mental health system, 440–441
    in psychology, 550
Radicalisation, 463–464, 468, 472
Rascality, 4
Real Talk, 168–169
Reciprocal determinism, 181
"Recognition trauma", 550
Reflections on becoming 'leaders'
    Romana Farooq, 324–327
    Tânia Rodrigues, 327–330
Reflexivity, 383
    in clinical and leadership practice, 306–307
    working within insider/outsider position, 382–383
Rehabilitation Act, 15, 268
Relational attribute, 210, 213
Religion, 299, 301, 307, 473
Resilience, 533
    training strategy for black youth, 261
Resiliency, 257
    addressing other health disparities, 262
    connectedness to positive people, places, and things to do, 259
    evaluation, 260–261
    faster recovery, 261
    higher purpose, 259
    improvisation, 259
    navigating systems, 260
    plans, 259
    primary prevention, 261
    sense of self, 258

take care of self/take care of
    others, 258
  trends in funding, 262
Respect, lack of, 253
Restraint(s), 38, 40, 42, 45, 49, 141,
    310, 447
'Reverse' transracial placement,
    397–398
Richard Reid case study, 464–467
  potential explanations for terrorist
    inclinations of, 468–474
Risk, 12, 42–43, 145, 419, 426, 553
  assessment, 152
  dementia, 422
  factors, 14–15, 119
  of relapse, 449
Royal College of Psychiatrists, 140

Safeguarding, 13, 154–155, 301, 509
Salafi-ism, 469
Schizophrenia, 431–432, 446, 448
  CaFI for, 450–453
  racialising and biased roots of,
    3–4
School Exclusion Risk Reduction
    Programme, 287–288
Schools, 352
Second generation socialisation,
    369–371
Segregation, 85
Self esteem, 5, 15, 73, 119, 133, 258,
    268, 273, 288, 401–404,
    549, 564
Self-agency of individuals, 509
Self-awareness, 9, 119, 258
Self-confidence/teacher efficacy, 210
Self-employment, 273–277
Self-esteem, 119
Self-identification, 469–470
Self-knowledge, 330–331
Self-organised learning (SOL),
    358–359
Self-reflection, 216–217
Self-reflexivity, 306, 512
Self-regulation, 485
Seni's Law, 141, 563

Sensory
  activities, 19
  diets, 485
  integration theory, 483
  modulation programmes, 486
  profile, 484–485
Sensory processing, 481
  Alert Programme strategies, 486
  behaviours indicating SPD,
    487–488
  disorder, 482–483
  expected response, 481
  explaining SPD to young people,
    parents and teachers,
    488–490
  occupational therapists, 483
  over responsive, 482
  under responsive, 482
  self-regulation, 485
  sensory integration theory, 483
  sensory modulation programmes,
    486
  sensory profile, 484–485
  SPD and Afro Caribbean
    Community, 486–487
  SPD vs. social anxiety, 484
  strategies to trying, 490–493
Sensory processing disorder (SPD),
    482–484
  and Afro Caribbean Community,
    486–487
  behaviours indicating, 487–488
  explaining to young people,
    parents and teachers,
    488–490
  indicators, 487
Service delivery, 109, 133, 179, 181,
    184–186, 189–190, 270
Service User Assessment, 450
Shadism, 529
Shame, 120, 555
Sharam, 19, 498–502, 509, 511–514
Shared learning, 450, 452
Shared testimony process, 541
Shelf test, 528
"Sit With Us" app, 244

Skin colour, 395
Slavery, 498, 437, 520
   alienation, 442, 468–469
Social
   anxiety, 484
   black children in social services care, 400–401
   construction, 306
   constructionism, 382
   determinants of health, 112–113
   and emotional development programs, 198–199
   exclusion, 135
   identity, 463
   justice, 211
   policy, 151
Social gender, race, religion, ability, culture, class, ethnicity, spirituality, and sexuality (Social GRRACCESS), 301
Socio-cultural
   concept, 554
   dichotomy, 549
   sociocultural/psychosocial model in education, 5
South Asian families, belief systems within, 500–501
Space or ability to control environment, 79–80
Special Hospital Service Authority (SHSA), 43
Spirit, 89, 302–304, 311
Spirit of Bermuda high seas program, 197
Spiritual reflexivity, 302–303
   representation, 304–305
Spiritual/supernatural forces, 450
Spirituality, 303, 307
   embodied spirituality within mental health journey, 311–312
   significance for black mental health professionals and service users, 299–302
   in systemic family therapy in communities, 526–527

Stafford Hospital, 149–150
Staff–student relations, 100
"Start-UP USA" projects, 275
Stereotyping, 181
Stigma, 8, 14, 110, 120, 135, 563–564
Strategic
   landscape, 162–164
   therapists, 528
Street 2 Boardroom program, 169
Streets, 250, 252
Strengths-based approaches, 147
Stressors, 248–250
Subjectification, 79, 180
Supervision process, 549, 557
Supervisory relationships
   breakdown, 89
   shift in, 96–97
Supervisory tool, 554
Support A Nation (SAN), 524
Supported employment, 272–273
Systematic failure, 447
Systemic family therapy, 519
   airport experience, 524–525
   attachment, 535–536
   class structure, 520–521
   community tasks, 536–537
   curiosity, 533
   Dominican Republic, 521
   expanding psycho-educative approach, 531–533
   eye contact and safe touch, 534–535
   family therapy in context of community, 527–531
   Haiti, 521
   Haitian family life, 525–526
   history of Caribbean, 520
   incorporating spirituality in systemic family therapy in communities, 526–527
   intervention, 533
   managing challenging teenagers, 537–538
   Mental Health Services, 523–524
   mission as vehicle for delivering family therapy within community, 524

pastors as counsellors and
translators, 541–544
political unrest, 521–523
thematic overview of work, 535
Vignettes, 538–539
working with families in
Dominican Republic,
539–541
working with fathers, 526
Systemic psychotherapy, 500, 513
Systemic racism, 48–49
big, bad and dangerous, 42–43
colonisation, 49–50
explanations, 51–52
inertia following inquires, 43–46
over-representation in mental Ill
health and custody, 39–41
post-colonial theory, 50
reasons for over representation,
41–42
Systemic thinking, 48

Take care of self/take care of others,
258
Talking therapy, 4
Targeted Intervention in Education,
283–294
Targeted therapy services and
training, need for, 183–187
Teacher Emotional Literacy Scale
(TELS), 205
Teachers/teaching, 531
empathy program, 14, 199–200,
205
explaining SPD to, 488–490
teacher–student relationships, 200
TELS score, 229–231
Terminology, 452
medical, 120
person-centred, 146
protective factors, 257
'Puwars', 92
impact of race and ethnicity,
160–161
Terrorism, 461, 463
Terrorist radicalisation

Carlos Bledsoe case study,
467–468
identity, 462–463
potential explanations for terrorist
inclinations of Reid and
Bledsoe, 468–474
radicalisation, 463–464
Richard Reid case study, 464–467
Western notions of terrorism,
461–462
Theories of mental illness, 462
Therapists' own racial identity status,
383–384
Trans-Atlantic slave trade, 437, 520
(*see also* Slavery)
Transcultural supervision, 550, 554
Transformative practice, creating
environment for, 308–311
Transgenerational healing, 519
Transgenerational trauma, 7,
527–531
Transnational minority ethnic
communities, 422
Transracial adoption, 17, 395
changes in law and political
backtracking, 396–400
looked after black children
in social services care,
400–401
mental health of looked after
children in UK, 401–409
skin colour difference in, 395–396
Trauma, 5, 73, 247, 257, 323, 529,
537, 551, 557, 559
childhood and adulthood, 446
effects of, 19
forms, 194
institutional, 253
racial and cultural, 6–8
urban, 250
Treatment-oriented approach, 256
Trust, lack of, 253

UK Psychiatric System
analysis, 345–346
being or becoming Ill, 336

Black Men in, 334
loss experiences, 339–340
persecutory framework development, 340–341
persecutory system, 336–339
recurrent and repeated themes, 334–335
wilderness, 341–344
UK social policy and modern mental health services development
asylums to community care, 146–147
categories of abuse, 155–156
debating poor outcomes, 148
one in four, 148–149
receiving care, 150–152
safeguarding, 154–155
staffing NHS, 147–148
Stafford Hospital, 149–150
staying involving, 153–154
working with mental health act–responsibilities and rights for relatives, 152–153
Unconscious perpetrators, 94
Underachievement, 352
Unintentional racism, 382
United Kingdom (UK), 445
mental health of looked after children in, 401–409
minority ethnic and migrant communities in, 420–421
school system, 284
United Nations (UN), 139
United States, minority ethnic and migrant communities and dementia in, 418–419
Urban black youth, 254
Urban trauma, 250
US Department of Labor, 275

Vascular dementia, 413
Video-recorded Goal Decision System, 305
Violence, 250, 474
Vocational rehabilitation services (VR services), 268

program, 268–269
recommendations, 272
self-employment, 273–277
services for African American with mental health diagnoses, 269–272
Voluntary and community sector, 164–165
Vulnerable population/groups, 5, 42, 101, 119, 145, 151, 155, 160, 164, 252, 285, 319–320, 323, 326, 527, 544

Wahhabi-ism, 469
Wellness, 3, 5, 66, 122, 124, 261
West Indian Psychosis, 136
West Indies, 497
Western notions of terrorism, 461–462
White British–black Caribbean achievement, 352
White Eurocentric models of health care, 8
White racial identity status, 372–374, 391–392
White therapists, 8
Whiteness, 372
Wilderness, 341–344
Windrush Generation, 369
Women of colour
in academy, 61
in critical studies, 65
Work-related stress, 60
Workforce Race Equality Scheme (WRES), 564
Workplace racism, 557
World Health Organization (WHO), 454

Young people, 159, 162, 165–166, 201
commissioning services, 164
explaining SPD to, 488–490
lack of data, 161–162
policy and strategic landscape, 162–164

impact of race and ethnicity terminology, 160–161
voluntary and community sector, 164–165
Youth culture, 211

Youth Information Advice and Counselling Service (YIACS), 159–160, 165

Zazi, 167–168